D1747357

AIDS and Infections of Homosexual Men
Second Edition

AIDS and Infections of Homosexual Men
Second Edition

Edited by

Pearl Ma, Ph.D.
Chief, Clinical Microbiology
St. Vincent's Hospital and Medical Center of New York
Assistant Professor of Clinical Pathology
New York University Medical Center

Donald Armstrong, M.D.
Chief, Infectious Disease Service
Memorial Sloan Kettering Cancer Center
Professor of Medicine
Cornell University Medical College

Butterworths
Boston London Singapore Sydney Toronto Wellington

Copyright © 1989 by Butterworth Publishers, a division of Reed Publishing (USA) Inc. All rights reserved.

No part of this publication may be reproduced, stored in a retrieval system, or transmitted, in any form or by any means, electronic, mechanical, photocopying, recording, or otherwise, without the prior written permission of the publisher.

Every effort has been made to ensure that the drug dosage schedules within this text are accurate and conform to standards accepted at time of publication. However, as treatment recommendations vary in the light of continuing research and clinical experience, the reader is advised to verify drug dosage schedules herein with information found on product information sheets. This is especially true in cases of new or infrequently used drugs.

Library of Congress Cataloging-in-Publication Data

AIDS and infections of homosexual men / edited by Pearl Ma, Donald Armstrong.—2nd ed.
    p. cm.
    Rev. ed of: The Acquired immune deficiency syndrome and infections of homosexual men.
    Includes bibliographies and index.
    ISBN 0-409-90161-X
    1. Sexually transmitted diseases.   2. AIDS (Disease)
3. Homosexuals, Male—Diseases.   I. Ma, Pearl, 1928–   . II. Armstrong, Donald, 1931–   .
III. Acquired immune deficiency syndrome and infections of homosexual men.
    [DNLM: 1. Acquired Immunodeficiency Syndrome.
2. Homosexuality.   3. Sexually Transmitted Diseases.
WD 308 A186]
RC200.1.A28   1989
616.97'92—dc19
DNLM/DLC
for Library of Congress   88-14631
                                                CIP

British Library Cataloguing in Publication Data

AIDS and infections of homosexual men.—2nd ed.
1. Male homosexuals, Sexually transmitted diseases
616.95'1'008806642

ISBN 0-409-90161-X

Butterworth Publishers
80 Montvale Avenue
Stoneham, MA 02180

10 9 8 7 6 5 4 3 2 1

Printed in the United States of America

To Gay Morgulas
for her guidance and tireless work on the
first edition of this book,
and for her friendship

Contents

Contributing Authors		xi
Preface	*David J. Sencer*	xvii
Introduction	*Pearl Ma and Donald Armstrong*	xix

Part I   Sexually Transmitted Diseases: Nondiarrheal   1

1. Overview of Sexually Transmitted Diseases in Homosexual Men   *Anne Rompalo and H. Hunter Handsfield*   3

2. Syphilis   *Lewis M. Drusin*   13

3. The Relationship of HIV Infections to Infections with Pathogenic *Neisseria* in Homosexual Men
   Franklyn N. Judson   25

4. Proctitis due to *Chlamydia trachomatis*
   Walter E. Stamm   39

Part II   Sexually Transmitted Diseases: Diarrheal   47

5. Gay Bowel Syndrome: An Overview   *Bruce S. Gingold*   49

6. Bacterial Diarrhea in Homosexual Men
   Anthony P. Lopez and Sherwood L. Gorbach   59

7. Parasitic Infectious Diseases as Sexually Transmitted Infections   *Daniel C. William*   69

8. Cryptosporidiosis, Isosporiasis, and Microsporidiosis
   Pearl Ma and Philip D. Marsden   77

Part III   Other Sexually Transmitted Diseases   97

9. Hepatitis B Virus Transmission between Homosexual Men: A Model for AIDS   *Miriam J. Alter and Donald P. Francis*   99

10. Herpes Simplex Virus Infections in Homosexual Men
   Carlos Lopez — 109

11. Cytomegalovirus Infection in Healthy and Immune Deficient Homosexual Men   W. Lawrence Drew and Lawrence Mintz — 119

12. Laboratory Diagnosis of Sexually Transmitted Diseases and Opportunistic Infections of AIDS   Pearl Ma — 131

Part IV   Infectious and Neoplastic Complications of AIDS — 203

13. The Etiologic Agent of AIDS   David W. Archibald and M. Essex — 205

14. Revision of the CDC Surveillance Case Definition for AIDS   Reported by Council of State and Territorial Epidemiologists; AIDS Program, Center for Infectious Diseases, Centers for Disease Control — 223

15. AIDS and HIV Infection: Surveillance and Epidemiology in the United States, 1981–1985   Richard M. Selik and James W. Curran — 237

16. Clinical Manifestations of Kaposi's Sarcoma   Bijan Safai — 251

17. Neurology in AIDS   Michael Grundman, Mitchell S. Felder, Hyman Donnenfeld, and Joseph C. Masdeu — 265

18. Case Presentations of AIDS in the United States
   AIDS in Prostitutes   Joyce Wallace — 285
   AIDS in Children   Anthony B. Minnefor and James M. Oleske — 296
   AIDS in Prisoners   Gary P. Wormser — 305

19. AIDS in Europe, and the Immunodeficiency of AIDS   Bo Hofmann, Jan Gerstoft, and Bjarne Ørskov Lindhardt — 311

20. Opportunistic Infections in AIDS Patients   Jonathan W. M. Gold and Donald Armstrong — 325

21. Treatment of Opportunistic Infections in Patients with AIDS   Jeffrey Kocher and Richard B. Roberts — 337

22. Treatment of Kaposi's Sarcoma   Patricia L. Myskowski and Bijan Safai — 355

| Part V | Immunologic Evaluation Methods and Controls | 371 |

23. Analysis of Mechanisms of Immune Suppression in AIDS
    Susanna Cunningham-Rundles — 373

24. Immunologic Responses in AIDS
    Patricia Fitzgerald-Bocarsly, Carlos Lopez, and Frederick P. Siegal — 383

25. Epidemiologic Observations of Immunologic Abnormalities in Homosexual Men *Michael Lange, Hardy Kornfeld, Elena Klein, Robert A. Vande Stouwe, and Michael H. Grieco* — 391

26. Immunogenetic Findings in Patients with Epidemic Kaposi's Sarcoma *Pablo Rubinstein, Mary Walker, Norman Mollen, Linda J. Laubenstein, and Alvin E. Friedman-Kien* — 403

27. Significance of Endogenous Interferon and Interferon-Induced Enzymes in Patients with AIDS
    Olivia T. Preble, M. Elaine Eyster, Edward P. Gelmann, and James J. Goedert — 419

28. Approaches to Therapy of AIDS *Frederick P. Siegal* — 433

| Part VI | Diagnostic Perspective | 447 |

29. AIDS: An Explanation for Its Occurrence among Homosexual Men *Joseph A. Sonnabend* — 449

30. AIDS: An Overview *B. H. Kean* — 471

Appendixes

A. Recommendations for Prevention of HIV Transmission in Health Care Settings *MMWR Supplement* — 479

B. Biosafety Level Criteria: Laboratory and Vertebrate Animal *MMWR Supplement* — 495

C. CDC Cautionary Notice for all Human-Serum-Derived Reagents Used as Controls *MMWR Supplement* — 505

Index — 507

Contributing Authors

Miriam J. Alter, Ph.D., Chief, Viral Hepatitis Surveillance, Hepatitis Branch, Division of Viral Diseases, Center for Infectious Disease, Centers for Disease Control, Atlanta, Georgia

David W. Archibald, D.M.D., D.Sc., Assistant Professor, Oral Pathology, University of Maryland Dental School, Baltimore, Maryland

Donald Armstrong, M.D., Chief, Infectious Disease Service, Memorial Sloan Kettering Cancer Center; Professor of Medicine, Cornell University Medical College, New York, New York

Susanna Cunningham-Rundles, Ph.D., Associate Professor of Immunology, Department of Pediatrics, The New York Hospital, Cornell University Medical Center, New York, New York

James W. Curran, M.D., M.P.H., Director, AIDS Program, Centers for Disease Control, Atlanta, Georgia

Hyman Donnenfeld, M.D., Associate Professor of Neurology, New York Medical College; Attending Neurologist and Neuropathologist, St. Vincent's Hospital and Medical Center, New York, New York

W. Lawrence Drew, M.D., Ph.D., Associate Professor of Medicine and Laboratory Medicine, In Residence, University of California, San Francisco; Director, Clinical Microbiology and Infectious Diseases, Departments of Pathology and Laboratory Medicine and Medicine, Mount Zion Hospital and Medical Center, San Francisco, California

Lewis M. Drusin, M.D., M.P.H., Professor of Clinical Public Health and Associate Professor of Clinical Medicine, Cornell University Medical College; Director, Department of Epidemiology, and Associate Attending Physician, The New York Hospital, New York, New York

M. Essex, D.V.M., Ph.D., Professor and Chairman, Department of Cancer Biology, Harvard School of Public Health; Chairman, Harvard AIDS Institute, Boston, Massachusetts

M. Elaine Eyster, M.D., Chief, Division of Hematology, M.S. Hershey Medical Center, Hershey, Pennsylvania

Mitchell S. Felder, M.D., Chief Resident, Department of Neurology, St. Vincent's Hospital and Medical Center, New York, New York

Patricia Fitzgerald-Bocarsly, Ph.D., Assistant Professor, Department of Pathology, University of Medicine and Dentistry of New Jersey, New Jersey Medical School, Newark, New Jersey

Donald P. Francis, M.D., D.Sc., AIDS Advisor, Centers for Disease Control, California Health Department, Berkeley, California

Alvin E. Friedman-Kien, M.D., Assistant Professor of Dermatology and Microbiology, and Attending Physician, Department of Dermatology, University Hospital, New York University Medical Center, New York, New York

Edward P. Gelmann, M.D., Chief, Division of Oncology, Georgetown University School of Medicine, Lombardi Cancer Center, Washington, DC; formerly, Senior Investigator, Medicine Branch, National Cancer Institute, National Institutes of Health, Bethesda, Maryland

Jan Gerstoft, M.D., Teacher of Clinical Medicine, Department of Infectious Diseases, University of Copenhagen; Senior Registrar, Department of Infectious Diseases, Rigshospitalet, Copenhagen, Denmark

Bruce S. Gingold, M.D., Assistant Clinical Professor of Surgery, Mount Sinai Medical School of Medicine; Attending Surgeon, St. Vincent's Hospital and Medical Center, New York, New York

James J. Goedert, M.D., Cancer Expert, Family Studies Section, Environmental Epidemiology Branch, National Cancer Institute, National Institutes of Health, Bethesda, Maryland

Jonathan W. M. Gold, M.D., Associate Professor of Clinical Medicine, Cornell University Medical College; Associate Attending Physician, Department of Infectious Disease Service, Memorial Sloan Kettering Cancer Center, New York, New York

Sherwood L. Gorbach, M.D., Professor of Community Health and Medicine, Tufts University School of Medicine, Boston, Massachusetts

Michael H. Grieco, M.D., Chief, Division of Allergy, Immunology and Infectious Diseases, St. Luke's–Roosevelt Hospital Center; Professor of Clinical Medicine, Columbia University, College of Physicians and Surgeons, New York, New York

Michael Grundman, M.D., Assistant Professor of Neurology, New York Medical College; Attending Neurologist, St. Vincent's Hospital and Medical Center, New York, New York

H. Hunter Handsfield, M.D., Professor of Medicine, Adjunct Professor of Epidemiology, University of Washington, Seattle; Director of Sexually Transmitted Disease Control Program, Seattle–King County Department of Public Health, Seattle, Washington

Bo Hofmann, M.D., Visiting Postdoctoral Research Fellow, Department of Microbiology and Immunology, University of California School of Medicine, Los Angeles, California

Franklyn N. Judson, M.D., Professor, Departments of Medicine (Infectious Diseases) and Preventive Medicine, University of Colorado Health Sciences Center; Director, Denver Public Health, Denver, Colorado

B. H. Kean, M.D., Clinical Professor (Emeritus) of Tropical Medicine and Public Health, Department of Medicine, Division of International Medicine, Cornell University Medical College; Attending Physician, The New York Hospital, New York, New York

Elena Klein, M.D., Director, Clinical Virology Laboratory, St. Luke's–Roosevelt Hospital Center; Associate Professor of Pediatrics, Clinical Virology, Columbia University, College of Physicians and Surgeons, New York, New York

Jeffrey Kocher, M.D., Associate Attending Physician, Department of Medicine, Englewood Hospital, Englewood, New Jersey

Hardy Kornfeld, M.D., Assistant Professor of Medicine, Pulmonary Center, Boston University School of Medicine, Boston, Massachusetts

Michael Lange, M.D., F.R.C.P.(C.), Associate Professor of Clinical Medicine, Columbia University, College of Physicians and Surgeons; Assistant Chief, Division of Infectious Diseases, St. Luke's–Roosevelt Hospital Center, New York, New York

Linda J. Laubenstein, M.D., Assistant Professor of Clinical Medicine, and Attending Physician, Departments of Oncology and Hematology, New York University Medical Center, New York, New York

Bjarne Ørskov Lindhardt, M.D., Research Associate, Laboratory of Tumor Virology, Fibiger Institute, Copenhagen, Denmark

Anthony P. Lopez, M.D., Chief, Infectious Diseases, Emerson Hospital, Concord, Massachusetts

Carlos Lopez, Ph.D., Director, Virology Research, Lilly Research Laboratories, Eli Lilly and Company, Indianapolis, Indiana

Pearl Ma, Ph.D., Assistant Professor of Clinical Pathology, New York University Medical Center; Chief, Clinical Microbiology, Department of Laboratories, St. Vincent's Hospital and Medical Center, New York, New York

Philip D. Marsden, M.D., Professor of Medicine and Chief, Department of Tropical Medicine and Nutrition, University of Brazil, Brazilia, Brazil

Joseph C. Masdeu, M.D., Professor of Neurology, New York Medical College; Director and Chairman of Neurology, St. Vincent's Hospital and Medical Center, New York, New York

Anthony B. Minnefor, M.D., Assistant Vice President for Medical Affairs and Chief, Division of Infectious Disease, St. Joseph's Hospital and Medical Center, Paterson, New Jersey

Lawrence Mintz, M.D., Associate Clinical Professor of Medicine, University of California, San Francisco; Hospital Epidemiologist and Co-Director, Infectious Diseases Service, Departments of Pathology and Laboratory Medicine and Medicine, Mount Zion Hospital and Medical Center, San Francisco, California

Norman Mollen, Senior Research Assistant, Laboratory of Immunogenetics, The Lindsley F. Kimball Research Institute of the New York Blood Center, New York, New York

Patricia L. Myskowski, M.D., Assistant Professor of Medicine, Cornell University Medical College; Associate Attending Physician, Medicine and Dermatology Service, Memorial Sloan Kettering Cancer Center, New York, New York

James M. Oleske, M.D., Professor and Director, Division of Allergy, Immunology and Infectious Diseases, Department of Pediatrics, University of Medicine and Dentistry of New Jersey and Children's Hospital of New Jersey, Newark, New Jersey

Olivia T. Preble, Ph.D., Health Scientist Administrator, AIDS Review Section, Program and Project Review Branch, National Institute of Allergy and Infectious Diseases, National Institutes of Health, Bethesda, Maryland; formerly, Department of Pathology, Uniformed Services, University of the Health Sciences, Bethesda, Maryland

Anne Rompalo, M.D., Research Associate, Division of Infectious Diseases, Johns Hopkins University, School of Medicine, Baltimore, Maryland

Richard B. Roberts, M.D., Professor and Vice Chairman, Department of Medicine, Cornell University Medical College; Attending Physician, Department of Medicine, The New York Hospital, New York, New York

Pablo Rubinstein, M.D., Director of Immunogenetics and Senior Investigator, The Lindsley F. Kimball Research Institute of the New York Blood Center, New York, New York

Bijan Safai, M.D., Professor of Medicine, Cornell University Medical College; Chief, Dermatology Service, Department of Medicine, Memorial Sloan Kettering Cancer Center, New York, New York

Richard M. Selik, M.D., Medical Epidemiologist, AIDS Program, Centers for Disease Control, Atlanta, Georgia

David J. Sencer, M.D., M.P.H., Management Sciences for Health, Boston, Massachusetts

Frederick P. Siegal, M.D., Head, Section of Hematology Research, Division of Hematology/Oncology, Long Island Jewish Medical Center, New Hyde Park, New York

Joseph A. Sonnabend, M.B., M.R.C.P., Associate Research Scientist, Department of Pediatrics, St. Luke's–Roosevelt Medical Center, New York, New York

Walter E. Stamm, M.D., Professor of Medicine, University of Washington School of Medicine, Seattle; Head, Infectious Diseases, Harborview Medical Center, Seattle, Washington

Robert A. Vande Stouwe, M.D., Ph.D., Fellow in Allergy and Immunology, R.A. Cooke Institute of Allergy, St. Luke's–Roosevelt Hospital Center, New York, New York

Mary Walker, Manager, Laboratory of Immunogenetics, The Lindsley F. Kimball Research Institute of the New York Blood Center, New York, New York

Joyce Wallace, M.D., Clinical Assistant Professor of Medicine, Department of Neoplastic Diseases, Mt. Sinai Medical School; President, Foundation for Research on Sexually Transmitted Diseases, Inc., and Associate Attending Physician, Department of Medicine, St. Vincent's Hospital and Medical Center, New York, New York

Daniel C. William, M.D., Instructor in Clinical Medicine, Department of Medicine, Columbia University College of Physicians and Surgeons; Assistant Attending Physician, Department of Medicine, St. Luke's–Roosevelt Hospital Center, New York, New York

Gary P. Wormser, M.D., Chief, Division of Infectious Diseases, Professor of Medicine and Pharmacology, New York Medical College; Chief of Infectious Diseases, Westchester County Medical Center, Valhalla, New York

Preface

When asked to write a Preface to this Second Edition, I reread the first. *The new material is italicized*, and the old in brackets.

*   *   *

New York City has the distressing distinction of being the home for the largest number of patients with acquired immunodeficiency syndrome (AIDS) of any geographical area in the world. It also has the good fortune of being the home of thousands of dedicated health care professionals working together to ease the burdens of those ill and attempting to find *a prophylaxis and cure* [the cause] and thereby prevent this syndrome.

Fifteen thousand nine hundred ninety nine [1049] cases of AIDS have been diagnosed in New York City since the first cluster of Kaposi's sarcoma was observed in 1979. Today *326* [218] cases and suspected cases are hospitalized in over *30* [34] hospitals. Unfortunately, *8187* [391] are known to be dead and over *350* [60] new cases are being diagnosed each month.

Fortunately, scores of research institutions in New York City are deeply committed to the research efforts that are necessary for a timely solution to the problem. The scientific community of New York City did not await a call from Washington naming AIDS as the nation's number one health priority. Concern for the persons with AIDS and those at risk were the driving factors that brought the scientific community of the city together to share their talents, recognizing that the complexities of the syndrome were such that no single investigator, laboratory, or institution could solve the problem alone.

The scientific inquiries have been made more difficult because of the personal circumstances surrounding persons with the syndrome and those at risk. The personal and professional sensitivity needed to deal with the problems of homosexuality, illicit drug use, and illegal immigration have added to the complexity but have been managed, *albeit imperfectly*.

The publication of this book provides an opportunity for the reader to note the ever-increasing interdependence of investigators in today's search for solutions to health problems. It also provides scientists the opportunity to review in their accepted format the facts in full, rather than as presented in the public media.

xviii   *AIDS and Infections of Homosexual Men*

*   *   *

It is both encouraging and discouraging to note the similarities between editions—discouraging because the epidemic continues, yet encouraging because our early knowledge of the methods of spread are re-enforced, not changed; discouraging because we have no vaccine or cure, yet encouraging because the infecting agent has been identified, which brings both prevention and cure closer.

David J. Sencer

Introduction

The first edition of *AIDS and Infections of Homosexual Men* was published in 1984, before human immunodeficiency virus (HIV), the retrovirus that causes acquired immunodeficiency syndrome (AIDS), was discovered. During the past five years, a great deal of progress has been made in combating the ever-increasing AIDS epidemic, necessitating a second edition to inform physicians, other health care workers, and the public of these advances.

Although AIDS has spread to such heterosexual populations as drug addicts, sexual partners of drug addicts, and children of drug addicts, 62% of cases are found in homosexual and bisexual men. Education on "safe sex" has led to the gradual decrease of certain sexually transmitted diseases, including gonorrhea, syphilis, and AIDS-related diarrhea, although the incidence of neurosyphilis and tuberculosis has increased.

The list of opportunistic infections continues to increase as well. One sees disseminated infections with skin lesions, such as *histoplasmosis,* and epithelioid angiomatosis marked by horrible pedunculated nodules (causative agent—cat-scratch disease bacillus). Other rare opportunistic infections are *Acanthamoeba* and *Prototheca* (algae) meningoencephalitis and microsporidiosis. *Pneumocystis carinii* pneumonia remains the most common opportunistic infection in AIDS patients, and azidothymidine (AZT) is the drug of choice to treat afflicted individuals.

New chapters in the second edition address HIV, central nervous system AIDS, and AIDS in prison; the book includes updated guidelines of the revised definition of AIDS by the Centers for Disease Control and safety measures for those working with high volume of the AIDS virus.

The goal of this book is to present the latest, rapid methods of diagnosing AIDS and opportunistic infections and attempts to illuminate our understanding of the pathogenesis of AIDS. New advancements in laboratory diagnosis are seen in, for instance, detection of a high incidence of *Mycobacterium avium intracellulare* and *M. tuberculosis,* with improved specimen collection systems. One rapid method in vogue is the gene probe (nucleic probe), which can demonstrate DNA/RNA in clinical specimens, especially in tissue for *Mycobacteria* and HIV. The gloomy message for AIDS diagnosis is the silent period in the disease course, when standard procedure may miss the diagnosis unless in situ hybridization is used.

Treatment for AIDS patients remains discouraging apart from AZT. A possible vaccine is years away. And death remains inevitable for all individuals with AIDS and AIDS-related complex (ARC).

We hope that this book will serve to guide all those who so unselfishly give their time and energy to combat AIDS. We thank all the contributors, many of whom completely rewrote their chapters to reflect changes in knowledge and treatment of AIDS. Finally, we are most grateful to Ms. Kathleen Benn McQueen and Ms. Barbara Murphy and their staffs at Butterworths for guiding this manuscript through editing and production.

Pearl Ma
Donald Armstrong

PART I
Sexually Transmitted Diseases: Nondiarrheal

Chapter 1

Overview of Sexually Transmitted Diseases in Homosexual Men

Anne Rompalo
H. Hunter Handsfield

Throughout the 1970s and early 1980s homosexual men were known to be at high risk of acquiring sexually transmitted diseases (STDs). In the 1980 Annual Summary Report from the Centers for Disease Control, over half the reported cases of infectious syphilis occurred in homosexual men.[1] Gonorrhea, hepatitis A and B, cytomegalovirus (CMV) infection, and anorectal warts also occurred more commonly in homosexual men than in heterosexual men or women. Intestinal or rectal infections with *Shigella* species, *Entamoeba histolytica*, *Giardia lamblia*, and other enteric pathogens were hyperendemic among homosexual men in many communities.[2-4] Nongonococcal urethritis (NGU), other chlamydial infections, herpes genitalis, genital warts, scabies, and pediculosis pubis also were extremely common in this population, but apparently less so than among heterosexuals, at least in populations studied in STD clinics.[2] The incidence of many of these STDs has declined recently with the greater emphasis on education and "safer" sexual practices due to the fear of acquired immunodeficiency syndrome (AIDS).[5,6,7] Cases of anorectal gonorrhea and syphilis have declined among young unmarried men in the United States and the United Kingdom.[5,6] Homosexual men are reporting fewer partners and less frequent sexual exposure.[8,9] Despite these behavioral changes and increased counseling about safer sexual practices, STDs remain a major health problem among homosexual men. This chapter will focus not on AIDS, which is reviewed in detail elsewhere, but on other STDs. It should be stressed that regardless of an individual's human immunodeficiency virus (HIV) antibody status, acute STDs still may be contracted and spread, and that acute rectal and enteric infections in gay men can be easily mistaken for AIDS-related syndromes. Most of these infections resolve when appropriately recognized and treated. Therefore, in the midst of the increasing number of AIDS cases, STDs among homosexual men should not be forgotten or missed.

"Maleness," homosexuality, and multiple sexual partners may be evaluated separately as distinct risk factors for STD.[10,11] The male urethra is a significant factor because during sexual contact it may be exposed to deep-seated pathogens in the rectum and mouth. Its ability to penetrate into cavities, combined with the forceful ejaculation of semen, makes the male urethra an excellent transmitter of infection. Certain sexual behaviors that are especially common among homosexual men, especially those involving direct or indirect contact with feces, specifically increase the risk of sexual transmission of enteric infections. Similarly, behaviors that may result in mucosal trauma are more common among homosexual men than heterosexuals, probably contributing to an elevated risk of hepatitis B[12] and perhaps infection with CMV or other pathogens as well. Some homosexual men regularly have multiple sexual partners, which increases STD risk. The risk is further enhanced by the anonymity of partners, a former common feature of homosexual behavior.[13] Such anonymity makes it nearly impossible to interrupt disease transmission through contact tracing and epidemiologic treatment.

It is important for health care providers to recognize and address these special, unique problems. This chapter discusses the etiology and epidemiology of STDs in this population and elucidates the personal and public health problems associated with these infections.

GASTROINTESTINAL INFECTIONS

Sexually transmitted pathogens can cause several clinically distinct gastrointestinal syndromes that include some of the most common problems affecting homosexual men. Proctitis, by definition, is inflammation limited to the rectal mucosa. The predominant symptoms and signs are mucopurulent or bloody discharge (often manifested only by a coating of exudate on the stools), anorectal pain or pruritus, tenesmus, and, in severe cases, constipation. Colitis is defined by inflammation proximal to the rectosigmoid junction and causes low abdominal pain, cramps, and diarrhea that commonly contains blood or leukocytes. It is often associated with fever, malaise, or other systemic signs. Enteritis, or small intestinal inflammation, causes nausea, bloating, and abdominal pain. Diarrhea is occasionally absent, but when it is present it usually is not apparently inflammatory. Syndromes involving more than one anatomic site are designated by such terms as proctocolitis and enterocolitis.[14]

The distinctions among these syndromes are important because they provide diagnostic information and guidance in evaluating patients.[15] *G. lamblia,* for example, is the predominant sexually transmitted cause of enteritis[15,16]; *Campylobacter fetus* and related organisms also usually cause enteritis or enterocolitis.[15,17] *E. histolytica* or *Shigella* species are the usual causes of colitis.[15,18] *Neisseria gonorrhoeae, Chlamydia trachomatis,* herpes simplex virus (HSV), and *Trepo-*

nema pallidum typically are associated with proctitis or, in severe cases, proctocolitis.[15] For these reasons, the collective designation of all enteric or rectal infections in this population as "gay bowel syndrome" is inappropriate, and clinical series that report the prevalence of various pathogens in populations in which the specific syndromes are not delineated provide little information of use to the clinician.

The pathogens that cause proctitis or proctocolitis usually result in typical anoscopic or proctoscopic findings. *N. gonorrhoeae* and most strains of *C. trachomatis* cause mild mucosal erythema or friability and small to moderate amounts of mucopurulent exudate, often localized to the anal crypts; HSV commonly causes severe mucosal inflammation, with many discrete ulcers; the lymphogranuloma venereum (LGV) strains of *C. trachomatis* cause proctocolitis with marked erythema, edema, and friability, typically with large amounts of purulent exudate; and syphilis often causes discrete intrarectal chancres or tumorlike mass lesions.[14] Thus, anoscopy or proctoscopy should be routine in homosexual men with symptoms of proctitis or proctocolitis.

GONORRHEA

Among homosexual men, the pharyngeal, urethral, and rectal mucosae all are commonly infected with *N. gonorrhoeae*. Although the overall prevalence of gonorrhea was previously greater in homosexual than heterosexual men,[2,19] (the incidence of gonorrhea in gay men has recently been declining). The rectal mucosa is infected by direct inoculation during receptive anal intercourse. Rectal infection has been reported to occur in 35% to 50% of homosexual men with gonorrhea, and to be the only infected site in about 40%.[20,21] The prevalence of gonorrhea was reported as between 6% and 8% in homosexual men attending steam baths and between 13% and 45% in those seen at an STD clinic.[17] Behavioral responses to AIDS prevention recommendations, however, have affected gonorrhea rates in some cities. Gonorrhea rates in homosexual men in Denver declined by 32% from 1979–1985.[7] In Seattle, a decline of 57% was reported, while in San Francisco rates decreased 63% from 1979 to 1985.[23,24]

Unlike the situation among heterosexual men, in whom asymptomatic urethral gonococcal infections are not rare, virtually all urethral infections in homosexual men cause overt symptomatic urethritis.[21] By contrast, anorectal gonorrhea in homosexual men may be symptomatic or asymptomatic. When symptoms are present, they are usually mild,[14] often consisting of only mild anorectal pain, pruritus, and mucopurulent discharge coating the stools. Less commonly, overt perianal irritation, tenesmus, and secondary constipation occur. The findings on proctoscopy are nonspecific, often limited to mucosal friability of distal mucosa or mucopus in the anal crypts.[14]

Pharyngeal infections have been seen in 10% to 25% of homosexual men with gonorrhea, but this is the sole infected site in less than 5%. The infection is usually asymptomatic.[25] The clinical and epidemiologic significance of pharyngeal gonorrhea is uncertain at present. Most cases resolve spontaneously, and most reports suggest that transmission from the pharynx is rare[25]; however, conflicting results have been reported,[26] and further studies are needed.

SYPHILIS

Primary syphilis in homosexual men commonly occurs perianally or in the anorectal mucosa. Rectal chancres, like classic penile chancres, are often painless and are easily overlooked by the patient and physician. Anorectal chancres have been recognized in 50% of primary cases of syphilis in homosexual men in Great Britain but in only 15% of primary cases in the United States[27]; this difference may reflect both improved recognition (due to more routine use of anoscopy or proctoscopy in Britain) and earlier detection (due to more effective contact tracing). Primary lesions or the condylomatous lesions of secondary syphilis are easily confused with nonspecific fissures, polyps, herpetic lesions, or anal warts. Occasionally, a rectal chancre is painful or causes symptoms of bloody diarrhea, constipation, tenesmus, or bleeding.

HERPES SIMPLEX VIRUS

Genital herpes is a common STD in both heterosexually and homosexually active persons, although it appears more common in the former, at least among patients attending STD clinics.[2] On the other hand, in a large survey,[13] 4% of homosexual men gave histories of symptomatic genital herpes and in several etiologic studies, herpes simplex virus was the most common cause of nongonococcal rectal infection in gay men.[14,28,30] Many reports have implicated *herpes simplex* virus (HSV) as a cause of anorectal disease in homosexual men,[14,28,31,32] but the diagnosis still is commonly missed. Goodell et al.[31] documented HSV as the most common cause of acute nongonococcal proctitis, isolating the virus from 15 (29%) of 52 such patients. Of these isolates, 13 were HSV type 2 strains and two were HSV type 1, suggesting that anogenital contact may be a more frequent method of acquiring anorectal HSV than is oroanal contact. Primary herpes rectal infections are characterized by severe anal pain, tenesmus, constipation, and rectal discharge, usually accompanied by constitutional symptoms such as fever, chills, malaise, and headache.[15,29,30] In fact, primary herpes causes some of the most severe forms of acute proctitis.[15,29] Recurrent rectal or perianal herpes, similar to recurrent genital herpes, usually causes mild symptoms.

CONDYLOMA ACUMINATA

Anal warts are common in persons who practice anal intercourse. In one series, 134 (52%) of 260 homosexual men seen in a proctology practice had anal warts.[33]

These are caused by human papilloma virus, usually type 6. They appear in the perianal area as raised pink-to-brown papules usually occurring in clusters but occasionally in large cauliflowerlike masses. They commonly are resistant to all forms of therapy and are among the most frustrating of all STD problems in homosexual men. Anal warts must be differentiated from condyloma lata, the moist, flat papules of secondary syphilis. Penile warts also are common in this population, but somewhat less so than in heterosexual men.[2]

NONGONOCOCCAL URETHRITIS AND CHLAMYDIAL INFECTIONS

In STD clinic populations, NGU is significantly less prevalent in homosexual than heterosexual men; in one study,[2] the prevalence of NGU in these groups was 14.6% and 36.4%, respectively. The authors speculated that the difference might be because the anal canal is less susceptible than the female genital tract to *C. trachomatis* or other causes of NGU, or that the anal mucosa is less able to transmit these organisms.[34] However, rectal *C. trachomatis* infections are common in homosexual men.[34] In a large survey of homosexual men, however, more gave past histories of NGU than of gonorrhea—the reverse of the situation in STD clinics.[13] It is probable, therefore, that the relatively low frequency of NGU among homosexual men in STD clinics does not reflect its incidence in the general population, although the reasons for the discrepancy are unknown.

C. trachomatis has been isolated from the urethras of 5% and the anal canals of 8% of homosexual men in an STD clinic.[34] The LGV strains of *C. trachomatis* typically cause acute proctocolitis with severe tenesmus, bloody diarrhea, fever, malaise, and weight loss.[15] The non-LGV strains, in contrast, usually cause asymptomatic infection or mild proctitis, mimicking anorectal gonorrhea.[15,35,36] *C. trachomatis* is the third most prevalent pathogen associated with acute proctitis, following *N. gonorrhoeae* and HSV.[14,15,37] The importance of culturing for *C. trachomatis* in homosexual men with colonic or anorectal symptoms cannot be overemphasized. For example, acute LGV proctocolitis may be clinically indistinguishable from acute shigellosis, amebiasis, or inflammatory bowel disease; in addition, on rectal biopsy, this disease is histologically indistinguishable from Crohn's disease.[38]

HEPATITIS A AND B

The opportunity during many homosexual practices for direct or indirect fecal-oral contamination explains the high rate of hepatitis A in this population.[39] Because saliva, urine, and semen commonly contain hepatitis B virus in patients or carriers of this agent, in theory infections may occur through anal sex, anilingus, fellatio, or mouth-to-mouth transmission of saliva.[40,41] The predominant mode of acquisition, however, probably is receptive anal intercourse.[40] From the standpoint of overall morbidity and potential complications, hepatitis B is among the most important of all STDs in homosexual men. The hepatitis B vaccine has the potential to bring this epidemic under control.[37]

INTESTINAL PARASITES

Sexual transmission of amebiasis was initially suggested in reports of cutaneous amebiasis of the penis and perineal area.[42,43] Subsequently both amebiasis and giardiasis have been found to be epidemic in homosexual men, and in New York City in the late 1970s E. *histolytica,* G. *lamblia,* or both were found in up to 40% of homosexual men attending STD clinics.[44,45] Similar prevalence figures have been reported in San Francisco, Seattle, and Cleveland.[18,46,48] *Enterobius vermicularis, Iodamoeba bütschlii, Dientamoeba fragilis,* and other nonpathogenic intestinal protozoa also have been described.[48,49] Anilingus is believed to be the major mode of transmission.

Amebiasis frequently results in a diffuse inflammation and ulceration of the distal colon that easily can be confused with Crohn's colitis or shigellosis.[45] Giardiasis can produce a severe enteritis with symptoms ranging from acute diarrhea to chronic malabsorption. Most infections with either of these pathogens, however, probably are asymptomatic. Complications of amebiasis, such as hepatic abscess, are apparently uncommon in the population; the reasons for this are unknown, but hypotheses include attenuation of the organism through repeated passage and development of a protective immune response following repeated exposure.

ENTERIC BACTERIAL PATHOGENS

During the late 1970s and early 1980s about 30% of indigenous shigellosis in the Seattle area occurred in homosexual men, and a similar phenomenon had been reported in San Francisco and New York.[44,45] C. *fetus* subspecies *jejuni,* reclassified as C. *jejuni,* recently has been recognized as a cause of acute enteritis in this population.[17] In addition, other campylobacter species, C. *cinadei* and C. *fennelliae,* have been associated with bacteremia and proctocolitis in gay men.[50,51] Quinn et al.[15] recovered C. *fetus* or campylobacterlike organisms (CLOs) from 24% of symptomatic homosexual men and 10% of asymptomatic homosexual men presenting to an STD clinic. *Shigella, Campylobacter,* and probably G. *lamblia* are the three most frequent causes of sexually transmitted enteritis.[15] Anecdotal reports also have implicated the occasional sexual transmission of *Salmonella* species.[52]

CONCLUSION

From this review it should be clear that homosexual men have a high risk of acquiring STDs. Numerous factors such as sexual practice, multiple partners, and anonymity interact to make the presentation and problems of STDs in homosexual men unique. With a better understanding of the etiology, incidence, and epidemiology of these STD syndromes, health care providers can better recognize and treat these personal and public health problems.

REFERENCES

1. Centers for Disease Control. Annual summary 1980. Reported morbidity and mortality in the United States. Morbid Mortal Weekly Rep 1981;29:72.
2. Judson FN, Penley KA, Robinson ME, Smith JK. Comparative prevalence rates of sexually transmitted disease in heterosexual and homosexual men. Am J Epidemiol 1980;112:836.
3. Phillips SC, Mildvan D, William DC, et al. Sexual transmission of enteric protozoa and helminths in a venereal disease clinic population. N Engl J Med 1981;305:603.
4. Baker RW, Peppercorn MA. Gastrointestinal ailments of homosexual men. Medicine 1982;61:290.
5. Carne CA, Weller IUO, Johnson AM, et al. Prevalence of antibodies to human immunodeficiency virus (HIV), gonorrhea rates and altered sexual behavior in homosexual men in London. Lancet 1987;8534:656–658.
6. Centers for Disease Control. Declining rates of rectal and pharyngeal gonorrhea among males—New York City. MMWR 1984;33:295.
7. Judson FN. Fear of AIDS and gonorrhea rates in homosexual men. Lancet 1983;253:1417.
8. Golubjatnikov R, Pfister J, Tillosten T. Homosexual promiscuity and the fear of AIDS. Lancet 1983;ii:681.
9. McKusick ML, Horstman W, Coates JJ. AIDS and sexual behavior reported by gay men in San Francisco. Am J Public Health 1985;75:493.
10. Henderson RH. Improved sexually transmitted disease health services for gays: A national prospective. Sex Transm Dis 1977;4:58.
11. Owen WF. Sexually transmitted disease and traumatic problems in homosexual men. Ann Intern Med 1980;92:805.
12. Schreeder MT, Thompson SE, Hadler KR, et al. Hepatitis B in homosexual men: Prevalence of infection and factors related to transmission. J Infect Dis 1982;146:7.
13. Darrow WW, Barrett D, Jay K, Young A. The gay report on sexually transmitted diseases. Am J Public Health 1981;71 (suppl):1004.
14. Quinn TC, Corey L, Chaffer RG, et al. The etiology of anorectal infections in homosexual men. Am J Med 1981;71:395.
15. Quinn TC, Stamm WE, Goodell SE, et al. The polymicrobial origin of intestinal infections in homosexual men. N Engl J Med 1983;309:576.
16. Kean BH, William DC, Luminais SK. Epidemic of amoebiasis and giardiasis in a biased population. Br J Vener Dis 1979;55:375.
17. Quinn TC, Corey L, Chaffee RG, et al. Campylobacter proctitis in a homosexual man. Ann Intern Med 1980;93:458.
18. Dritz SK, Ainsworth TE, Garrard WF, et al. Patterns of sexually transmitted enteric diseases in a city. Lancet 1977;2:3.
19. Handsfield HH. Gonorrhea and nongonococcal urethritis. Recent advances. Med Clin North Am 1978;62:925.
20. Klein EJ, Fisher LS, Chow AW, et al. Anorectal gonorrhea infection. Ann Intern Med 1977;86:340.

21. Handsfield HH, Knapp JS, Diehr PK, Holmes KK. Correlation of auxotype and penicillin susceptibility of *Neisseria gonorrhoeae* with sexual preference and clinical manifestations of gonorrhea. Sex Transm Dis 1980;7:1.
22. Judson FN, Miller KG, Schaffnet TR. Screening for gonorrhea and syphilis in the gay baths, Denver, Colorado. Am J Public Health 1977;67:740.
23. Handsfield HH. Decreasing incidence of gonorrhea in homosexually active men—minimal effect on risk of AIDS. West J Med 1985;143:469.
24. Zenilman JM, Cates W Jr, Morse SA. *Neisseria gonorrhoeae:* An old enemy rearms. Infect Dis Med Let Obstet Gynecol 1986;7:2.
25. Wiesner PJ, Tronca E, Bonin P, et al. Clinical spectrum of pharyngeal gonococcal infection. N Engl J Med 1973;288:181.
26. Tice AW, Rodriquez UL. Pharyngeal gonorrhea. JAMA 1981;246:2717.
27. Bennet JH, Holmes KK. Epidemiology of syphilis and the non-venereal treponema. In: Johnsen RC, ed. The biology of parasitic species. New York: Academic Press, 1976;157.
28. Goldmeier R. Proctitis and herpes simplex virus in homosexual men. Br J Vener Dis 1980;56:111.
29. Goodell SE, Quinn TC, Mkrtichian EE, et al. Herpes simplex virus proctitis in homosexual men: clinical, sigmoidoscopic, and histopathological features. N Engl J Med 1983;308:868.
30. Rompalo AM, Mertz GJ, Davis LG, et al. A double-blind study of oral acyclovir for the treatment of first episode herpes simplex virus proctitis in homosexual men. JAMA 1988;259:2879.
31. Jacobs E. Anal infections caused by herpes simplex virus. Dis Colon Rectum 1976;19:151.
32. Waugh MA. Anorectal herpes virus hominis in man. J Am Vener Dis Assoc 1976;3:68.
33. Sohn N, Robilotti JG. The gay bowel syndrome: A review of colonic and rectal conditions in 200 male homosexuals. Am J Gastroenterol 1977;67:478.
34. Stamm WE, Koutsky L, Cole B, et al. Chlamydial urethritis in men: Epidemiology, diagnosis and treatment. Proceedings of the 12th International Congress of Chemotherapy. Washington, DC: American Society of Microbiology, 1982:268.
35. Stamm WE, Quinn TC, Mkrtichian E, et al. *Chlamydia trachomatis* proctitis. In: Chlamydial infections, Proceedings of the Fifth International Symposium on Human Chlamydial Infections. Amsterdam: Elsevier Biomedical Press, 1982:111.
36. Rompalo AM, Price CB, Roberts PL, et al. Potential value of rectal screening culture for *Chlamydia trachomatis* in homosexual men. J Infect Dis 1986;153:888.
37. Szmuness W, Sterons CE, Harley EJ, et al. Hepatitis B vaccine: Demonstration of efficacy in a controlled clinical trial in a high-risk population in the United States. N Engl J Med 1980;303:833.
38. Quinn, TC, Goodell SE, Mkrtichian E, et al. *Chlamydia trachomatis* proctitis. N Engl J Med 1981;305:195.
39. Corey L, Holmes KK. Sexual transmission of hepatitis A in homosexual men: Incidence and mechanism. N Engl J Med 1980;302:435.
40. Heathcote J. Hepatitis B antigen in saliva and semen. Lancet 1974;1:71.
41. Villarjos VM, Vesona KA, Gruterrez A, Rodriquez A. Role of saliva, urine and feces in the transmission of type B hepatitis. N Engl J Med 1974;291:1375.
42. Thomas JA, Anthony AJ. Amoebiasis of the penis. Br J Med 1976;48:269.
43. Cooke RA. Cutaneous amoebiasis involving the anogenital region. J Med Assoc Thai 1973;56:354.

44. William DC, Felman YM, Mau JS, Shookhoff HB. Sexually transmitted enteric pathogens in male homosexual populations. NY State J Med 1977;77:2050.
45. Pittman FE, Wenleed KB, Pittman JC. Studies of human amebiasis. Gastroenterology 1973;65:581.
46. Bader M, Pederson AHB, Wiliams R, et al. Venereal transmission of shigellosis in Seattle-King county. Sex Transm Dis 1977;4:89.
47. Kazal HL, Sohn N, Carrasco JI. The gay bowel syndrome: Clinicopathologic correlation in 260 cases. Assoc Clin Lab Sci 1976;6:184.
48. Shookhoff HB. Parasite transmission. JAMA 1972;222:1310.
49. Waugh MA. Threadworm infestation in homosexuals. Trans Johns Hopkins Dermatol Ser 1972;58:224.
50. Quinn TC, Goodell SE, Fennell CL, et al. Infections with *Campylobacter jejuni* and *Campylobacter*-like organisms in homosexual men. Ann Intern Med 1984;101:187.
51. Fennell CL, Totten PA, Quinn TC, et al. Characterization of Campylobacter-like organisms isolated from homosexual men. J Infect Dis 1984;149:58.
52. Drusin LM, Generrt G, Topf-Olstum B, et al. Shigellosis: Another sexually transmitted disease? Br J Vener Dis 1976;82:348.

Chapter 2

Syphilis

Lewis M. Drusin

Recently, infectious syphilis has become a disease primarily affecting homosexual males. Between 1967 and 1979, cases among white males reported by public clinics increased by 351%, and the percentage of these patients with early syphilis who reported at least one male sex partner increased from 38% in 1969 to 70% in 1979.[1] The male to female ratio was 3:1. Fear secondary to the dramatic increase in the reported cases of AIDS has caused homosexual men to adopt safer sexual practices. This trend has in large part been responsible for a 14.9% diminution in reported cases of syphilis between 1982 and 1984 (33,613 to 28,607 cases).[2]

From 1987 to 1988 there has been a 25% increase in reported cases of primary and secondary syphilis.[3] This new outbreak is mostly in women and heterosexual men who are either black or hispanic. A diminution in reported cases in white males was attributed to the continuing decreased incidence in homosexual men secondary to their change in sexual practices aimed at diminishing their risk for AIDS. In a prevalence study of sexually transmitted diseases on a university campus that we did in the early 1970s,[4] there were four cases of syphilis and four cases of syphilis with gonorrhea reported in a population of about 15,000 during the six-month study period. After the study ended, there was a cluster of seven cases of syphilis in a small group of homosexual men.

CASE PRESENTATIONS

As syphilis has become less frequent in the general population, physicians have become less familiar with its clinical manifestations. Over an eight-year period, we have seen 20 cases of primary and secondary syphilis (Table 2–1) admitted to The New York Hospital–Cornell Medical Center and Memorial Sloan-Kettering Cancer Center as diagnostic problems because the correct diagnosis was not obvious to the referring physicians.[5–7] Of these patients, 16 were male; 14 of the 16 were homosexual. Eight patients who had rectal chancres initially consulted surgeons. In six patients, diagnoses of hemorrhoids, fistulas, or ab-

13

Table 2-1 Summary of 20 patients with primary and secondary syphilis who were admitted as diagnostic problems. (Reprinted with permission from Arch Intern Med 1979;139:901–904. Copyright 1979, American Medical Association.)

Service	Patients (N)	Admission Diagnosis and Plan	Correct Diagnosis
Surgery			
General	6	Abscess, fistula, hemorrhoids; 3 were excised	Rectal chancre
General	2	Malignant lymphoma: staging for radiation and/or chemotherapy	Rectal chancre with secondary skin lesions
General	1	Carcinoma of rectum: referred for possible radical surgery	Rectal chancre with secondary skin lesions
General	1	Carcinoma of tongue: referred for possible radical surgery	Chancre of tongue (VDRL test negative)
General	1	Incarcerated femoral hernia: surgically explored	Primary chancre, left inguinal adenopathy
Ear, nose, and throat	1	Meniere's syndrome	Secondary: meningeal (eighth nerve) signs without skin lesions
Urology	1	Chronic lesions of foreskin, patient circumcised	Primary chancre with secondary lesions on foreskin and head of penis
Medicine	3	Hepatitis	Secondary: hepatic signs, one patient without skin lesions
	1	Lymphosarcoma	Secondary: skin lesions with generalized adenopathy
Neurology	1	Intracranial neoplasm	Secondary: headache and papilledema with skin lesions
	1	Carcinomatous meningitis	Rectal chancre, secondary with skin lesions, meningeal signs and carcinomatous meningitis
Obstetrics/gynecology	1	Multiple sclerosis	Secondary: optic neuritis
	1	Carcinoma of vagina: patient scheduled for radical vulvectomy	Vaginal chancre

scesses were made, and three of these patients had surgical resections.[5] Three of these patients complained of painful chancres, and two also complained of painful inguinal adenopathy. Chancres and lymphadenopathy are usually relatively painless in primary syphilis; however, rectal chancres are usually infected. We attributed pain from these lesions to secondary infection. Two patients were referred to cancer surgeons for management of presumed malignancies.[6] One patient was already scheduled for surgery when his qualitative venereal disease research laboratory (VDRL) test, done on admission, was found strongly positive. The diagnosis of syphilis was confirmed by a positive dark-field examination of the rectal lesion. The other man[7] was undergoing a staging procedure before treatment for malignant lymphoma when both his admission VDRL (1:64) and fluorescent treponemal antibody absorption (FTA-ABS) tests were reported positive. A lymphangiogram performed as part of this evaluation showed enlarged granular retroperitoneal lymph nodes, suggesting widespread involvement with lymphoma. Following appropriate therapy with penicillin, flat plates of the abdomen repeated at two months and two years showed a marked diminution in the size of the two lymph nodes, which remained opacified.

Three men with secondary syphilis were admitted to the medical service with severe hepatitis. Two of them had skin lesions characteristic of secondary syphilis, but one had only the signs and symptoms of hepatitis. Syphilitic hepatitis is characterized by a very high alkaline phosphatase that is greatly elevated compared with the transaminases. Signs and symptoms of hepatitis show rapid resolution following adequate penicillin therapy.[8-10]

Two patients presented with neurologic manifestations of secondary syphilis. One was admitted for evaluation of headache, unilateral papilledema, and generalized adenopathy. A normal carotid arteriogram and brain scan eliminated the possibility of an intracranial neoplasm. Following an admission VDRL of 1:128 with a positive FTA-ABS test, he was treated with adequate penicillin intramuscularly (IM) and recovered completely.[6] The other patient was admitted with meningitis considered to be metastasis from reticular cell sarcoma of the small intestine. Physical examination revealed abnormalities of cranial nerves III and VI, skin lesions on the face, and a rectal chancre. Cytologic examination of the cerebrospinal fluid (CSF) initially revealed inflammatory cells; however, following a course of intravenous (IV) penicillin, the inflammatory cells disappeared and only the malignant cells remained.[11] The patient had both primary and secondary syphilis. Because they did not put the patient in a position where they could look at the rectum when they performed the rectal examination, four house officers missed the rectal chancre.

A 27-year-old man was admitted to the ear, nose, and throat (ENT) service for management of Meniere's syndrome after complaining of intermittent vertigo and hearing loss, particularly on the left side, for ten days. During an outpatient clinic visit before admission, the patient's Rinné test showed diminished hearing in the left ear, Weber test revealed lateralization to the left, and audiogram showed hearing loss bilaterally, left greater than right with no airborne difference (Figure 2–1). He was treated with a standard regimen including IV histamine

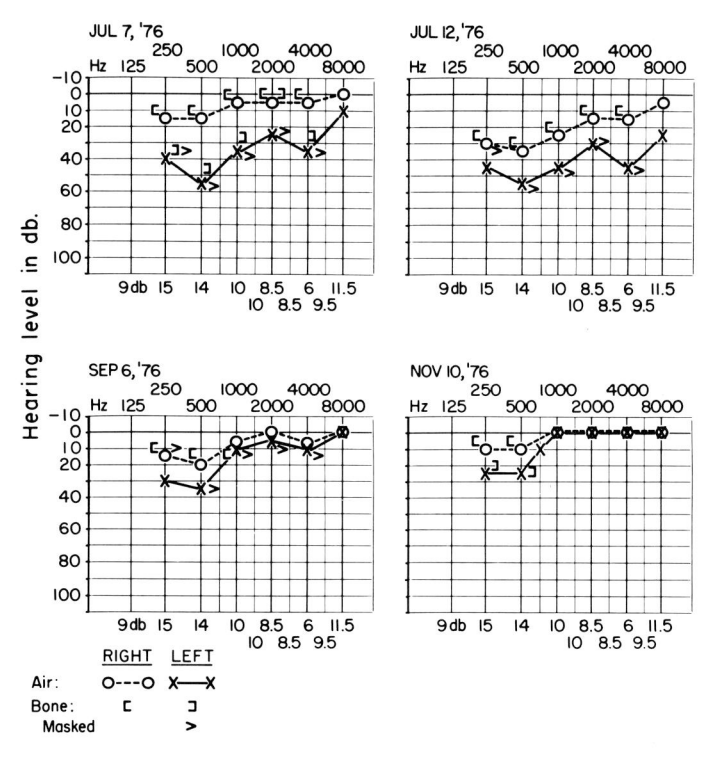

FIGURE 2–1 *Audiograms demonstrating eighth nerve involvement with secondary syphilis and recovery following treatment.*

and oral nicotinic acid. Although he thought his hearing had improved, repeat audiograms five days later showed further diminution in hearing, especially on the right side. The patient's admission VDRL was 1:8 with a positive FTA-ABS. Examination of the CSF revealed a pleocytosis (white blood cell count of 335, 98% lymphocytes), elevated protein (103 mg/dl), and a VDRL of 1:8. Since he was allergic to both penicillin and tetracycline, the patient was treated with 30 g of oral erythromycin and corticosteroids. He experienced complete resolution of his clinical abnormalities. Follow-up audiograms (Figure 2–1) confirmed his recovery of normal hearing. Since a repeat examination of the CSF at five months showed a slightly elevated protein, the patient was given a second course of erythromycin. A repeat examination of the CSF six months later was normal. Wilcox and Goodwin[12] reported a series of three homosexual men with eighth nerve involvement as a part of secondary syphilis. Two had persistence of their chancres. All three had careers in music, which made them acutely aware of changes in their hearing. All had a gradual improvement in their hearing within 18 to 24 months following treatment with antibiotics and corticosteroids.

CLINICAL MANIFESTATIONS

Treponema pallidum can enter the patient through an intact mucous membrane or a small break in cornified epithelium. Following an incubation period of 10 to 90 days (an average of 21 days), the chancre of primary syphilis forms at the site of inoculation as a small papule, which breaks down to form a clean, indurated ulcer. Although the chancre is relatively painless compared with other genital lesions, it can be very painful if it is secondarily infected or in an area of possible trauma, as are rectal lesions. Common sites for the chancre include the genitalia, mouth, or rectum or inside the urethra. A single lesion is usually seen, but multiple lesions can occur if several organisms penetrate the skin at approximately the same time. The chancre lasts approximately three to 12 weeks but may not be obvious because of its location or because it may disappear as a result of partial treatment with antibiotics given for another illness. The chancre may not appear in patients who have had previous infections with syphilis[13]; these patients may present initially with manifestations of a later stage of the disease. This immunity changes the clinical presentation of the disease but does not prevent reinfection. Primary syphilis is accompanied by unilateral or bilateral lymphadenopathy (round, rubbery, freely movable, not usually tender, and without erythema), which begins three or four days following the appearance of the chancre in the regional lymph nodes draining the area containing the chancre. Systemic signs might include fever, malaise, and pharyngitis.

Secondary syphilis appears approximately six weeks to six months (an average of six to eight weeks) after the appearance of the primary lesion. A few patients have persistence of the chancre into the secondary stage (Figure 2–2). If the chancre has healed, often a small scar is visible at the site. The skin lesions, which are occasionally pruritic but almost always bilaterally symmetrical, in-

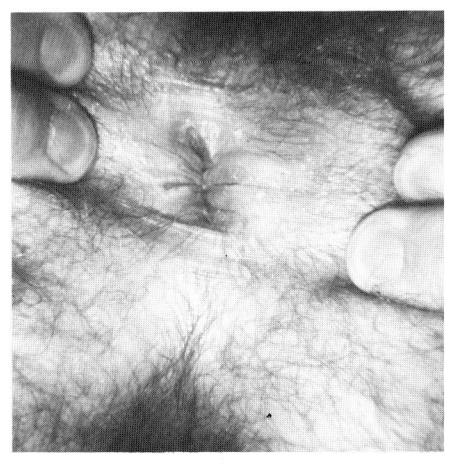

FIGURE 2–2 *An indurated rectal chancre in a homosexual male who had persistence of his chancre into the secondary stage.*

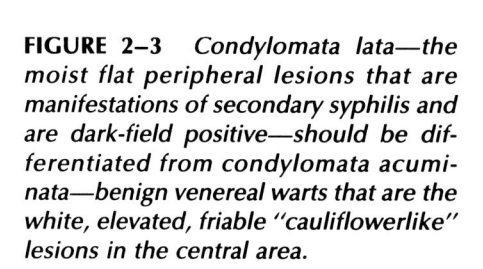

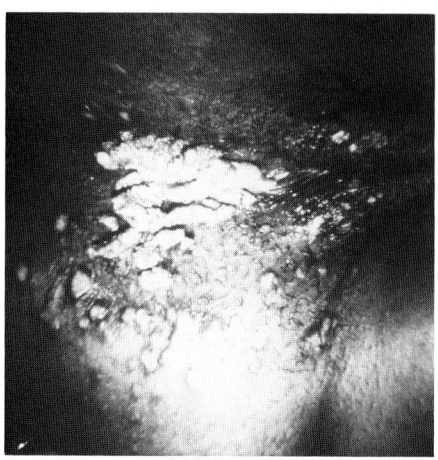

FIGURE 2–3 *Condylomata lata—the moist flat peripheral lesions that are manifestations of secondary syphilis and are dark-field positive—should be differentiated from condylomata acuminata—benign venereal warts that are the white, elevated, friable "cauliflowerlike" lesions in the central area.*

clude a broad range of dermatologic findings but are not bullous or vesicular (Figures 2–3 and 2–4). Bullous or vesicular lesions are usually found only in early congenital syphilis. Patients may also complain of recent hair loss before a patchy alopecia is noticeable on physical examination. In secondary relapsing syphilis, lesions are sometimes asymmetrical and somewhat indurated. As described earlier, systemic manifestations of secondary syphilis could include hepatic changes or abnormalities of the central nervous system (CNS). Signs of renal involvement might include mild asymptomatic proteinuria or transient nephrotic syndrome.[14] There is usually a generalized lymphadenopathy. The lymph nodes are similar to the enlargement seen with primary syphilis—round, rubbery, not usually tender, freely movable, and without erythema.

FIGURE 2–4 *A split papule in the nasolabial fold is seen in secondary syphilis.*

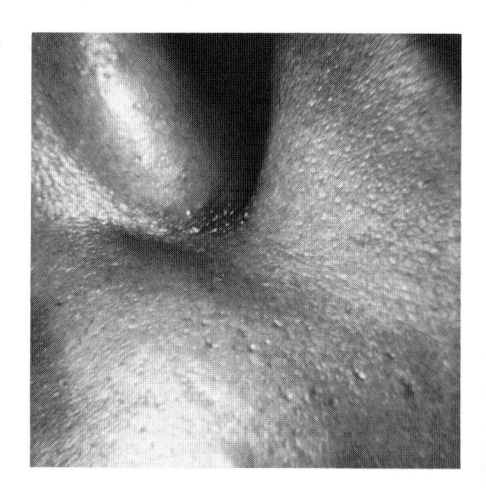

LABORATORY DIAGNOSIS

Dark-field examination is the most important diagnostic test for primary syphilis.[15] A small sample of serosanguinous fluid from the base of the chancre is observed under a dark-field microscope by an experienced microbiologist. *T. pallidum* is identified by both its characteristic morphology and motion. It is a spirochete 6 to 14 μm long (average 10 μm) that rotates on its long axis. As it moves longitudinally across the microscopic field, it demonstrates a unique twisting motion that resembles a coiled spring snapping back into shape after it has been released. Because only a small percentage of patients have a positive serologic test when the chancre first appears, the dark-field examination may be the only method of making a positive diagnosis of syphilis in the earliest stage of the disease. The dark-field examination is more difficult to perform in secondary syphilis because many of the lesions are dry and must be scraped with a scalpel. Dark-field microscopy cannot be performed reliably on mouth lesions because the mouth contains saprophytes, which are normal flora that may be morphologically indistinguishable from *T. pallidum*. In this situation, the organism can be positively identified by injecting a small amount of sterile saline into an enlarged regional lymph node and immediately aspirating material to examine by the dark-field technique.

Serologic tests for syphilis include both nontreponemal tests—such as the VDRL, rapid plasma reagin (RPR), and the automated reagin test (ART)—and treponemal tests—such as the FTA-ABS and the microhemagglutination (MHA) tests. Nontreponemal tests measure nonspecific antibodies associated with both syphilis and a variety of other diseases. When the test is positive in a patient who does not have syphilis, the result is called a biologic false-positive (BFP) reaction. Acute BFP reactions present for less than six months are usually associated with acute febrile illnesses and smallpox vaccinations. Chronic BFP reactions that remain positive for longer than six months are associated with aging, leprosy, collagen vascular diseases, autoimmune diseases, and neoplasia.[15] It is a mistake to assume that BFP reactions are associated only with low VDRL titers. One report discussed a patient with lymphosarcoma who had a prozone reaction with a titer of 1:256,[16] and we have seen one patient with Waldenstrom's macroglobulinema who had a titer in the range of 1:16,000 to 1:32,000.[17] A positive VDRL, therefore, supports a diagnosis of syphilis only when the patient has an appropriate history and physical examination.

There are two clinical situations where a treponemal test is necessary for diagnosis. The first is a patient who has a positive routine VDRL but has a normal physical examination and denies a history of syphilis. The second is a patient who has a BFP reaction but may also be at risk for syphilis. The best example of the latter is a heroin addict, as reported in studies of patients in New York City.[18,19] The treponemal test of choice has been the FTA-ABS. This is an indirect fluorescent antibody reaction performed with slides containing heat-fixed Nichol's strain of *T. pallidum* and the patient's serum. Most laboratories are performing an MHA test, which has the same sensitivity as the FTA-ABS except in primary syphilis. It is easier to perform and also displays fewer false-positive results. Chapter 13 presents more information on laboratory diagnosis.

It is important to realize that none of these tests can differentiate syphilis from the other treponemal diseases—yaws, pinta, and bejel. The FTA-ABS can be considered specific for syphilis among native-born North Americans because they are infrequently exposed to other treponemal diseases; however, it is always important to determine if a patient with positive tests that are otherwise unexplainable may have been exposed to another treponemal disease.

Even after treatment, the patient will have a positive FTA-ABS for life, except in very few cases where patients treated during the early primary stage may return to seronegativity.[20,21] The VDRL, on the other hand, is useful in following the course of disease after treatment and for evaluating reinfection. Within one year after treatment for primary syphilis, the VDRL returns to negative in nearly all patients. By the end of two years, almost all patients adequately treated for secondary syphilis will return to seronegativity. In early latent syphilis, those patients who will revert to seronegativity with treatment do so by the end of four years.[22] Patients treated for late latent syphilis generally demonstrate a diminution in titer; however, they usually remain serofast for life.

TREATMENT

The Centers for Disease Control (CDC) have issued revised guidelines for syphilis therapy.[23] The recommendations for primary, secondary, and latent syphilis of less than one year's duration are unchanged. Penicillin G benzathine, 2.4 million units given intramuscularly (IM) once, is still the regimen of choice. People allergic to penicillin should receive tetracycline, 500 mg orally four times daily for 15 days. Patients allergic to both penicillin and tetracycline can be treated with erythromycin, 500 mg orally four times daily for 15 days.

For latent syphilis of greater than one year's duration and cardiovascular and late benign syphilis, penicillin G benzathine 2.4 million units given IM once a week for three weeks remains the preferred regimen. Patients allergic to penicillin may be treated with tetracycline, 500 mg orally four times daily for 30 days. For patients allergic to both penicillin and tetracycline, erythromycin, 500 mg orally four times daily for 30 days, is an acceptable regimen. To rule out asymptomatic neurosyphilis, examination of the CSF before treatment is recommended for all patients who have had syphilis for longer than one year. This examination is especially important in patients who are not treated with penicillin, because data to support the effectiveness of the alternate regimens are not extensive. It is always important to remember that there is some risk of noncompliance with oral regimens.

Some recent reports in the literature[24-27] have suggested that penicillin G benzathine in the recommended doses does not always provide adequate therapeutic levels in the CSF; therefore, the CDC have provided several alternative regimens for treating neurosyphilis. Aqueous crystalline penicillin G, 2 to 4 million units IV every four hours for ten days, followed by penicillin G benzathine, 2.4 million units IM once weekly for three weeks, is a schedule recommended for inpatients. Outpatients may be treated with both aqueous penicillin G procaine, 2.4 million units IM daily, and probenecid, 500 mg orally four times daily, for 10 days. This should be followed by penicillin G benzathine, 2.4 million units weekly for three weeks. Another alternative is the previously recommended schedule of penicillin G benzathine, 2.4 million units IM at weekly intervals for a total of three weeks.

Follow-up should include repeat quantitative VDRL tests at 3, 6, 9, 12, 18, and 24 months following treatment to document a fall in titer. A greater than fourfold rise in titer or failure to observe a fourfold drop in titer over the year strongly suggests reinfection and requires clinical evaluation. It is usually an indication for retreatment.

It is clear from the controversy generated by several anecdotal reports[28-34] that much more data is necessary before definite conclusions can be drawn about the natural history of a dual infection with HIV and *T. pallidum*. CDC suggests that until more factual information is available patients with syphilis should be tested for HIV and vice versa.[35] Because results of serologic tests may not always be reliable in patients with both infections,[36] CDC recommends more frequent use of dark-field microscopy and direct fluorescent antibody staining for *T. pallidum*. Neurosyphilis should always be considered in the differential diagnosis of HIV-infected patients with neurologic complaints. Standard treatment schedules as described above are appropriate. Careful CSF examination prior to treatment in patients infected for longer than one year and serologic follow-up after therapy as described above are both especially important for managing patients with a dual infection.

REFERENCES

1. Fichtner RR, Arol SO, Blount JH, et al. Syphilis in the United States: 1967–1979. Sex Transm Dis 1983;10:77.
2. Centers for Disease Control. Division of Venereal Disease Control. Sexually transmitted disease (STD) statistical letter, calendar year 1984. Issue 134, Washington, DC: U.S. Department of Health and Human Services.
3. Centers for Disease Control. Syphilis and congenital syphilis—United States 1985–1988. MMWR 1988;37:486.
4. Drusin LM, Magagna J, Yano K, Ley AB. An epidemiologic study of sexually transmitted diseases on a university campus. Am J Epidemiol 1974;100:8.
5. Drusin LM, Homan WP, Dineen P. The role of surgery in primary syphilis of the anus. Ann Surg 1976;184:65.
6. Drusin LM, Singer C, Valenti AJ, Armstrong D. Infectious syphilis mimicking neoplastic disease. Arch Intern Med 1977;137:156.
7. Drusin LM, Topf-Olstein B, Levy-Zombek E. The epidemiology of infectious syphilis at a tertiary hospital. Arch Intern Med 1979;139:901.

8. Baker AL, Kaplan MM, Wolfe HJ, McGowan JA. Liver disease associated with early syphilis. N Engl J Med 1971;284:1422.
9. Lee RV, Thornton GF, Conn HO. Liver Disease associated with secondary syphilis. N Engl J Med 1971;284:1423.
10. Keisler DS, Starke W, Looney DJ, Mark WW Jr. Early syphilis with liver involvement. JAMA 1982;247:1999.
11. Drusin LM. Syphilis and other sexually transmitted diseases. Cutis 1981;27:286.
12. Willcox RR, Goodwin PG. Nerve deafness in early syphilis. Br J Vener Dis 1971;47:401.
13. Magnuson HJ, Thomas EW, Olansky S, et al. Inoculation syphilis in human volunteers. Medicine 1956;35:33.
14. Bhorade MS, Carag HB, Lee HJ, et al. Nephropathy of secondary syphilis. JAMA 1971;216:1159.
15. Drusin LM. The diagnosis and treatment of infectious and latent syphilis. Med Clin North Am 1972;56:11.
16. Wuepper KD, Tuffanelli DL. False positive reaction to VDRL test with prozone phenomena associated with lymphosarcoma. JAMA 1966;195:868.
17. Drusin LM, Litwin SD, Armstrong D, et al. Waldenstrom's macroglobulinemia in a patient with a chronic biologic false positive serologic test for syphilis. Ann J Med 1974;56:429.
18. Kaufman RE, Weiss S, Moore JD, et al. Biological false positive serological tests for syphilis among drug addicts. Br J Vener Dis 1974;50:350.
19. Tuffanelli DL. Narcotic addiction with a false positive reaction for syphilis: Immunologic studies. Acta Derm Venereal (Stockh) 1968;48:542.
20. Schroeter AL, Lucas JB, Price EV, et al. Treatment for early syphilis and reactivity of serologic tests. JAMA 1972;221:471.
21. Kampmeir RH, Sweeney A, Quinn RW, et al. A survey of 251 patients with acute syphilis treated in the collaborative penicillin study of 1943–1950. Sex Transm Dis 1981;8:266.
22. Fiumara NJ. Reinfection of primary, secondary and latent syphilis. The serologic response after treatment. Sex Transm Dis 1980;7:111.
23. Centers for Disease Control. 1985 STD treatment guidelines. MMWR (Suppl);34:4S.
24. Yoder FW. Penicillin treatment of neurosyphilis. Are recommended dosages sufficient? JAMA 1975;232:270.
25. Mohr JA, Griffiths W, Jackson R, et al. Neurosyphilis and penicillin levels in cerebrospinal fluid. JAMA 1976;236:2208.
26. Tramont EC. Persistence of *Treponema pallidum* following penicillin G therapy. Report of two cases. JAMA 1976;236:2206.
27. Greene BM, Miller NR, Bynum TE. Failure of penicillin G benzathine in the treatment of neurosyphilis. Arch Intern Med 1980;140:1117.
28. Carter JB, Hamill RJ, Matoba AV. Bilateral syphilitic optic neuritis in a patient with a positive test for HIV. Arch Ophthalmol 1987;105:1485.
29. Kleiner RC, Najarian L, Levenson J, Kaplan HJ. AIDS complicated by syphilis can mimic uveitis and Crohn's disease. Arch Ophthalmol 1987;105:1486.
30. Berry CD, Hooton TM, Collier AC, et al. Neurologic relapse after benzathine penicillin therapy for secondary syphilis in a patient with HIV infection. New Engl J Med 1987;316:1587.
31. Johns DR, Tierney M, Felsenstein D. Alteration in the natural history of neurosyphilis by concurrent infection with the human immunodeficiency virus. N Engl J Med 1987;316:1569.

32. Beck-Sague CM, Alexander ER, Jaffe HW. Neurosyphilis and HIV infection. Letter to the editor. N Engl J Med 1987;317:1473.
33. Jordan KG. Neurosyphilis and HIV infection. Letter to the editor. N Engl J Med 1987;317:1473.
34. Johns DR, Tierney M, Parker SW. Pure motor hemiplegia due to meningovascular neurosyphilis. Arch Neurol 1987;44:1062.
35. Centers for Disease Control. Recommendations for diagnosing and treating syphilis in HIV infected patients. MMWR 1988;37:600.
36. Hicks CB, Benson PM, Lupton GP, et al. Seronegative secondary syphilis in a patient infected with human immunodeficiency virus (HIV) with Kaposi sarcoma. Ann Intern Med 1987;107:492.

Chapter 3

The Relationship of HIV Infections to Infections with Pathogenic *Neisseria* in Homosexual Men

Franklyn N. Judson

Even early asymptomatic infection with HIV can lead to a broad array of immunologic abnormalities.[1] Theoretically, HIV-induced defects in bactericidal antibody production and in neutrophil and macrophage function could predispose individuals infected with the pathogenic *Neisseria* to more severe and prolonged local infections as well as to higher rates of disseminated disease. Although selective defects in soluble antigen recognition,[2] depressed B-cell proliferative responses both to T-cell-dependent and T-cell-independent mitogens,[3,4] depressed antibody responses to pneumococcal polysaccharide vaccine,[5] defective polymorphonuclear leukocyte chemotaxis,[6] and impaired macrophage function[7] have been described in homosexual men with acquired immunodeficiency syndrome (AIDS) or generalized lymphadenopathy syndrome, thus far there is no evidence that individuals with HIV infections of any level of severity are experiencing immunologic difficulties with *Neisseria* infections. Nonetheless, because of recent reports in AIDS patients of an excess of severe bacterial diseases including pneumonia caused by *Haemophilus influenzae*,[8,9] a bacterium closely related to the gonococcus, continued surveillance of *Neisseria* infections in homosexual men seems prudent.

This chapter will broadly review the subject of pathogenic *Neisseria* as they affect homosexual men. In particular, it will provide an update on the use of gonococcal incidence rates to monitor indirectly occurrence of sexual behavior at high risk of transmitting HIV.

There are ten recognized species within the genus *Neisseria*, but only two—*N. gonorrhoeae* and *N. meningitidis*—are well-known pathogens of human beings. Undoubtedly the products of a lengthy evolutionary divergence, the meningococcus and the gonococcus remain very similar in terms of colonial and cellular morphology, nutritional requirements, susceptibility to antibiotics, exclusive human host, mucous membrane ecologic niches, and disease spectra. Their most striking differences are epidemiologic, yet even here the distinctions are blurred.

In the general population, the prevalence of colonization with *N. meningitidis* is much higher than with *N. gonorrhoeae* and is not restricted to young, sexually active individuals. The predominant site for colonization is the nasopharynx, where carriage rates may exceed 20% during some winter months. In a 32-month study of families from Syracuse, NY, prevalence rates for nasopharyngeal infections with *N. meningitidis* ranged from 4.9% to 10.6%, affecting all age groups.[10] The primary mode of meningococcal transmission is through nasopharyngeal secretions, either by direct contact or through respiratory droplets.

The primary mode of gonococcal transmission is through infectious secretions of genital mucous membranes that are shared during vaginal intercourse. Consequently, most reported cases of gonorrhea are endocervical or urethral infections in heterosexual men and women. Nonetheless, it is now clear that the ecologic niche for *N. gonorrhoeae* is far larger than originally thought and comprises, in addition, the transitional or columnar epithelial linings of numerous genital and perigenital glands, the anorectum, and the oropharynx. Likewise, the meningococcus has recently been found outside its customary nasopharyngeal habitat and has been isolated with variable frequency from the endocervix, urethra, and anal canal.

The gonococcus is far more likely than the meningococcus to produce local symptomatic disease and suppurative complications, particularly of the urethra, epididymis, salpinx, and Bartholin's glands. Neither species causes symptoms very often when infecting the anorectum or oropharynx. Dissemination from any mucosal surface into the blood or cerebrospinal fluid (CSF) is a rare but well-recognized complication of infection with either species. Among homosexual men who attend public clinics for the treatment of sexually transmitted diseases, infection rates from both *N. meningitidis* and *N. gonorrhoeae* are significantly higher than for their heterosexual male counterparts, often by a factor of 2 or more.[11,12] Very high carriage rates (e.g., 40% to 50% for *N. meningitidis* and 10% to 15% for *N. gonorrhoeae*) have also been noted in homosexual men who patronize commercial steam baths to engage in recreational sex.[13,14] Apart from these high-risk settings, little is known about comparative *N. meningitidis* colonization rates in homosexual men within the general population because surveillance studies have not attempted to determine sexual preference.

EPIDEMIOLOGY

Neisseria gonorrhoeae

Table 3–1 presents mucosal-site-specific prevalence rates for gonococcal infections in 8278 homosexual men who made initial visits (i.e., for a new problem)

Table 3–1 Results of urethral, anal canal, and pharyngeal cultures for N. gonorrhoeae in 8278 homosexual men who made initial visits to the Denver Metro Health Clinic, July 1, 1978, to June 30, 1980

Culture Site(s)	Positive (N)	Tested Men Positive (%)	Infected Men Positive (%)
Urethra only	1225	14.8	44.3
Anal canal only	1014	12.2	36.6
Pharynx only	161	2.0	5.8
Urethra and anal canal	209	2.5	7.6
Urethra and pharynx	59	0.7	2.1
Anal canal and pharynx	71	0.9	2.6
Urethra, anal canal, and pharynx	28	0.3	1.0

to the Denver Metro Health Clinic during a two-year period (July 1, 1978, to June 30, 1980). The review was facilitated by a computerized records system supported by the Centers for Disease Control (CDC), Atlanta, GA. Overall, 2767 or 33.4% of homosexual men were infected at one or more sites, including the urethra in 1521 (18.4%), the anal canal in 1322 (16.0%), and the pharynx in 319 (3.8%). During the same period, the corresponding urethral infection rate for heterosexual male patients matched for age and race was 14.8%. Wiesner et al. noted pharyngeal infection rates of 1.4% (3/217) in male heterosexual patients compared with 9.9% (14/143) in male homosexual patients at a venereal disease clinic.[15] Thus, most of the excess prevalence of gonococcal infections in homosexual men is accounted for by infections of the additional at-risk anal canal and pharyngeal sites.

Of 2767 homosexual men from whom N. gonorrhoeae was isolated from any site, the urethra was infected in 1521 (55.0%), the anal canal in 1322 (47.8%), the pharynx in 319 (11.5%), two sites in 339 (12.3%), and three sites in 28 (1.0%). Importantly, a mutual exclusion did not exist between infections of the active urethral site and the passive anal canal and pharyngeal sites, because 296 (19.5%) of 1521 men with urethritis also had involvement of a passive site. This can be explained either by infection with different strains acquired from different partners or by active and passive transmission during anilingus. Evidence has shown that both are possible.[16] The therapeutic implication is that homosexual men diagnosed as having gonorrhea on the basis of a urethral discharge should not be assumed to be infected at only one site and should not be treated with an ampicillin or tetracycline regimen known to be suboptimal for anorectal or pharyngeal infection.

Gonorrhea incidence rates specific for sexual preference (per 100,000 men) cannot be determined accurately because (1) the proportion of the male population that is homosexual in a given community is not known and (2) gonorrhea cases are not reported by sexual preference in the United States. However, if we accept that (1) homosexual and heterosexual men of the same age are equally likely to attend the Denver Metro Health Clinic based on health care needs, (2) 10% of men in Denver are homosexual, and (3) 30% of male visits are made by homosexual men,[11] we may calculate that the relative gonorrhea incidence rate in homosexual men is 6.8 times greater than in heterosexual men in Denver.

In 1982, coverage of AIDS by medical journals and by national and local news media mushroomed, and by the end of 1982, most homosexual men in Denver, Colorado, knew that they comprised about 85% of all AIDS cases, that AIDS was probably caused by a sexually transmitted agent, and that the major risk factor for AIDS appeared to be the number of male sexual partners per year. It was to be expected that fear of acquiring an untreatable, ultimately fatal disease would influence sexual behavior. This has proved true.

Rates of infection with *N. gonorrhoeae* is a sensitive indicator of changing sexual behavior because this infection is so common in homosexual men, it is easy to detect and to treat, and the incubation period is short. Table 3–2 compares the seroprevalence of HIV antibody and the number of cases of gonorrhea in homosexual men who attended the Denver Metro Health Clinic with the number of new cases of AIDS in Colorado from 1980 to 1988. The 95% decline in yearly incidence of gonorrhea from 1809 cases in 1982 to 92 cases in 1988 clearly indicates that most homosexual men have opted for more conservative sexual life styles.

Neisseria meningitidis

The oropharynx is the preferred habitat of the meningococcus in both homosexual and heterosexual men; however, as with the gonococcus, carriage rates appear to be much higher in homosexual men. Table 3–3 presents the comparative isolation rates of *N. meningitidis* and *N. gonorrhoeae* from posterior pharyngeal specimens of 10,436 homosexual men who made initial visits to the Denver Metro Health Clinic during an 18-month period (Jan. 1, 1981, to June 30, 1982). *N. meningitidis* was isolated nearly six times as often as *N. gonorrhoeae* (35.6% vs 6.5%). Meningococcal isolation rates did not vary much on a seasonal basis and ranged from 31.7% to 38.3% during the six periods of three months each that were analyzed.

Because routes of transmission for and susceptibility to the meningococcus and gonococcus are very similar, it was to be expected that the meningococcus would be found in anorectal and urethral sites of homosexual men. In an earlier study,[16] we isolated *N. meningitidis* from the anal canals and urethras, respectively, of 2.1% and 0.4% of 731 male homosexuals. *N. meningitidis* comprised, respectively, 15.0% and 3.5% of total *Neisseria* isolates from these sites. Janda et al.[12] took cultures from 815 homosexual men over a 12-month period and noted similar carriage rates: oropharynx, 42.5%; anal canal, 2.0%; and urethra, 0.7%. It is not known how long meningococcal carriage at the anorectum or urethra is sustained, but it is at least a number of days to weeks in some pa-

Table 3–2 Seroprevalence of HIV antibody[a] and number of cases of gonorrhea in homosexual men who attended the Denver Metro Health Clinic and number of new cases of AIDS in Colorado, 1980 to 1988

	Year								
	1980	1981	1982	1983	1984	1985	1986	1987	1988
Seroprevalence of HIV antibody	1%	[b]	[b]	[b]	52%	49%	49%	38%	47%
Number of cases of AIDS	0	0	7	23	41	85	177	248	274
Number of cases of gonorrhea	[b]	[b]	1809	1149	898	785	270	166	92

[a]Litton Bionetics ELISA; positives confirmed by Western blot.
[b]Not studied.

Table 3–3 Comparative isolation rates of *N. meningitidis* and *N. gonorrhoeae* from posterior pharyngeal specimens from 10,436 homosexual men who made initial visits to the Denver Metro Health Clinic, Jan. 1, 1981, to June 30, 1982

Species Isolated	Positive (N)	% of Total
N. meningitidis	3635	34.8
N. gonorrhoeae	591	5.7
Both	86	0.8
Neither	6124	58.7

tients,[16] although higher positivity rates in the anal canals of men tested at bathhouses could imply shorter terms of carriage for others.[14]

We have speculated that most meningococcal anal canal infections result from contact with infectious saliva, either directly through anilingus or indirectly off the penis following fellatio or when applied to the anal area as a lubricant.[16] Urethral infection is much less common and could occur during either fellatio or anal intercourse.

A number of investigators have shown that homosexual men who have *N. meningitidis* isolated from the oropharynx are 1.8 to 2.7 times more likely to have *N. gonorrhoeae* isolated from an anogenital area.[11,17] Conversely, men with genital gonorrhea are two to six times more likely to have pharyngeal cultures positive for *N. meningitidis*.[11,18,19] Undoubtedly, this association is again owing to similar susceptibility and sexual activity factors. Of the two risk factors, current opinion favors sexual activity as the key.

CLINICAL SPECTRUM

The clinical spectra of *N. meningitidis* and *N. gonorrhoeae* are nearly identical at the various potential sites of infection. Almost all gonococcal urethral infections are symptomatic at some time. Janda et al.[12] reported that all 270 men with urethral gonorrhea had symptoms. This high rate of symptoms has been attributed to the selection, in homosexual men under antibiotic pressure, of a population of gonococcal strains characterized by lower susceptibility to antibiotics and lower rates of the arginine, hypoxanthine, and uracil (AHU) requiring nutritional auxotype.[20] The antibiotic pressure is, in turn, probably the result of more frequent treatment of homosexual men with penicillin and tetracycline because of their more frequent contact or infection with *N. gonorrhoeae* and *Treponema pallidum*. The use of long-acting penicillin G benzathine for syphilis may be a particularly effective selective pressure favoring accumulation of relatively resistant gonococci.

Meningococcal urethritis has not been studied extensively enough to determine symptomatic rates, but Janda et al.[12] noted urethral discharge in five of six patients. We reported urethral discharge in two of three homosexual men with *N. meningitidis* infection.[16]

The natural history of either gonococcal or meningococcal anorectal infection in homosexual men has not been well studied, and the duration of infection without treatment is unknown. Both infections are believed to be largely asymptomatic, but no study has followed a sufficiently large number of infected men using a full complement of diagnostic tests for other rectal pathogens to define symptomatic rates and clinical spectra adequately.

An early study by Owen and Hill concluded that similar rectal symptoms in men with and without rectal gonorrhea suggested that symptoms are not directly related to gonorrheal infection.[21] This may be valid as a general rule, yet most experienced venereologists are quite familiar with the homosexual man who complains of recent onset of anorectal symptoms, who is found to have a purulent anal discharge diagnostic for *Neisseria* on Gram's stain (i.e., gram-negative intracellular diplococci within abundant polymorphonuclear leukocytes), whose cultures are subsequently positive for *N. gonorrhoeae*, and whose symptoms respond rapidly to treatment (e.g., ceftriaxone, 125–250 mg intramuscularly [IM]). Both we[16] and Janda et al.[12] found anorectal meningococcal infections to be largely asymptomatic, but neither study had sufficient patients to rule out low rates of symptomatic proctitis.

The clinical spectrum of pharyngeal gonococcal infection closely resembles anorectal infection in that the preponderance of infections are asymptomatic. Wiesner et al.,[15] in a study of pharyngeal gonorrhea that included 14 infected homosexual men, concluded that symptoms of pharyngitis correlated with the practice of fellatio but not with gonococcal pharyngeal infection. Wallin and Siegel[22] went so far as to follow—without treatment—17 initially asymptomatic men and women with pharyngeal gonorrhea to learn the natural history of this infection. All the subjects became culture negative over 12 weeks, and none transmitted infection to a sexual partner through mouth-to-mouth contact. This study does not, however, preclude transmission through saliva, and data from our clinic indicate that caution with oral secretions is advisable because 67% of patients with pharyngeal cultures positive for *N. gonorrhoeae* also had positive saliva cultures.

As in anorectal infection, the gonococcus can occasionally cause pharyngeal symptoms. Symptomatic gonococcal pharyngitis has been a well-recognized clinical entity for many years.[23] Even Wiesner et al.[15] noted that *N. gonorrhoeae* did appear responsible for symptoms of pharyngitis in selected patients. In contradistinction, no one has yet shown that the meningococcus causes symptoms of pharyngitis.

Both *N. gonorrhoeae* and *N. meningitidis* may rarely disseminate from mucosal sites. Although it has been thought that dissemination of *N. gonorrhoeae* may occur more readily from the pharynx than from other sites, site-specific rates of dissemination have not been determined. Considering the very high prevalence and incidence rates for gonococcal infection in homosexual men, dissemination may actually be relatively less frequent per infected site than in heterosexual men and women. Again, this may be due to the high proportion of strains isolated from homosexual men that do not have the biologic characteristics of strains prone to disseminate.[20]

Disseminated meningococcal disease is rare in sexually active young adults and is not reported by sexual preference. There is, however, not even suggestive evidence that incidence rates are higher in homosexual than in heterosexual men. Dissemination from the very commonly colonized pharyngeal mucosa must be extraordinarily unusual, even in men infected with HIV.

DIAGNOSTIC CONSIDERATIONS

This section will not constitute a full review of procedures used in the diagnosis of infections with *N. gonorrhoeae* and *N. meningitidis* but rather will present a few selected recommendations I have found useful.

When properly performed, a urethral gram-stained smear should be approximately 98% sensitive and 98% specific in diagnosing a gonorrheal discharge.[24] Because almost all gonococcal urethritis in homosexual men results in a discharge, cultures are seldom necessary, particularly if a recommended ceftriaxone (125–250 mg IM) regimen is used. If a urethral culture is performed, speciation of *Neisseria* isolates is not indicated on a cost-benefit basis because only a few percent will be *N. meningitidis* and the epidemiologic, clinical, and treatment implications may be the same.[16]

With anorectal gonorrhea, unless pus is actually exuding from the anal canal, gram-stained smears are of low sensitivity and specificity due to the diagnostic difficulties encountered in sorting through complex fecal cellular constituents.

An anal canal culture is the most sensitive diagnostic test available, yet the actual sensitivity has never been determined. It is probably no more than 70% to 80% sensitive and may even be much lower when specimen collection and culture techniques are suboptimal.[24] Fortunately, anal canal specimens taken blindly seem to perform as well as rectal specimens taken through a proctoscope.[25] A convenient approach to specimen collection is for a seated clinician—aided by good lighting—to ask the patient to "Turn around, bend over, spread your cheeks, and bear down slightly." The clinician is then free to guide a cotton-tipped swab, using a rotary motion, several centimeters into the protruding anal canal, allowing about five seconds for absorption of the specimen. Unless it contains gross feces, the specimen then can be directly plated onto selective medium (e.g., Thayer-Martin, Martin-Lewis, or New York City). Speciation of anal canal *Neisseria* isolates is advisable for microbiologic accuracy because up to 20% will be *N. meningitidis*.[12,14,16]

Gram-stained smears of posterior pharyngeal specimens are of no value in diagnosing either gonococcal or meningococcal infections. There are too few polymorphonuclear leukocytes, and gonococci cannot be distinguished from meningococci or the far more numerous nonpathogenic *Neisseria*. The culture sensitivity of a single, well-directed, vigorously swabbed posterior pharyngeal specimen can only be inferred. Based on our results from repetitive cultures taken from infected men before treatment, I estimate that a single positive culture is 60% to 70% reproducible. It can easily be much less if the most careful culturing technique is not used. Following are detailed guidelines for optimizing pharyngeal culture sensitivity:

1. Pharyngeal cultures should be inoculated directly onto a selective media (e.g., Thayer-Martin or New York City) that has been warmed to room temperature. Immediate plating will reduce loss of organisms due to drying or exposure to fatty acids that may be present if cotton swabs are used.
2. Inoculated plates should always be cross streaked. This will reduce exposure of *N. gonorrhoeae* or *N. meningitidis* to inhibitory substances or other bacteriocin-producing organisms that may be present in the inoculum. Pharyngeal cultures will often contain yeasts or gram-negative rods that have not been inhibited by the media. Cultures from patients who frequent bathhouses tend to have gram-negative rods such as *Flavobacterium* and *Pseudomonas* species, which seem to thrive in a humid environment.
3. Plates should be placed with little delay in an incubator with a temperature of 35° to 36.5°C. If 37°C is used, fluctuations to 37.5°C may inhibit the growth of some heat-sensitive strains of gonococci. The atmosphere should contain from 3% to 10% CO_2, and the humidity should be at least 70%.
4. Plates should be incubated for a minimum of 48 hours. *Neisseria* appearing at 24 hours are usually meningococci. Gonococci are seldom readily apparent on pharyngeal cultures before 48 hours.
5. Plates are examined for the presence of oxidase-positive, gram-negative diplococci. Colonies of *N. gonorrhoeae* tend to be smaller than those of *N. meningitidis*. Meningococcal colonies will often give a greenish cast to the medium beneath the colony. When freshly cultured, meningococcal colonies will have a smooth, entirely round edge. Gonococcal colonies may also appear this way or have an irregular edge. Frequently, gonococci will demonstrate different colony types on the same plate. Care must be taken to identify each colony type by confirmatory tests because mixtures of gonococci and meningococci are not uncommon in pharyngeal cultures. Portions of colonies with morphology suggestive of *Neisseria* should be tested for an oxidase-positive reaction. If no *Neisseria* colonies are detected after incubation for 48 hours, the plates should be flooded with oxidase-indicator solution to detect small numbers of inhibited colonies of *Neisseria*. If the Thayer-Martin or Martin-Lewis media are overly inhibitory, *N. gonorrhoeae* may appear as small, pinpoint colonies. Colonies should be subcultured immediately before they turn black and nonviable. All oxidase-positive colonies should have their morphology confirmed by Gram's smears.
6. All oxidase-positive, gram-negative diplococci should be speciated by an appropriate confirmatory method such as acid production from carbohydrates, fluorescent antibody, or coagglutination. The rapid fermentation test, based on preformed enzyme in a heavy inoculum, is fast and reliable and has

bypassed some of the problems encountered when using carbohydrate degradation in cystine-tryptic digest agar-base media. Specific commercial fluorescent antisera that will accurately distinguish between gonococci and meningococci are not readily available. Commercially available coagglutination tests do not react with all strains of gonococci, and specificity can be a problem. Colony morphology and technician experience should be the guide. If the results of one confirmatory test do not correlate with the appearance of the colonies, a second method should be used to confirm the results. Kraus has succinctly summarized the challenge: "The ability of a laboratory to isolate the gonococcus relates to the quality of the reagents and media, and the technician's expertise, time, and interest."[27]

TREATMENT CONSIDERATIONS

Treatment recommendations for gonococcal infections have been recently reviewed by Washington.[26] For a comprehensive approach to treatment, the reader is referred to this paper as well as to the CDC's *Sexually Transmitted Diseases Treatment Guidelines 1985*.[28] Herein, I will discuss a few special considerations in the therapy of anogenital and pharyngeal gonorrhea in homosexual men.

Although urethral infections probably can be cured with any of the CDC's recommended treatment regimens,[28] my treatment of choice for most gonococcal infections of homosexual men is ceftriaxone, 125 mg in 0.5 ml of diluent, injected into a deltoid muscle. This is because gonorrhea is not infrequently a multiple site infection, and ceftriaxone achieves maximal cure rates at all three potentially infected sites with minimal discomfort and no risk of toxic procaine reactions.[29] In addition, ceftriaxone is highly active against the increasingly prevalent strains of *N. gonorrhoeae* that are relatively resistant to penicillin, based on plasmid-mediated penicillinase production or chromosomally mediated resistance.

Tetracycline and, to a lesser extent, ampicillin regimens have high failure rates (e.g., 5% to 30%) in patients with anorectal gonorrhea.[26] Tetracycline probably fails more often in men than in women because isolates from men tend to be more resistant to penicillin and tetracycline. Table 3–4, which compares susceptibility to ampicillin and tetracycline of anorectal isolates from 178 homosexual men and 44 heterosexual women seen at the Denver Metro Health Clinic, supports this explanation. The geometric mean minimal inhibiting concentration (MIC) of tetracycline was nearly two times higher for anorectal isolates from men (0.524 µg/ml) than for anorectal isolates from women (0.283 µg/ml).

It is possible that higher resistance could be overcome with larger daily doses of tetracycline, but predictably at a cost of greater gastrointestinal intolerance. There seems to be little reason to study tetracycline further in homosexual men because its major advantage in the treatment of gonorrhea is its efficacy against concomitant *Chlamydia trachomatis* infections in heterosexual men and women. Nongonococcal urethritis, postgonococcal urethritis, and culture-positive chla-

Table 3–4 Geometric mean MIC (μg/ml) of ampicillin and tetracycline for pretreatment anorectal N. gonorrhoeae isolates from 178 homosexual men and 44 heterosexual women who attended the Denver Metro Health Clinic, 1982

		Geometric Mean MIC (μg/ml)	
Patients	Isolates (N)	Ampicillin	Tetracycline
Homosexual men	178	0.156	0.524
Heterosexual women	44	0.124	0.283

mydial urethritis are all markedly less common in homosexual men, who, in addition, play little role in the most important chlamydial complications: pelvic inflammatory disease and neonatal infections. Sands and Sellers found that if oral therapy is desired, repeating the standard ampicillin regimen (3.5 g plus 1 g of probenecid) in 8 to 14 hours reduced the anorectal failure rate to 1.6%, an efficacy comparable to the aqueous penicillin G procaine regimen.[30] Limited clinical data indicate that anorectal N. meningitidis infections should respond to the same treatment regimens effective in gonorrhea.[16]

Both single-dose spectinomycin (2 g IM) and ampicillin regimens have high failure rates in pharyngeal gonorrhea,[26] although an extended ampicillin regimen consisting of a single oral 3.5 g dose plus 1 g of probenecid followed by 500 mg of ampicillin four times a day for two more days (total ampicillin dose of 7.5 g) resulted in only three failures (3.9%) of 77 trials in men and women.[31] Currently ceftriaxone, 125–250 mg should be the treatment of choice for pharyngeal gonorrhea.

Except for ceftriaxone, 125 mg, which eradicated N. meningitidis from the posterior pharynx of 29 of 29 homosexual men and heterosexual women,[32] there have been no other published studies on the efficacy of recommended gonorrhea treatment regimens in eradicating pharyngeal meningococcal carriage. However, at this time there is no reason to treat asymptomatic pharyngeal carriage with endemic strains. Moreover, on the basis of susceptibility to ampicillin and tetracycline, it is likely that pharyngeal N. meningitidis would respond similarly to N. gonorrhoeae. Table 3–5 presents our susceptibility results for pharyngeal isolates from homosexual men.

Table 3–5 Geometric mean MIC (μg/ml) of ampicillin and tetracycline for pretreatment pharyngeal N. gonorrhoeae and N. meningitidis isolates from homosexual men who attended the Denver Metro Health Clinic, 1982

		Geometric Mean MIC (μg/ml)	
Species	Isolates (N)	Ampicillin	Tetracycline
N. gonorrhoeae	41	0.102	0.639
N. meningitidis	101	0.099	0.604

IMPLICATIONS FOR AIDS AND OTHER HIV INFECTIONS

It is highly unlikely that mucous membrane colonization or infection with *N. gonorrhoeae* or *N. meningitidis* plays any direct part in the pathogenesis of AIDS. Although there is a cell-mediated immune response to gonococcal infections, which includes lymphocyte transformation,[33,34] its significance in overall host defense is not known but is probably minor. The most important immune responses to *Neisseria* infections involve antibody production[35] and polymorphonuclear phagocytic function.[36] Until AIDS patients are terminal, they seem to have normal or increased antibody levels and normal numbers of circulating phagocytes.

There have been no reports, to date, of severe gonococcal infections in HIV infections at any level of severity or of disseminated infection with either *N. gonorrhoeae* or *N. meningitidis*, despite the extremely high rates with which pathogenic *Neisseria* infections occur in sexually active homosexual men. The only apparent role left for *Neisseria* infections would seem to be as nonetiologic risk markers for HIV infection.

REFERENCES

1. Nicholson KA, McDougal JS, Jaffee HW, et al. Exposure to human T-lymphotropic virus type III/lymphadenopathy associated virus and immunologic abnormalities in asymptomatic homosexual men. Ann Intern Med 1985;103:37.
2. Lane CH, Depper JM, Greene WC, et al. Qualitative analysis of immune function in patients with the acquired immunodeficiency syndrome. Evidence for a selective defect in soluble antigen recognition. N Engl J Med 1985;313:79.
3. Lane HC, Masur H, Edgar LC, et al. Abnormalities of B-cell activation and immunoregulation in patients with the acquired immunodeficiency syndrome. N Engl J Med 1983;309:453.
4. Pahwa SG, Quilop MTJ, Lange M, et al. Defective B-lymphocyte function in homosexual men in relation to the acquired immunodeficiency syndrome. Ann Intern Med 1984;101:757.
5. Ammann AJ, Schiffman G, Abrams D, et al. B-cell immunodeficiency in acquired immunodeficiency syndrome. JAMA 1984;251:1447.
6. Valone FH, Payan DG, Abrams DI, Goetzl EJ. Defective polymorphonuclear chemotaxis in homosexual men with persistent lymph node syndrome. J Infect Dis 1984;150:267.
7. Murray HW, Rubin BY, Masur H, Roberts RB. Impaired production of lymphokines and immune (gamma) interferon in the acquired immunodeficiency syndrome. N Engl J Med 1984;310:883.
8. White S, Tsou E, Waldhorn RE, Katz P. Life-threatening bacterial pneumonia in male homosexuals with laboratory features of the acquired immunodeficiency syndrome. Chest 1985;87:486.
9. Polsky B, Gold JWM, Whimbey E, et al. Bacterial pneumonia in patients with the acquired immunodeficiency syndrome. Ann Intern Med 1986;104:38.

10. Greenfield S, Scheehe PR, Feldman HA. Meningococcal carriage in a population of "normal" families. J Infect Dis 1971;123:67.
11. Judson FN, Penley KA, Robinson ME, Smith JK. Comparative prevalence rates of sexually transmitted diseases in heterosexual and homosexual men. Am J Epidemiol 1980;112:836.
12. Janda WM, Bohnhoff M, Morello JA, Lerner SA. Prevalence and site-pathogen studies of *Neisseria meningitidis* and *N. gonorrhoeae* in homosexual men. JAMA 1980;244:2060.
13. Judson FN, Miller KG, Schaffnit TR. Screening for gonorrhea and syphilis in the gay baths—Denver, Colorado. Am J Public Health 1977;67:740.
14. Carlson BL, Fiumara NJ, Kelly JR, McCormack WM. Isolation of *Neisseria meningitidis* from anogenital species of homosexual men. Sex Transm Dis 1980;7:71.
15. Wiesner PJ, Tronca E, Bonin P, et al. Clinical spectrum of pharyngeal gonococcal infection. N Engl J Med 1973;288:181.
16. Judson FN, Ehret JM, Eichoff TC. Anogenital infection with *Neisseria meningitidis* in homosexual men. J Infect Dis 1978;137:458.
17. Willcox RR, Spenser RC, Ison C. Which *Neisseria*? Br J Vener Dis 1977;53:394.
18. Rufli J. Which *Neisseria*? Br J Vener Dis 1978;54:352.
19. Odegaard K, Gedde-Dahl TW. Frequency of simultaneous carriage of *Neisseria gonorrhoeae* and *Neisseria meningitidis*. Br J Vener Dis 1979;55:334.
20. Janda WM, Morella JA, Lerner SA, Bohnhoff M. Characteristics of pathogenic *Neisseria* sp. isolated from homosexual men. J Clin Microbiol 1983;17:85.
21. Owen RL, Hill JL. Rectal and pharyngeal gonorrhea in homosexual men. JAMA 1972;220:1315.
22. Wallin J, Siegel MS. Pharyngeal *Neisseria gonorrhoeae:* Colonizer or pathogen? Br Med J 1979;1:1462.
23. Fiumara NJ. Pharyngeal infection with *Neisseria gonorrhoeae*. Sex Transm Dis 1979;6:264.
24. Judson FN. A clinic-based system for monitoring the quality of techniques for the diagnosis of gonorrhea. Sex Transm Dis 1978;5:141.
25. Kolator B, Rodin P. Comparison of anal and rectal swabs in the diagnosis of anorectal gonorrhea in women. Br J Vener Dis 1979;55:186.
26. Washington AE. Update on treatment recommendations for gonococcal infections. Rev Infect Dis 1981;4(suppl):758.
27. Kraus SJ. Culture methods for *Neisseria gonorrhoeae*. Arch Androl 1979;3:343.
28. Centers for Disease Control. Sexually transmitted diseases treatment guidelines 1985. Morbid Mortal Weekly Rep (Suppl); 1985;34:8.
29. Judson FN, Ehret JM, Handsfield HH. Comparative study of ceftriaxone and spectinomycin for treatment of pharyngeal and anorectal gonorrhea. JAMA 1985;253:1417.
30. Sands M, Sellers T. Therapy of anorectal gonorrhea in men. Efficacy of oral antibiotic regimens. West J Med 1980;133:469.
31. DiCaprio JM, Reynolds J, Frank G, et al. Ampicillin therapy for pharyngeal gonorrhea. JAMA 1978;239:1631.
32. Judson FN, Ehret JM. Single-dose ceftriaxone to eradicate pharyngeal *Neisseria meningitidis*. Lancet 1984;2:1462.
33. Grimble AS, McIllmurray MB. Cell-mediated immune response in gonorrhea. Br J Vener Dis 1973;49:446.
34. Wyle FA, Rowlett C, Blumenthal T. Cell-mediated immune response in gonococcal infections. Br J Vener Dis 1977;53:353.

35. Broude AI. Resistance to infection with the gonococcus. J Infect Dis 1982;145:623.
36. Densen P, Mandell GL. Gonococcal interactions with polymorphonuclear neutrophils. Importance of the phagosome for bactericidal activity. J Clin Invest 1978; 62:1161.

Chapter 4
Proctitis due to *Chlamydia trachomatis*

Walter E. Stamm

Chlamydia trachomatis rectal infection occurs both in women and homosexual men,[1-4] with clinical manifestations ranging from no symptoms to acute but usually mild proctitis. Rectal infection with *C. trachomatis* lymphogranuloma venereum (LGV) strains has typically been associated with indolent chronic disease characterized by fistula formation[5,6] and, more recently, with acute proctocolitis.[4] Recent studies have helped to delineate the incidence and spectrum of *C. trachomatis* rectal infection in homosexual men.

Our studies of chlamydial urethritis among 540 consecutive heterosexual and homosexual men attending a sexually transmitted disease (STD) clinic in 1980 (Table 4–1) demonstrated a significantly higher isolation rate of *C. trachomatis* from the urethras of heterosexual men (14% versus 5%, $P < 0.01$) but a higher prevalence of antibody to *Chlamydia* as assessed by the microimmunofluorescence assay among homosexual men (52% versus 45%).[7] The ratio of seropositive to culture-positive patients was thus 10.4:1 for homosexual men compared with 3.3:1 for heterosexual men. These data suggested that homosexual men probably had acquired antichlamydial antibody secondary to infections at sites other than the urethra, most likely the rectum. To better define the prevalence, clinical manifestations, histopathology, and treatment of chlamydial proctitis, we studied populations of homosexual men who were either referred because of proctitis symptoms or were randomly selected for study.

METHOD

Men with symptoms of proctitis and enteritis seen in our STD clinic in 1980–1981 were referred for evaluation as part of an ongoing study. In addition to *C. trachomatis* cultures and serology, these men underwent anoscopy and, in consenting cases, sigmoidoscopy and rectal biopsy. All referred patients underwent clinical and microbiologic evaluation for other causes of proctitis, including *Neis-*

Table 4–1 Prevalence of *C. trachomatis* urethral infection in men attending an STD clinic in 1980

Patients	Culture Positive (%)	Seropositive (%)	Ratio of Seropositive to Culture Positive
Heterosexuals (N = 329)	14	46	3.3
Homosexuals (N = 114)	5	52	10.4

seria gonorrhoeae, *Campylobacter*, herpes simplex virus, *Giardia*, *Entamoeba*, *Salmonella*, *Shigella*, and *Clostridium difficile* toxin. In the same clinic population, randomly selected consenting homosexual men, who did not have gastrointestinal symptoms, provided rectal swab specimens that were evaluated for *C. trachomatis* and the other pathogens listed above.

Specimens for isolation of *C. trachomatis* were collected using type 3 calcium alginate swabs inserted into the rectal canal either directly or through anoscopy. Swabs were placed in 0.2 m sucrose-phosphate transport medium containing gentamicin (5 µg/ml), vancomycin (12.5 µg/ml), and nystatin (12.5 µg/ml) and were refrigerated during and after transport to the laboratory. Within 24 hours of collection, all specimens were inoculated onto cycloheximide-treated McCoy cells in a microtiter system as previously described.[8] Iodine or immunofluorescence staining was used to identify inclusions. Studies of millipore filtration of rectal specimens used a filter with pores of 0.8 µm, while sonication of rectal specimens employed a sonicator probe placed into the transport vial for 15 to 30 seconds. Methods used for immunotyping and serologic studies have been described previously.[9]

RESULTS

Despite the routine use of antibiotics in both transport and cell-culture media, bacterial contamination or toxicity of McCoy cell monolayers hindered recovery of *Chlamydia* from rectal specimens in prior studies. Sonication proved superior to millipore filtration as a means of reducing contamination and improving isolation of *Chlamydia* from rectal swabs (Table 4–2). When millipore filtration was used on 303 rectal specimens collected over a 60-day period, 3% were positive and 2% were contaminated. Of 415 specimens collected over another 60-day period and sonicated before inoculation, 6.5% grew *C. trachomatis* ($P < 0.05$ versus filtration) and 3% were contaminated. No increase in the rate of isolation of *Chlamydia* from unsonicated male urethral specimens (1851 cultured) or female cervical specimens (888 cultured) occurred during the second 60-day period. Of 150 rectal swabs obtained from homosexual men and processed in duplicate using both sonication and millipore filtration, 7% of sonicated specimens and 3% of filtered specimens grew *C. trachomatis* ($P < 0.05$).

Table 4-2 Sonication vs millipore filtration of rectal specimens[a]

Specimens Tested (N)	Sonication		Millipore	
	Positive (%)	Contamin (%)	Positive (%)	Contamin (%)
303	—	—	3	2
415	6	3	—	—
150	7	2	3	2

[a] $P < 0.05$, percent positive in sonicated versus filtered specimens.

We isolated *C. trachomatis* from the rectums of 17 of 154 (11%) homosexual men referred for evaluation of proctitis and from 4 of 75 (5%) asymptomatic homosexual men. Five of the 17 isolates from symptomatic men were of the L_2 (LGV) immunotype; no LGV strains were isolated from the asymptomatic men. Coexistent chlamydial infection at other sites was noted in only one patient, who also had conjunctivitis. Simultaneous rectal infection with other pathogens was found in 6 of the 17 symptomatic patients and 2 of the 4 asymptomatic patients. Leukocytes were present on rectal Gram's smears obtained from all the patients with symptomatic *C. trachomatis* proctitis and from 92% of the asymptomatic patients with chlamydial rectal infection but from only 19% of asymptomatic homosexual men without chlamydial infection.

Isolates from five of the symptomatic patients were immunotyped as L_2 strains. All five of these patients had clinically severe proctitis manifested by anal discharge, hematochezia, and anorectal pain. In addition, tenesmus, abdominal pain, constipation, fever, and inguinal adenopathy were all found significantly more often in the patients with LGV-strain infection than in patients infected with other immunotypes. On anoscopic and sigmoidoscopic examinations, all patients with L_2 infection had mucopurulent discharge and friable rectal mucosa with multiple discrete ulcerations and hemorrhage. In two of the three cases, sigmoidoscopic abnormalities were found above 15 cm (i.e., above the rectum). Biopsies of rectal mucosa were obtained in three patients with LGV infection, and two of these three showed diffuse inflammation with crypt abscesses, granulomas, and giant cells (Figure 4-1). All three had broadly reactive IgG antibody to *C. trachomatis* in titers between 1:512 and 1:2048, but none had IgM antibody (Table 4-3).

Isolates from the remaining 12 symptomatic and from all four asymptomatic men were immunotyped as non-LGV strains. Symptoms in these men consisted mainly of mild to moderate rectal discharge, rectal pain, and hematochezia. Anoscopy and sigmoidoscopy (Figure 4-2) exhibited a mucopurulent discharge, erythema, and localized friability (manifested as a positive wipe test), and biopsies showed a polymorphonuclear infiltrate with the lamina propria. Although IgG antibody to *Chlamydia* was present in 15 of the 16 patients who were tested, none had titers ≥ 512 (Table 4-3).

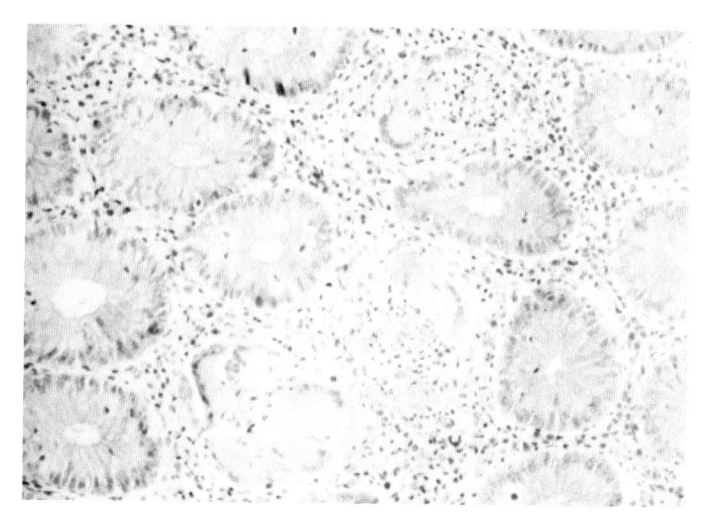

FIGURE 4–1 Rectal biopsy from a patient with LGV-strain proctitis, characterized by granulomatous inflammation and giant cell formation.

All the symptomatic patients were treated with tetracycline, 500 mg by mouth (PO) qid for 7 to 14 days, and all were culture negative for *C. trachomatis* at posttreatment follow-up visits; all had resolution of symptoms and fecal leukocytes as well. Asymptomatic patients were treated with the same regimen; all were culture negative after treatment, and their fecal leukocytes had resolved.

COMMENT

These data indicate that chlamydial proctitis occurred commonly in homosexual men in the pre-AIDS era in Seattle. Subsequent studies have indicated young age (particularly adolescence) and multiple sexual partners to be the most important factors associated with an increased risk of *C. trachomatis* rectal infection in gay men.[10] Transmission presumably occurs through receptive rectal intercourse with a partner who harbors urethral infection. All our patients with chlamydial proc-

Table 4–3 Microimmunofluorescence antibody titers in homosexual men with chlamydial rectal infections

	IgG	IgM	Titer Rise or Fall[a]	Titer ≥512
LGV strains	5/5	0/5	4/5	5/5
Non-LGV strains	15/16	2/16	3/14	0/16

[a]Eightfold change.

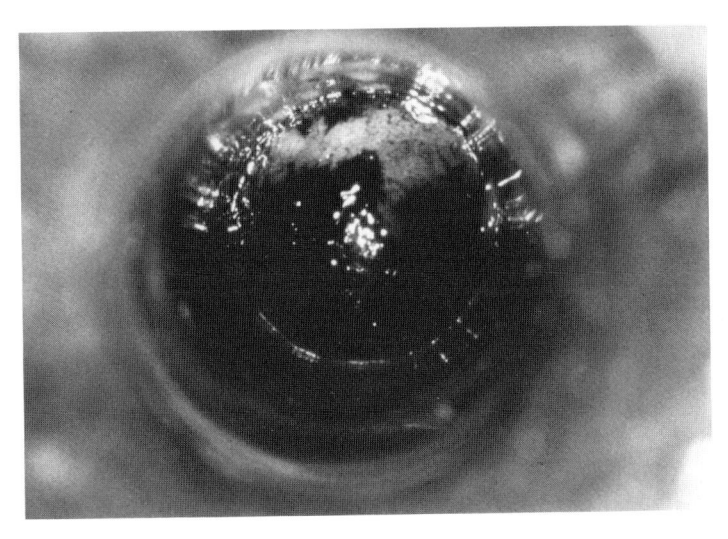

FIGURE 4–2 *Anoscopic examination in a patient with non-LGV strain C. trachomatis proctitis demonstrating a mucopurulent discharge.*

titis gave a history of rectal intercourse, but we were unable to evaluate their partners in most instances. Clinical manifestations range from asymptomatic infection to severe, acute proctitis manifested by rectal pain, mucopurulent discharge, hematochezia, abdominal pain, and diarrhea or loose stools. Patients infected with LGV strains manifested severe proctitis clinically and sigmoidoscopically. Similar results have been reported by Bolan et al.[11] Both their report and this study emphasize that LGV strains produce an ulcerative proctitis or proctocolitis that closely resembles herpetic proctitis clinically. Both produce ulcers, rectal pain, purulent discharge, constipation, hematochezia, fever, and adenopathy in some cases. Signs of sacral radiculopathy (urinary retention, severe constipation, and radiating leg pains) suggest herpes infection. Histopathologically, our patients with LGV infection had findings consistent with Crohn's disease. Infection with strains of the non-LGV immunotypes were associated with milder or no symptoms and with less marked findings on anoscopic examination. However, most asymptomatic patients were found to have fecal leukocytes on rectal Gram's smear, and those from whom biopsies were obtained had an inflammatory infiltrate in the lamina propria on histologic examination.

There is no evidence that *C. trachomatis* proctitis occurs more frequently or is of unusual severity in patients with AIDS, AIDS-related complex (ARC), or serologic evidence of HIV infection. In fact, recent studies suggest that both gonococcal and chlamydial proctitis may now be less frequent among gay men due to altered sexual practices in the AIDS era.[12]

Chlamydial proctitis should be suspected in homosexual men who exhibit the clinical findings outlined above, particularly when gonococcal infection has been ruled out by culture or when symptoms persist after treatment of gonococcal infection. Anoscopy should be performed routinely in these patients; the findings of leukocytes on a rectal Gram's smear further supports the diagnosis. The diagnosis should be confirmed by culture or by the newer direct slide tests utilizing fluorescein-conjugated monoclonal antibodies for visualization of chlamydial elementary bodies.[13] Mild or asymptomatic cases are best detected by chlamydial culture. Serodiagnosis appears useful in men with LGV-strain infection in that all our cases and all those reported by Bolan et al.[11] developed titers ≥ 512 using the microimmunofluorescent assay. In another population, however, Schachter reported antibody titers in this range in some homosexual men with non-LGV-strain proctitis,[3] and thus further assessment of LGV serodiagnosis in the setting of acute proctocolitis is needed. Serodiagnosis appears to have little value in non-LGV proctitis because of the high background prevalence of antibody in this population and the apparent absence of changing titers or IgM antibody in most patients.

Tetracycline therapy was successful in most of our patients. At least 14 days of treatment should probably be provided for LGV-strain infection, while seven days may be adequate for milder or asymptomatic infections. Further systematic studies of treatment are needed.

ACKNOWLEDGMENT

This work was supported in part by Research Grants AI 12192, AI 16222, AI 17805, EY 00219, and AM 16059 from the National Institutes of Health and Project Grant SEA 80-06-72 from the Bureau of Medical Services, Public Health Service, U.S. Department of Health and Human Services.

REFERENCES

1. Dunlop EMC, Hare MJ, Darougar S, Jones BR. Chlamydial isolates from the rectum in association with chlamydial infection of the eye or genital tract. II. Clinical aspects. In: Nichols RL, ed. Trachoma and related disorders. New York: Excerpta Medica, 1971;507.
2. Goldmeier D, Darougar S. Isolation of *Chlamydia trachomatis* from throat and rectum of homosexual men. Br J Vener Dis 1977;53:184.
3. Schachter J. Copnfirmatory serodiagnosis of lymphogranuloma venereum proctitis may yield false-positive results due to other chlamydial infections of the rectum. Sex Transm Dis 1981;8:26.
4. Quinn T, Goodell S, Mikrichian E, et al. *Chlamydia trachomatis* proctitis. N Engl J Med 1981;305:195.
5. Grace AW. Anorectal lymphogranuloma venereum. JAMA 1943;122:74.
6. Schachter J. Chlamydial infections. N Engl J Med 1978;298:490.
7. Stamm WE, Koutsky L, Benedetti JK, et al. *Chlamydia trachomatis* urethral infections in men. Prevalence, risk factors, and clinical manifestations. Ann Intern Med 1984;100:47.

8. Yoder BL, Stamm WE, Koester CM, Alexander ER. A microtest procedure for isolation of *Chlamydia trachomatis*. J Clin Microbiol 1981;14:325.
9. Wang SP, Grayston JT, Kuo CC, et al. Serodiagnosis of *Chlamydia trachomatis* infection with micro-immunofluorescence test. In: Hobson D, Holmes KK, eds. Nongonococcal urethritis and related infections. Washington, DC: American Society for Microbiology, 1977;237.
10. Rompalo AM, Price CB, Roberts PL, Stamm WE. Potential value of rectal screening cultures for *Chlamydia trachomatis* in homosexual men. J Infect Dis 1986;153:888.
11. Bolan RK, Sands M, Schachter J, et al. Lymphogranuloma venereum and acute ulcerative proctitis. Am J Med 1982;72:703.
12. Rompalo AM, Price CB, Roberts PL, Stamm WE. Anorectal and enteric infections in homosexual men pre- and post AIDS. Proceedings of the 25th Interscience Conference on Antimicrobial Agents and Chemotherapy, Minneapolis, 1985.
13. Stamm WE, Harrison HR, Alexander ER, et al. Diagnosis of *Chlamydia trachomatis* infection by direct immunofluorescence staining of genital secretions—a multicenter trial. Ann Intern Med 1984;101:638.

PART II

Sexually Transmitted Diseases: Diarrheal

Chapter 5

Gay Bowel Syndrome: An Overview

Bruce S. Gingold

The term *gay bowel syndrome* was first used by Kazal et al.[1] to describe a group of proctologic problems occurring in homosexual males. These disorders are not exclusive to the gay community but are seen more frequently in this population. However, several problems exist concerning the use of this term. First, many if not most of these entities can also be found in the nongay population. The common denominator appears to be either anal or oral-genital sexual contact. In these days of so-called sexual liberation, many heterosexual couples engage in these activities and, as a result, subject each other to possible undesirable consequences. Condyloma acuminatum, while still overwhelmingly seen in males, is being seen more often in women, and gonorrheal proctitis can likewise be seen in females. Although these and other sexually transmitted diseases are most commonly encountered in the gay community, the term *gay bowel syndrome* implies a situation specific to that community and this is certainly not the case. Second, the term *bowel* is similarly inaccurate because many of the problems described involve the perianal skin, such as anal fissures, external hemorrhoids, condyloma acuminata, and herpes simplex type 2 infection. Third, the term *syndrome*, according to *Dorland's Medical Dictionary*[2] is defined as "a set of symptoms which occur together."

The fact that these entities are seen in members of the gay community does not mean that they all occur together in any single individual. Perhaps the term *sexually related problems of the gay community* might be preferred to the *gay bowel syndrome,* since it is more precise, although admittedly less catchy a phrase. The clinical diagnoses of the more prevalent sexually related diseases of the gay community are outlined below. An overview of these problems will be discussed in the remaining sections of this chapter. More detailed discussions are presented in subsequent chapters.

Clinical diagnoses of some sexually related diseases seen in homosexuals
I. Trauma
   A. Fissure

B. Laceration
        C. Foreign body
 II. Infections
        A. Bacteria
            1. Gonorrhea
            2. Shigellosis
            3. Salmonellosis
            4. Campylobacteriosis
            5. Syphilis
            6. Nongonococcal urethritis
            7. Lymphogranuloma venereum
        B. Viruses
            1. Condyloma acuminata
            2. Hepatitis B infection
            3. *Herpes simplex* infection
        C. Parasites
            1. Strongyloidiasis
            2. Amebiasis
            3. Giardiasis
III. Nonspecific proctitis
IV. AIDS Related
        A. Lymphadenopathy
        B. *Pneumocystis carinii* pneumonia
        C. Cytomegaloviral infection
        D. *Herpes simplex* infection
        E. Cryptosporidiosis
        F. Isosporiasis
        G. Microsporidiosis
        H. Mycobacterium avium intracellulare (MAI)
        I. Kaposi's sarcoma

TRAUMA

Anal fissure is one of the most common and painful disorders seen in proctology. It is by no means limited to the gay community. Any sudden dilatation of the anal canal can split the anoderm and produce a fissure. Most fissures are caused by straining at defecation and are usually superficial. They are commonly seen in patients with inflammatory bowel disease. Anal fissures may be divided into two types: acute and chronic. Although sexual distribution is approximately the same for males and females, there is a 10% incidence of anterior fissures in females as opposed to a 1% incidence in males. The most common location for both sexes is the posterior midline. This is seen in approximately 75% of patients.[3] Typical acute fissures are quite painful and may often be diagnosed simply by eliciting a history of painful defecation with discomfort lasting from a few minutes to several hours following completion of a bowel movement. If the patient is too uncomfortable to allow digital rectal examination, a small cotton swab may be inserted into the rectum. If the physician withdraws the swab slowly, a linear streak of blood will often coat the swab and thus reveal the corresponding site of the fissure. In a high percentage of patients, acute fissures heal spontaneously if the patient uses stool softeners, bulk laxatives or bran, and witch hazel and cotton to keep the perianal skin clean and, above all, avoids straining at defecation. Approximately 50% of acute fissures will not heal. Many will close temporarily but will reopen with the first hard bowel movement or attempt at anal sex. In most cases, if the fissure has not healed within two months, the simple medical regimen outlined above will not prove fruitful. At this point, I usually recommend a lateral internal sphincterotomy. If enough scar tissue is found at the site of the fissure, a partial fissurectomy is performed. The scar tissue is excised but not the base, which may be curetted. This can usually be performed quite simply as an office or ambulatory surgical procedure. It takes approximately 20 minutes and can be done under local anesthesia. The success rate has been found to be better than 95%. It usually takes three to four weeks for the operative site to completely heal. The technique is similar to that described by Portin et al.[4]

A more serious result of anal trauma is laceration of the anal canal. This is most commonly caused by insertion of a large object or clenched fist. Lacerations can be of different degrees. Superficial lacerations may result in severe pain and serious hemorrhage. These should be debrided and, if the patient is seen soon after the actual trauma, may occasionally be sutured closed primarily. If any questions exist with regard to timing, or if healing is questionable, it is far better to debride the area, cauterize or ligate all the bleeding vessels, and allow the defect to granulate. A full-thickness laceration is a far more difficult problem to manage, even when seen early, and may result in permanent fecal incontinence. Because of the circumferential nature of the sphincter muscle fibers, it is difficult for these tissues to hold sutures. A not uncommon situation is to obtain a fairly gratifying initial result with a sphincter muscle repair, only to have the patient subsequently have a large or hard bowel movement or engage in anal sex and have incontinence recur. A possible method for solving this problem involves creating a new anal sphincter mechanism by using a gracilis muscle transplant.

A third type of traumatic problem seen in the gay community is that of a retained foreign body. Commonly a vibrator is found. However, the variety of objects recovered can be quite extensive. If no injury to the colon is suspected, the objects can usually be removed in the office or in the hospital emergency room with a vaginal speculum. The anus can usually be dilated and the lowest end of the object thus exposed. A Parks retractor can also be used for the same purpose. This is not an uncommon problem. Barone et al. reported 23 patients with retained foreign bodies over a five-year period.[5] Sohn and Weinstein[6] reported removal of 100 foreign bodies from the rectum. In addition to the insertion of rigid objects, insertion of fists into the rectum was at one time an increasingly common type of injury. Sohn et al.[7] reported 11 patients with injuries of this type. Four patients suffered perforation of the rectosigmoid requiring laparotomy, and one patient sustained a severe laceration with resultant complete fecal incontinence. With the increased awareness of the transmissibility of acquired immunodeficiency syndrome (AIDS), this practice has apparently diminished in the past six or seven years.

INFECTIONS

Salmonella and *Shigella* infections are by no means limited to homosexuals. Most of the cases are not serious and produce transient nausea, vomiting, and diarrhea with blood streaking. Similar findings are present with other bacterial enteric pathogens. A culture specimen of freshly passed stool frequently identifies these organisms, and treatment in most cases consists of oral antibiotics, selected according to the susceptibility.

Gonorrheal proctitis is by far the most common bacterial infection seen in the gay community, although it is being seen somewhat more often in heterosexual females engaging in anal sex.

The mucosa of the lower 5 to 6 cm of the rectum appear edematous, friable, and beefy red with a purulent exudate. Crypts may also appear edematous with pus exuding from them as well. Unlike urethral gonorrhea, which is usually quite susceptible to 4.8 M units of procaine penicillin (although resistant strains are emerging), rectal gonorrhea is less sensitive. We treat this entity with 4 g of spectinomycin given intramuscularly at time of diagnosis, without waiting for culture reports in most cases. Most patients report marked improvement within a few days and almost complete resolution in two weeks. Should there be no significant improvement within one week, penicillin is then added to the regimen. If there is still no improvement, lymphogranuloma venereum, which in its early (i.e., prestricture) phase often looks identical to gonorrheal proctitis, should be considered. The most common viral condition with the exception of hepatitis seen in gay men is condyloma acuminata (Figure 5–1). It is caused by a papova (DNA) virus and is almost always transmitted by direct sexual contact. It appears to have an incubation period of six weeks to eight months. Although occasionally warts may be seen only on the perianal skin, the majority of them are seen both externally and internally, extending approximately 3 cm above the anal verge. As a result, the application of podophyllin or bichloracetic acid is usually not a satisfactory initial treatment, since when either of these medications is applied to warts, it must be washed off five to six hours after application, otherwise the chemical process will continue and a patient may be subjected to painful burns in the area of application. It is extremely difficult to apply podophyllin accurately inside the anal canal and likewise wash this material off at the proper time. Consequently, I prefer not to use it as a primary treatment. Occasionally, isolated external recurrences may be treated in this manner. A more effective method is to electrocoagulate these lesions, both internally and externally. With this technique, at least 90% of patients may be treated in the office or minor surgery

Gay Bowel Syndrome: An Overview 53

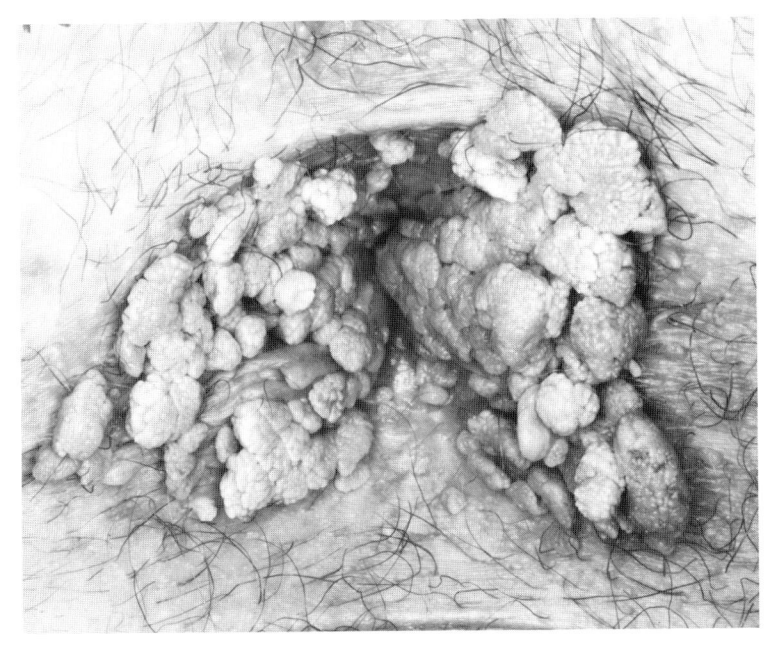

FIGURE 5–1 *Perianal condyloma acuminata in a homosexual man.*

unit under local anesthesia. Generally, 5 to 10 ml of 0.25% Marcaine (without epinephrine) is used. A ball-tipped or needle probe is used with the machine set to "spark-gap." The patient is not grounded. Most patients will require at least one, and many will require two or more, follow-up treatments at monthly intervals. The patients are informed in advance and thus are not surprised when recurrent warts are found at follow-up examination. However, in recent years, the incidence of condylomata in the gay community appears to have diminished. This may be due to a change in sexual behavior—decreased number of sexual partners and increased use of condoms. Another viral infection seen frequently in the gay community is hepatitis B. Since it does not involve the bowel, it is not included in this discussion. However, 80% of gay men have circulating antibody to this virus, and this usually results in generalized lymphadenopathy.

Herpes simplex type 2 is not limited to homosexuals by any means. It is a painful, recurrent, incurable viral infection that causes great misery without regard to sexual orientation. It is usually a self-limiting infection, and although no cures are available, it appears that acyclovir is an effective medication for symptomatic relief. This virus is also seen in patients who are immunoincompetent from AIDS, leukemia, or chemotheraphy or in transplant patients who take antirejection medication; it may become widespread in this setting and may require systemic acyclovir for palliation.

Syphilis is caused by the spirochete *Treponema pallidum* and is likewise not limited to the gay community. Primary syphilis presents as a small painful ulceration whether on the glans of the penis, in the perianal region, or in the mouth. The organism can be easily identified during the primary stage by darkfield examination of the lesion. The primary chancre generally heals spontaneously between 10 and 40 days. The patient is then asymptomatic from two to six months before multiple secondary lesions are seen on the skin and mucous membranes. These lesions last from three weeks to three months and then generally disappear but may recur three months to a year later.

Generalized lymphadenopathy is also associated with this condition. A prolonged latent period then ensues. If left untreated, the patient will progress to the tertiary phase. Manifestations of tertiary syphilis involve gumma formation, aneurysms of the aorta, and central nervous system (CNS) involvement, including paresis and tabes dorsalis.

Lymphogranuloma venereum (LGV) is caused by *Chlamydia trachomatis*. In its earliest stages it may be clinically indistinguishable from gonorrheal proctitis. The rectal mucosa is beefy red with a purulent exudate but without ulcerations. Culture specimens are very difficult to obtain with this organism, and the best available method of diagnosis in most hospitals at present is by complement fixation with a titer of 1:64 or a fourfold rise in titer considered a positive result. Treatment is tetracyline or erythromycin by mouth for four weeks. If LGV is diagnosed early, symptoms are entirely reversible, and no long-lasting effects may ensue. However, if treatment is delayed, patients frequently develop enlarged lymph nodes that may suppurate and require drainage. As the process continues, a patient may develop fibrosis of the entire anal canal and rectum with marked stricture and fistula formation. Although the organism may be obliterated by using the appropriate antibiotics, the fibrosis is usually irreversible, and extensive reconstructive procedures such as abdominoperineal pull-through may be required.

The most common parasites seen in the gay community are *Entamoeba histolytica, Giardia lamblia,* and *Strongyloides stercoralis,* which will be discussed further in subsequent chapters.

Nonspecific proctitis can also be seen and must be distinguished from the above-mentioned infections as well as that due to ulcerative and Crohn's proctitis. A patient may present with a history of recent onset of diarrhea, perirectal irritation, inflammation, and some streaking of blood. Proctologic examination will reveal friable mucosa, but biopsy does not reveal any evidence of granulomata, results of cultures and examination for ova and parasites will be negative, and the entity may disappear over days or weeks without any teatment other than symptomatic relief. This entity is usually self-limited and may be related to stress.

ACQUIRED IMMUNODEFICIENCY SYNDROME

AIDS is a potentially catastrophic occurrence that at present appears to lead to a fatal outcome in virtually all cases. It will be discussed in more detail in subsequent chapters. Although it does not directly involve the bowel, certain aspects will be discussed here. AIDS was unheard of ten years ago. Now, most physicians who deal with proctologic problems as well as most members of the gay community are only too well aware of its existence. It is caused by the HIV virus and is transmitted by an exchange of body fluids (e.g., blood or semen) or contaminated needles. One of the earliest manifestations may be the development of generalized lymphadenopathy. Note that 80% of the gay men seen in my office have enlarged nodes on physical examination. Although the mere presence of enlarged lymph nodes in the neck, axillae, and groins does not indicate AIDS per se, a patient previously noted not to have lymphadenopathy who subsequently develops it without apparent cause (i.e., hepatitis B, syphilis) must be watched very carefully for the development of other manifestations of AIDS and should have T4:T8 lymphocyte ratios determined and HIV antibody screening. *Pneumocystis carinii* and cytomegalovirus (CMV) are serious manifestations of AIDS and are usually treated by antibiotics; in most cases they can be temporarily arrested. However, in the debilitated patient with advanced AIDS or Kaposi's sarcoma, the outcome is often fatal. Herpes simplex type 2, as previously mentioned, is a painful chronic incurable condition involving lesions in the genital and perianal areas. However, when complicated by AIDS, it may lead to dissemination and eventually death (Figure 5–2). Siegal et al.[8] reported four

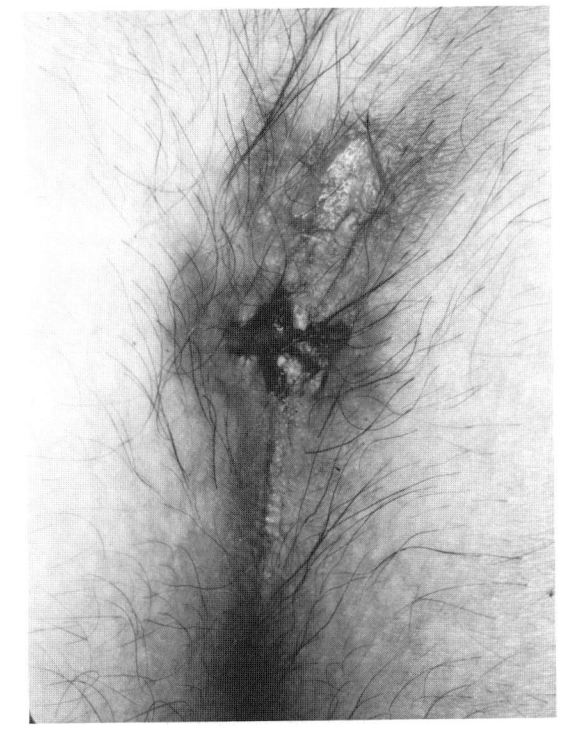

FIGURE 5–2 *Perianal herpes simplex Type 2 in gay male with AIDS.*

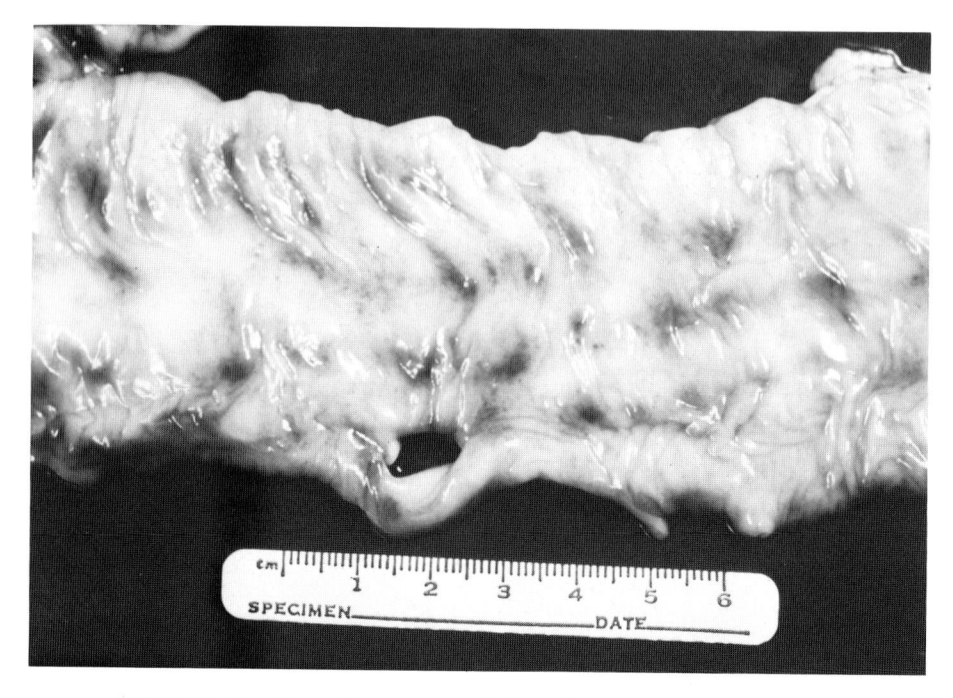

FIGURE 5–3 *Kaposi's sarcoma of the colon in homosexual man.*

patients who developed herpes simplex in the presence of AIDS; three of these patients died. I have seen two patients with herpes associated with AIDS, one of whom died following plasmaphoresis in an attempt to gain control of this process. Cryptosporidiosis, a parasitic infection normally seen in farm animals, is not usually seen in humans. However, patients who are immunocompromised may contract this entity, which produces persistent continuous watery diarrhea and inevitably leads to death. Despite hyperalimentation and massive doses of medication to slow down bowel motility, these patients become so dehydrated and wasted that they succumb to a variety of opportunistic infections. *Mycobacterium avium intracellulare*, *Isospora belli*, and *Microsporidia* spp. are also seen as opportunistic infections in immunocompromised patients and are causes of diarrhea as is CMV.

Kaposi's sarcoma is also seen as part of the AIDS syndrome (Figures 5–3 through 5–5). There is no definitive treatment at present. One problem is that if chemotherapy is given, thus suppressing the lesions, the individual becomes even more immunocompromised and is thus susceptible to other entities that may prove to be even more devastating than Kaposi's sarcoma.

CONCLUSION

This has been an overview of bowel manifestations seen in the gay population, both HIV and non-HIV related. As more homosexuals seek medical treatment

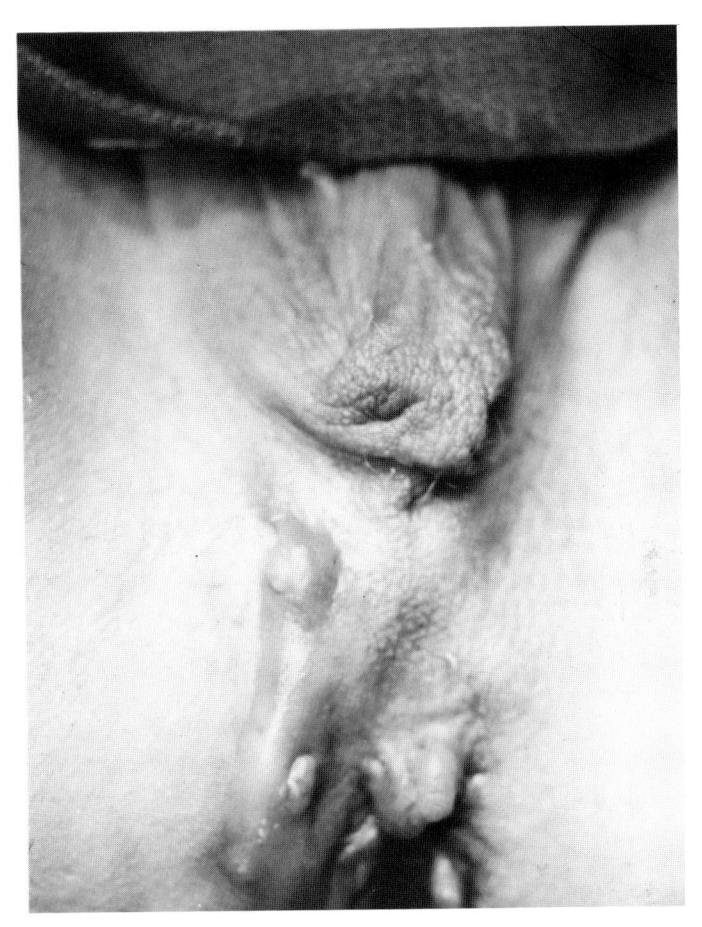

FIGURE 5–4 *Kaposi's sarcoma of perineum in homosexual man (preoperative).*

for HIV and associated conditions, many if not most of these entities are being seen more frequently. However, if current trends continue, at some point the incidence of HIV in the gay community should level off due to changes in lifestyle and behavior. At that time, the highest risk group will become IV drug abusers and their sex partners.

REFERENCES

1. Kazal HL, Sohn N, Carrasco J, et al. The gay bowel syndrome. Clinico-pathologic correlation in 260 cases. Ann Clin Lab Sci 1976;16:184.
2. Dorland's Medical Dictionary, 27th ed. Philadelphia: Saunders, 1988.
3. Mazier W, DeMoraes R, Dignan R. Anal fissure and anal ulcers. Surg Clin North Am 1978;58:479.

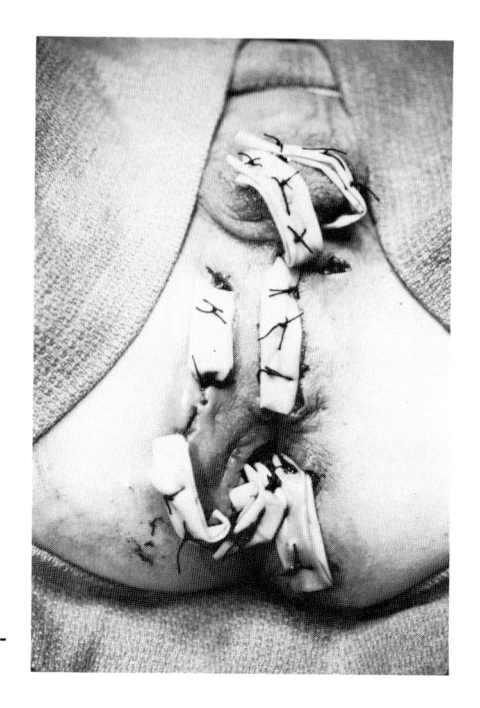

FIGURE 5–5 *Patient in Figure 5–4 (postoperative).*

4. Portin B, Bernhoft W, Teitler R, Boehmke F. Sphincterotomy for anal fissure: An outpatient procedure. Presented at the 78th annual convention, American Society of Colon and Rectal Surgeons, Atlanta, June 14, 1979.
5. Barone J, Sohn N, Nealon T. Perforations and foreign bodies of the rectum. Ann Surg 1976;184:601.
6. Sohn N, Weinstein M. Office removal of foreign bodies in the rectum. Surg Gynecol Obstet 1978;146:209.
7. Sohn N, Weinstein M, Gonchor J. Social injuries of the rectum. Am J Surg 1977;134:611.
8. Siegal FP, Lopez C, Hammer GS, et al. Severe acquired immunodeficiency in male homosexuals manifested by chronic perianal ulcerative *herpes simplex* lesions. N Engl J Med 1981;305:1439.
9. Antony MA, Brandt LJ, Klein RS, et al. Infectious diarrhea in patients with AIDS. Dig Dis Sci 1988;33:1141.

Chapter 6

Bacterial Diarrhea in Homosexual Men

Anthony P. Lopez
Sherwood L. Gorbach

Acute and chronic gastrointestinal illnesses occur commonly in male homosexuals.[1-10] The awareness of sexual transmission of enteric disease dates from 1968 with the initial description in New York City.[11] Although this early report involved protozoan infections, other observers noted the association soon after with bacterial pathogens.[2,6,12-15] Various organisms have been reported, including *Salmonella, Shigella, Campylobacter,* and *Chlamydia*.[1,2,13,16-23] *Clostridium difficile* has also been observed,[24] but homosexual men do not appear to be at increased risk of this infection. This chapter will discuss the bacterial pathogens with respect to their microbiology, epidemiology, and clinical characteristics in homosexual men.

Fecal-oral exposure is felt to be the route of transmission of bacterial intestinal pathogens among homosexual males. Multiple sexual partners accelerate the spread of these organisms. Also, the high infectivity of a relatively small inoculum, combined with short-term asymptomatic fecal carriage, facilitates the spread of these bacteria in this population.

Shigella has clearly been implicated as a major cause of bowel disease in gay males.[1,2,13,17-19,24] *Salmonella* has also been found in symptomatic and asymptomatic homosexual men and their contacts[13,14]; initial reports focused on typhoidal strains but more recent studies, primarily in acquired immunodeficiency syndrome (AIDS) patients, have emphasized nontyphoidal strains causing bacteremia and enteritis.[25-27] Recent evidence also points to an increased rate of *Campylobacter* infection in homosexual men, including *Campylobacter jejuni, C. fetus* subsp. *fetus,* as well as *Campylobacter*-like organisms (CLOs).[24] Two new species, *C. cinaedi* and *C. fennelliae,* have been proposed from four groups of CLOs found in several studies from Seattle.[28] Although there are important differences among all these organisms, a common property is the initiating event of mucosal invasion and tissue replication in the pathogenesis of diarrhea.

SHIGELLA

Shigella is the classic cause of bacterial dysentery, a disease of worldwide significance whose regional incidence mirrors prevailing standards of sanitation and whose clinical impact is most frequent in the pediatric population.[29] The responsible organism is a nonmotile gram-negative rod of the family *Enterobacteriaceae*, which may be distinguished from *Escherichia coli* by its inability to ferment lactose and from *Salmonella* species by its lack of gas production in glucose. Strains of *Shigella* are characterized by specific cell-wall antigens and are subdivided into the following four species, all of which produce invasive human disease:

Group A: *Sh. dysenteriae*, 10 serotypes
Group B: *Sh. flexneri*, 6 serotypes
Group C: *Sh. boydii*, 15 serotypes
Group D: *Sh. sonnei*, 1 serotype

Although *Sh. flexneri* is the most common isolate in developing countries, *Sh. dysenteriae* 1, also known as Shiga's bacillus, produces the most virulent clinical disease; in Central America, a five-country pandemic of the latter strain caused over 10,000 deaths in 1968 through 1972, mostly in young children.[30] In the United States, *Sh. sonnei* has gained preeminence over *Sh. flexneri* as the most common domestic species. This trend is reflected in the 1980 Centers for Disease Control (CDC) tabulation attributing 70% of 19,041 U.S. cases to *Sh. sonnei* in that year.[31]

Shigellae are highly host-adapted bacteria, natural pathogens only of humans and a few higher primates. As a consequence, one human infection is always theoretically traceable to another human source, although the route may deviate through contaminated food or liquid. Studies of volunteers indicate that an oral dose of 10^5 Shigella organisms produces a 75% attack rate, but experimental infection has been established with as few as 10 to 200 viable bacilli of virulent *Sh. dysenteriae* 1 or *Sh. flexneri* 2a strains.[32,33] Once introduced to the intestinal tract, disease results only when the organisms adhere to the mucosal surface by a specific receptor mechanism, then penetrate epithelial cells and multiply, often spreading laterally from cell to cell. A sharp drop-off in bacteria and inflammation at the submucosa level probably accounts for the rarity of bloodstream invasion, although the luminal concentration of *Shigella* reaches 10^{10}/ml during active disease. Since acutely symptomatic patients can excrete up to 10^8 viable shigellae per gram of stool, and convalescent patients from 10^2 to 10^3 organisms per gram of stool, it is easy to imagine how readily transmission can be accomplished by intimate association in a household or by oroanal sexual contact. Although most infected individuals will cease to excrete the pathogen within three to four weeks of the onset of diarrhea, a rare, chronic *Shigella* carrier state has been described. Unlike long-term excretors of *Salmonella*, the patients who harbor *Shigella* tend to have intermittent recurrence of enteric symptoms. A totally asymptomatic carrier state beyond one year has also been reported for *Sh. sonnei* and *Sh. flexneri* 2a in two institutionalized individuals.[34]

The classic clinical presentation of bacillary dysentery includes the acute onset of abdominal cramps, rectal burning, and fever associated with the passage of multiple, small-volume stools containing blood and mucus; nonetheless, only a minority of patients manifest this distinctive constellation. As with other forms of bacterial diarrhea, there are probably more subclinical than overt cases.[35] The most common findings in symptomatic shigellosis are abdominal pain and diarrhea, followed in three to five days by the invasive colitic phase. The early secretory stage is felt to reflect the action of a heat-labile, protein enterotoxin, which has now been purified from all *Shigella* species.[36,37] Direct intracecal inoculation of *Sh. flexneri* 2a in Rhesus monkeys circumvents this initial phase of watery diarrhea but still produces invasive disease,[38] an observation that suggests the feasibility of rectal implantation as a route of introduction in homosexual males. In contrast, live oral challenge with nonpenetrating, toxin-positive mutants of *Sh. dysenteriae* failed to elicit overt illness in humans and monkeys,[39] once again emphasizing the critical contribution of invasion to the pathogenesis of shigellosis. Although the average length of intestinal symptoms in adults is less than seven days, severe cases may extend three to four weeks, raising potential confusion with idiopathic ulcerative colitis. Following natural clearance of *Shigella* organisms by the host, lingering mucosal injury may cause a persistence of colitic symptoms.

The apparent high risk of homosexuals to contract and transmit *Shigella* was first publicized by Dritz and Back in 1974, when they described a largely homosexual outbreak of more than 50 cases of *Sh. flexneri* in San Francisco.[13] Kazal et al. subsequently reported a 2.3% incidence of shigellosis in 260 homosexual males presenting to a large private practice with a variety of proctologic complaints.[1] In 1976, another New York–based survey of 113 hospitalized patients with documented shigellosis revealed that homosexuals comprised 45% of males over the five-year review period.[17] Additional confirmation of the venereal transmission of shigellosis comes from the description of an 18-month outbreak in the homosexual community of Seattle, where fellatio, oroanal contact, or both were reported by 90% of the infected men[18]; isolates were divided between *Sh. sonnei* and a strain of *Sh. flexneri* 3 that was new to the Seattle area.

Other studies from Seattle have confirmed the importance of this organism,[24] with *Sh. flexneri* found in 3 of 119 symptomatic and 1 of 75 asymptomatic homosexual men. *Shigella*, along with *Campylobacter* and occasionally *Entamoeba histolytica*, are more often seen in men with proctocolitis, an entity defined by abnormal sigmoidoscopic findings beyond 15 cm.

CAMPYLOBACTER

Campylobacter fetus, formerly known as *Vibrio fetus*, has long been recognized as a major veterinary pathogen responsible for septic abortion, hepatitis, and enteritis in a wide range of farm animals. It was not until the late 1970s, however, that human campylobacteriosis was perceived as more than a medical rarity and the subspecies *fetus, intestinalis,* and *jejuni* were routinely differentiated. *C. jejuni,* now designated as a separate species,[40] has subsequently emerged as a leading cause of human diarrhea and is estimated to account for 3% to 14% of unselected cases of gastroenteritis in North America and Europe.[41] This once-obscure agent is a curved, highly motile, oxidase-positive, gram-negative rod whose optimal culture conditions were defined in 1972, thus permitting accurate prevalence surveys in humans and animals. As with other species of *Campylobacter,* successful isolation depends on the use of specific antibiotic-supplemented media and incubation in a microaerophilic, capneic (5% to 10% CO_2) environment. In addition, *C. jejuni* can be distinguished from the only other human pathogen, *C. fetus* subsp. *fetus* (a tissue and bloodstream opportunist with vascular tropism), and the human oral commensal *C. sputorum* subsp. *sputorum* by its relative thermophilia. *C. jejuni* grows best at 42°C and poorly, if at all, in room temperature.

Few zoonotic pathogens better illustrate the important interface between veterinary flora and human disease than *C. jejuni*. Animal reservoirs are now known to include swine,[42] cattle,[42] sheep,[42] horses,[43] and goats.[44] Of special note is the fecal excretion of *C. jejuni* by 30% to 100% of avian species.[41] Other animals may develop a diarrheal illness in association with intestinal colonization, including lambs, calves, and young dogs and cats.[45,46] Contamination of commercial poultry, beef, lamb, and pork carcasses at seaports has been well documented as a result of this ubiquitous carriage,[41,47] and environmental isolation of *C. jejuni* from fresh and salt water has also been reported.[48,49] Humans may consequently encounter this organism in a vast array of settings, as indicated by the proliferation of clinical cases in the last five years attributed to different modes of exposure. Numerous outbreaks of human *Campylobacter* diarrhea have now been linked to primary contamination of animal foodstuffs, public water supplies, and raw milk,[41] and direct fecal transmission from infected pets and incontinent young children has also been demonstrated.[50,51] In contrast, no secondary propagation from one adult to another has yet been proved, either in the setting of an ongoing outbreak or an asymptomatic index source.

The infective human dose of *C. jejuni* organisms has been examined in only two isolated volunteer studies to date, where separate oral inocula of 10^6 and 500 viable bacteria in milk each produced a characteristic self-limited illness. Significant fecal excretion of the organism was noted over the ensuing one to four weeks.[52,53] The inability of *C. jejuni* to replicate in milk, coupled with the dilutional effect of the large storage tanks associated with many milkborne outbreaks in England, has also been cited as indirect evidence for a low inoculum requirement; nonetheless, a milk vehicle, by virtue of gastric acid neutralization, may favor infection by the organism.

Symptomatic intestinal infection with *C. jejuni* generally follows within one to seven days of successful oral exposure. The clinical complaints of fever, cramps, and often bloody diarrhea reflect the associated tissue injury, which may involve the entire jejunum, ileum, and colon. Although *Campylobacter* infection can clinically resemble any other bacterial diarrhea, a distinctive constitutional prodrome, with fever as the most prominent feature, may precede and even overshadow the enteric phase in some patients. The actual pathogenesis of human campylobacteriosis is still debated. Although cellular infiltration on biopsy specimens and the occasional detection of bacteremia strongly suggest a primary tissue invasion, enterotoxin activity has been described in tissue culture and rat ileal loops and, as in shigellosis, may contribute to the development of diarrhea.[54]

During active infection, patients often excrete 10^6 to 10^9 *C. jejuni* organisms per gram of stool,[48] a concentration that could at least theoretically promote secondary cases by sexual contact, based on our scant knowledge of the minimum infective inoculum. Perhaps the more relevant questions concerning transmission by homosexual males involve duration of convalescent excretion and potential asymptomatic carriage in humans. Blaser and Reller, summarizing data from six studies totaling 495 untreated patients of all ages, found a two- to three-week median duration of fecal isolation and a three-month limit for universal clearing.[41] Following the institution of effective antibiotic therapy, fecal excretion of organisms is reduced to a mean of 1.1 days.[55] Posttreatment relapse after an initial five-day course of erythromycin was not detected in nine patients followed with three sequential stool cultures over two weeks.[56] Although a symptomatic infection has been described in several large outbreaks, carriage in healthy control subjects is virtually absent in studies from North America and Europe. In contrast, surveys in South Africa and Bangladesh reveal that 40% of children aged nine to 24 months excrete *C. jejuni*,[57,58] implying that substandard hygiene and nutrition may prolong the duration of asymptomatic fecal carriage in children following primary exposure.

In the absence of an outbreak in the homosexual community with contact verification, definite evidence linking *Campylobacter* with a sexual mode of transmission will be difficult in light of the vast environmental reservoir of this pathogen. *C. jejuni* proctitis in homosexual men has been described in case reports,[20,21] but more suggestive evidence comes from a prospective study of 194 homosexual men seen at the Seattle–King County Sexual Transmitted Disease Clinic.[24] In this population, 7% of symptomatic men with proctitis or protocolitis had *Campylobacter* isolated from stool. Seven of these were *C. jejuni* and one was *C. fetus* subsp. *fetus*. Three percent of asymptomatic men attending the same STD Clinic also harbored *C. jejuni*. In contrast, a prospective survey of 50 homosexual men undergoing rectal culture for *Neisseria gonorrhoeae* in Britain and 168 asymptomatic homosexual men in Denver, Colorado, failed to yield any *Campylobacter* isolates.[48,59] It is unclear whether this discrepancy reflects regional differences in endemic carriage and transmission or whether other factors are important.

An interesting new development was the recent discovery of campylobacter-like organisms (CLOs) isolated from 25 of 158 (16%) symptomatic and 6 of 75 asymptomatic homosexual men in Seattle.[24,28] The CLOs were isolated on *Campylobacter*-selective medium and incubated at 37°C for seven days in a reduced O_2 atmosphere. These *Campylobacter* are catalase- and oxidase-positive, asaccharolytic, microaerophilic, motile, curved, gram-negative rods. The CLOs, however, differed from other *Campylobacter* in colony morphology, some biochemical tests, and temperature required for growth. Genetically, the CLOs were divided into four groups: CLO-1A, 1B, 2, and 3. Three of these strains (CLO-1B, 2, and 3) were only isolated from symptomatic men, and one (CLO-1A) was found in both symptomatic and asymptomatic men. Clinically, men infected with these organisms tended to have abnormal sigmoidoscopic findings, acute inflammation on rectal biopsy, and increased numbers of fecal leukocytes. These strains have also been isolated from blood cultures of two homosexual men,[60] but they have not been found in heterosexual men or in women. Some of these CLOs have been tentatively assigned to two new species: *C. cinaedi*, made up of CLO-1 strains, and *C. fennelliae*, comprised of CLO-2 strains. The remaining CLO-3 strain could not be assigned to any group. Further clinical, epidemiologic, and taxonomic studies are required to define these organisms' role in human disease.

SALMONELLA

The three species of *Salmonella*—*S. typhi*, *S. cholera-suis*, and *S. enteritidis*—are worldwide enteric pathogens responsible for a spectrum of human disease that encompasses typhoid fever, septicemia with or without focal suppuration, acute gastroenteritis, and asymptomatic carrier states. *S. typhi* is remarkably host-adapted to humans, who represent the only natural reservoir of infection. In contrast, the almost 2000 serotypes of *S. enteritidis* that cause the majority of cases of *Salmonella* gastroenteritis are widely prevalent in domestic and natural animal populations as well as sewage, river water, and seawater. Food and fluid vehicles such as poultry, eggs, milk, and drinking water are most commonly implicated in the transmission of *S. enteritidis*, although infection may be traced to another human host.

Microbiologic characteristics of the *Salmonella* genus include their classification in the family *Enterobacteriaceae* and possession of flagellar motility. Like *Shigella*, the salmonellae are facultative anaerobes that ferment glucose but not lactose or sucrose. They can be distinguished from the shigellae by positive H_2S and lysine decarboxylase reactions. A complex system of biochemical properties and serologic tests for capsular (K), somatic (O), and flagellar (H) antigens serves to further differentiate the major *Salmonella* species and *S. enteritidis* serotypes.

The minimum inoculum necessary to establish infection with *S. typhi* is 10^5 organisms, as determined by studies with the virulent Quailes strain in volunteers.[61] In contrast, the infectivity of *S. enteritidis* varies with serotype and inoculum size; for example, 10^5 *S. enteritidis* serotype *newport* produced illness in some subjects, whereas 10^9 *S. enteritidis* serotype *pullorum*, a strain that is highly adapted to its natural host, the chicken, was *unable* to produce human disease.[62,63] Age, gastric acidity, and composition of normal bacterial flora are additional host factors that influence the infectious human dose of all *Salmonella* organisms. The importance of the latter parameter is best illustrated in experimental animal studies, which indicate that the number of bacteria required for infection can be significantly reduced by pretreatment of the host with antibiotics.

The clinical features of typhoid fever reflect the pathogen's remarkable ability to invade bowel mucosa, disseminate to lymphatic foci within the gastrointestinal tract, and, following several days of intracellular replication in reticuloendothelial tissue, produce sequential waves of bacteremia that then establish more distant sites of infection. Nontyphoidal salmonellosis is a more purely gastrointestinal disease marked by short incubation (6 to 48 hours), nausea, vomiting, abdominal cramps, and diarrhea of 3 to 4 day's duration with fever present in only 50% of affected individuals. Histologic abnormalities and the relative frequency of bacteremia bespeak primary tissue invasion even in the gastroenteritis syndrome. From a public health standpoint, the variable propensity for chronic intestinal carriage following active *Salmonella* infection in either of these clinical settings has potential relevance for both naturally and sexually acquired disease. Six weeks after the onset of illness approximately 50% of typhoid victims are still shedding organisms in their feces, although this figure progressively declines to a 5% to 10% rate at 3 months and a 1% to 3% chronic carriage at 1 year.[64,65] Chronic carriers of *S. typhi* are statistically most likely to be older patients, with a 3:1 female predominance; preexisting biliary disease in these individuals allows persistent colonization of the gallbladder. The overall carrier rate following nontyphoidal salmonellosis is estimated as between 2 and 6 per 1000 symptomatically or asymptomatically infected patients, with a bimodal predilection for children (especially neonates) and patients over 60 with cholelithiasis or nephrolithiasis.[66]

The acquisition of typhoid fever in two homosexual men from sexual partners who were asymptomatic carriers illustrates the role of fecal-oral transmission.[14] Newer studies have also emphasized the occurrence of *S. enteritis* and bacteremia in AIDS patients, most of whom were homosexual men.[25–27] Many of these patients had disease due to *S. typhimurium* consisting of severe, recurrent enteritis and bacteremia.

CONCLUSION

The toll of human misery related to diarrhea spans the millennia of recorded history. From the time of Moses there has been consciousness of the importance to the public health of careful fecal disposal.[67] The increase in transmission of intestinal infections among homosexual males offers new challenges in preventive medicine for physicians who care for these patients. Although these pathogens may be widespread, the behavioral changes of the male homosexual population in response to the AIDS epidemic, which has led to a decrease in gonococcal infections, may also diminish the incidence of intestinal disease.[68]

REFERENCES

1. Kazal HL, Sohn N, Carrasco JI, Robilotti JG Jr, Delaney WE. The gay bowel syndrome: Clinicopathologic correlation in 260 cases. Ann Clin Lab Sci 1976;6:184.
2. Sohn N, Robilotti JG Jr. The gay bowel syndrome: A review of colonic and rectal conditions in 200 male homosexuals. Am J Gastroenterol 1977;67:478.
3. William DC, Felman YM, Marr JS, Shookhoof HB. Sexually transmitted enteric pathogens in male homosexual population. NY State J Med 1977;77:2050.
4. Owen RL, Dritz SK, Wibbelsman CJ. Venereal aspects of gastroenterology. West J Med 1979;130:236.
5. Felman YM, Riccardi NB. Sexually transmitted enteric diseases. Bull NY Acad Med 1979;55:533.
6. Dritz SK, Goldsmith RS. Sexually transmissable protozoal bacterial and viral enteric infections. Compr Ther 1980;6:34.
7. Owen WF. Sexually transmitted diseases and traumatic problems in homosexual men. Ann Intern Med 1980;92:805.
8. Heller M. The gay bowel syndrome. A common problem of homosexual patients in the emergency department. Ann Emerg Med 1980;9:487.
9. Quinn TC, Corey L, Chaffee RG, et al. The etiology of anorectal infections in homosexual men. Am J Med 1981;71:395.
10. Quinn TC. Clinical approach to intestinal infections in homosexual men. Med Clin North Am 1986;70:611.
11. Most H. Manhattan: A tropic isle? Am J Trop Med Hyg 1968;17:333.
12. Dritz SK, Ainsworth TE, Back A, et al. Patterns of sexually transmitted enteric diseases in a city. Lancet 1977;2:3.
13. Dritz SK, Back AF. Shigella enteritis venereally transmitted (letter). N Engl J Med 1974;291:1194.
14. Dritz SK, Braff EH. Sexually transmitted typhoid fever (letter). N Engl J Med 1977;296:1359.
15. Blaser MJ, Berkowitz ID, LaForce FM. *Campylobacter* enteritis: Clinical and epidemiologic features. Ann Intern Med 1979;91:179.
16. Dritz SK. Medical aspects of homosexuality (editorial). N Engl J Med 1980;302:463.
17. Drusin LM, Genvert G, Topf-Olstein B, Levy-Zombek E. Shigellosis: Another sexually transmitted disease? Br J Vener Dis 1976;52:348.
18. Bader M, Pedersen AHB, Williams R, et al. Venereal transmission of shigellosis in Seattle–King County. Sex Transm Dis 1977;4:89.
19. Mildvan D, Gelb AM, William D. Venereal transmission of enteric pathogens in male homosexuals. JAMA 1977;238:1387.
20. Carey PB, Wright EP. *Campylobacter jejuni* in a male homosexual (letter). Br J Vener Dis 1979;55:380.
21. Quinn TC, Corey L, Chaffee RG, et al. *Campylobacter* proctitis in a homosexual man. Ann Intern Med 1980;93:458.
22. Quinn TC, Goodell SE, Mikrichian EE, et al. Etiology of proctitis and enteritis in homosexual men (abstr.). Clin Res 1981;29:534A.
23. Quinn TC, Goodell SE, Mikrichian E. *Chlamydia trachomatis* proctitis. N Engl J Med 1981;305:195.
24. Quinn TC, Stamm WE, Goodell SE. The polymicrobial origin of intestinal infections in homosexual men. N Engl J Med 1983;309:576.

25. Jacobs JL, Gold JWM, Murray HW. Salmonella infections in patients with the acquired immune deficiency syndrome. Ann Intern Med 1985;102:186.
26. Glaser JB, Morton-Kute L, Berger SR. Recurrent *Salmonella typhimurium* bacteremia associated with the acquired immune deficiency syndrome. Ann Intern Med 1985;189:207.
27. Smith PD, Macher AM, Bookman MA. *Salmonella typhimurium* enteritis and bacteremia in the acquired immune deficiency syndrome. Ann Intern Med 1985;102:207.
28. Totten PA, Fennell CL, Tenover FC. *Campylobacter cinaedi* (sp. nov.) and *Campylobacter fennelliae* (sp. nov.): Two new *Campylobacter* species associated with enteric disease in homosexual men. J Infect Dis 1985;151:131.
29. Keusch GT. *Shigella* infections. Clin Gastroenterol 1979;8:645.
30. Mata LJ, Gangarosa EJ, Caceres A, et al. Epidemic Shiga bacillus dysentery in Central America: I. Etiologic investigations in Guatemala. J Infect Dis 1969;122:170.
31. Centers for Disease Control. Annual summary 1980. Reported morbidity and mortality in the United States. Morbid Mortal Weekly Rep 1981;29:76.
32. Levine MM, Dupont HL, Formal SB, et al. Pathogenesis of *Shigella dysenteriae* 1 (Shiga) dysentery. J Infect Dis 1973;127:261.
33. Dupont HL, Hornick RB, Snyder MJ, et al. Immunity in shigellosis: II. Protection induced by oral live vaccine or primary infection. J Infect Dis 1972;125:12.
34. Levine MM, Dupont HL, Khodabandelou M, Hornick RB. Long-term *Shigella*-carrier state. N Engl J Med 1973;288:1169.
35. Watt J, Hardy AV. Studies of the acute diarrheal diseases: XIII. Cultural surveys of normal population groups. Public Health Rep 1945;60:261.
36. Keusch GT, Grady GF, Mata IJ, Melver J. The pathogenesis of *Shigella* diarrhea: I. Enterotoxin production by *Shigella dysenteriae* 1. J Clin Invest 1972;51:1212.
37. Keusch GT, Jacewicz M. Pathogenesis of *Shigella* diarrhea: VI. Toxin and anti-toxin in *Sh. flexneri* and *Sh. sonnei* infections in humans. J Infect Dis 1977;135:522.
38. Kinsey MD, Formal SB, Dammin GJ, Giannella RG. Fluid and electrolyte transport in rhesus monkeys challenged intracecally with *Shigella flexneri* 2a. Infect Immun 1976;14:368.
39. Gemski P, Takeuchi A, Washington O, Formal SB. Shigellosis due to *Shigella dysenteriae* 1. Relative importance of mucosal invasion versus toxin production in pathogenesis. J Infect Dis 1972;126:523.
40. Sherman VBD, McGowan V, Sneath PHA, eds. Approved lists of bacterial names. Inst J Syst Bacteriol 1980;30:225.
41. Blaser MJ, Reller BL. *Campylobacter* enteritis. N Engl J Med 1981;305:1444.
42. Smibert RM. The genus *Campylobacter*. Annu Rev Microbiol 1978;32:674.
43. Atherton JG, Ricketts SW. *Campylobacter* infection from foals (letter). Vet Rec 1980;107:264.
44. Dobbs EM, McIntyre RW. A case report of vibrionic abortion in a goat herd. Calif Vet 1951;4:19.
45. Firehammer BD, Myers LL. *Campylobacter fetus* subsp. *jejuni*: Its possible significance in enteric disease of calves and lambs. Am J Vet Res 1981;42:918.
46. Blaser MJ, LaForce FM, Wilson NA, Wang WLL. Reservoirs for human campylobacteriosis. J Infect Dis 1980;141:665.
47. Stern NJ. Recovery rate of *Campylobacter fetus* ssp. *jejuni* on eviscerated pork, lamb and beef carcasses. J Food Sci 1981;46:1291.
48. Blaser MJ, Hardesty HL, Powers B, Wang WLL. Survival of *Campylobacter fetus* subsp. *jejuni* in biologic milieus. J Clin Microbiol 1980;11:309.

49. Knill M, Sucklin WG, Pearson AD. Environmental isolation of heat-tolerant *Campylobacter* in the Southhampton area. Lancet 1978;2:1002.
50. Blaser M, Cravens J, Powers BW, Wang WL. *Campylobacter* enteritis associated with canine infection. Lancet 1978;2:979.
51. Blaser MJ, Waldman RJ, Barrett T, Erlandson AL. Outbreaks of *Campylobacter* enteritis in two extended families: Evidence for person to person transmission. J Pediatr 1981;98:254.
52. Steele TW, McDermott S. *Campylobacter* enteritis in South Australia. Med J Aust 1978;2:404.
53. Robinson DA. Infective dose of *Campylobacter jejuni* in milk. Br Med J 1981; 282:1584.
54. Ruiz-Palacios GM, Escaimilla E, Torres J, Torres N. Production of enterotoxins by *Campylobacter jejuni*. Paper presented at the Twenty-Second Interscience Conference on Antimicrobial Agents and Chemotherapy, Miami Beach, Oct. 4–6, 1982.
55. Pitkaneen T, Pettersson T, Ponka A, Kosunen TV. Effect of erythromycin on the fecal excretion of *Campylobacter fetus* subspecies *jejuni*. J Infect Dis 1982;145:128.
56. Blaser MJ, Cheko P, Bopp C, et al. *Campylobacter* enteritis associated with food-borne transmission. Am J Epidemiol 1982;116:886.
57. Bokkenheuser VD, Richardson NJ, Bryner JH, et al. Detection of enteric campylobacteriosis in children. J Clin Microbiol 1979;9:227.
58. Blaser MJ, Glass RI, Huq MI, et al. Isolation of *Campylobacter fetus* ssp. *jejuni* from Bangladeshi children. J Clin Microbiol 1980;12:744.
59. Simmers PD, Tabaqchali S. *Campylobacter* species in male homosexuals (letter). Br J Vener Dis 1979;55:66.
60. Pasternak J, Bolivar R, Hopfer RL. Bacteremia caused by *Campylobacter*-like organisms in two male homosexuals. Ann Intern Med 1984;101:339.
61. Hornick RB, Greiseman SE, Woodward TE, et al. Typhoid fever: Pathogenesis and immunological control. N Engl J Med 1970;283:686.
62. McCullough NB, Eisele CW. Experimental human salmonellosis: III. Pathogenicity of strains of *Salmonella newport, Salmonella derby* and *Salmonella bareilly* obtained from spray-dried whole egg. J Infect Dis 1951;89:209.
63. McCullough NB, Eisele CW. Experimental human salmonellosis: IV. Pathogenicity of strains of *Salmonella pullorum* obtained from spray-dried whole eggs. J Infect Dis 1951;89:259.
64. Hoffman TA, Ruiz CJ, Counts GW, et al. Water-borne typhoid fever in Dade County, Florida: Clinical and therapeutic evaluations of 105 bacteremic patients. Am J Med 1975;59:481.
65. Kaye D, Merselis JG, Connolly CS, Hook EW. Treatment of chronic carriers of *Salmonella typhosa* with ampicillin. Ann NY Acad Sci 1967;145:429.
66. Musher DN, Rubenstein AD. Permanent carriers of nontyphosa salmonellae. Arch Intern Med 1973;132:869.
67. Deut. 23:12–13.
68. Curran JW, Morgan WM, Hardy AM. The epidemiology of AIDS: Current status and future prospects. Science 1985;229:1352.

Chapter 7

Parasitic Infectious Diseases as Sexually Transmitted Infections

Daniel C. William

Until only 14 years ago, the sexual transmission of enteric protozoans was an unrecognized part of these diseases' epidemiology. Public health measures ensuring clean food and water had largely eliminated these infections from developed countries in the 19th and early 20th centuries. Enteric protozoan infections were seen only where failures of public health existed.

Dr. Most is credited with the first written account (in 1968) noting the association between sexual behavior and enteric protozoa infection. By 1982, it was recognized that these diseases were hyperendemic in the urban, sexually active, homosexual male population. Several surveys have demonstrated point prevalence rates of 20% to 31% for amebiasis and 4% to 18% for giardiasis in this population. Mixed infections with both agents have occurred in up to 10% of surveyed men. Since none of these point prevalence surveys relied on multiple stool examinations of the study populations, they all would be expected to have underestimated the true disease prevalence.

Why had these diseases become hyperendemic in this population? The functional overlap between the genitourinary and gastrointestinal tracts during some sexual activities among homosexuals had permitted direct person-to-person transfer of a variety of enteric protozoans. Analingus, or oral-rectal contact, is the most obvious mode of transmission. Now, with homosexual patients' increased awareness of the inherent disease risks, analingus probably accounts for a smaller percentage of infections than in the past. Currently, indirect exposure represents the major mode of disease acquisition. This can occur whenever oral sex takes place in the presence of fecal contamination. Although anal intercourse in itself is devoid of this hazard, resultant genital soiling and later genital-oral or genital-hand-oral contact can eventually result in the ingestion of enteric pathogens. This condition is facilitated by group sex encounters. Because protozoa cysts remain viable for prolonged times, often measured in days, fomites such as contaminated rectal tubes as well as towels, mats, walls, floors, and other environmental surfaces are also responsible for some disease spread.

One described outbreak of amebiasis occurred secondary to a contaminated colonic irrigation system. This suggests that rectal-rectal transmission may also occur with the sharing of enema nozzles or rectal douches or in group sex situations. Since many infected patients lack significant symptoms, a large reservoir of infected, sexually active carriers may unknowingly transmit their infection to their sexual partners.

The risk of potential exposure for an individual patient is further determined by the total number of different sexual partners and the frequency of sexual contact. Because of the high disease prevalence of amebiasis, however, even nonpromiscuous homosexual men are at significant risk of disease acquisition whenever they engage in at-risk behavior with nonmonogamous sexual partners. Hence, it is not surprising that many patients currently being treated for enteric protozoa have a history of infection and are at significant risk for future disease.

AIDS AND ENTERIC PROTOZOA

In the initial case control studies of homosexual men with acquired immunodeficiency syndrome (AIDS), amebiasis as well as other sexually transmitted diseases were more often associated with AIDS patients compared with controls. This association is now thought to be a surrogate for sexual behaviors allowing for the transmission of human immunodeficiency virus (HIV). Moreover, amebiasis and possibly other enteric protozoa may be cofactors in the progression of HIV infection to full-blown AIDS.

AMEBIASIS

Amebiasis is the most common sexually transmitted enteric protozoan. The life cycle of *Entamoeba histolytica* begins with ingestion of *E. histolytica* cysts. The cysts disintegrate in the small bowel, releasing immature amebas. These amebas migrate down into the large intestine, where mature adult amebic trophozoites produce new infective cysts. These are in turn passed in the feces. In many cases, the amebas exist commensally, living freely in the intestinal lumen. Unless the amebas invade the mucosa, significant disease symptoms will be absent. Although any portion of the large bowel can be affected, the cecum and rectosigmoid colon are common sites of involvement.

The incubation period for symptomatic disease following ingestion of cysts is one week or longer. Commonly, symptoms begin insidiously and are frequently overlooked by those infected. Bowel habits typically change. Stools may become flaky, poorly formed, or soft. Some patients have increased frequency of movements; others complain of tenesmus or constipation. In still others, symptoms wax and wane. Bloating, cramping, flatulence, fecal mucus, and fatigue are also commonly seen with amebiasis. Symptoms of amebic dysentery, including bloody diarrhea, weight loss, and fever, are uncommon.

The pathogenicity of amebiasis is determined by a variety of factors. The dose of the inoculum, the virulence of the infective strain, and the host's general nutritional status all influence the severity of the infection. Patients with poor nutritional status and chronic wasting illness, including AIDS, are more likely to be severely ill with amebic infections. Because the normal intestinal flora provide necessary nutrients for amebic survival, antibiotics such as tetracycline, erythromycin, and the sulfonamides tend to ameliorate the symptoms of intestinal amebiasis by changing the normal flora. Amebic infection should therefore be suspected in patients with nonspecific bowel symptoms who favorably respond to these drugs when medicated for unrelated conditions.

The metastatic spread of venereal amebic infections into the liver, lungs, or other vital organs has to date been notably rare. Possible explanations for the infrequency of complications include the protective value of high-protein diets seen in these patients or the nonpathogenicity of many strains of *E. histolytica* seen in homosexual men.

Diagnosis

On physical examination, patients with amebiasis may be completely normal. Increased bowel sounds and lower abdominal tenderness are common nonspecific findings. Examination of the patient with an anoscope may show small punctate ulcerations within the rectum in more severe disease.

The accurate diagnosis of intestinal amebiasis remains a major clinical dilemma. In the absence of tissue-invasive disease, serologic tests are insensitive and therefore not recommended. Direct examination of bowel scrapings obtained through an anoscope or sigmoidoscope can reliably diagnose disease only when performed by a skilled and well-trained clinician. All too frequently, however, macrophages and nonpathogenic protozoa are misread as pathogens. The same problem can occur when stool examinations are performed by inexperienced laboratory personnel. Because viable trophozoites are found only in fresh liquid specimens, any delay in stool examination can produce false-negative test results. The immediate preservation of fresh stool specimens with polyvinyl alcohol and formalin, for example, may circumvent problems associated with delays in laboratory examination. Examination of formed movements for protozoa cysts may require collection of several specimens over several days because cyst production may occur only sporadically. A more sensitive test is the examination of freshly purged stool obtained by administering a saline cathartic. Purging increases the sensitivity by providing the possibility of finding both trophozoites and cysts in a fresh liquid stool. Though time consuming and unpleasant, purged-stool testing, performed in a licensed parasitology laboratory, has become a common outpatient test for diagnosis of intestinal amebiasis. Because no single test is 100% sensitive, repeated examinations may be indicated where clinical suspicion exists. The finding of nonpathogenic protozoa, including *E. coli, Endolimax nana, Iodamoeba butschlii, E. hartmanni,* and *Trichomonas hominis* represents a marker for past fecal-oral exposure. When carefully retested, more than 50% of these patients will concurrently harbor a pathogenic protozoan.

A further factor decreasing the sensitivity of all stool testing is the presence of interfering substances. Bismuth of alkaline salt—including kaolin, nonabsorbable antacids, tetracycline, erythromycin, sulfonamides, barium sulfate, mineral oil, and castor oil—can produce false-negative test results. Patients should refrain from using any of these substances for as long as two weeks before a stool test.

Treatment

The effective treatment of amebiasis remains a complicated problem for all clinicians. No drug is uniformly effective. Many drugs have annoying side effects and require prolonged use; others are costly or have potentially serious side effects. For these reasons, the proliferation of treatment schedules and combinations of drugs has been seemingly endless.

Iodoquinol (Diiodohydroxyquin) has remained one of the mainstays of therapy for intestinal amebiasis. The drug is prescribed as 650 mg three times daily for 20 days. Common side effects include headache, various gastrointestinal symptoms, and anal pruritus. When given to children on a long-term basis, the drug has caused optic atrophy and blindness. Because the drug contains iodine, the furunculosis of iodines is a contraindication to its use. Iodoquinol is also radiopaque and may interfere with x-ray studies of the abdomen. The drug is especially useful in eliminating amebic cysts from carriers.

Metronidazole (Flagyl) is effective in both intestinal and extraintestinal amebic infections. The dose is 750 mg three times daily for five to ten days. Unfortunately, the majority of patients taking this dose of drug will experience a variety of unpleasant reactions, including nausea, metallic taste, dark urine, fatigue, headache, paresthesia, and depression. Alcohol is contraindicated when a patient is taking metronidazole because of a potential disulfiram (Antabuse)-like reaction. Metronidazole has been mutagenic in bacteria and carcinogenic in rodents. Neither effect has been documented in humans.

Paromomycin (Humatin) is a nonabsorbable antibiotic not unlike neomycin. In the absence of significant colitis (where absorption may occur), the drug has an excellent safety record. Like neomycin, however, the drug is both ototoxic and nephrotoxic when absorbed. Various gastrointestinal disturbances are the major adverse reactions encountered with paromomycin. The dose is 25 mg/kg/day in divided doses for 5 to 12 days. Paromomycin is expensive, costing $35 to $75 per treatment course.

Diloxanide furoate, available only from the Parasitic Division of the Centers for Disease Control (CDC), is also effective for asymptomatic cyst carriers. This drug is safe and usually well tolerated. Flatulence is the most common reaction. The dose is 500 mg three times daily for ten days.

Tetracycline and erythromycin, and their various analogs, are often useful adjuncts to therapy. They are, however, of necessity combined with other drugs to effect a therapeutic cure.

Carbarsone (Pulvule) is an arsenical, the usefulness of which is limited by potentially severe reactions including cholestatic jaundice and hemorrhagic encephalitis. The slow elimination of arsenicals also mandates adequate "rest periods" between courses of therapy. Emetine, dehydroemetine, and chloroquine are rarely used in uncomplicated intestinal infections and will not be discussed.

For the average patient with symptomatic intestinal amebiasis, a reasonable drug schedule would be the combination of iodoquinol and paromomycin. All patients so treated should have one or more follow-up stool examinations to ensure clinical cure.

GIARDIASIS

Next to amebiasis, giardiasis is the most common venereally transmitted enteric protozoa pathogen. Like *E. histolytica*, *Giardia lamblia* has both a trophozoite and cyst stage. Following ingestion, the cysts undergo excystation in the duodenum. These flagellated *Giardia* trophozoites then attach by sucking disks to an intestinal epithelial cell. Except when severe diarrhea is present, *G. lamblia* trophozoites are rarely present in the stool. The exact pathogenic mechanisms causing symptoms of giardiasis are unknown.

Following an incubation period of one to two weeks, giardiasis often abruptly begins with nausea, anorexia, and explosive diarrhea. Severe, foul-odored flatulence, often associated with epigastric distention, are prominent components of giardiasis. Some patients complain of eructation. Mild constitutional symptoms, including headache and low-grade fever, may be present. The foul-smelling stools seen with giardiasis suggest steatorrhea. Blood and pus are notably absent from stool specimens. Rarely, parasites may ascend the biliary tree, causing signs and symptoms of gallbladder disease.

Diagnosis

On physical examination, patients with giardiasis may have epigastric distention or tenderness. The diagnosis of giardiasis can only occasionally be confirmed by finding trophozoites or cysts in the stool. Cyst formation is sporadic, and chronically infected patients may have multiple negative stool examinations. Unlike amebiasis, purging is not a reliable mechanism for eliciting trophozoites in the stool of patients with giardiasis. Duodenal specimens obtained by aspiration, biopsy, or "enterotest" probably are the most sensitive tests for the diagnosis of giardiasis. Unfortunately, their cost, time, and discomfort preclude their adoption as routine testing procedures. For these reasons, many clinicians will clinically diagnose giardiasis without identifying the parasite in a patient's specimen.

Treatment

The treatment of choice for giardiasis is quinacrine hydrochloride (Atabrine), 100 mg three times daily after meals for five to ten days. Quinacrine hydrochloride is inexpensive. It commonly causes lightheadedness, headache, insomnia, and nausea. A reversible, acute toxic psychosis is the most common severe adverse reaction. This often is preceded by inappropriate mood swings and bizarre dream content. As a dose-related reaction, toxic psychosis more likely occurs toward the end of therapy. Quinacrine hydrochloride frequently discolors the skin to an icteric-like yellow and can severely exacerbate psoriasis. Hemolysis can be precipitated by quinacrine in G6PD-deficient patients. As with metronidazole, alcohol should be avoided during a quinacrine regimen because of a potential disulfiram-like reaction.

Metronidazole (Flagyl), 250 mg three times daily for seven to ten days, is an effective alternative to quinacrine hydrochloride.

Patients with giardiasis often develop lactase deficiency, which persists long after cure. These patients will continue to complain of bloating, flatulence, and diarrhea unless lactose-containing foods are diligently eliminated from their diet.

OTHER PARASITES

Dientamoeba fragilis is a large bowel parasite lacking a cyst stage. Although not invasive, this parasite often causes diarrhea, flatulence, and distention. Treatment with a 20-day course of iodoquinol (diiodohydroxyquin) or a ten-day course of tetracycline is said to be effective. Since the AIDS epidemic began, parasites considered as potential STD pathogens are *Cryptosporidium* and *Isospora belli*, which are presented in Chapters 8 and 12.

PATIENT EDUCATION

When treating any patient with sexually acquired parasitic infection, the most important function a clinician must provide is adequate information to allow one's patient a choice to remain disease free. As with any chronic infectious disease, the size of the infected pool is a function of the rate of new infections minus the rate of therapeutic and spontaneous cures.

Given even the best of circumstances, the medical diagnosis and treatment of patients with enteric protozoa will have only a negligible impact on the overall disease rates unless there is a concurrent diminution of new infections. To prove this point, let us follow 100 hypothetical homosexual men unknowingly infected with *E. histolytica*. Only half these patients (or 50 men) will have symptoms; the rest will be asymptomatic carriers. Few, if any, of these carriers will be tested for parasites.

Of the 50 men with symptoms, probably only 40 will seek medical attention. Those patients with symptoms who fail to seek care may believe their symptoms are caused by diet or, perhaps, "nerves." Others cannot afford the time or money necessary for medical evaluation. Of the 40 men who are evaluated by a physician, perhaps in only 30 men will the diagnosis of amebiasis be considered. (This is probably overly generous, since many homosexual men will "pass" as heterosexual and the symptoms of amebiasis may be attributed to irritable bowel syndrome or nonspecific gastroenteritis.) Probably fewer than 20 of the 30 men suspected of having amebiasis will actually be diagnosed, given the expense, time, and insensitivity of stool examinations. Since treatment is not always successful, perhaps only 15, or 15%, of the original 100 patients will ultimately be cured.

The total cost of each cured patient will probably exceed $200 not counting lost time from work for office visits and testing.

Therefore, even under the best of circumstances, only a small percentage of patients infected can be medically removed from the reservoir of infection.

CONCLUSION

For those patients lucky enough to be cured, the only hope to prevent reinfection is to understand how to remain disease free. Patients must realize how direct and indirect sexual exposure can frequently result in disease acquisition. The patient who says he does not understand how he has become reinfected usually is telling the truth. A complete understanding by patients of the biology and epidemiology of their disease will go a long way in preventing recurrences and, one hopes, in controlling these diseases for all.

REFERENCE

1. Krogstad D.J. Isoenzyme patterns and pathogenicity in amebic infection (editional). N Eng J Med 315:390–391.

Chapter 8
Cryptosporidiosis, Isosporiasis, and Microsporidiosis

Pearl Ma
Philip D. Marsden

In the first edition we reviewed the human intestinal Coccidia in general, including *Isospora belli* and the two human species of *Sarcocystis*. However, since that time *Cryptosporidium* infections have assumed the importance that we predicted, and several reviews of cryptosporidiosis have appeared.[1-4] Also, it has become clear that in immunocompetent individuals, especially children, cryptosporidiosis is a relatively common cause of self-limiting diarrhea. If the correct techniques are used in investigating childhood diarrhea, this infection can be found.[5] Since infection with human immunodeficiency virus (HIV), the virus associated with acquired immunodeficiency syndrome (AIDS), has spread worldwide, its geographical distribution based on epidemiologic studies becomes important because cryptosporidial infection in immunodeficient individuals is frequently fatal. There have been reports of isosporiasis in patients with AIDS.[6-8] However, it was often a chance finding in stool surveys and not associated with symptoms. Like cryptosporidiosis, isosporiasis in AIDS patients is usually associated with symptoms.[9] Perhaps the most interesting report is from Haiti, where 15% of 31 AIDS patients with diarrhea were found to be infected with *I. belli*.[7] Since no animal reservoir is known, this implies that human fecal contamination of the environment affects infection. The protozoan, *Microsporidia*,[10] rarely known in clinical medicine, has also been diagnosed in AIDS patients.[10-13] A brief description of this protozoan is included in this chapter.

CRYPTOSPORIDIUM

Taxonomy and Life Cycle

The taxonomic position of *Cryptosporidium* sp. in its relationship to other protozoans is shown in Figure 8–1. The species differentiation of the genus

	Protozoa		
Phylum	*Sarcomastigophora* (Amoeba, Flagellates) *Ciliophora* (Ciliates)	*Apicomplexa*	*Microspora*
Class		*Sporozoasida*	*Microsporea*
Subclass		*Coccidiasina*	
Order		*Eucoccidiorida*	*Microsporidia*
Family	*Eimeriidae*	*Sarcocystidae*	*Cryptosporidiidae*
Genus	*Isospora* *Eimeria*	Sarcocystis Toxoplasma	Cryptosporidium	Nosema Encephalitozoon Enterocytozoon Pleistophora

FIGURE 8–1 *Taxonomic classification of protozoa. Adapted from Levine ND et al. A newly revised classification of the Protozoa. J Protozool 1980;27(1):37–58; and Current WL. The biology of cryptosporidium. Am Soc Microbiol News 1988;54:605.*

Cryptosporidium is confusing. Levine[14] has suggested that *Cryptosporidium* species be limited to four, depending on the host involved: mammal, bird, reptile, or fish. Certainly cryptosporidiosis of calves and lambs has been successfully transmitted to humans, and vice versa.[15] It has been proposed that there are at least two species in mammals (*C. parvum* and *C. muris*) and two species in birds (*C. baileyi* and *C. meleagridis*).[16] Studies are in progress to solve the classification of *Cryptosporidium*.

Coccidia are *Sporozoa* with both asexual and sexual cycles of multiplication. Usually multiplication occurs in the epithelium of the intestinal tract (Figure 8–2)[1–4] and rarely in the respiratory tract.[3,4,17–22] The AIDS epidemic[1,22] has fostered increased awareness of cryptosporidial infections in other sites, such as laryngotracheitis,[23] esophagitis,[24] cholecystitis,[25] and hepatitis,[26] as well as disseminated infections involving multiple sites.[27,28] The sexual multiplication produces a resistant oocyst form, which sporulates to contain infective sporozoites within the host. *Cryptosporidium* produces an oocyst with four naked sporozoites and no evident sporocyst wall. Failure to recognize this until recently was due to the organisms' minute size on intestinal biopsy or in stool specimens.

Pathology reveals asexual and sexual stages of the parasite embedded in the microvillar border of the small intestinal columnar cells. They are so superficial as to appear to be on the surface of the mucosa. The spherical trophozoites, meronts, and gametes are very tiny (2 to 4 μm) and appear smaller because of histologic processing. They are visible by hematoxylin-eosin, Giemsa, or toluidine blue stains. To someone not familiar with this protozoan, unless the small bowel biopsies are looked at under oil-immersion lens, the protozoa may be mistaken for artifacts. They are attached to the host cell membrane and are now believed to be intracellular[29] but extracytoplasmic. Electron microscopy reveals a complex ultrastructure.[30–33] Recent advances using thin section and freeze frac-

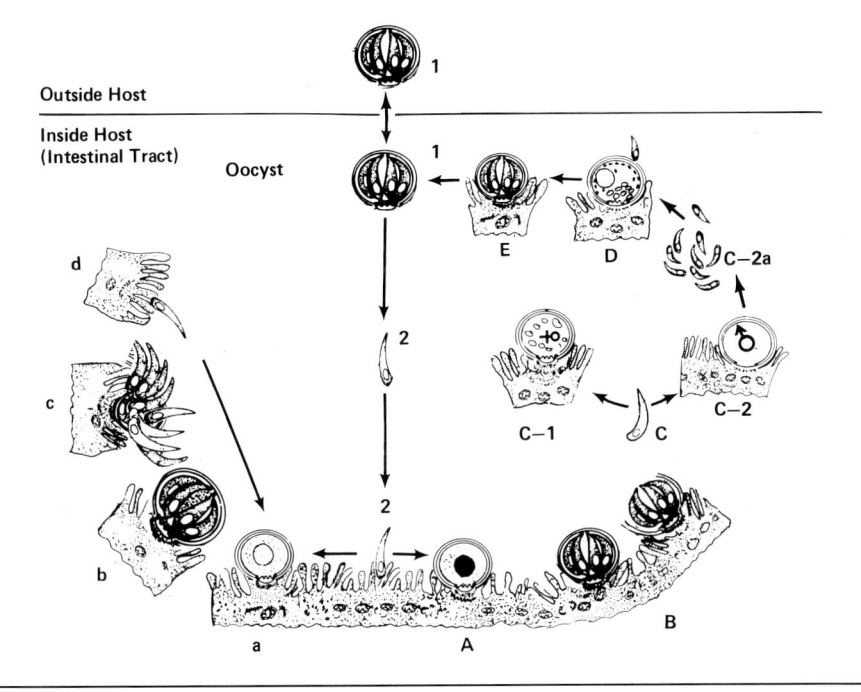

Asexual	Sexual
1. Infective oocyst	1. Infective oocyst
2. Sporozoite	2. Sporozoite
a. Trophozoite	A. Trophozoite
b. First generation meront	B. Second generation meront
c. First generation merozoite	C. Second generation merozoite
d. First generation merozoite attached to microvilli	1. Macrogamont
	2. Microgamont
	a. Microgamete
	D. Zygote (C-1 to C-2a)
	E. Sporulated oocyst

FIGURE 8–2 *Schematic life cycle of* Cryptosporidium *Spp. Reprinted by permission from Ma P. Cryptosporidiosis and immune enteropathy: a review. In: Remington JS, Swartz MN, eds. Current clinical topics in infectious diseases. New York: McGraw-Hill, 1987;8:99–153.*

ture techniques demonstrate the presence of cryptosporidial antigen in the cytoplasm of the host cell.[34] As the trophozoite matures, an attachment organ of membranous folds develops in the host cell cytoplasm.[30–33] Oocysts can sporulate and liberate sporozoites within the intestine, causing autoinfection. If the host's immune response is defective, merogony and gametogony may proceed through many cycles.

On entering a host cell, the sporozoite induces an asexual meront with eight merozoites. This stage is called the first generation–type 1 meront. The meront reinfects other mucosal cells, producing the second generation–type 2 meront in merogony, and proceeds to form the male or female gamete in gametogony of the sexual cycle. Fertilization occurs, leading to the production of the oocyst, which undergoes sporulation to produce four naked sporozoites—the infective stage. Matured oocysts are acid-fast and are best detected with acid-fast stain, such as the modified cold kinyoun stain.[35–37] The staining procedure takes only 1 minute for fresh stool and 5 to 15 minutes for stool specimen with preservatives such as formalin and polyvinyl alcohol added. Also, it is cost effective. Another rapid procedure is the sucrose flotation on coverslipped slide,[37] which allows the oocysts to float in the sucrose directly below the coverslip. One must do the direct preparation from tissue, since oocysts extruded into the intestinal lumen are mature and thus easily dislodged or washed away during processing.[38] Direct fluorescent antibody testing using monoclonal antibody has been used to identify the oocyst in stool specimens.[39] Laboratory diagnosis is further detailed in Chapter 12.

The oocysts have been reported to infect the entire gastrointestinal tract, with predominant infection of the small intestine and, rarely, the stomach. Other sites are involved in chronic infections, especially in the terminal stage of the disease. Complications have been reported showing endogenous stages in the gallbladder,[25] liver,[26] alveolar spaces of the bronchi,[20] lung proper,[17–21,28] and laryngotracheal area.[23] Another interesting case is one associated with perinatal infection.[40] Review of our unpublished data also shows cases of cryptosporidiosis in newborns of a Haitian mother.

Cryptosporidiosis in Immunocompetent Individuals

The incubation period of cryptosporidiosis appears to be about one week after cyst ingestion.[1–4] Most outbreaks are due to traveler's diarrhea[41–44] or are found in day-care centers,[45–48] small communities,[47–49], or hospitals.[50,51] About 50 publications address the clinical picture of cryptosporidiosis in otherwise healthy subjects.[1–4] In such immunocompetent individuals, cryptosporidiosis is a self-limiting internal illness usually characterized by watery diarrhea lasting one to two weeks with varying degrees of abdominal pain and weight loss.[52–54] Periodically, it may extend to six weeks. Eosinophilia is sometimes present. The oocysts are detectable in the stool, ranging from those with no cellular exudate to semisolid stool with or without mucus. The stool is distinctly nonbloody. Small bowel or rectal biopsy shows the microvilli altered to atrophied, shortened, and fused during the phase of symptomatic disease, with endogenous stages embedded in the microvilli. However, recovery must occur rapidly and the transient malabsorption resolve spontaneously, as seen in immunocompetent homosexual, bisexual and heterosexual individuals.[52–54] Investigation of affected individuals in a day-care center revealed that oocysts were not related to the symptomatology of the infections and persisted even after the symptoms subsided.[53]

Cryptosporidiosis in Immunocompromised Individuals (non-AIDS)

Increasing numbers of publications[1-4] have dealt with cryptosporidiosis in immunocompromised hosts who do not have AIDS. The underlying conditions include bullous pemphigoid[55,56] and ulcerative colitis for which steroid therapy was given, leukemia,[57] organ[58] or bone marrow transplantation,[59,60] cancer treatment,[61] hypogammaglobulinemia,[58,62] and multiple opportunistic infections such as cytomegalovirus (CMV), Epstein-Barr virus (EBV), and disseminated toxoplasmosis similar to that seen in AIDS patients.[63] In some cases, the diarrhea had persisted for months or even years,[62,63] leading to a high fatality rate. One case of spontaneous remission was reported in a child with acute lymphocytic leukemia.[64]

Two cases of disseminated cryptosporidiosis have been reported.[28,60] One occurred in a double-immunocompromised infant who might have acquired the infection from his mother, who had similar diarrhea symptoms two weeks before the infant's infection appeared. The infant failed to survive despite multiple therapeutic regimens, including a thymus transplant. The endogenous stages of *Cryptosporidium* were demonstrated in the infant's pancreatic duct, small intestine, and bronchioles.[28]

The other case was a seven-year-old girl with severe combined immunodeficiency who failed to thrive after receiving a bone marrow transplant from her father. She suffered voluminous diarrhea. At autopsy, the organism was present in the jejunum, ileum, colon, rectum, and bronchial tree.[60] Other patients showed remission on cessation of immunosuppressive therapy for the underlying diseases,[55-57] which may represent possible activation of latent infection,[56] although spontaneous remission was seen in a child with acute lymphocytic leukemia.[64]

Acquired Immunodeficiency Syndrome

The majority of AIDS patients with cryptosporidiosis had persistent watery diarrhea resisting available therapy.[1,35,65,66] Thus, the Centers for Disease Control (CDC) definition of AIDS has included cryptosporidiosis for more than a month as an indication of AIDS in a high-risk population. However, we have occasionally found cryptosporidial oocysts in AIDS or AIDS-related complex (ARC) patients without diarrheal symptoms, which may represent transient oocyst excretion in a carrier state. Our investigation of cryptosporidiosis in AIDS and ARC patients since 1981 led us to conclude that, in general, diarrhea is more severe (as measured by number of bowel movements each day and duration of diarrheal symptoms) in AIDS patients than in ARC patients.[67] The difference is statistically significant. On the other hand, the watery consistency of the diarrhea may wax and wane with few to many oocysts in some patients during hospitalization. AIDS patients received multiple therapy, and although it did not eradicate the parasite, treatment did temporarily change stool consistency from watery to semisolid or formed with none or fewer oocysts in rare cases.[68,107]

Both monoinfection or mixed infections with *Cryptosporidium* and pathogens such as *Giardia lamblia*,[52–54] *Entamoeba histolytica, I. belli, Mycobacterium avium intracellulare* complex, *Shigella* sp., and *Campylobacter* sp. are seen in AIDS patients, but these companion pathogens have not been consistently present.[1] In fact, the generally regarded commensal protozoans such as *Endolimax nana, Iodamoeba butschlii,* and *Blastocystis hominis* are frequently detected, indicating enteric contamination. The AIDS patient has a malabsorption type of diarrhea. Complications are more common in the AIDS group, and infection extends to the gallbladder, liver, bronchi, and lung proper. Frequently, CMV and enteric gram-negative bacilli such as *Enterobacter, Klebsiella,* and *Pseudomonas* were isolated from the same sites. In the lung and bronchi, *Legionella,* CMV, gram-negative bacteria, and *Candida* have been detected with *Cryptosporidia*.[17,21,69] In 1983, we encountered a newborn with AIDS suffering from persistent cryptosporidiosis and candidiasis (unpublished data).

Transmission

Animal handlers and farm workers may be exposed to special risk of acquiring cryptosporidiosis from young infected farm animals (e.g., calves, lambs, kids, foals, piglets). Today we believe that the majority of new infection is the result of person-to-person transmission, such as occurs in day-care centers and among family members, especially those known to have changed the diapers of an infected child.[42,53] In our survey in the New York City area, travel to warm climates appears to be a risk factor for *Cryptosporidium* in men with AIDS.[67] Seasonal difference in incidence is reported in some areas and not in others.[1–4] More severe symptoms tend to occur in younger children. A high incidence has been seen in malnourished children from poor villages in Jerusalem (personal communication, Irmgard Schid, Ph.D., Caritas Baby Hospital, Jerusalem), and in a day-care center[46] (41% and 64%, respectively). Various incidence reports are shown in Figure 8–3. The list may not be complete at time of publication.

The mode of transmission is believed to be oral-fecal.[1–4] No respiratory case without intestinal involvement has been diagnosed, although this is common in turkeys. Since the oocysts are extremely light, it may only be a matter of time before a primary case of cryptosporidial pneumonia without intestinal involvement is diagnosed. The possibility of aerosol transmission exists, but to date all cases of documented respiratory cryptosporidiosis in humans have been associated with intestinal infection.[17–21,28,69] Since the oocysts are so resistant, they may contaminate milk[48] or water supplies.[41,70] There is little evidence at present that heterosexual genital sexual transmission is possible, since among homosexuals, contamination with oocysts may be high and they may be ingested by mouth. A similar situation must occur in large animal breeding centers. However, the incidence of cryptosporidiosis in the New York City area shows a decrease of

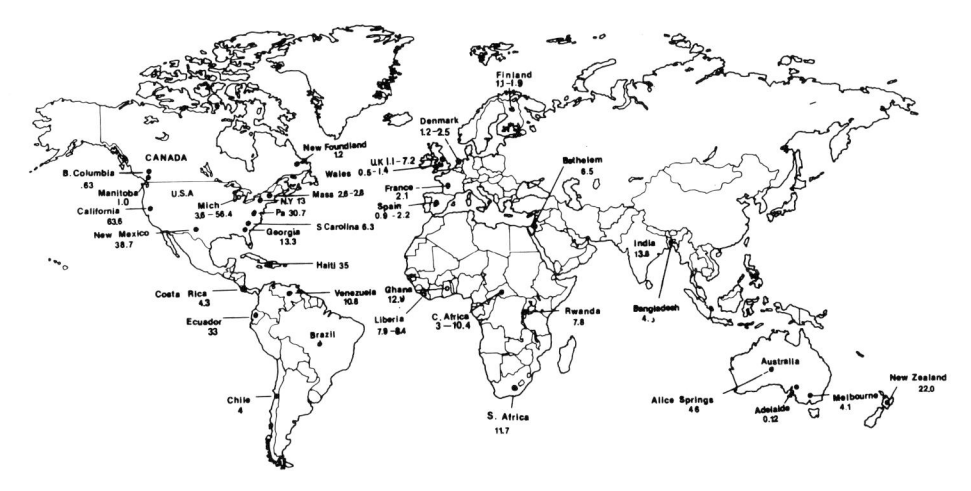

FIGURE 8–3 *Global distribution of* Cryptosporidium spp.

cases, parallel to the decreased incidence of gonorrhea in the city. Whether this phenomenon results from homosexual men's changed life style requires further investigation, but it suggests that cryptosporidiosis may be transmitted by oral-genital or oral-anal contact.

Pathogenesis

The immune defect in homosexual men with AIDS is now believed to be caused by the human T cell lymphotrophic virus type III (HTLV-III)–lymphadenopathy-associated virus (LAV), renamed in 1986 the human immunodeficiency virus (HIV).[71] The immune dysfunction of the T4 lymphocyte appears to allow the parasite multiplicative cycle to continue unchecked. The degree of parasitic infection seen on small bowel biopsies must considerably reduce the absorptive gut surface, with resultant malabsorption.

The fact that cryptosporidiosis is a self-limiting disease in immunocompetent individuals indicates the importance of immune determinants in the outcome of the infection. There is evidence that both T and B cell immune deficiencies are involved in the persistence of intestinal infection that occurs with AIDS. Such an infection occurred in an immunosuppressed renal transplant patient with IgA deficiency.[58] In our prospective study of the host immune response in cryptosporidiosis, lack of IgM and IgA antibodies in AIDS patients *suggests* that infection may be related to the host's inability to clear the oocysts in chronic infections, while immunocompetent individuals with cryptosporidiosis who have IgM and IgA antibodies usually have self-limited infections.[72,73] The detection of enterotoxinlike activity has been reported.[74]

Epidemiology

Figure 8–3 reveals that incidences of infection vary greatly in different parts of the world, but these distributions are more apparent than real because some studies concentrate on AIDS patients and others are concerned with children with diarrhea. What is clear is that human infections extend to all five continents and that cryptosporidiosis should be thought of as a cause of diarrhea, particularly in small children and immunosuppressed individuals.

Many cases of cryptosporidiosis in humans probably pass undetected and resolve spontaneously. One infection was associated with vomiting, abdominal colic, watery diarrhea, lethargy, weakness, sweating, and persistent headache. The symptoms resolved and the parasite disappeared from the patient's stools after seven days. The daughter of this patient had similar symptoms for just two days.[75] Young lambs develop severe infections, suggesting that children could be more symptomatic than adults.[42,45] After a symptomatic case occurred in an Alabama calf handler, 7 of 12 animal handlers had cryptosporidial oocysts in their stools; only 2 were asymptomatic. All had normal globulins and lymphocyte blastogenesis.[76]

In the initial few patients reported in the literature, the parasite was found in bowel biopsy specimens. Because of its small size, electron microscopic confirmation of the parasite's nature was recommended. The oocyst (4 to 5 μm) is so small that it is best recognizable under oil-immersion lens, as with other *Coccidia*. Salt or sucrose flotation is the best way of concentrating the oocysts. However, recent investigation has indicated that the standard formalin-ether concentration procedure can be modified for use in the clinical laboratory, especially if the stool specimen is semisolid.[77] One caution is to eliminate the ether step, since it can cause the oocyst to become less acid-fast.[36,37,78] This is discussed in more detail in Chapter 12. Since these techniques are well known in most clinical laboratories, more than 100 publications on cryptosporidiosis have appeared in the last three years. It will be important to establish the normal pattern of oocyst shedding in humans.[53,54] In the presence of an intact immune response, this is probably quite short. One study reported that 15% of immunocompetent individuals continued to shed oocysts for two weeks or more after diarrhea ceased.[53] In calves, oocyst shedding began 5 to 12 days after birth and continued for 3 to 12 days. If such a brief period exists, detecting the true prevalence of human cryptosporidial infections will be difficult. Experimental data of cryptosporidiosis in Syrian golden hamster neonates indicated that oocyst shedding occurred as early as day 2 after oral inoculation of oocysts, reached a peak on day 6, and started to decline on day 8; negative or minimum oocyst shedding was observed at day 26.[79]

In immunosuppressed patients, oocyst excretion may continue for months or years.[1,62] The study conducted at St. Vincent's Hospital and Medical Center of New York from 1981 to 1985 totaled 145 cases.[72] The cases consist of AIDS and ARC patients with chronic cryptosporidiosis and non-AIDS (homosexual or bisexual individuals and some heterosexuals) patients with acute or intermittent diarrhea with cryptosporidiosis. In the AIDS group, most patients died even with treatment, while in the non-AIDS groups, most cases were self-limited, except two ARC patients with persistent oocysts in their stool whose disease progressed to AIDS within a year. Some patients had intermittent positive stool examinations in the absence of clinical symptoms. Undoubtedly carrier state must exist in this group, as in the immunocompetent group.[53,68]

Certainly stool surveys using flotation techniques to detect oocysts will be time consuming because they involve centrifugation. This can be overcome by using coverslipped preparation *without* centrifugation. Most hospitals are using the acid-fast stained techniques and auramine-rhodamine fluorescent technique with other methods of concentration with success.[35-37] Recently, indirect fluorescent antibody (IFA) testing has been used to monitor detection of cryptosporidial oocysts in community outbreaks.[47]

Another approach relates to the observation of persistent infection in gammaglobulin-deficient subjects, suggesting such globulins may be important in limiting human infection. A study using an IFA test with frozen sections of infected lamb small intestine as antigen detected infections in most of 225 sera tested at a serial dilution of 1:10. Controls included uninfected lamb small intestine as antigen, which gave negative results. Conversion to seropositivity was noted in experimentally infected animals.[80] Positive rates were 86% of 23 men; 80% for dogs; 87% for cats; 100% for cattle, sheep and deer; 95% for pigs; and 88% for chickens. Eleven pools of mice sera were negative.

Recent study of cryptosporidial enzyme-linked immunosorbent assay (ELISA) tests[81] indicated that patients without AIDS showed an early rise and fall of IgM and later of IgG, with some patients producing IgM and all patients producing IgG. Titers remained positive for 12 months. In our study using fecal oocysts as antigen in the IFA test, patients without AIDS had detectable IgA and IgM levels, in contrast to minimal or no detectable level of both specific classes of immunoglobulins in AIDS patients. Lack of IgG was noted in three of eight immunocompetent individuals, even though their IgA and IgM titers were positive in consecutive serial multiple sera tested. IgA and IgM titers in immunocompetent individuals disappeared within three to eight months after onset of symptoms.[72] Casemore, using a similar IFA technique, reported that IgG response in primary infections of immunocompetent individuals is poor.[73]

Treatment

An effective drug is needed to arrest debilitating diarrhea in the immunosuppressed patient with cryptosporidial infection. Or, if we treat the underlying disease, namely, the HIV infection, we might change our management techniques, as shown in one case when the patient was treated with recombinant interleukin-2 for AIDS and the diarrhea subsided for three months with no detection of oocysts.[82] This debilitating diarrhea is difficult to control in AIDS and other severely immunocompromised patients. The majority of them die. No drug therapy seems to be effective.[83] Trimethoprim and sulfamethoxazole or furazolidone—the drugs normally recommended for *Isospora* infections—have little effect, and therapy with amprolium, quinine, clindamycin, and dapsone has been unsuccessful. Spiramycin, a macrolide with an antimicrobial activity similar to erythromycin, was given to 13 AIDS patients in an adult dose of 1 g three or four times a day. After three to four weeks, three patients had no parasites in stool and intestinal biopsy examination; although parasites persisted in three others, symptomatic improvement occurred.[84] On the other hand, treatment failures did occur.[1,83,85,86] A controlled clinical trial is needed to determine the efficacy of spiramycin for treating cryptosporidiosis in AIDS patients. The latest advances that appear most promising are the treatment regimens with hyperimmune colostrum.[85-87] Tzipori et al. treated three AIDS patients with hyperimmune bovine colostrum infected with *Cryptosporidia* with good remission within as early as three days after treatment.[85,86]* This treatment is currently being conducted at St. Vincent's Hospital in a double-blind study. Preliminary results appear encouraging.[107]

Isospora INFECTION

I. belli infections are often self-limiting in immunocompetent individuals,[88,89] but not in isosporiasis in the presence of AIDS infection characterized with chronic watery diarrhea and weight loss[6-10,89,90] or in immunocompromised patients without AIDS.[91]

In the first edition, we mentioned two infections with relatively mild symptoms in homosexual men. With the awareness of this enteric pathogen and the application of a simple three-step stool examination (iodine, modified cold Kinyoun, and sucrose flotation)[35-37] and auramine-rhodamine preparation,[6,37,38] AIDS-associated isosporiasis began to emerge in publications, leading CDC to include diarrhea lasting more than a month with *I. belli* as one of the opportunistic infections in AIDS diagnosis.

Isospora infections have been reviewed elsewhere.[88,89] Only one human species is generally accepted: *I. belli*. Laboratory diagnosis is similar to the one used for cryptosporidiosis, since *Isospora* is also acid-fast positive by modified cold Kinyoun and auramine-rhodamine staining procedures. It also appears with a pink hue in the sucrose flotation method. The technologist will have no difficulty differentiating *Isospora* from *Cryptosporidium* oocysts because they differ in morphology and size.[6,7,9] Like cryptosporidiosis, transmission is by infective sporulated oocysts in fecal-contaminated situations.[6-10] Where fecal transmission is intense (e.g., mental institutions), minor outbreaks have occurred.

The life cycle of *Isospora* (Figure 8–4) is very similar to that of *Crypto-

---

*This treatment is being set up at St. Vincent's Hospital and Medical Center of New York, 158 W. 12th St. New York City, N Y. 10011 (212) 790-8415.

Cryptosporidiosis, Isosporiasis, and Microsporidiosis   87

Asexual life cycle
A. Sporogony
B. Excystation
C. Merogony

Sexual life cycle
D. Gametogony
E. Fertilization

Various stages
1. Sporoblast (immature)
2. Sporoblast (mature) undergoing divisions
3. Sporocysts
4. Sporocysts (mature)
4a. Sporozoites (free)
5. Sporozoites (invade)
6. Meront (type 1)
7. Merozoite (type 1)
8. Microgamont
9. Microgametocyte
10. Microgamete
11. Macrogamont
12. Macrogamete
13. Zygote
14. Oocyst (unsporulated)

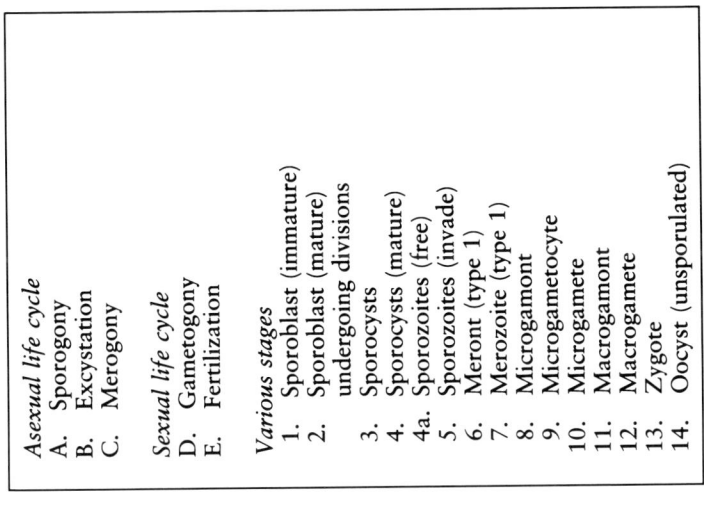

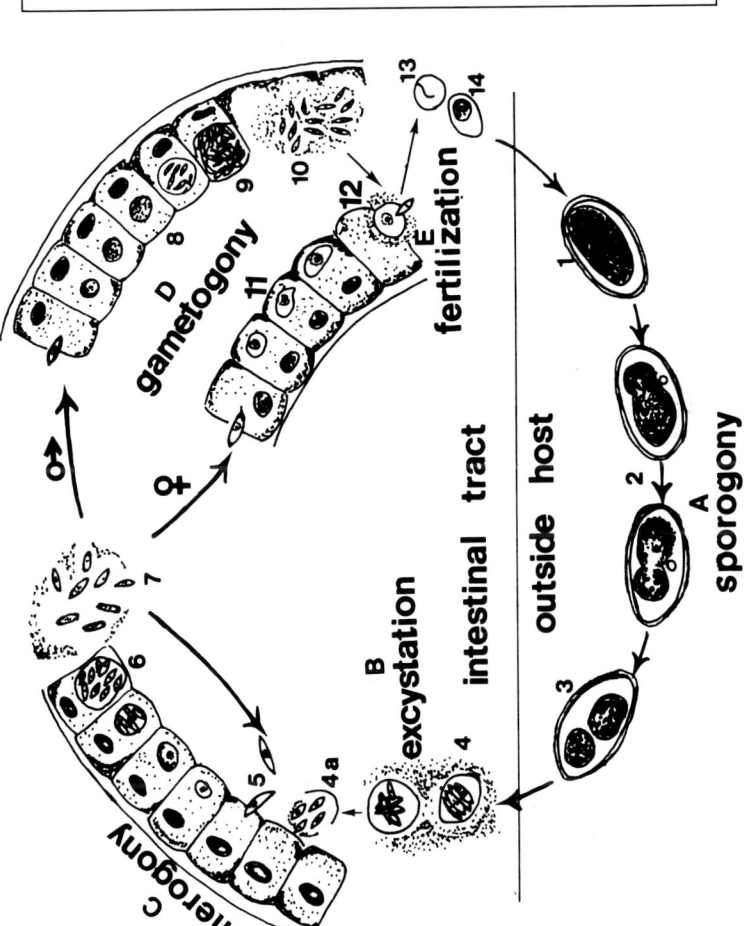

FIGURE 8–4   Life cycle of Isospora belli.

sporidium (Figure 8–2). It has an alternation of sexual and asexual reproductive life cycles that take place in the host cytoplasm, which differs from the extracytoplasmic location in *Cryptosporidium*. The oocyst measures 31 to 33 × 14 to 15 μm and is 10 times larger than *Cryptosporidium*.

Isospora excyst in the presence of trypsin and bile in the stomach, giving rise first to two *sporocysts* each containing four sporozoites. The sporozoites, when liberated, will infect uninfected host cells by rounding up to become the trophozoites and establishing themselves within a parasitophorus vacuole, where they undergo asexual divisions to give rise to merozoites (exact number unknown). These are then liberated and infect other host cells, thus repeating the cycle. This may explain the situation in chronic infection.

At some point, the trophozoites undergo sexual reproduction and differentiate into male (microgamont) or female (macrogamont). The macrogamont matures to become the macrogametocyte, while the microgamont gives rise to microgametes (number unknown). Fertilization takes place between microgamete and macrogamete to give rise to a zygote. Soon a wall is formed around the zygote and becomes the oocyst. All these endogenous stages are visible *in* the cytoplasm of columnar epithelia of the small intestine.

Unlike *Cryptosporidium,* the *Isospora* oocyst is *not infectious* inside the host. When liberated in the environment, the oocyst, in the sporoblast stage, will undergo sporogony to give rise to two sporocysts, each of which gives rise to four banana-shaped sporozoites, representing the infective stage. This may take place in the environment within 48 hours. Also, the number of oocysts detected in the stool is few compared with a positive fecal sample of cryptosporidiosis. Probably many infections are short term and asymptomatic. Patients often only have mild diarrhea and transient passage oocysts. However, more severe forms are known to cause intractable diarrhea in infants and malabsorption syndrome in AIDS patients. Eosinophilia is a frequent finding. Charcot-Leyden crystals are detectable in some specimens. One patient had diarrhea for 20 years, malabsorption and eosinophilia for 7 years, and *I. belli* oocysts in the stool detectable for 10 months.

The determinants of these different clinical patterns are not clear, but more and more severe cases have been reported in AIDS patients. Isosporiasis was found in 15% of a group of AIDS patients in Haiti.[7] These symptoms promptly responded to oral trimethoprim (160 mg) and sulfamethoxazole (80 mg), four times a day for ten days and then twice daily for three weeks. However half the patients relapsed, although they responded to further similar treatment. Success has been reported using this regimen in other patients.[7] At St. Vincent's Hospital, eight AIDS patients with isosporiasis all succumbed to infection, including one with combined cryptosporidiosis and isosporiasis.[6,9,90] Two homosexual men, one immunocompetent, responded to atabrine within one week of therapy, while the other, who had ARC, showed delayed response after one month of therapy.[6]

It is clear that treating the underlying disease, namely, AIDS, will be the most promising approach in curbing both cryptosporidiosis and isosporiasis.

MICROSPORIDIA

Besides *Cryptosporidium* sp. and *I. belli*, the two *Coccidia* commonly associated with AIDS-associated diarrhea, another rare protozoan that has presented itself in various AIDS patients is *Microsporidia*.[10–13,92–95,107] Before the AIDS epidemic, only seven human cases had been reported.[95–101] All cases were diagnosed by biopsied materials from intestine,[96,97,100] cornea,[98,99] and brain.[101] Antibody titer to *Encephalitozoon cuniculi* has been noted in homosexual men in Sweden.[102] Most of the publications of microsporidiosis dealt with animals, especially insects, fish, and rodents. *Microsporidia* is a protozoan classified as follows: phylum, Microspora; class, Microsporea; order, Microsporidia; genus *Nosema, Encephalitozoon, Enterocytozoon, Pleistophora* (see Figure 8–1). The life cycle of *Nosema* is shown in Figure 8–5. The characteristic stage is the spore, which is oval, uninucleated, thick walled, and refractile and measures 2.7 to 3.0 × 1.2 to 1.8 μm. It has a spirally coiled tubular filament and a prominent polar vacuole visible by electron microscopy. There are no mitochondria. It stains positively with Gram, Grocott, and Weil-Weigert stains, and some strains stain with Ziehl-Neelsen stain.[10,95,96,99] When ingested or inhaled, the spore invades the intestinal epithelium by discharging its contents (sporoplasm) into the host cell through its

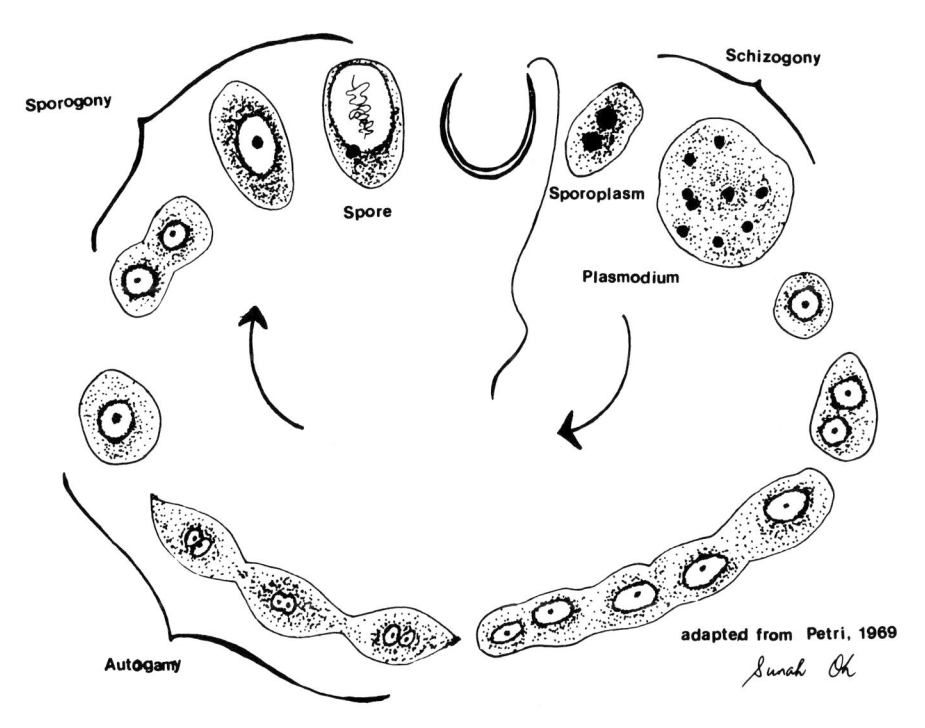

FIGURE 8–5 *Schematic life cycle of microsporidia. Adapted from Petri, 1969.*

extruded tubular filament. Within the cell, the injected sporoplasm divides by binary fission to form uninucleated or multinucleated sporonts, uninucleated sporoblasts with two to six nuclei. They split into unicellular organisms (meronts); these then secrete a rigid capsule. The fully formed spore measures about 2.5 × 1.5 μm. The cell eventually ruptures, and the cycle repeats itself. A sexual phase in which the nuclei of binuclear stages fuse ("autogamy") has been reported.[98] All AIDS-related cases of microsporidiosis were diagnosed by small bowel biopsies,[10,12,92–95] one case of myositis by muscle biopsy,[11] and one case of hepatitis by liver biopsy.[13]

The first case was reported in a 29-year-old Haitian with a five-month history of diarrhea, weight loss, fever, and epigastric pain.[10] He had been living in France for four years. He denied any homosexual practice, drug addiction, or blood transfusion. Hematoxylin-eosin preparation of duodenal biopsy revealed numerous small (1 to 5 μm) round or ovoid basophilic bodies in the enterocytes, mostly in the apical area of the villus. They were located in the supranuclear portion of the cytoplasm.[10] None had been detected in stool specimen. The organism was identified as *Microsporidia,* characterized by multinucleated plasmid and mononucleated sporoblast and a polar filament in electron microscopy. The species was characterized as *Enterocytozoon bieneusi.*[103] The stool examination was reported negative.

The second case was an AIDS patient with unexplained chronic diarrhea. Intestinal biopsy revealed intracellular *Microsporidia* with multiple disk-shaped densities and multiple nuclei enclosed within a single plasma membrane without a cell wall. There were no mitochondria on electron microscopy, but the formalin-fixed paraffin-embedded sections stained with hematoxylin-eosin preparation or with Goodpasture's tissue and gram stain failed to reveal the organism.[92]

Similar failure to demonstrate the organism by light microscopy with hematoxylin-eosin stain was reported in a 45-year-old man with severe weight loss and intractable diarrhea. Jejunal biopsy showed nonspecific villus shortening and leukocyte infiltration. Electron microscopy of enterocytes showed multiple, mature 1 μm *Microsporidia* spores with characteristic coiled polar tubules. Enterocytes with swelling and vesiculation indicating cell damage contained the organism in sporogenic dividing stages. Although infiltration of the epithelium by the organism was extensive, none was detected by light microscopy with hematoxylin-eosin, Giemsa, acid-fast, periodic acid–Schiff (PAS), and Brown-Brenn tissue Gram's stain.[12] In contrast, light microscopy of intestinal biopsies, reported in three cases, demonstrated the organisms as hyaline with pale blue cytoplasm and reddish purple nuclei varying from one to many by Giemsa stain. The extracellular stages ranged from 2 to 9 μm in diameter. The nuclei were highly irregular, appearing as rounded, triangular, or elongated.[93]

The single case of hepatitis reported revealed various endogenous stages and a late sporont containing a singe nucleus and five cross-sections of the coiled polar tube on each side of the posterior region of this parasite. The parasite was enclosed within a parasitophorus vacuole.[13] In the patient with myositis, atrophic and degenerating muscle fibers were infiltrated by spores in clusters of at least

12, each held together by enclosing membranes. Individual spores or groups of two or three spores appeared to be in phagocytic cells. The spores were oval, 2.8 by 3.2 to 3.4 μm, and had a dark center and relatively unstained ends on hematoxylin-eosin preparation. A dot or line was present in the anterior, unstained end. Many spores were brilliantly acid-fast with Ziehl-Neelsen stain but stained variably with Brown-Hopps stain. A PAS-positive granule was seen inside the spores on electron microscopy. Accurate identification of *Microsporidia* depends on electron microscopy[104–106] and was tentatively classified as *Pleistophora* sp.[93] Chapter 12 continues this discussion.

ACKNOWLEDGMENT

We thank Ms. Sunah Oh, premedical student, Cornell Medical College, New York, for her excellent drawings, and Ms. Lisa Feldman, St. Vincent's Hospital and Medical Center, New York, for her photographs.

REFERENCES

1. Ma P. Cryptosporidiosis and immune enteropathy: a review. In: Remington JS, Swartz MN, eds. Current clinical topics in infectious diseases. McGraw-Hill, 1987;8:99–153.
2. Fayer R, Ungar BLP. *Cryptosporidium* spp. and cryptosporidiosis. Microbiol Rev 1986;50:458–483.
3. Tzipori S. Cryptosporidiosis in perspective. Advances in Parasitology 1988;27:63–129.
4. Crawford FG, Vermund SH. Human cryptosporidiosis. CRC Crit Rev Microbiol 1988;16:113.
5. Mata L, Bolanos H, Pezarro D, Vives M. Cryptosporidiosis in children from some highland Costa Rican rural and urban areas. Am J Trop Med Hyg 1984;33:24–29.
6. Ma P, Kaufman D, Montana J. *Isospora belli* diarrheal infection in homosexual men. AIDS Res 1984;1:327–338.
7. DeHovitz JA, Pape JW, Boncy M, Johnson WD. Clinical manifestations and therapy of *Isospora belli* infection in patients with the acquired immunodeficiency syndrome. N Engl J Med 1986;315:87–90.
8. Forthal DN, Guest SS. *Isospora belli* enteritis in three homosexual men. Am J Trop Med Hyg 1984;33:1060–1064.
9. Ma P. *Cryptosporidium* spp. and *Isospora belli*. In: Leoung GS, Mills J, eds. Opportunistic infections in patients with the acquired immunodeficiency syndrome. New York: Marcel Dekker, pp. 355–377.
10. Modigliani R, Bories C, Le Charpentier Y, et al. Diarrhoea and malabsorption in acquired immune deficiency syndrome: A study of four cases with special emphasis on opportunistic protozoan infestations. Gut 1985;26:179–181.
11. Ledford DK, Overman MD, Gonzalvo A, et al. Microsporidiosis myositis in a patient with the acquired immunodeficiency syndrome. Ann Intern Med 1985;102:628–630.

12. Owen RL. Intestinal *Microsporidia* infection in humans: Clinical description and diagnostic approach (abstr. J18). Program of the 87th Annual Meeting of the American Society for Microbiology, Atlanta, March, 1987.
13. Terada S, Rajender R, Jeffers LJ, et al. Microsporidian hepatitis in the acquired immunodeficiency syndrome. Ann Intern Med 1987;107:61–62.
14. Levine MD. Taxonomy and review of the coccidian genus *Cryptosporidium* (Protozoa, Apicomplexa). J Prozool 1984;31:94–98.
15. Tzipori S, Angus KW, Campbell I, Gray EW. Experimental infection of lambs with *Cryptosporidium* isolated from a human patient with diarrhoea. Gut 1982;23:71–74.
16. Moon HW, Woodmansee DB. Cryptosporidiosis. J Am Vet Med Assn 1986;189:643–646.
17. Ma P, Villanueva TG, Kaufman D, Gillooley JF. Respiratory cryptosporidiosis in the acquired immune deficiency syndrome. Use of modified cold Kinyoun and hemacolor stains for rapid diagnoses. JAMA 1984;252:1298–1301.
18. Ma P, Villanueva TG, Kaufman D, Gillooley JF. Cryptosporidiose respiratoire au cours du SIDA. Utilisation de la solution froide modifiée de kinyoun et de l'hemacolor pour un diagnostic rapide. French JAMA 1984;89:848–850.
19. Ma P, Villanueva TG, Kaufman D, Gillooley JF. Respiratory cryptosporidiosis in the acquired immune deficiency syndrome. Japan JAMA 1985;5:33–35.
20. Forgacs P, Tarshis A, Ma P, et al. Intestinal and bronchial cryptosporidiosis in an immunodeficient homosexual man. Ann Intern Med 1983;99:793–794.
21. Brady EM, Margolis ML, Korzeniowski OM. Pulmonary cryptosporidiosis in acquired immune deficiency syndrome. JAMA 1984;252:89–90.
22. Ma P. *Cryptosporidium* and the enteropathy of immune deficiency (editorial). J Pediatr Gastroenterol Nutr 1984;3:488–489.
23. Harari MD, West B, Dwyer B. *Cryptosporidium* as cause of laryngotracheitis in an infant (letter). Lancet 1986;1:1207.
24. Kazlow PG, Shah K, Benkov KJ, et al. Esophageal cryptosporidiosis in a child with acquired immune deficiency syndrome. Gastroenterology 1986;91:1301–1303.
25. Blumberg RS, Kelsey P, Perrone T, et al. Cytomegalovirus- and *Cryptosporidium*-associated acalculous gangrenous cholecystitis. Am J Med 1984;76:1118–1123.
26. Kahn DG, Garfinckle JM, Klonoff DC, et al. Cryptosporidial and cytomegaloviral hepatitis and cholecystitis. Arch Pathol Lab Med 1987;111:879–881.
27. Gross TL, Wheat J, Bartlett M, O'Connor KW. AIDS and multiple system involvement with *Cryptosporidium*. Am J Gastroenterol 1986;81:456–458.
28. Kocoshis SA, Cibull ML, Davis TE, et al. Intestinal and pulmonary cryptosporidiosis in an infant with severe combined immune deficiency. J Pediatr Gastroenterol Nutr 1984;3:149–157.
29. Iseki M. *Cryptosporidium felis sp n* (Protozoa: Eimeriorina) from the domestic cat. Jpn J Parasitol 1979;28:285–307.
30. Vetterling JM, Takeuchi A, Madden PA. Ultrastructure of *Cryptosporidium wrairi* from the guinea pig. J Protozool 1971;18:248–268.
31. Bird RG, Smith MD. Cryptosporidiosis in man: Parasite life cycle and fine structural pathology. J Pathol 1980;132:217–233.
32. Pearson GR, Logan EF. Scanning and transmission electron microscopic observations on the host-parasite relationship in intestinal cryptosporidiosis of neonatal calves. Res Vet Sci 1983;34:149–154.

33. Lefkowitch JH, Krumholz S, Chen KF, et al. Cryptosporidiosis of the human small intestine. A light and electron microscopic study. Hum Pathol 1984;15:746–752.
34. Marcial MA, Madara JL. *Cryptosporidium:* Cellular localization, structural analysis of absorptive cell-parasite membrane, membrane interactions in guinea pigs, and suggestion of protozoan transport by M cells. Gastroenterology 1986;90:583–594.
35. Ma P, Soave R. Three-step stool examination for cryptosporidiosis in 10 homosexual men with protracted watery diarrhea. J Infect Dis 1983;147:824–828.
36. Ma P. Laboratory diagnosis of coccidiosis. In: Leive L, Schlessinger D, eds. Microbiology 1984. Washington, D.C.: American Society for Microbiology, 1984;224–231.
37. Ma P. *Cryptosporidium*—biology and diagnosis. In: Actor P, Evangelista A, Poupard J, Hinks E, eds. Infections in the immunocompromised host. Adv Exper Med Biol 1986;202:135–152.
38. Pohlenz J, Moon HW, Cheville NF, Bemrick WJ. Cryptosporidiosis as a probable factor in neonatal diarrhea of calves. J Am Vet Med Assoc 1978;172:452–457.
39. Garcia LS, Brewer TC, Bruckner DA. Fluorescence detection of *Cryptosporidium* oocysts in human fecal specimens by using monoclonal antibodies. J Clin Microbiol 1987;25:119–121.
40. Lahdevirta J, Jokipii MM, Sammalkorpi K, Jokipii L. Perinatal infection with *Cryptosporidium* and failure to thrive. Lancet 1987;1:48–49.
41. Ma P, Kaufman DL, Helmick CG, et al. Cryptosporidiosis in tourists returning from the Caribbean (letter). N. Engl J Med 1985;312:647–648.
42. Soave R, Ma P. Cryptosporidiosis: Traveler's diarrhea in two families. Arch Intern Med 1985;145:70–72.
43. Jokipii LS, Pohjola S, Jokipii A. Cryptosporidiosis associated with traveling and giardiasis. Gastroenterology 1985;89:838–842.
44. Sterling CR, Seegar K, Sinclair NA. *Cryptosporidium* as a causative agent of traveler's diarrhea. J Infect Dis 1986;153:380–381.
45. Alpert G, Bell LM, Kirkpatrick CE, et al. Outbreak of cryptosporidiosis in a daycare center. Pediatrics 1986;77:152–157.
46. Combee CL, Collinge ML, Britt EM. Cryptosporidiosis in a hospital-associated day care center. Pediatr Infect Dis 1986;5:528–532.
47. D'Antonio RG, Winn RE, Taylor JP, et al. A waterborne outbreak of cryptosporidiosis in normal hosts: I. Ann Intern Med 1985;103:886–888.
48. Casemore DP, Jessop EG, Douce D, Jackson FB. *Cryptosporidium* plus *Campylobacter:* An outbreak in a semi-rural population. J Hyg Camb 1986;96:95–105.
49. Ribeiro CD, Palmer SR. Family outbreak of cryptosporidiosis. Br Med J 1986;292:377.
50. Baxby D, Hart CA, Taylor C. Human cryptosporidiosis: A possible case of hospital cross infection. Br Med J 1983;287:1760–1761.
51. Dryjanski J, Gold JW, Ritchie MT, et al. Cryptosporidiosis. Case report in a health team worker. Am J Med 1986;80:751–752.
52. Wolfson JS, Richter JM, Waldron MA, et al. Cryptosporidiosis in immunocompetent patients. N Engl J Med 1985;312:1278–1282.
53. Stehr-Green JK, McCaig L, Remsen HM, et al. Shedding of oocysts in immunocompetent individuals infected with *Cryptosporidium.* Am J Trop Med Hyg 1987;36:338–342.

54. Jokipii L, Jokipii MM. Timing of symptoms and oocysts excretion in human cryptosporidiosis. N Engl J Med 1986;315:1643–1647.
55. Meisel JL, Perera DR, Meligro BC, Rubin CE. Overwhelming watery diarrhoea associated with a *Cryptosporidium* in an immunosuppressed patient. Gastroenterology 1976;70:1156–1160.
56. Holley HP, Thiers BH. Cryptosporidiosis in a patient receiving immunosuppressive therapy. Possible activation of latent infection. Dig Dis Sci 1986;31:1004–1007.
57. Miller RA, Holmberg RE Jr, Clausen CR. Life-threatening diarrhea caused by *Cryptosporidium* in a child undergoing therapy for acute lymphocytic leukemia. J Pediatr 1983;103:256–259.
58. Weisburger WR, Hutcheon DF, Yardley JH, et al. Cryptosporidiosis in an immunosuppressed renal-transplant recipient with IgA deficiency. Am J Clin Pathol 1979;72:473–478.
59. Collier AC, Miller RD, Joel D, Meyers MD. Cryptosporidiosis after marrow transplantation: person-person transmission and treatment with spiramycin. Ann Intern Med 1984;101:205.
60. Manivel C, Filipovich A, Snover DC. Cryptosporidiosis as a cause of diarrhea following bone marrow transplantation. Dis Colon Rectum 1985;28:741–742.
61. Mead GM, Sweetenham JW, Ewins DL, et al. Intestinal cryptosporidiosis: A complication of cancer treatment. Cancer Treat Rep 1986;70:769–770.
62. Sloper KS, Dourmashkin RR, Bird RB, et al. Chronic malabsorption due to cryptosporidiosis in a child with immunoglobulin deficiency. Gut 1982;23:80–92.
63. Stemmerman GN, Nayashi T, Glober GA, et al. *Cryptosporidiosis:* Report of a fatal case complicated by disseminated toxoplasmosis. Am J Med 1980;69:637–642.
64. Stine KC, Harris JS, Lindsey NJ, Cho CT. Spontaneous remission of cryptosporidiosis in a child with acute lymphocytic leukemia. Clin Pediatr 1985;24:722–724.
65. Pitlik SD, Fainstein V, Garza D, et al. Human cryptosporidiosis: Spectrum of disease. Report of six cases and review of the literature. Arch Intern Med 1983;143:2269–2275.
66. Whiteside ME, Barkin JS, May RG, et al. Enteric coccidiosis among patients with the acquired immunodeficiency syndrome. Am J Trop Med Hyg 1984;33:1065–1072.
67. Ma P, Vermund SH, Cunin JR, et al. Travel to warm climate countries as a risk factor for *Cryptosporidium* in men with AIDS in New York City. The 35th Annual Meeting of the American Society of Tropical Medicine and Hygiene. Poster 148, Denver, Dec. 7–11, 1986.
68. Zar F, Geiseler PJ, Brown VA. Asymptomatic carriage of *Cryptosporidium* in the stool of a patient with acquired immunodeficiency syndrome (letter). J Infect Dis 1985;151:195.
69. Ma P. Cryptosporidiosis: A new AIDS opportunist. Reply to a letter. J Respir Dis 1986;7:10–11.
70. Ongerth JE, Stibbs HH. Identification of *Cryptosporidium* oocysts in river water. Appl Environ Microbiol 1987;53:672–676.
71. Coffin J, Haase A, Levy JA, et al. Human immunodeficiency viruses (letter). Science 1986;232:697.
72. Ma P, Tsaihong J. Immune response of AIDS and non-AIDS individuals to *Cryptosporidium*. Session 72, Abstract 833. In the 27th Interscience Conference on Antimicrobial Agents and Chemotherapy, New York, Oct 6, 1987.

73. Casemore DP. The antibody response to *Cryptosporidium:* Development of a serological test and its use in a study of immunologically normal persons. J Infect 1987;14:125–134.
74. Garza DH, Fedorak RN, Soave R. Enterotoxin-like activity in cultured cryptosporidia: Role in diarrhea (abstr.). Gastroenterology 1986;90:1424.
75. Tzipori S, Angus KW, Gray EW, Campbell I. Vomiting and diarrhea associated with cryptosporidial infection (letter). N Engl J Med 1980;303:818.
76. Current WL, Reese NC, Ernst JV, et al. Human cryptosporidiosis in immunocompetent and immunodeficient persons. N Engl J Med 1983;308:1252–1257.
77. McNabb SJN, Hensel DM, Welch DF, et al. Comparison of sedimentation and flotation techniques for identification of *Cryptosporidium* sp oocysts in a large outbreak of human diarrhea. J Clin Microbiol 1985;22:587–589.
78. Tsaihong J, Ma P. The effect of preservatives and formalin-ether procedure on the properties of *Cryptosporidium* oocysts (submitted for publication).
79. Kim CW. Research brief. *Cryptosporidium* sp.: Experimental infection in Syrian golden hamsters. Exp Parasitol 1987;63:243–246.
80. Tzipori S, Campbell I. Prevalence of *Cryptosporidium* antibodies in 10 animal species. J Clin Microbiol 1981;14:455–456.
81. Ungar BLP, Soave R, Fayer R, Nash TE. Enzyme immunoassay detection of immunoglobulin M and G antibodies to *Cryptosporidium* in immunocompetent and immunocompromised persons. J Infect Dis 1986;153:570–578.
82. Kern P, Toy J, Dietrich M. Preliminary clinical observations with recombinant interleukin-2 patients with AIDS or LAS. Blut 1985;50:1–6.
83. Rolston KV, Fainstein V. Cryptosporidiosis. Eur J Clin Microbiol 1986;5:135–137.
84. Portnoy D, Whiteside ME, Buckley E, Macleod CL. Treatment of intestinal cryptosporidiosis with spiramycin. Ann Intern Med 1984;101:202–204.
85. Tzipori S, Roberton D, Chapman C. Remission of diarrhoea due to cryptosporidiosis in an immunodeficient child treated with hyperimmune bovine colostrum. Br Med J 1986;293:1275–1277.
86. Tzipori S, Roberton D, Cooper DA, White L. Chronic cryptosporidial diarrhea and hyperimmune cow colostrum. Lancet 1987;2:344–355.
87. Kotler DP. Preliminary observations of the effect of cow's milk globulin upon intestinal cryptosporidiosis in AIDS (abstr. THP 148). Third International Conference on AIDS, Washington, D.C., June 1–5, 1987.
88. Sun T. Coccidiosis. In: Sun T, ed. Pathological and clinical features of parasitic disease. New York: Masson, 1982;99.
89. Soave R, Warren J. *Cryptosporidium* and *Isospora belli.* J Inf Dis 1988;157:225–229.
90. Ma P, Kaufman D, Miglietta L, et al. A four-year follow-up of cryptosporidiosis and isosporiasis in AIDS and non-AIDS individuals of the Greater New York area. Poster 547, p 65. International Conference on AIDS, Paris, June 25, 1986.
91. Kitsukawa K, Kamihira S, Kinoshita K, et al. An autopsy case of T-cell lymphoma associated with disseminated varicella and malabsorption syndrome due to *Isospora belli* infection. Rinsho Ketsueki 1981;22:258–265.
92. Dobbins WO, Weinstein WM. Electron microscopy of the intestine and rectum in acquired immunodeficiency syndrome. Gastroenterology 1985;88:738–49.
93. Rijpstra AC, Canning EU, Van Ketel RJ, et al. Use of light microscopy to diagnose small-intestinal microsporidiosis in patients with AIDS. J Infect Dis 1988;157:827.

94. Lucas S, Wamukota S. HIV and the local African population. In: Pounder RE, Chiodini PL, eds. Advanced medicine 23. London: Bailliere Tindall, 1987:102–111.
95. Shadduck JA. Human microsporidia and AIDS (in press.)
96. Strano AJ, Cali A, Neafie RC. Microsporidiosis. In: Binford CH, Connor DH, eds. Pathology of tropical and extraordinary diseases. Washington, D.C.: Armed Forces Institute of Pathology, 1976;336–339.
97. Margileth AM, Strano AJ, Chandra R, et al. Disseminated nosematosis in immunologically compromised infant. Arch Pathol 1973;95:145–150.
98. Ashton N, Wirasinha PA. Encephalitozoonosis (nosematosis) of the cornea. Br J Opthalmol 1973;57:669–674.
99. Pinnolis M, Egbert PR, Font RL, Winter FC. Nosematosis of the cornea. Arch Ophthalmol 1981;99:1044–1047.
100. Matsubayashi H, Koike T, Mikata I, et al. A case of *Encephalitozoon-like* body infection in man. Arch Pathol 1959;67:181–187.
101. Wolf A, Cowen D. Granulomatous encephalomyelitis due to an encephalitozoon (encephalitozoic encephalomyelitis). Bull Neurol Inst NY 1937;6:306–371.
102. Bergquist R, Morfeldt-Mansson L, Pehrson PO, et al. Antibody against *Encephalitozoon cuniculi* in Swedish homosexual men. Scand J Infect Dis 1984;16:389–391.
103. Desportes I, Le Charpentier Y, Galian A, et al. Occurrence of a new microsporidian: *Enterocytozoon bieneusi* n.g. n sp, in the enterocytes of a human patient with AIDS. J Protozool 1985;32:250–254.
104. Cali A. Morphogenesis in the genus *Nosema*. In: Proceedings of the Fourth International Colloquium of Insect Pathology. College Park, M.D.: Society for Invertebrate Pathology, 1971;431–438.
105. Canning EU, Hollister WS. Microsporidia of mammals—widespread pathogens or opportunistic curiosities. Parasitology Today 1987;3:267.
106. Current WL, Owen RL. Cryptosporidiosis and microsporidiosis. In: Farthing MJG, Keusch GT, eds. Enteric infection: mechanisms, manifestations, and management. London: Chapman and Hall, 1988.
107. Nord J, Ma P, Tacket CO, et al. Treatment of AIDS associated cryptosporidiosis with hyperimmune colostrum from cows vaccinated with cryptosporidium. Submitted to V International Conference on AIDS, June 4–9, 1989.

BIBLIOGRAPHY

AIDS Program. Resision of the CDC surveillance case definition for acquired immunodeficiency syndrome, MMWR supplement. Atlanta: Center for Infectious Diseases, Centers for Disease Control, 1987;36:1S.

PART III

Other Sexually Transmitted Diseases

Chapter 9

Hepatitis B Virus Transmission between Homosexual Men: A Model for AIDS

Miriam J. Alter
Donald P. Francis

Until recently, groups recognized as being at high risk of acquiring infection with hepatitis B virus (HBV) were those who were traditionally associated with apparent percutaneous needle exposures, such as blood transfusion recipients (before donor screening for HBV), intravenous drug users, and health care workers. In the last decade, additional observations of other individuals with HBV infection have suggested that other types of exposures, particularly sexual contact with HBV-infected individuals, may play an important role in the transmission of this disease.

In 1971, Hersh et al.[1] reported the transmission of HBV to the female sexual partners of six men with acute or chronic HBV infection. Although the index patients all had a history of percutaneous needle exposure, none of the sexual partners had a history of any exposure other than contact with the infected patient. Subsequent reports on the prevalence of HBV infection among household contacts of hepatitis B surface antigen (HBsAg) carriers revealed that these contacts had a higher prevalence of HBV serologic markers than did household contacts of noncarriers.[2,3] Furthermore, spouses or other sexual partners in these studies had a higher prevalence of HBV infection than did other members of the household[3,4] (Table 9–1).

Additional evidence of HBV transmission between heterosexual persons was gleaned from investigating cases of acute hepatitis B. In a study of patients with acute HBV infection who had no history of percutaneous exposure, 44% were found to have a history of sexual contact with an HBsAg-positive or jaundiced person.[5] In a small outbreak of HBV infections in a nursing home, the only exposure identified for two of the three cases was sexual contact with an HBsAg carrier.[6] Prospective studies on the secondary attack rates for susceptible heter-

Table 9–1 Prevalence of HBV infection among household contacts of HBsAg carriers

Relationship of Contact	Reference	Number of Positive/ Number Tested (%)	
		HBsAg[a]	HBsAg/ Anti-HBs[b]
Spouse or sexual partner	3	2/22 (9.1)	8/22 (36.4)
Others in household		1/32 (3.1)	6/32 (18.8)
Spouse or sexual partner	4	0/17	10/17 (58.8)
Children in household		2/35 (5.7)	6/35 (17.1)

[a]Hepatitis B surface antigen.
[b]Anti-HBs-antibody to HBsAg.

osexual partners of persons with acute hepatitis B found that 20% to 42% became infected[7-9] (Table 9–2).

In addition to heterosexual partners of patients with acute hepatitis B and carriers, homosexual men were also found to be at high risk of acquiring HBV infection. In London, Heathcote et al.[5] found that 45% of men with acute hepatitis B who had no known history of exposure to HBV were either homosexual or bisexual. Others found that among patients attending sexually transmitted disease (STD) clinics, 3.9% of the homosexual men were HBsAg-positive compared with 0.19% of the heterosexual men[10] and that the overall rate of HBV infection was 22% for homosexual men compared with 5% for heterosexual men.[11] In studies in the United States, 4% to 6% of the homosexual men were found to be HBsAg-positive compared with 1% of the heterosexual men attending STD clinics and 0.3% to 0.9% of controls (blood donors or men undergoing preemployment physical examinations).[12-14] The overall prevalence of HBV infection among these three groups ranged from 40% to 60%, 4% to 18%, and 4% to 7%, respectively (Table 9–3). Until recently, in some areas of the country, 21% of the reported cases of acute hepatitis B were in homosexual men,[14a] and prospective studies from the late 1970s reported an annual incidence of HBV among this group of 16% to 28%.[15-17]

How is HBV transmitted through sexual contact? The HBsAg has been detected in saliva,[18,19] semen,[18] and vaginal secretions[20]; however, the transmission

Table 9–2 Incidence of HBV infection for susceptible heterosexual partners of patients with hepatitis B

Reference	Follow-up Period (mo.)	Number Infected/ Number Followed (%)
7	12	3/13 (23.1)
8	3–12	2/10 (20.0)
9	5	14/33 (42.4)

Table 9–3 Prevalence of HBV infection among groups of males with different sexual behaviors

		Percent Positive	
Group	Reference	HBsAg	HBsAg/Anti-HBs
Homosexual STD clinic men	10	3.9	ND[a]
Heterosexual STD clinic men		0.19	ND
Blood donors		0.1	ND
Homosexual STD clinic men	11	3.25	21.75
Heterosexual STD clinic men		2.6	5.1
Blood donors		0.2	0.6
Homosexual men	12	4.3	48.1
Heterosexual STD clinic men		1.3	17.9
Blood donors		0.3	7.3
Homosexual men	13	5.6	39.6
Heterosexual STD clinic men		0.9	4.5
Controls (routine physical examination)		0.9	4.5
Homosexual STD clinic men	14	6.1	61.5[b]

[a]Not done.
[b]Includes testing for antibody to hepatitis B core antigen.

of HBV involving these body fluids appears to occur because they contain blood or serum and only when percutaneous exposure or trauma to mucosal surfaces is involved. In experimental settings, Bancroft et al.[21] were able to infect gibbons with whole mouth saliva positive for HBsAg injected subcutaneously but not when administered orally. The saliva was positive for occult blood. Similarly, Scott et al.[22] were also able to infect gibbons with saliva administered through the subcutaneous route but did not produce infection with saliva administered orally. In addition, these investigators were able to demonstrate transmission of HBV infection to gibbons with HBsAg-positive semen introduced by both the subcutaneous and the intravaginal route. Both saliva and semen preparations were positive for occult blood and were donated by an HBsAg carrier who was also hepatitis B e antigen (HBeAg) positive. HBeAg has been shown to be associated with increased DNA polymerase activity and the presence of whole virus particles, indicators of more active ongoing HBV replication and, therefore, increased infectivity.[23,24]

Both experimental and epidemiologic observations suggest that effective transmission involving body fluids such as saliva and semen occurs only when they contain blood or serum. HBV does not originate from the salivary gland but is expressed in serum-derived intracravicular fluid.[21] In natural settings, no infection could be demonstrated in susceptible persons directly exposed to HBsAg-positive saliva although the infected individual's serum was HBeAg-positive.[25]

In parts of the world where hepatitis B infection during infancy and childhood is uncommon, sexual transmission is an important mechanism in the spread of this disease.[26] In the United States, historically, homosexual men have had a higher prevalence of HBV infection than any other single group. Szmuness et al.[12] investigated the types of sexual behavior associated with their acquiring HBV infection. Compared with heterosexual men attending an STD clinic, homosexual men were more likely to have had 10 or more sexual partners in the previous 6 months (mean 20; range up to 60) and were more likely to engage in anal intercourse. Among the homosexual men, factors found to be related to prevalence of HBV infection included history of multiple episodes of venereal disease, large numbers of sexual partners, long duration of homosexual activity, and engaging in anal intercourse. The history of multiple episodes of venereal disease and the long duration of homosexuality may actually reflect large numbers of sexual partners and be only indirectly related to the acquisition of HBV. Other investigators have found that homosexual men who frequent gay bathhouses and bars and who attend STD clinics (and therefore are presumably more promiscuous) have higher rates of HBV infection than homosexual men who do not.[13,17] Schreeder et al.[14] found the same associations described above but further defined the risk of acquiring HBV infection as being related to the frequency of passive anal-genital intercourse, active oral-anal intercourse, and rectal douching (Table 9–4). Importantly, this study found no association of HBV infection with kissing or oral-genital intercourse. In addition, these investigators noted that 65% of the HBsAg-positive carriers were HBeAg-positive.[14,27] In studies of transmission between heterosexual partners, HBsAg carriers who were HBeAg-positive were significantly more likely to transmit infection than carriers who were HBeAg-negative.[28,29]

In light of these specific sexual activities being identified as related to acquiring HBV infection and in light of other investigators noting that homosexual

Table 9–4 Factors most highly correlated with hepatitis B virus infection among homosexual men[a]

Factor	Relative Risk	P Value
Long duration of regular homosexual activity	19.912	<0.0001
Interaction of number of nonsteady male partners and frequency of passive anal-genital intercourse with nonsteady male partners	5.590	<0.0001
Duration of all homosexual activity	3.986	0.0022
Rectal douching before or after sexual activity	3.243	<0.0001
Interaction of frequency of active anal-genital intercourse and active oral-anal intercourse	2.448	<0.0001
Frequency of passive anal-genital intercourse with nonsteady partners	2.282	0.0069

[a]Source: Schreeder et al.[14]

men have a high frequency of genital sores and lesions,[10,12] Seeff et al.[33] conducted a study of HBV-infected homosexual men to identify the specific mechanisms of HBV transmission between homosexual men. Thirteen (59%) of the 22 HBsAg-positive homosexual men in this study had rectal mucosal lesions. Twelve of these lesions consisted of multiple punctate bleeding points within 6 cm of the anal verge. HBsAg was recovered (in decreasing order of frequency) from gingiva, rectal lesions, feces, normal rectal mucosa, and anal sphincter. The frequency with which HBsAg was recovered by site generally paralleled the frequency of site-specific contamination with blood. Furthermore, specimens taken from sites adjacent to visible mucosal lesions were likely to be HBsAg-positive, suggesting that normal rectal mucosa adjacent to a rectal lesion could serve as a source of HBV transmission as a result of the lesion's weeping blood or serous exudate. In addition, this study found that individuals with HBsAg serum endpoint titers of $\geq 10^5$ were more likely to have HBsAg recovered from rectal lesions or mucosa, and 77% of the men in this study were HBeAg-positive. The authors concluded that exposure to infectious virus in the presence of urethral or rectal mucosal defects would result in transmission of HBV.

Transmission to and from open mucous membrane lesions appears to be the most likely mechanism of spread for HBV between homosexual men. The excesss prevalence of infection in this group is a result of a combination of factors including an HBsAg positivity rate 40 to 60 times higher than that of the general population; a high proportion of HBsAg-positive individuals being HBeAg-positive; a high frequency of nonsteady sexual partners that may range as high as 1000 lifetime partners, resulting in a high probability of contact with an HBsAg, HBeAg carrier; and participation in sexual activities that efficiently transmit HBV.

The similarities between the epidemiologic patterns of HBV and the human immunodeficiency virus (HIV) are striking. Qualitatively, the groups at risk of the two infections are very similar (Table 9–5). Individuals whose behavior involves multiple sexual partners or sharing of injection paraphernalia are at marked increased risk for infection by both viruses. As a result, the occurrence of both diseases is heavily weighted toward homosexual men and intravenous drug users. Homosexual men are more heavily represented in AIDS than in hepatitis B,

Table 9–5 Percent of all patients with hepatitis B and AIDS belonging to specific patient groups, 1985

Group	% Hepatitis B	% AIDS
Homosexual men	24	78
IV drug users	14	15
Heterosexual contact	14	1
Health care worker	4	0
Household contact (nonsexual)	2	0
Miscellaneous	2	2
Unknown	40	7

Source: Centers for Disease Control.

because AIDS has not reached an epidemiologic steady state in the United States. Its introduction, or at least its major amplification in the United States, has been in the homosexual community and, because the entire epidemic is a relatively recent occurrence, the continuing prominence of AIDS in the homosexual community is not surprising. Whether, given time, it will broaden epidemiologically, more like hepatitis B, is a major question.

The virologic reasons that explain the epidemiologic similarity, and dissimilarity, between hepatitis B and AIDS are becoming quite clear. Both viruses are blood borne. HBV is found primarily free in the plasma but may also replicate in lymphocytes.[31] AIDS virus is lymphocytotropic but is also found free in plasma. Thus, the blood-borne transmission of the two viruses (either through sharing of needles and syringes for illicit drug use or through the therapeutic use of blood or blood product transfusions) is not surprising. Of epidemiologic interest is the difference in titers found in blood. HBV is found in extremely high titers in blood,[24] whereas AIDS virus appears to replicate in lower concentrations.[32] The resulting transmission by small quantities of blood appears to be appreciably affected by this difference, at least in the needle-stick setting. In one large study, over one-third of hospital staff exposed percutaneously (including some direct mucous membrane exposure) to HBsAg-positive patients were infected with HBV.[33] In contrast, infection rates below 1% appear to be the case for hospital personnel exposed in a similar manner to the AIDS virus.[34]

Both viruses are effectively transmitted by sexual contact. The experimental and epidemiologic data for HBV have been presented above. For AIDS virus, which has been isolated from semen,[35,36] several epidemiologic studies among homosexual men have associated receptive anal intercourse as a risk factor for infection.[37-39] Like HBV, the AIDS virus has spread very effectively among homosexual men. In a cohort of homosexual men from San Francisco, the prevalence of AIDS virus infection has risen from 3% in 1978 to over 70% in 1985.[40,41] Experimental studies have shown that cell-free virus will infect chimpanzees when given intravaginally or intravenously but not orally.[32,32a] The overall rates of transmission from infected men or women to their sexual partners may be quite similar for HBV and the AIDS virus[7,9,42-45a] (Table 9–6).

Table 9–6 Comparative prevalence of infection in sexual contacts of hepatitis B virus and AIDS virus-infected people

Direction of Transmission	Number/Total (%) Positive Serologic Markers			
	HBV	Reference	AIDS Virus	Reference
Male to female	3/13 (23)	7	2/21 (10)	42
	22/34 (65)	9	7/17 (41)	43
			13/22 (59)	44
Female to male	30/68 (44)	45	2/ 6 (33)	44
	4/10 (40)	9	3/19 (16)	45a

Despite the similarities between HBV and the AIDS virus, there is a major virologic difference between these two agents that could have a profound epidemiologic effect. The difference is the proportion of infected individuals who become persistent carriers and, thus, form the reservoir of infection for others. For HBV it is well accepted that approximately 10% of infected adults will develop persistent, often lifelong, infection. For the AIDS virus the proportion is much higher—probably over two-thirds.[46] This high rate of persistently infectious individuals has made and will continue to make interruption of transmission of the AIDS virus difficult. A case in point has been the homosexual male community, where concern about AIDS has resulted in a considerable decrease in the number of sexual partners, yet until recently the concomitant increase in the number of infectious people left the risk of exposure essentially unchanged. In contrast, such modification of behavior resulted in a significant decrease in the incidence of hepatitis B in this group beginning in 1986.[14a]

REFERENCES

1. Hersh T, Melnick JL, Goyal RK, Hollinger FB. Nonparenteral transmission of viral hepatitis type B (Australia antigen-associated serum hepatitis). N Engl J Med 1971;285:1363–1364.
2. Szmuness W, Prince AM, Hirsch RL, Brotman B. Familial clustering of hepatitis B infection. N Eng J Med 1973;289:1162–1166.
3. Heathcote J, Gateau PH, Sherlock S. Role of hepatitis-B antigen carriers in nonparenteral transmission of the hepatitis-B virus. Lancet 1974;2:370–372.
4. Irwin GR, Allen AM, Bancroft WH, et al. Hepatitis B antigen and antibody. Occurrence in families of asymptomatic HBAg carriers. JAMA 1974;227:1012–1013.
5. Heathcote J, Sherlock S. Spread of acute type B hepatitis in London. Lancet 1973;1:1468–1473.
6. Wright RA. Hepatitis B and the HBsAg carrier. An outbreak related to sexual contact. JAMA 1975;232:717–721.
7. Koff RS, Slavin MM, Connelly LJD, Rosen DR. Contagiousness of acute hepatitis B. Secondary attack rates in household contacts. Gastroenterology 1977;72:297–300.
8. Peters CJ, Purcell RH, Lander JJ, Johnson KM. Radioimmunoassay for antibody to hepatitis B surface antigen shows transmission of hepatitis B virus among household contacts. J Infect Dis 1976;134:218–223.
9. Redeker AG, Mosley JW, Gocke DJ, et al. Hepatitis B immune globulin as a prophylactic measure for spouses exposed to acute type B hepatitis. N Engl J Med 1975;193:1055–1059.
10. Jeffries DJ, James WH, Jefferies FJG, et al. Australia (hepatitis-associated) antigen in patients attending a venereal disease clinic. Br Med J 1973;2:455–456.
11. Fulford KWM, Dane DS. Australia antigen and antibody among patients attending a clinic for sexually transmitted diseases. Lancet 1973;1:1470–1473.
12. Szmuness W, Much MI, Prince AM, et al. On the role of sexual behavior in the spread of hepatitis B infection. Ann Intern Med 1975;83:489–495.
13. Dietzman DE, Harnisch JP, Ray CG, et al. Hepatitis B surface antigen (HBsAg) and

antibody to HBsAg. Prevalence in homosexual and heterosexual men. JAMA 1977;238:2625–2626.
14. Schreeder MT, Thompson SE, Hadler SC, et al. Hepatitis B in homosexual men: prevalence of infection and factors related to transmission. J Infect Dis 1982;146:7–15.
14a. Centers for Disease Control. Changing patterns of groups at high risk for hepatitis B in the United States. MMWR 1988;37:429–432, 437.
15. Szmuness W, Stevens CE, Harley EJ, et al. Hepatitis B vaccine. Demonstration of efficacy in a controlled clinical trial in a high-risk population in the United States. N Engl J Med 1980;303:833–841.
16. Francis DP, Hadler SC, Thompson SE, et al. The prevention of hepatitis B with vaccine. Report of the Centers for Disease Control multi-center efficacy trial among homosexual men. Ann Intern Med 1982;97:362–366.
17. Coutinho RA, Schut BJT, Albrecht–Van Lent N, et al. Hepatitis B among homosexual men in the Netherlands. Sex Transm Dis 1981;8:333–335.
18. Heathcote J, Cameron CH, Dane DS. Hepatitis B antigen in saliva and semen. Lancet 1974;1:71–73.
19. Villarejos M, Visona KA, Gutierrez A, et al. Role of saliva, urine and feces in the transmission of type B hepatitis. N Engl J Med 1974;291:1375–1378.
20. Darani M, Gerber M. Hepatitis B antigen in vaginal secretions. Lancet 1974;2:1008.
21. Bancroft WH, Snitbhan R, Scott RM, et al. Transmission of hepatitis B virus to gibbons by exposure to human saliva containing hepatitis B surface antigen. J Infect Dis 1977;135:79–85.
22. Scott RM, Snitbhan R, Bancroft WH, et al. Experimental transmission of hepatitis B virus by semen and saliva. J Infect Dis 1980;142:67–71.
23. Hindman SH, Gravelle CR, Murphy BL, et al. "e" antigen, dane particles, and serum DNA polymerase activity in HBsAg carriers. Ann Intern Med 1976;85:458–460.
24. Shikata T, Karasawa T, Abe K, et al. Hepatitis B e antigen and infectivity of hepatitis B virus. J Infect Dis 1977;136:571–576.
25. Osterholm MT, Bravo ER, Crosson JT, et al. Lack of transmission of hepatitis B to humans after oral exposure to hepatitis B surface antigen-positive saliva. Morbid Mortal Weekly Rep 1978;27:247–248.
26. Grady GF. Strategies for prevention of hepatitis B as a sexually transmitted disease. Sex Transm Dis 1981;8:344–348.
27. Murphy BL, Schreeder MT, Maynard JE, et al. Serological testing for hepatitis B in male homosexuals: special emphasis on hepatitis B e antigen and antibody by radioimmunoassay. J Clin Microbiol 1980;11:301–303.
28. Perrillo RP, Gelb L, Campbell C, et al. Hepatitis B e antigen, DNA polymerase activity, and infection of household contacts with hepatitis B virus. Gastroenterology 1979;76:1319–1325.
29. Bernier RH, Sampliner R, Gerety R, et al. Hepatitis B infection in households of chronic carriers of hepatitis B surface antigen: Factors associated with prevalence of infection. Am J Epidemiol 1982;116:199–211.
30. Reiner NE, Judson FN, Bond WW, et al. Asymptomatic rectal mucosal lesions and hepatitis B surface antigen at sites of sexual contact in homosexual men with persistent hepatitis B virus infection. Ann Intern Med 1982;96:170–173.
31. Romet-Lemonne J-L, McLane MF, Elfassi E, et al. Hepatitis B virus infection in cultured human lymphoblastoid cells. Science 1983;221:667–669.
32. Fultz PN, McClure HM, Swenson RB, et al. Persistent infection of chimpanzees with

human T lymphotrophic virus type III/lymphadenopathy-associated virus: A potential model for acquired immunodeficiency syndrome. J Virology 1986;58:116–124.
32a. Fultz PN, McClure HM, Daugharty H, et al. Vaginal transmission of human immunodeficiency virus (HIV) to a chimpanzee. J Infect Dis 1986;154:896–900.
33. Seeff LB, Wright EC, Zimmerman HG, et al. Type B hepatitis after needle-stick exposure: Prevention with hepatitis B immune globulin. Final report of the Veterans Administration Cooperative Study. Ann Intern Med 1978;88:285–293.
34. Hirsch MS, Wormser GP, Schooley RJ. Risk of nosocomial infection with human T-cell lymphotropic virus III (HTLV-III). N Engl J Med 1985;312:1–4.
35. Ho DD, Schooley RT, Rota TR, et al. HTLV-III in the semen and blood of a healthy homosexual man. Science 1984;226:451–3.
36. Zagury D, Bernard J, Leibowitch J, et al. HTLV-III in the cells cultured from semen of two patients with AIDS. Science 1984;226:449–51.
37. Jaffe HW, Choi K, Thomas PA, et al. National case-control study of Kaposi's sarcoma and *Pneumocystis carinii* pneumonia in homosexual men: I. Epidemiologic results. Ann Intern Med 1983;99:145–51.
38. Goedert JJ, Sarngadharan MG, Biggar RJ, et al. Determinants of retrovirus (HTLV-III) antibody and immunodeficiency conditions in homosexual men. Lancet 1984;2:711–16.
39. Marmor M, Friedman-Kien AE, Laubenstein L, et al. Risk factors for Kaposi's sarcoma in homosexual men. Lancet 1982;1:1083–1087.
40. Jaffe HW, Darrow WW, Echenberg DF, et al. The acquired immunodeficiency syndrome in a cohort of homosexual men. A six year follow-up study. Ann Intern Med 1985;103:210–214.
41. Centers for Disease Control. Update: Acquired immunodeficiency syndrome in the San Francisco cohort study, 1978–1985. Morbid Mortal Weekly Rep 1985;34:573–575.
42. Kreiss JK, Kitchen LW, Prince HE, et al. Antibody to human T-lymphotropic virus type III in wives of hemophiliacs. Evidence of heterosexual transmission. Ann Intern Med 1985;102:623–626.
43. Redfield RR, Markham PD, Salahuddin SZ, et al. Frequent transmission of HTLV-III among spouses of patients with AIDS-related complex and AIDS. JAMA 1985;253:1571–1573.
44. Luzi G, Engoli B, Turbessi G, et al. Transmission of HTLV-III infection by heterosexual contact. Lancet 1985;2:1018.
45. Inaba N, Ohkawa R, Matsuura A, et al. Sexual transmission of hepatitis B surface antigen. Infection of husbands by HBsAg carrier state-wives. Br J Ven Dis 1979;55:366–368.
45a. Padian NS. Heterosexual transmission of acquired immunodeficiency syndrome: international perspectives and national projections. Rev Infect Dis 1987;9:947–960.
46. Francis DP, Jaffe HW, Fultz PN, et al. The natural history of LAV/HTLV-III infection. Ann Intern Med 1985;103:704–709.

Chapter 10

Herpes Simplex Virus Infections in Homosexual Men

Carlos Lopez

During the past 30 years, genital herpes simplex virus (HSV) infection has emerged as a major public health problem. These infections are associated with significant morbidity in otherwise healthy individuals and are especially severe in patients with primary or secondary cell-mediated immunodeficiency disorders. Major advances have been achieved in our understanding of the molecular biology of HSV types 1 and 2 and the natural history, epidemiology, and immunobiology of these infections.

THE VIRUSES

Morphologically, herpes simplex virions (Figures 10-1 and 10-2) are composed of an electron-dense core, an icosahedral capsid with 162 capsomers that encloses the core, an amorphous tegument surrounding the capsid, and an enveloping membrane that has an outer surface covered with small spikes.[1] The core contains the linear, double-stranded DNA that encodes the genetic information of the virus.[2] When susceptible cells in culture are infected with HSV, 50 or more virus-specified polypeptides are made.[3] Host cell macromolecular synthesis is turned off, and a well-controlled cascade of viral proteins ensues.[4] The first set of viral polypeptides (termed alpha gene products) regulates production of the second set (termed beta gene products). The alpha proteins wrest control of the infected cell, while the beta proteins are required for viral DNA synthesis. The last set of viral proteins, called gamma gene products, is regulated by beta gene products and make up the structural components of the virus particles.

The genomes of HSVs have a molecular weight of approximately 100 million[5] and are found as four equimolar populations differing from each other in the orientation of unique-long and unique-short DNA segments, which invert rela-

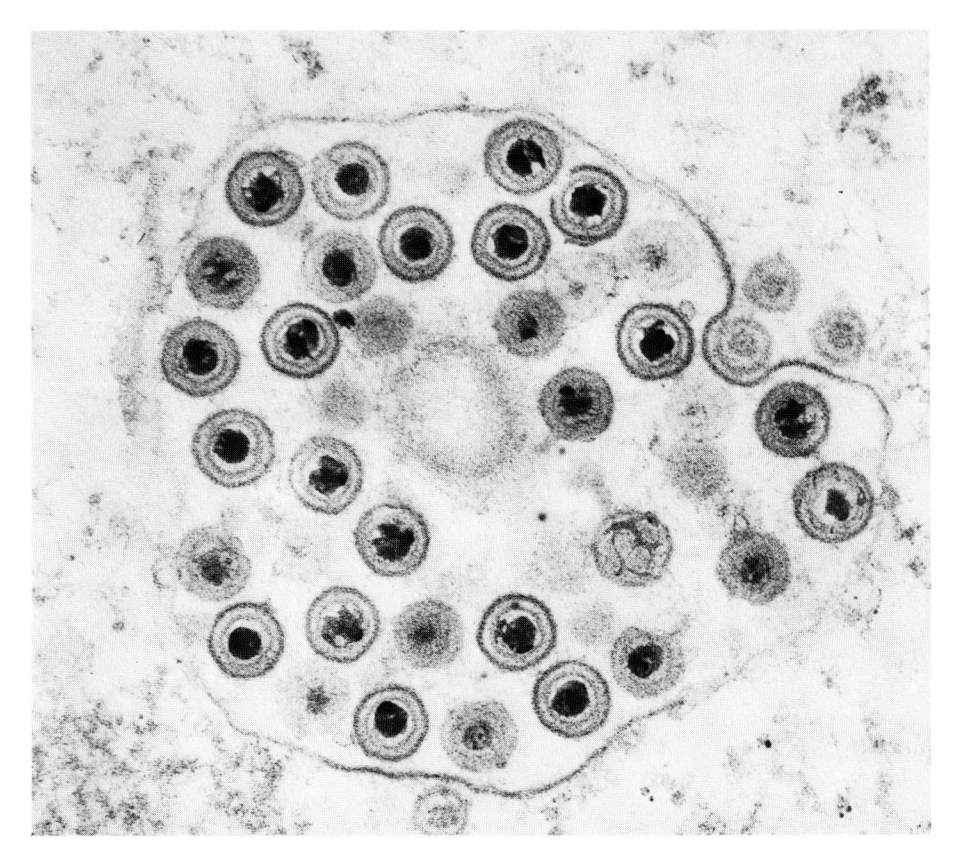

FIGURE 10–1 *Electronphotomicrograph of HSV-1-infected MA 104 cells. Vacuole containing mature virions with electron-dense cores. Black line represents 100 nM. (Courtesy Dr. Erskin Palmer.)*

tive to each other.[4] These inversions appear to result from the mechanism by which viral DNA is synthesized in infected cells.[4] All four isomeric arrangements appear to be biologically active, and, in fact, inversion between the short and long components is not necessary for virus viability in cell culture.[6]

Nahmias and Dowdle[7] first reported that two major types of HSV could be identified by neutralization tests. Further studies showed that most genital infections were caused by HSV type 2 (HSV-2), while most oral-labial infections were caused by HSV type 1 (HSV-1).[8] More recent studies have shown that HSV-1 and HSV-2 are closely related viruses whose DNA is colinear; they share about 50% of their sequences with good matching of base pairs but with differing locations for many restriction enzyme cleavage sites.[4] The latter have been used to distinguish HSV-1 and HSV-2 isolates; however, even within these two types, sufficient differences among restriction enzyme cleavage sites exist to differen-

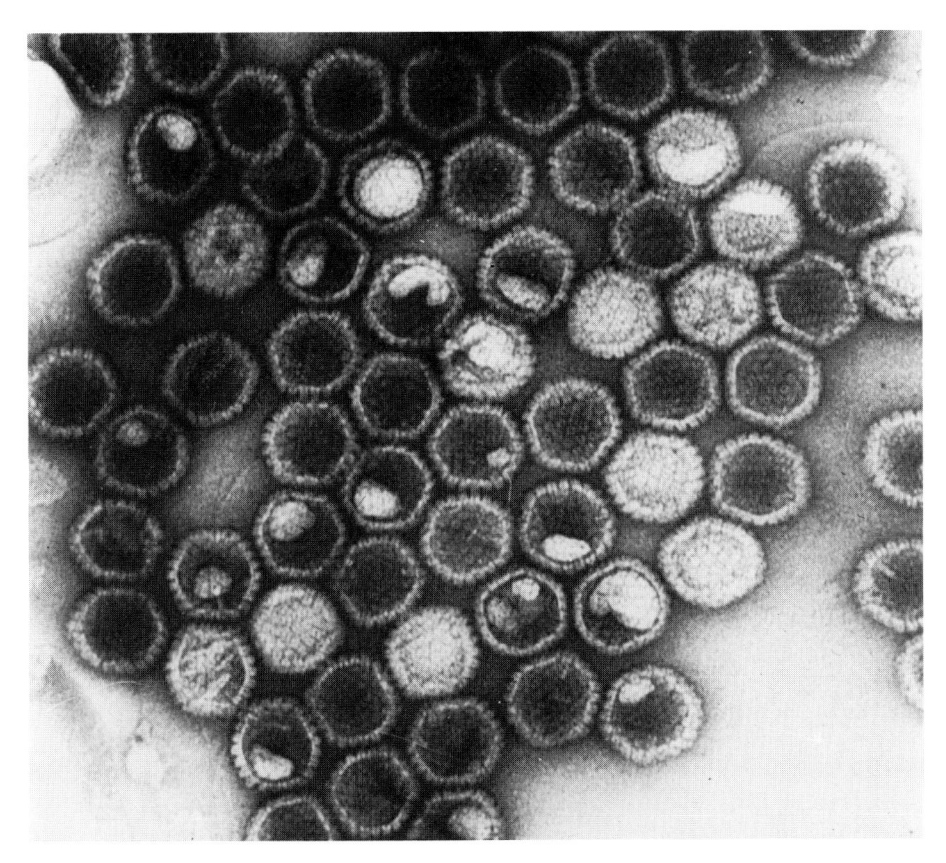

FIGURE 10–2 *Electronphotomicrograph of negatively stained preparation of purified HSV-1 nucleocapsides. Black line represents 100 nM. (Courtesy Dr. Erskin Palmer.)*

tiate as many as 10^{23} subtypes.[9] Since these viruses do not change readily on passage from one individual to the next, these small differences in cleavage patterns have been used to trace the spread of infection epidemiologically.

Selective antiviral chemotherapy is based on developing drugs that are preferentially used by enzymes encoded for by the virus rather than by the comparable cellular enzymes.[10] For example, acyclovir is a potent and selective drug used against HSV because the pyrimidine nucleotide kinase specified by the virus can activate (phosphorylate) the drug more efficiently than can the cellular enzyme. Furthermore, the activated (triphosphated) acyclovir interacts much better with viral DNA polymerase than with any of the cellular DNA polymerases. These preferential interactions lead to the drug's inhibiting the replication of the virus while having little or no effect on uninfected cells that lack these viral enzymes.

EPIDEMIOLOGY

The prevalence of genital herpes infection depends on the patient populations studied and the tests used to study them. HSV has been isolated from women much more frequently than from men attending sexually transmitted disease (STD) clinics.[11] Furthermore, clinically diagnosed genital herpes infection is more prevalent in white than nonwhite populations.[11]

In many populations throughout the United States and the world, the incidence of genital HSV infections has been increasing. The rate of increase has ranged from about 8%[11] to 100%[12] per year. However, this rate has not increased in some populations, notably those with an already high incidence.[13]

Because of the great antigenic cross-reactivity between HSV-1 and HSV-2, routine serologic tests have not always been able to distinguish past exposure to HSV-2 from past exposure to HSV-1 or to both viruses. Sufficient type specificity has been detected, however, to estimate past experience with each virus.[11] Antibodies to HSV-2 are usually not found in sera until puberty, and prevalence of specific antibody depends on sexual activity.[14] Also, in one study adults of lower socioeconomic status had a higher incidence of anti-HSV-2 antibodies than did those of higher status.[15]

PATHOGENESIS

Genital herpes infections are usually acquired during sexual intercourse. Although some genital infections are caused by HSV-1, most (>85%) are caused by HSV-2.[8] Most HSV-2 infections are subclinical, and transmission from asymptomatic partners is common. Even so, a 1985 study indicates that the risk of transmitting HSV is much higher when the source contact has lesions.[11] Women have also been shown to be at higher risk of acquiring infection than men, and the risk was three times higher for seronegative persons than for those with preexisting antibody to HSV.[11]

The severity of clinical disease and the recurrence rate are determined by host factors and virus type (Tables 10–1 and 10–2). When genital HSV-2 infections occur in persons without antibody to HSV-1 or HSV-2, infections are often associated with systemic symptoms and prolonged duration of viral shedding and lesions.[8,11] Prior exposure to HSV-1, however, results in a milder infection with HSV-2. Infection without preexisting antibody to HSV-1 or HSV-2 results in a true primary infection, while infection in the face of antibody to HSV-1 results in a first episode of disease (Table 10–1). Genital HSV-1 infections are generally milder than HSV-2 infections and are less often associated with recurrent disease. Another host factor affecting genital infections is patient gender: A higher percentage of females experience constitutional symptoms than do males, and the symptoms last longer in females than in males.[11]

After primary or first-episode genital infection, whether symptomatic or asymptomatic, HSV-2 almost invariably establishes a latent infection in the sac-

Table 10–1 Clinical HSV-2 infections

Type of Infection	Clinical Disease	Prior Antibody to HSV
Primary infection	Usually symptomatic Local and systemic Worse in women Many patients have CNS[a] and other complications	None
First episode	Often symptomatic Usually local only Shorter lasting disease Fewer complications	HSV-1 or HSV-2
Recurrent	Mild, often symptomatic Local disease Shorter duration of disease Prodromal symptoms More severe in women Few complications	HSV-2

[a]CNS, central nervous system

ral ganglia.[16] By mechanisms that are still poorly understood, latent infections can be reactivated later and lead to asymptomatic shedding of virus or symptomatic clinical disease. Little is known about what triggers reactivation of a latent infection or the immune mechanisms required for sequestering the recurrent disease. Clinical lesions and symptoms, when they occur, are much milder than those associated with primary infection (see Tables 10–1 and 10–2).[8]

CLINICAL DISEASE

HSV has been demonstrated to be a major cause of proctitis in homosexual men (Table 10–3). The virus has been isolated from 15/52 (29%) of those with nongonococcal proctitis, 23/102 (23%) of those with proctitis, and 5/77 (6%) of

Table 10–2 Clinical symptoms and signs of genital herpes infection[11]

Clinical Symptoms	Type of Infection (Duration, in days)		
	Primary	First Episode	Recurrent
Pain	9 to 12	6 to 9	3 to 6
Viral shedding	9 to 12	6 to 9	3 to 6
Time to healing	18 to 21	15 to 18	9 to 12

Table 10-3 Incidence of HSV proctitis

15/52 (29%) HSV isolated from homosexual men with nongonococcal proctitis[17]
23/102 (23%) HSV isolated from homosexual men with proctitis[22]
5/77 (6%) HSV isolated from homosexual men with clinical proctitis of unknown cause[19]

those with clinical proctitis of unknown cause.[17-23] Both HSV-1 and HSV-2 have been isolated from rectal mucosa and rectal biopsies in men with symptoms of rectal pain and discharge.[21,23] Clinical findings that characterized HSV proctitis (Table 10-4), rather than proctitis caused by other organisms, included severe pain, fever, systemic symptoms, constipation, and evidence of sacral neuritis.[22] Acute HSV proctitis usually lasts two to three weeks and is treated only symptomatically. Sigmoidoscopic examination reveals mucosal friability that is common to all forms of infectious proctitis. Vesicular or pustular rectal lesions and diffuse ulceration of the distal rectum were associated with HSV proctitis.[22]

Symptomatic HSV proctitis usually occurs as a first episode of rectal HSV-2 infection.[23] Thus, the acute-phase sera from most patients are found to contain no antibodies to HSV-1 or HSV-2 or antibodies only to HSV-1. However, asymptomatic rectal shedding of HSV has also been documented in a seronegative individual, indicating that not all first-episode HSV infections of the rectum cause painful disease.

As noted in other chapters of this book, acquired immunodeficiency syndrome (AIDS) is caused by a lentivirus called lymphadenopathy-associated virus/human T-lymphotropic virus type III (LAV/HTLV-III, now called human immunodeficiency virus [HIV]). Over a period of years, the virus induces a profound deficiency of host defense that allows certain malignancies and opportunistic

Table 10-4 Signs and symptoms of HSV proctitis in homosexual men[22]

Infection	Asymptomatic (%)
Primary	50
First episode or recurrent	80
Symptoms	Positive (%)
Pain	100
Tenesmus	100
Constipation	78
Perianal ulcers	70
Inguinal lymphadenopathy	57
Fever	48
Difficulty urinating	48
Sacral paresthesias	26

infections to flourish.[24] Clinically, patients are characterized as being (1) asymptomatic, (2) slightly symptomatic but with few symptoms of AIDS, (3) with Kaposi's sarcoma but without opportunistic infections, or (4) with opportunistic infections. Prevalence of antibody to HSV among homosexuals is high; about 90% have antibody when first studied, and the calculated incidence of seroconversion to HSV-2 positivity is 0.05 per person-month.[23,25] Isolation of HSV is much higher among patients with AIDS and opportunistic infections than those with Kaposi's sarcoma but without opportunistic infections or patients with lymphadenopathy only.[25] Since patients with AIDS and opportunistic infections are significantly more immunosuppressed than either patients with Kaposi's sarcoma alone or those with lymphadenopathy, isolation of HSV documents the host's inability to deal with a reactivated infection.

Four percent of newly diagnosed AIDS patients have as their presenting sign chronic HSV infection.[24-27] In AIDS patients, as in certain other patients with deficiencies of cell-mediated immunity, HSV infections present as painful, indolent, and gradually enlarging shallow ulcers in the perineum and intergluteal regions or around the mouth and nose.[24] These lesions are often associated with hematochezia, fever, and a wasting syndrome. Most of these patients have a history suggesting that these chronic HSV infections represent recurrent disease rather than first-episode or primary infections. Chronic HSV infections may lead to visceral infections and may provide portals of entry for other microorganisms.

Acyclovir is a potent and selective drug against HSV.[10] It is remarkably effective against severe mucocutaneous HSV infections in immunosuppressed patients when used intravenously.[10] Acyclovir is thus the treatment of choice for AIDS patients with chronic HSV infections.[24] Patients should be treated for five to ten days with doses appropriate for surface area and renal function. In most patients, such treatments result in prompt response, with rapid reepithelization of previously infected lesions. Usually, patients are pain free after five days and epithelization is well established within ten days.[24] In many AIDS patients, a recurrence of their HSV infection results in chronic, ulcerative disease in the same site within weeks or months of clearing of earlier lesion.[24] Retreatment of these patients results in effective control of HSV infection without evidence of viral resistance to this drug. More recently, oral acyclovir has been used as prophylaxis against recurrent HSV infections in immunodeficient patients.[28] The number and severity of reactivated infections were reduced significantly. Although resistance to the drug has not been observed, patients receiving oral acyclovir must be followed closely for such a possibility.

HSVs are among the microorganisms that can devastate AIDS patients, whose immunity has been obliterated by persistent HIV infection. Treatment of HSV or any other opportunistic infection represents no more than treating the symptoms of an almost uniformly fatal disease. If the patient manages to recover from chronic HSV infection with the help of acyclovir, another opportunistic, life-threatening agent will at some point infect the patient. In the end, a treatment must be developed to rid the patient of HIV and reestablish the host defense systems. Efforts to achieve this end are ongoing in many centers.

REFERENCES

1. Spear PG. Composition and organization of herpesvirus virions and properties of some of the structural proteins. In: Rapp F, ed. Oncogenic herpesviruses, vol. I. Boca Raton, FL: CRC Press, 1980;53.
2. Furlong D, Swift H, Roizman B. Arrangement of herpesvirus deoxyribonucleic acid in the core. J Virol 1972;10:1071.
3. Spear PG, Roizman B. Proteins specified by herpes simplex virus: V. Purification and structural proteins of herpesvirus. J Virol 1972;9:431.
4. Roizman B. Structural and functional organization of herpes simplex virus genomes. In: Rapp F, ed. Oncogenic herpesviruses, vol I. Boca Raton, FL: CRC Press, 1980;19.
5. Kieff ED, Bachenheimer SL, Roizman B. Size, composition and structure of the DNA of subtypes 1 and 2 herpes simplex virus. J Virol 1971;8:125.
6. Poffenberger KL, Roizman B. Non-inverting genome of a viable herpes simplex virus 1: Presence of head-to-tail linkages in packaged genomes and requirements for circularization after infection. J Virol 1985;53:587.
7. Nahmias AJ, Dowdle WR. Antigenic and biologic differences in herpesvirus hominis. Prog Med Virol 1968;10:110.
8. Corey L, Holmes KK. Genital herpes simplex virus infection: Current concepts in diagnosis, therapy, and prevention. Ann Intern Med 1983;98:973.
9. Bachman TG, Simpson T, Nosal C, et al. The structure of herpes simplex virus DNA and its application to molecular epidemiology. Ann NY Acad Sci 1980;354:179.
10. Whitley RJ. A perspective on the therapy of human herpesvirus infections. In: Roizman B, Lopez C, eds. The herpesviruses. Immunobiology and prophylaxis of human herpesvirus infections, vol. 4. New York: Plenum Press, 1985;339.
11. Corey L. The natural history of genital HSV. In: Roizman B, Lopez, C, eds. The herpesviruses. Immunobiology and prophylaxis of human herpesvirus infections, vol. 4. New York: Plenum Press, 1985;1.
12. Britto E, Dikshit SS, Naylor B. Herpes virus simplex infection of the female genital tract. Univ Mich Med Bull 1976;42:152.
13. Nahmias AJ, Keyserling HL, Kerrick GM. Herpes simplex virus. In: Remington JS, Klein JO, eds. Infectious diseases of the fetus and newborn infant. Philadelphia: W. B. Saunders, 1983;642.
14. Duenas A, Adam E, Melnick JL, Rawls WE. Herpesvirus type 2 in a prostitute population. Am J Epidemiol 1972;95:483.
15. Nahmias AJ, Josey WE, Naib ZM, et al. Antibodies to herpesvirus hominis types 1 and 2 in humans. Am J Epidemiol 1970;91:539.
16. Hill TJ. Herpes simplex virus latency. In: Roizman B, ed. The herpesviruses, vol. 3. New York: Plenum Press, 1985;175.
17. Quinn TC, Corey L, Chafee RG, et al. The etiology of anorectal infections in homosexual men. Am J Med 1981;71:395.
18. Samarasinghe PL, Oates JK, MacLennan IPB. Herpetic proctitis and sacral radiomyelopathy—a hazard for homosexual men. Br Med J 1979;2:365.
19. Goldmeier D. Proctitis and herpes simplex virus in homosexual men. Br J Vener Dis 1980;56:11.
20. Guttman D, Raymond A, Gelb A, et al. Virus-associated colitis in homosexual men: Two case reports. Am J Gastroenterol 1983;78:167.
21. Heller M, Dix RD, Baringer JR, et al. Herpetic proctitis and meningitis: Recovery of two strains of herpes simplex virus type 1 from cerebrospinal fluid. J Infect Dis 1982;146:584.

22. Goodell SE, Quinn TC, Mkritichian PAC, et al. Herpes simplex proctitis in homosexual men. Clinical, sigmoidoscopic, and histopathological features. N Engl J Med 1983;308:868.
23. Mann SL, Meyers JD, Holmes KK, Corey L. Prevalence and incidence of herpesvirus infections among homosexually active men. J Infect Dis 1984;149:1026.
24. Siegal FP, Lopez C, Hammer G, et al. Severe acquired immunodeficiency in male homosexuals, manifested by chronic perianal ulcerative herpes simplex lesions. N Engl J Med 1981;305:1439.
25. Quinnan GV, Masur H, Rook AH, et al. Herpesvirus infections in acquired immune deficiency syndrome. JAMA 1984;252:72.
26. Gerstaft J, Malchow-Moller A, Bygbjerg I, et al. Severe acquired immunodeficiency in European homosexual men. Br Med J 1982;285:17.
27. Centers for Disease Control. Update: Acquired immunodeficiency syndrome: United States. MMWR 1986;35:17.
28. Straus SE. Oral acyclovir for recurrent herpesvirus infections. In: Lopez C, Roizman B, eds. Human herpesvirus infections: Pathogenesis, diagnosis, and treatment. New York: Raven Press, 1986:93–101.

Chapter 11

Cytomegalovirus Infection in Healthy and Immune Deficient Homosexual Men

W. Lawrence Drew
Lawrence Mintz

In the past several years, increasing attention has been focused on cytomegalovirus (CMV) infections in homosexual men and the role these infections might play in the pathogenesis of acquired immunodeficiency syndrome (AIDS) and Kaposi's sarcoma (KS). The initial documentation of high rates of CMV infection in homosexual men resulted from prevalence studies we performed at the San Francisco City Clinic in 1979.[1] Urinary excretion of CMV was noted in 14 of 90 (7.4%) homosexual men but in none of 101 heterosexual men attending the same sexually transmitted disease (STD) clinic (P <0.005). Similarly, antibody to CMV was detected in 130 of 139 (93.5%) homosexual men but in only 38 of 70 (54.3%) heterosexual men (P <0.005).

In a subsequent prospective study[2] of 237 homosexual men participating in the Western Study Group Hepatitis Vaccine Trial at the San Francisco City Clinic, we again noted a high prevalence of CMV IgG serum antibody—206 of 237 (86.9%). Of the 31 men lacking CMV antibody on initial testing, 22 experienced seroconversion within 9 months of follow-up, for an attack rate of 71% during this time period.

During a mean follow-up period of 14.3 months (range, 2 to 20) 66 of the 206 initially seropositive men (32%) excreted CMV in their urine on one or more occasions. Both a urine and a semen specimen were obtained during a single visit from 52 of the homosexual men. CMV was recovered from 18 of the

---

This work was supported in part by the State of California and allocated on recommendations of the Universitywide Task Force on AIDS. It was also supported by grants from the John Kerner Foundation, the Ernest H. Rosenbaum Cancer Research Fund, and the Alan B. Glassberg Cancer Research Fund, Mount Zion Hospital and Medical Center, San Francisco, California, and by the NIH (San Francisco Men's Health Study, NIH-N01-AI-82515).

semen specimens but from only 3 of the 18 corresponding urine samples. Specimens from a single individual grew CMV from the urine but not from the semen. Semen therefore appears to be nearly five times as sensitive as urine in detecting the presence of CMV. Clearly, the widespread occurrence of CMV viruria and "virusemenia" in this population makes exposure to the virus all but inevitable and accounts for the extraordinarily high attack rate of CMV infections among seronegative homosexual men.

Data on the prevalence of CMV IgM antibody further suggest that homosexual men experience repeated episodes of CMV infection. CMV IgM antibody was detected on one or more occasions in the sera of more than 90% of the homosexual men and tended to appear, disappear, and reappear over time.[2] In contrast, IgM antibody to CMV was detected in only 3.8% of 103 serum specimens randomly collected from volunteer male blood donors. Among the homosexual men there was no temporal correlation between the presence of CMV viruria and serum IgM antibody titers. CMV IgM antibody was detected in a significantly ($P < 0.05$) higher proportion of serum samples from the 206 initially seropositive men (67% of 1136 samples) than in the postconversion samples obtained from the 22 seroconverters (53% of 86 samples). These data are summarized in Table 11–1. The higher prevalence of CMV IgM antibody in longstanding seropositive men than in recent seroconverters suggests that the former group is continually being reexposed to (and possibly reinfected with) exogenous strains of the virus. Earlier studies in women and their infants have shown that individuals can be serially infected with different strains of CMV.[3] Two other studies have demonstrated that different strains of CMV can be isolated simultaneously from multiple sites in patients with AIDS.[4,5] Since CMV infection alone (i.e., in the absence of concomitant human immunodeficiency virus [HIV] infection) can cause sustained suppression of CD4/CD8 ratios,[6] we believe that multiple exogenous reinfections of homosexual men with differing strains of CMV may result in protracted suppression of host immunity, thus facilitating subsequent infection with HIV.

Questionnaires concerning demographic data, clinical histories, and sexual practices were completed by 78 subjects (54 of whom were initially seropositive

Table 11–1 Presence of CMV IgM antibody in 237 prospectively studied homosexual men

Group	Subjects No. Positive/ No. Tested (%)	Serum Samples No. Positive/ No. Tested (%)
Seronegatives	0/9 (0)	0/54 (0)
Seropositives	196/206 (95)	765/1136 (67)
Seroconverts	20/22 (91)	46/86 (53)[a]

[a]Samples obtained after seroconversion.

and 24 of whom were initially seronegative, including 17 of the 22 seroconverters and 7 of the 9 who remained persistently seronegative). Among the men who were seropositive on initial testing, those who excreted CMV during the study period were significantly younger (mean age = 26.6) than those who did not (mean age = 32.7) ($P < 0.05$). This finding confirms our earlier observation that CMV excretion by healthy homosexual men rarely occurs beyond age 30[1] and suggests that viruria tends to decrease with time.

Information was obtained regarding the frequency of participation in the following sex practices: kissing, oral-anal contact (oral role), oral-anal contact (anal role), fellatio (oral role), fellatio (genital role), anal intercourse (active role), and anal intercourse (passive role). Only passive anal intercourse correlated with the initial presence of anti-CMV antibody or with seroconversion to this virus during the course of the study. Of 59 men who engaged in passive anal intercourse, CMV antibody was present in 96.6%, but of the 19 men who did not engage in this practice, antibody was present in only 73.7% ($P < 0.01$) (Table 11–2). The latter figure does not differ significantly from the prevalence of CMV antibody among heterosexual men attending a venereal disease clinic. These data suggest that exposure of the anorectal mucosa to CMV-infected semen constitutes the major route of acquisition of CMV infection by homosexual men.

ROLES OF CMV

In the remainder of this chapter, we shall address the contribution of CMV to AIDS, KS, and *Pneumocystis carinii* pneumonia in homosexual men.

In AIDS

Data from a number of studies suggest a possible cofactor role for CMV infection in AIDS. As noted above, CMV infection is highly prevalent both among ho-

Table 11–2 Prevalence of CMV antibody among homosexual and heterosexual men

Group	No. of Men	No. Positive (%)
1. Homosexual men: passive anal intercourse	59	57 (96.6)
2. Homosexual men: no passive anal intercourse	19	14 (73.7)
3. Heterosexual men	70	38 (54.3)

1 vs 2: $P < 0.01$
1 vs 3: $P < 0.001$
2 vs 3: not statistically significant

mosexual men and among patients with AIDS. Of 164 AIDS patients (including homosexual men, intravenous drug users, and hemophiliacs) tested by the Centers for Disease Control (CDC) for CMV antibody, 162 were positive.[7] The two with negative results may have been end-stage AIDS patients who, in our experience, are often unable to maintain antibody responses.

CMV is known to cause T cell dysfunction during the syndrome of acute CMV mononucleosis. Suppression of T helper lymphocytes and mitogen responses occur and then revert to normal after convalescence.[8,9] A review of the immunologic consequences of acute CMV mononucleosis has been published.[10]

Since CMV infects both B and T lymphocytes, it may therefore enhance subsequent infection of lymphocytes by AIDS-related retroviruses. Rice et al.[11] have reported in vitro infection of human peripheral blood T and B lymphocytes, natural killer cells, and monocytes by low-passage CMV isolated from patients with various clinical syndromes. Virus expression was limited to the synthesis of immediate-early CMV polypeptides; viral replication did not occur. "Wild" virus strains were more infective than laboratory adapted viruses, suggesting that the latter are highly adapted to fibroblasts whereas in "nature" CMV may be more lymphotropic. Immunocompetent mononuclear cells infected by CMV had diminished mitogen and antigen responses. These results correlate with previous observations of decreased lymphocyte proliferation responses to mitogens and antigens in patients with acute CMV infection.[12-14] The latter also show a transient defect in cytotoxic lymphocyte responses to allogeneic cells.

We have investigated the relationship between CMV serologic status and T cell imbalance in homosexual men.[15] Normal T helper/T suppressor ratios (>1.0) were found in 40 of 42 homosexual men without antibodies to CMV versus only 34 of 67 (51%) homosexual men with antibodies to the virus (P<0.001) (Table 11–3). In order to determine whether asymptomatic primary CMV infection in homosexual men induces immunologic abnormalities, 34 of the 42 CMV-seronegative men were enrolled in a prospective study to document the time of seroconversion and relate it to helper/suppressor ratio results. During an average follow-up period of 13.6 months, 12 (35%) seroconverted, 10 of whom were asymptomatic. All 12 had helper/suppressor ratios ≥1.0 in the month before seroconversion, and these ratios all dropped below 1.0 within 1 to 3 months following seroconversion (average nadir, 0.62). Helper/suppressor ratios have remained ≤1.0 for an average of 9.6 months. Of the seven seroconverters who

Table 11–3 Relationship of T cell ratio to CMV antibody status in 109 homosexual men without AIDS

CMV Antibody	No. (%) with Normal Helper/Suppressor Ratio
Present (n = 67)	34 (51)[a]
Absent (n = 42)	40 (95)[a]

[a]P <0.001.

have been followed for at least 12 months, 3 remain <1.0. The degree of abnormality of helper/suppressor ratio did not differ in the asymptomatic versus the symptomatic patients. Of 20 seronegative men whose initial helper/suppressor ratio was >1.0 and who have remained seronegative, only one developed a helper/suppressor ratio consistently below 1.0. Three of the men in this prospective study developed antibodies to HIV, but the magnitude and duration of T lymphocyte abnormalities in the HIV-positive patients did not differ from those who remained HIV negative.

Our results suggest that CMV is responsible for at least some of the immunologic abnormalities occurring in homosexual men. Even asymptomatic CMV infection induces profound disturbances in the ratio of helper to suppressor lymphocytes, and these may persist for prolonged periods. These abnormalities appear to occur before, and independent of, infection by the AIDS-associated retrovirus. In summary, we suspect that CMV infection may be an important cofactor in the genesis of AIDS and may enhance susceptibility to infection by HIV.[15] Of even greater importance, CMV infection may help convert HIV infection from a latent state to active viral replication. In vitro studies indicate that CMV can act to transactivate HIV.[16] CMV may not be unique in this regard, however, since other DNA viruses have been shown to enhance HIV replication similarly.[17]

In *P. carinii* Pneumonia

Evidence for CMV infection in ten homosexual patients with *P. carinii* pneumonia is presented in Table 11–4. A complete report on five of those patients has been described elsewhere.[18] In all ten patients evidence was found for either

Table 11–4 *P. carinii* pneumonia and CMV in homosexual men

Subject	ACIF[a]	IgM FA[b]	Cultures		
			Blood	Lung	Urine
1	1024	8	ND[c]	+	ND
2	256	32	ND	+	−
3	128	16	ND	ND	+
4	256	8	ND	−	−
5	512	128	−	+	−
6	128	<8	−	+	−
7	1024	16	−	ND	+
8	4096	32	−	+	+
9	1024	64	+	+	−
10	128	8	ND	+	−

[a]Anticomplement immunofluorescent assay for CMV IgG antibody.
[b]Fluorescent antibody assay for CMV IgM antibody.
[c]Not done.

past or present infection with CMV. All patients had CMV-specific IgG antibody, and nine had CMV-specific IgM antibody. The virus was recovered from lung tissue in seven of the eight patients in whom viral culture was attempted. In several instances we can infer that the virus was present in extremely high titer because it grew out in just one or two days. Recovery of CMV from lung tissue in 88% of homosexual men with *P. carinii* pneumonia suggests a possible association between these two infectious agents.

Coexistent CMV and pneumocystis pneumonia has been described previously. If CMV infection predisposes persons to pneumocystis infection, what is the mechanism? The alveolar macrophages of both man[19] and mouse[20] can be infected by CMV; in the mouse model, CMV has been shown to impair phagocytosis of bacteria.[20] Histologic studies suggest that the macrophage is an important component of the host response to *P. carinii*.[21] It may be that CMV infection of alveolar macrophages impairs their ability to interact with *P. carinii* pneumonia by impairing cell-mediated immune responses, as mentioned above.

In Kaposi's Sarcoma

The first evidence of an association between KS and CMV was presented by Giraldo and Beth in 1972.[22,23] They isolated a unique strain, K9V, from a cell line derived from a KS patient from Zaire. This strain shared significant homology with another transforming CMV strain, Mj, and was capable of inducing lymphadenopathy in young baboons. The following lines of evidence suggest a possible cofactor role for CMV in the genesis of KS.

Oncogenic Potential. As summarized in Table 11–5, CMV stimulates synthesis of cellular DNA, RNA, and enzymes in host cells.[24,25] The virus also trans-

Table 11–5 Oncogenic potential of human CMV in vitro

Stimulation of cellular macromolecules synthesis
Cellular DNA
Cellular RNA
Mitochondria DNA
Cellular enzyme
  DNA polymerase (alpha and beta)
  Thymidine kinase
  Ornithine decarboxylast
  Plasminogen activator
  DNA-dependent RNA polymerase
  Exonuclease
  Topoisomerase
Morphologic transformation of mammalian cell
  Hamster embryonic fibroblast
  Rodent cell
  Human fibroblast

forms human embryo fibroblasts, which then grow as sarcomatous tumors when transplanted to immunosuppressed or athymic mice.[26] Nelson et al.[27] have refined the latter observation by identifying the transforming segment of the CMV genome. Additionally, Stinski and Roehr[28] and Boshart et al.[29] have shown that the gene products responsible for immediate early (IE) antigen coding can activate transcription.

Serologic Association. The second line of evidence linking CMV to KS stems from work previously reported by Giraldo et al.[30] A significantly higher prevalence of CMV antibody was detected in 46 elderly European and American patients with KS than in two age-matched control groups without KS. This serologic difference was not seen with antibodies to Epstein-Barr virus (EBV) and herpes simplex and varicella-zoster viruses. No differences in serologic patterns were observed in African KS patients versus controls because of a high background of CMV seropositivity.[31]

Demonstration of CMV Genome and Antigens in KS Tissue. Further evidence for an association of CMV with KS derives from the demonstration of CMV nucleic acids and antigens in KS tumor biopsies. Reports of detection of CMV antigens and DNA or RNA in KS tissue are conflicting. Boldogh et al.[32] and Giraldo et al.[33] have reported the presence of CMV early antigens in tumor tissues from patients with classic and endemic forms of KS. We have detected CMV early antigens by a similar procedure in six of nine KS biopsy specimens from homosexual men with AIDS[34] and more recently have found this antigen in an additional nine of 18 cases examined. Biopsies of normal skin from 21 of 22 of our patients were negative for CMV antigens, and all KS biopsies were also negative for CMV by culture. The presence of CMV early antigens, coupled with the failure to detect CMV late antigens or whole virus in KS biopsies,[33,35] suggests that CMV genome is present in a nonreplicative (and hence more likely oncogenic) state and rules out the possibility that viral presence results simply from disseminated CMV infection or from a tropism of the virus for dermal or tumor tissue.

Boldogh et al.[32] have also detected CMV DNA in 6 of 12, and CMV RNA in 3 of 9, biopsies from African patients. EBV and HSV type 2 sequences were not detected. We reported the presence of CMV RNA by in situ hybridization in two of three KS biopsies from homosexual men whose tumor cultures were negative for replicating CMV.[34] Huang has also demonstrated viral nucleic acid in tumor cell foci in lymph nodes of KS patients by in situ nucleic acid hybridization using biotinylated DNA as probe.[24]

More recently, Spector et al.[37] have employed the technique of in situ hybridization to detect CMV DNA specifically within tumor cells of KS tissue specimens. Instead of whole virus genome, they used as probes subgenomic fragments of CMV DNA that had previously been shown not to cross-hybridize with host cell human DNA. With this technique they were able to detect CMV genetic sequences in tumor cells from six of ten available KS specimens but not in sections of uninvolved skin. Others have been unable to detect CMV DNA or RNA in KS tumor tissue.[37] In part this may stem from the use of procedures of differing sensitivity. For example, using a Southern blot procedure, Ruger et al. were not able to detect CMV DNA in six AIDS-related KS tissues they examined. In biopsies from eight African and one European KS patients they detected marginal hybridization in only two.[38]

Epidemiology. The epidemiologic evidence for CMV involvement in KS derives from the heightened prevalence of this tumor in two groups of individuals, renal transplant patients and homosexual men with AIDS, who share the dual features of immunosuppression and extremely high rates of active CMV infection.

To date, we have studied 57 homosexual men with KS for CMV antibody, and all are positive. Of 39 who have had appropriate secretion cultures, 24 (62%) have been positive. Zur Hausen[39] has stated that "it is likely that the epigenetic burden of persisting viral DNA increases with the number of infections and is therefore correlated with age and exposure." A quantitative estimate of the extent of CMV exposure among gay men can be inferred from the finding that, even on a single sample, the semen of 25% of homosexual men is CMV culture-positive.[42]

A most important epidemiologic clue linking CMV to KS has come to light during the current AIDS epidemic: the marked discrepancy in the incidence of KS cases among homosexual versus heterosexual AIDS patients. In New York City, KS occurs in 46% of AIDS cases among homosexual men but in only 3.8% of AIDS cases among heterosexual men.[40] This striking discrepancy suggests that a cofactor may be present in homosexual men that is not present in heterosexuals. This cofactor may be CMV infection, since intravenous (IV) drug users (most of whom are heterosexual) do not have unusually high rates of CMV infection. Of 143 IV drug users in San Francisco and New York City studied by us, only 92 (64%) were seropositive, a rate similar to that observed in the general population.[41] Marmor et al. have extended this observation to compare the prevalence of CMV antibody in IV-drug-using females (87%) versus males (42%).[42] This finding adds to the correlation of CMV antibody and KS prevalence, since KS is more common as the presenting manifestation of AIDS in female IV drug users (KS prevalence 12.5%) than in male IV drug users (3.8%).[40] Table 11–6, based on their report, shows that the prevalence of KS as a presenting manifestation of AIDS correlates with the prevalence of CMV antibody in the risk group,

Table 11–6 Relationship between CMV seropositivity and KS in AIDS patients

AIDS Risk Group	CMV Seropositive (%)	KS in Initial Diagnosis (%)
Homosexual	94[1]	46[40]
Females with IV drug use	87[42]	12.5[40]
Males with IV drug use	64[41]	3.8[40]

Note: Superscripts indicate reference numbers.

Table 11-7 Decline in prevalence of Kaposi sarcoma (KS) and cytomegalovirus (CMV) seroconversion in homosexual men

Year	Prevalence of KS as Presenting Manifestation of AIDS[a] (%)	Seroconversion of CMV Antibody in Cohorts of Initially CMV Seronegative Homosexual Men (%)
1981	63	71
1982	54	57
1983	46	25
1984	35	10
1985	24	4

[a]Drew WL, Mocarski ES, Sweet E, et al. Multiple infections with CMV in AIDS patients: documentation by southern blot hybridisation. J Infect Dis 1984;150:952.

although the use of CMV IgG antibody prevalence is an imperfect marker of the magnitude of CMV exposures in a group such as homosexual men. In this group, as documented previously, there may be multiple, repetitive exposures and even infection by the virus, yet antibody only measures a single exposure.[4]

A decline has been noted in KS as the presenting manifestation of AIDS in homosexual men. As shown in Table 11-7, we have been able to relate this decline to a similar decline in the acquisition of CMV infection among seronegative homosexual men. As mentioned previously, 22 of 31 (71%) homosexual men who were CMV seronegative acquired infection during the first 7 months of 1981. In contrast, only 1 of 26 CMV seronegative men acquired CMV during the 12 months of 1984. Correspondingly, the prevalence of KS as the presenting manifestation of AIDS in homosexual men has declined from 63% in 1981 to 24% in 1985.[43]

The reason for the decline in CMV infections is undoubtedly the reduction of STDs in general among homosexual men. At least in San Francisco, the rates of gonorrhea, amebiasis, and so on have diminished since 1986 in association with closure of bath houses and adoption of "safe sex" guidelines.

The decline in KS may reflect diminished exposure to any one or several STDs as well as to other putative cofactors, such as amyl nitrite (which is used to assist the frequency of sexual acts). Thus, the correlation of decreased KS with decreased CMV infection may be only coincidental. However, in view of the many threads of evidence implicating CMV in KS, the observation is provocative.

REFERENCES

1. Drew WL, Mintz L, Miner RC, et al. Prevalence of cytomegalovirus infection in homosexual men. J Infect Dis 1981;143:188–192.
2. Mintz L, Drew WL, Miner RC, Braff EH. Cytomegalovirus infections in homosexual men: An epidemiologic study. Ann Intern Med 1983;99:326–329.

3. Huang E-S, Alford CA, Reynolds DW, et al. Molecular epidemiology of cytomegalovirus infections in women and their infants. N Engl J Med 1980;303:958–962.
4. Drew WL, Sweet ES, Miner RC, Mocarski ES. Multiple infections by cytomegalovirus in patients with acquired immunodeficiency syndrome: Documentation by Southern blot hybridization. J Infect Dis 1984;150:952–953.
5. Spector SA, Hirata KK, Neuman TR. Identification of multiple cytomegalovirus strains in homosexual men with acquired immunodeficiency syndrome. J Infect Dis 1984;150:953–956.
6. Drew WL, Mills J, Levy J, et al. Cytomegalovirus infection and abnormal T-lymphocyte subset ratios in homosexual men. Ann Intern Med 1985;103:61–63.
7. Centers for Disease Control. Preliminary results reported at NIH Conference on AIDS. Bethesda, MD: May, 1983.
8. Rinaldo CR, Carney WP, Richter BS, et al. Mechanisms of immunosuppression in cytomegaloviral mononucleosis. J Infect Dis 1980;141:488–495.
9. Carney WP, Rubin RH, Hoffman RA, et al. Analysis of T lymphocyte subsets in cytomegalovirus mononucleosis. J Immunol 1981;126:2114–2116.
10. Hirsch MS, Felsenstein D. Cytomegalovirus-induced immunosuppression. In: Selikoff IJ, Teirstein AS, Hirschman SZ, eds. Acquired immune deficiency syndrome. Ann NY Acad Sci 1984;437:8–15.
11. Rice GPA, Schrier RD, Oldstone MBA. Cytomegalovirus infects human lymphocytes and monocytes: Virus expression is restricted to immediate early gene products. Proc Natl Acad Sci USA 1984;81:6134–6138.
12. Rinaldo CR, Black PH, Hirsch MS. Virus-leukocyte interactions in cytomegalovirus mononucleosis. J Infect Dis 1977;136:667–668.
13. Levin MJ, Rinaldo CR, Leary PL, et al. Immune response to herpes virus antigens in adults with acute cytomegalovirus mononucleosis. J Infect Dis 1979;140:851–857.
14. Carney WP, Iacoviello V, Hirsch MS. Functional properties of T lymphocytes and their subsets in cytomegalovirus mononucleosis. J Immunol 1983;130:390–393.
15. Drew WL, Mills J, Levy J, et al. Cytomegalovirus infection and abnormal T-lymphocyte subset ratios in homosexual men. Ann Intern Med 1985;103:61–63.
16. Davis MG, Kenny SC, Kaminer J. Immediate early gene region human cytomegalovirus transactivates the promoter of human immunodeficiency virus. Proc Natl Acad Sci 1987;84:8642–8646.
17. Gendelman HE, Phelps W, Feigenbaum L, et al. Trans-activation of the human immunodeficiency virus long terminal repeat sequence by DNA viruses. Proc Natl Acad Sci 1986;83:9759–9763.
18. Follansbee SE, Busch DF, Wofsy CB, et al. An outbreak of *Pneumocystis carinii* pneumonia in homosexual men. Ann Intern Med 1982;96:705–713.
19. Drew WL, Mintz L, Hoo R, Finley TN. Growth of herpes simplex and cytomegalovirus in cultured human alveolar macrophages. Am Rev Respir Dis 1979;119:287–291.
20. Shanley JD, Pesanti EL. Replication of murine cytomegalovirus in lung macrophages: Effect on phagocytosis of bacteria. Infect Immun 1980;29:1152–1159.
21. Hughes WT. *Pneumocystis carinii*. In: Mandell GL, Douglas RG, Bennett JE, eds. Principles and practice of infectious diseases. New York: John Wiley & Sons. 1979;2137–2142.
22. Giraldo G, Beth E, Coeur P, et al. Kaposi's sarcoma: A new model in the search for

viruses associated with human malignancies. J Natl Cancer Inst 1972;49:1495–1507.
23. Giraldo G, Beth E, Hagenau F. Herpes-type virus particles in tissue culture of Kaposi's sarcoma from different geographic regions. J Natl Cancer Inst 1972;49:1509–1513.
24. Huang ES. The role of cytomegalovirus infection in Kaposi's sarcoma. In: Friedman-Kien AE, Laubenstein LJ, eds. AIDS—the epidemic of Kaposi's sarcoma and opportunistic infections. Masson Publishing Co, 1984;111–126.
25. St Jeor SC, Albrecht TB, Frank FD, Rapp R. Stimulation of cellular DNA synthesis with human cytomegalovirus. J Virol 1974;13:353–362.
26. Geder L, Lausch R, O'Neill F, Rapp F. Oncogenic transformation of human embryo lung cells by human cytomegalovirus. Science 1976;192:1134–1137.
27. Nelson J, Fleckenstein B, Galloway DA, McDougall JK. Transformation of NIH 3T3 cells with cloned fragments of human cytomegalovirus AD-169. J Virol 1982;43:83–91.
28. Stinski MF, Roehr T. Activation of the major immediate early gene of human cytomegalovirus by cis-acting elements in the promoter regulatory sequence and by virus-specific trans-acting components. J Virol 1985;55:431–441.
29. Boshart M, Weber F, Gerhard J, et al. A strong enhancer is located upstream of an immediate early gene of human cytomegalovirus. Cell 1985;41:521–530.
30. Giraldo G, Beth E, Henle W, et al. Antibody patterns to herpesviruses in Kaposi's sarcoma: II. Serological association of American Kaposi's sarcoma with cytomegalovirus. Int J Cancer 1978;22:126–131.
31. Giraldo G, Beth E, Kourilsky FM, et al. Antibody patterns of herpesviruses in Kaposi's sarcoma: Serologic association of European Kaposi's sarcoma with cytomegalovirus. Int J Cancer 1975;15:839–848.
32. Boldogh I, Beth E, Huang E-S, et al. Kaposi's sarcoma: IV. Detection of CMV DNA, CMV RNA, and CMNA in tumour biopsies. Int J Cancer 1981;28:469–474.
33. Giraldo G, Beth E, Huang E-S. Kaposi's sarcoma and its relationship to cytomegalovirus (CMV): III. CMV DNA and CMV-early antigens in Kaposi's sarcoma. Int J Cancer 1980;26:23–29.
34. Drew WL, Conant MA, Miner RC, et al. Cytomegalovirus and Kaposi's sarcoma in young homosexual men. Lancet 1982;2:125–127.
35. Civantos F, Penneys NS, Haines H. Kaposi's sarcoma: Absence of cytomegalovirus. J Invest Dermatol 1982;79:79–80.
36. Stribling J, Weitzner S, Smith GV. Kaposi's sarcoma in renal allograft recipients. Cancer 1978;42:442–446.
37. Spector DH, Shaw SB, Hock LJ, et al. Association of human cytomegalovirus with Kaposi's sarcoma. In: Gottlieb MS, Groopman JE, eds. Acquired immune deficiency syndrome. New York: Alan R. Liss, 1984;109–126.
38. Ruger R, Burmester GR, Kalden JR, et al. Search for human cytomegalovirus DNA in Kaposi sarcomas and hematopoietic cells from homosexual men with AIDS or unexplained lymphadenopathy. In: Gottlieb MS, Groopman JE, eds. Acquired immune deficiency syndrome. New York: Alan R. Liss, 1984;127–137.
39. Zur Hausen H. The role of viruses in human tumors. Adv Cancer Res 1980;33:77–107.
40. Des Jarlais DC, Marmor M, Thomas P, et al. Kaposi's sarcoma among four different AIDS risk groups. N Eng J Med 1984;310:1119.

41. Brodie HR, Drew WL, Maayan S. Prevalence of Kaposi's sarcoma in AIDS patients reflects differences in rates of cytomegalovirus infection in high risk groups. AIDS Memorandum. 1984;1:12.
42. Marmor M, Des Jarlais DC, Spira T, et al. AIDS and cytomegalovirus exposure in New York City drug abusers (poster). International Conference on AIDS, Atlanta, April 1985.
43. Drew WL, Mills J, Hauer LB, et al. Declining prevalence of Kaposi's sarcoma in homosexual AIDS patients paralleled by fall in cytomegalovirus transmission (letter). Lancet 1988;2:9.

Chapter 12

Laboratory Diagnosis of Sexually Transmitted Diseases and Opportunistic Infections of AIDS

Pearl Ma

In the first edition, the laboratory diagnoses of sexually transmitted diseases with and without diarrhea were detailed without knowledge of the causative agent of acquired immunodeficiency syndrome (AIDS), a devastating sexually transmitted disease (STD). Now AIDS is known to be caused by a retrovirus called human immunodeficiency virus (HIV),[1] previously referred to as human T cell lymphotropic virus/lymphadenopathy virus (HTLV-III/LAV). Large-scale screening of blood donors for HIV antibody by enzyme immunoassay (EIA),[2] and the introduction in 1986 of the antigen test further increasing screening sensitivity and specificity,[3] have made detection of HIV possible. Statistics indicate that AIDS has spread to the heterosexual population[4,5] (intravenous [IV] drug users and their sex partners and newborns; blood transfusion recipients[6]; health care workers[7,8]; and research scientists exposed to an exceptionally high volume of virus-contaminated material),[9] but homosexual and bisexual men remain the group most affected—62% of 78,545 AIDS individuals as of Dec. 5, 1988.[4] On the other hand, New York City health officials have found that AIDS has killed more IV drug addicts than homosexuals in the city.[10] Despite attempts to alert the public to practice "safe sex" and to abstain from IV drug use to prevent the spread of AIDS, the epidemic continues to proceed with full force, and the Centers for Disease Control (CDC) predicts that 365,000 people will have AIDS by 1992.[6] Approximately 20% to 30% of individuals already infected who are asymptomatic or who have AIDS-related complex (ARC) will progress to full-

---

I would like to thank Sr. C. Sherry and Drs. J. Gillooley and L. King for their moral support, Ms. Lisa Feldman for the beautiful photography, and Ms. Michelle McPherson for her excellent secretarial skills.

blown AIDS in a few months to five years. A detailed description of HIV and AIDS is presented in Chapter 13. In this chapter, the laboratory diagnoses are divided into three sections: sexually transmitted diseases not associated with diarrhea, (Table 12–1), sexually transmitted diseases associated with diarrhea (Table 12–1), and opportunistic infections in AIDS (Table 12–2). The chapter is completely updated, since many advancements have been made for rapid diagnosis, especially in the use of monoclonal antibody, gene probe, and so on, not only for HIV but also for various agents for STDs and opportunistic infections (OIs). More opportunistic agents have surfaced, including *Microsporidia, Acanthamoeba, Cunninghamella,* and Cat Scratch Disease bacillus (CSDB).

SEXUALLY TRANSMITTED DISEASES WITHOUT DIARRHEA

Bacterial Infections

Pathogenic Neisseriae

Gonorrhea (Causative Agent—Neisseria gonorrhoeae). Since the beginning of the AIDS epidemic, vigorous educational programs launched in the homosexual community, about safe sex with the use of condoms and monogamous relationships instead of multiple sex partners, resulted in some reduction in the incidence of gonorrhea.[11] Although penicillinase-producing *N. gonorrhoeae* has caused worldwide outbreaks, the incidence remains low in anorectal mucosa.[12] Pertinent information for the laboratory diagnosis of gonorrhea is summarized in Tables 12–3 and 12–4. Successful laboratory diagnosis depends strongly on knowing the biologic properties of the causative agent and providing effective specimen collection, transport, and isolation.[13] For instance, *N. gonorrhoeae*(1) is sensitive to cold, and specimens and inoculated plates held at 4°C or 22°C for 24 hours before being incubated at 37°C would give a false-negative result; the test should be repeated in highly suspect cases, (2) is easily killed by drying, so medium or specimen collected on swabs should not be allowed to dehydrate, (3) requires 5% to 10% CO_2 to survive and grow, so this environment should be provided not only during incubation but also during transport to the laboratory by using a Neigen-Jembac (Figure 12–1) or Thayer-Martin plate placed in a candle jar, and (4) is a slow grower easily overgrown by normal flora from the skin, urethra, throat, or rectum; therefore one must minimize the presence of such normal flora contaminants from various sites during collection by using a tongue depressor, anoscope, or surface cleansing, depending on the site, as well as using media selective for *N. gonorrhoeae* and *N. meningitidis* (see Tables 12–3, 12–4). New York City medium containing lincomycin in lieu of vancomycin is useful in detecting the vancomycin-sensitive strain.[14] Specimen collection should also include multiple sites (endourethra, rectum/anus, and pharynx) concurrently because treatment differs based on site of infection.[15] Similarly, disseminated

Table 12–1 Infectious agents of STDs in AIDS

	Nondiarrheal		Diarrheal	
Group	Infection	Infectious Agent	Infection	Infectious Agent
Bacteria	Gonorrhea	Neisseria gonorrhoeae	Gonorrhea	Neisseria gonorrheae
	Meningococcal	Neisseria meningitidis	Shigellosis	Shigella spp.
	Nongonococcal urethritis	Chlamydia trachomatis (D-K) Ureaplasma urealyticum	Salmonellosis	Salmonella spp.
	Lymphogranuloma venereum	Chlamydia trachomatis, L_1-L_3	Campylobacteriosis	Campylobacter spp.
			Chlamydia proctitis	Chlamydia trachomatis
	Syphilis	Treponema pallidum		
	Chancroid	Hemophilus ducreyi		
	Donovanosis	Calymmatobacterium granulosis		
	Trichomoniasis	Trichomonas hominis		
Parasites	Pediculosis	Phthrirus pubis	Amebiasis	Entamoeba histolytica
	Scabies	Sarcoptes scabiei	Giardiasis	Giardia lamblia
			Coccidiosis	Isospora belli
				Cryptosporidium spp.
			Enterobiasis	Enterobius vermicularis
			Endolimaxiasis	Endolimax nana
			Microsporidiosis[b]	Microsporidia
Viruses	AIDS	Human immunodeficiency virus[a] (HIV-1 and HIV-2)	CMV infection	Cytomegalovirus (CMV)
	Hepatitis A, B, and non-A, non-B	Hepatitis A, B, and non-A, non-B virus		
	Rectal herpes	Herpes simplex virus types 1 and 2 (HSV-1, HSV-2)		
	Molluscum contagiosum	Pox virus		
	Condyloma acuminatum	Papilloma virus		

[a]Previously named human T cell lymphotropic virus III (HTLV-III), lymphadenopathy virus (LAV).
[b]Intestinal microsporidiosis is diagnosed only in homosexual men with AIDS and is possibly sexually transmitted.

Table 12-2 Infectious agents of OIs in AIDS

Group	Infection	Infectious Agent
Bacteria	Septicemia	*Salmonella* sp. (nontyphi), Staphylococci, *Streptococcus pneumoniae*, *Hemophilus influenzae*, *Listeria monocytogenes*, Gram-negative enteric bacilli, *Mycobacterium* spp.[a]
	CNS	*Streptococcus pneumoniae*, *Nocardia asteriodes*, *Listeria monocytogenes*, *Mycobacteria* spp.[a]
	Pneumonia	*Hemophilus influenzae*, *Legionella pneumophila*, *Mycobacterium* spp.[a]
	Skin	Cat-scratch disease bacillus
	Disseminated infection	MAI,[b] *M. kansasii*, *Campylobacter* spp.
Fungi	Pneumonia	*Histoplasma capsulatum*, *Cryptococcus neoformans*
	Esophagitis	*Candida* spp.
	CNS	*Cryptococcus neoformans*, *Pseudallescheria boydii*
	Skin lesion	*Histoplasma capsulatum*, *Aspergillus* spp.
	Disseminated infection	*C. neoformans*, *H. capsulatum*, *Aspergillus* spp., *Candida* spp., *Trichosporon* spp., *Cunninghamella bertholletiae*
Algae	CNS	*Prototheca wickerhamii*
Parasites	Pneumonia	*Pneumocystis carinii*, *Cryptosporidium* spp.
	Ocular	*Toxoplasma gondii*
	GI	*Cryptosporidium* spp., *Isospora belli*, *Microsporidia*, "nonpathogenic amoeba"
	CNS	*Toxoplasma gondii*, *Acanthamoeba* spp.
	Skin lesions	*Acanthamoeba* spp. *Toxoplasma*
	Myositis	*Microsporidia* spp.
	Hepatitis	*Cryptosporidium* spp., *Microsporidia*
Viruses	Pneumonia	CMV, adenovirus, HIV-1, EBV[c]
	CNS	Papovavirus (JC), HSV-1, HSV-2, varicella zoster, CMV, adenovirus, EBV, HIV-1
	Ocular	CMV, HSV, HIV-1
	Skin	HIV-1, HSV, V2, etc.
	Disseminated infections	CMV, adenovirus, HSV-1, HSV-2, varicella zoster, HIV-1

[a] *Mycobacterium tuberculosis* and atypical *Mycobacterium* sp. (MAI, *M. kansasii*, *M. fortuitum*).
[b] Mycobacterium avium intracellularis.
[c] Epstein-Barr virus.

Table 12-3 Laboratory diagnosis of STD—Gonorrhea (general information)

Biologic characteristics of *Neisseria gonorrhoeae*
    Extremely sensitive to cold, drying, and lack of CO_2. Slow grower, requires X and V factors for growth.
Specimen collection (see Table 12-4)
Growth media and transport conditions
    Selective primary isolation media
        Thayer-Martin medium—chocolate agar with vancomycin, colistin, nystatin, trimethoprim.
        New York City medium—chocolate agar with lincomycin, colistin, nystatin, trimethoprim.
    Atmospheric condition—5% to 10% CO_2 (Neigen-Jembac/candle jar)
    Optimal growth temperature—35° to 39°C.
    Incubation period—24 to 48 hours.
Identification profile
    Gram smear: gram-negative kidney-bean shaped diplococci 0.6 to 0.8 μm, intracellular (direct smear).
    Colony characteristics: small/pinpoint gray mucoid
    Presumptive test: oxidase (+).
    Definitive tests: coagglutination test:
        Phadebact Omni monoclonal & Gonogen—1 minute.[a]
        Gonozyme—20 minutes.[a]
        Rapid carbohydrate fermentation/utilization <5 mins. (RIM-N kit, quad Derm, RIN-test.)[b]
    Strain variation: T_1, T_2, T_3, T_4.
Antibiotic susceptibility tests
    Preliminary test: beta-lactamase test (+) indicates penicillinase producer (PPNG).
    Definitive test: agar dilution (μg/ml).
Test of cure
    Repeat cultures of various sites one week after treatment is stopped.

[a]Gonozyme (Abbott), Phadebact (Pharmacia), Gonogen (New Horizon Diagnostics).
[b]RIM-N Kit (Austin Biological Labs), quadFerm (API), RIN Test (Winfield Labs).

gonococcal infection requires culturing the blood, infected joint, and skin lesions. Conjunctiva swabs should be taken from purulent conjunctivitis and an early morning urine specimen in asymptomatic screening.

Preliminary identification of gonococci can be made from direct smears only from sites devoid of numerous microbial contaminants (see Table 12-4). A positive Gram's smear is characterized by numerous polymorphonuclear leukocytes containing gram-negative kidney bean-shaped diplococci with either no or few nongonococcal organisms. Although carbohydrate fermentation using cystine tryptophane peptone agar (BBL, CTA medium; Difco cystine tryptic agar) has been the standard procedure to identify gonococci, these procedures require overnight or longer incubation at 37°C and have been replaced by more rapid methods. In the first edition, we introduced the coagglutination tests: Phadebact (Pharmacia) and GonoGen (New Horizon Diagnostics). The Phadebact test involves adding the suspected oxidase-positive colonies to a suspension of *Staph*-

Table 12–4 Laboratory diagnosis of STD—Gonorrhea (specimen collection and transport)

Infective Site	Preparation	Collection-Transport System	Neigen-Jembac[c]	Transport Temperature (°C)	Direct Smear
Endourethra[a] (purulent discharge)	—	Ca alginate swab on thin wire	Neigen-Jembac[c]	22 to 25	Glass slide
Rectum/anus[a]	Anoscope examination	Cotton swab on stick	See above	See above	—
Pharynx[a]	Tongue depressor	See above	See above	See above	—
Urine	Cleanse genital area with soap and water	Clean catch	—	See above	Glass slide with sediment
Conjunctiva (purulent discharge)	Evert conjunctiva	See above	See above	See above	Glass slide
Epididymis	Local anesthesia	Aspirate with tuberculin syringe[d]	See above	See above	Glass slide
Skin lesion[b]	Cleanse with sterile saline	Aspirate with tuberculin syringe[d]	See above	See above	Glass slide
Joint fluid[b]	Cleanse surface with sterile saline	Aspirate with 5 ml syringe[c]	See above	See above	Glass slide with sediment
Blood[b]	Cleanse with I$_2$ preparation at venipuncture site.	Blood collecting unit	Blood culture bottle with CO_2 and in sterile tube Blood culture sets	See above	—

[a]Test concurrently.
[b]Test concurrently for disseminated gonococcal infection, in addition to X.
[c]Warm at room temperature before use, place CO_2 tablet in well, seal bag (Neigen-Jembac).
[d]Usually performed by urologist.

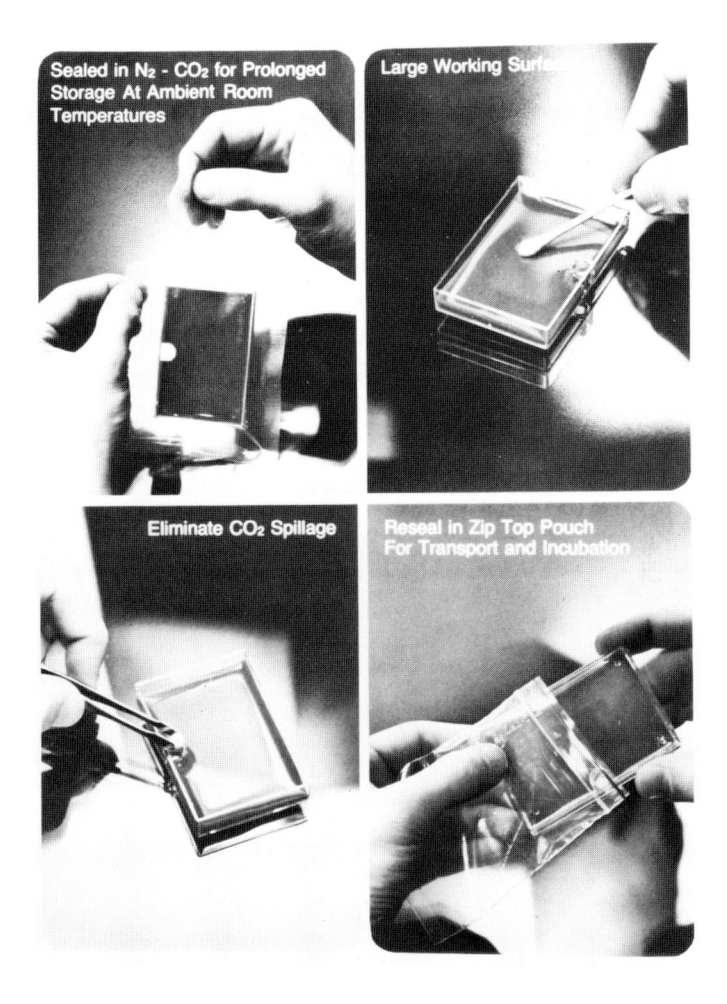

FIGURE 12–1 *Stepwise procedure of using Neigen-Jembac specimen collection-transport system.*

ylococcus aureus (previously sensitized to the gonococcal antibody) on a slide, causing *N. gonorrhoeae* to agglutinate within one minute. The GonoGen test is similar, except the antibody used is the murine monoclonal antibody to the protein 1 antigen from gonococci and the colonies require preheating for one minute for specific reactivity. One report indicates that heating is not required in the improved product.[16] Phadebact Omni Monoclonal, another new test, has been shown to be superior to the above tests.[17] Other rapid tests are two carbohydrate fermentation systems, RIM-N Kit (Austin Biological Labs) and quadFERM (API), and a preformed enzyme detection system, RIN-Test (Winfield Labs). The hands-on time requires three minutes for the first two and 4.5 minutes for the third test. Both quadFERM and RIM revealed 88% to 94% specificity and 100% sensitivity, but RIN has a low sensitivity of 63%.[17,18] Two other kits, Gonocheck (Dupont) and RapID NH (IDS), can identify a wider spectrum of organisms that, periodically, can grow on the Thayer-Martin plate, supposedly a selective medium for pathogenic *Neisseria*. These organisms are *N. lactamica, Branhamella catarrhalis, Kingella denitrificans,* and *N. mucosa*. Unfortunately, both systems may misidentify *N. mucosa* as *N. gonorrhoeae*.[19]

On the other hand, the Gonozyme[20] is designed to detect the gonococcal antigen directly from the specimen without culturing. Although this may be useful in screening positive cases, it will fail if it is used to test a cure, since it can detect both live and dead organisms. To conduct epidemiologic surveys of gonococcal isolates, they can be further differentiated into strains by auxotyping with the use of various nutritional exact media.[21]

Meningococcal Infection (Causative Agent—N. meningitidis). *N. meningitidis* from the oropharyngeal area has been implicated in the increasing incidence of anogenital lesions, due to oroanogenital sexual behavior.[22,23] Specimen collection, transport, and growth requirements are essentially the same as those listed in Tables 12–3 and 12–4. Meningococci differ from gonococci in that they can ferment glucose as well as maltose. Although identification has been done by serotyping using a slide test, group B serotype appears to present difficulties due to the presence of cross-reactions.

Chlamydial and Ureaplasmal Infections

Chlamydial Infection. Sexually transmitted chlamydial infections include nongonococcal urethritis (NGU), epididymitis, proctitis, and lymphogranuloma venereum (LGV) in homosexual and bisexual men. Pertinent information is shown in Table 12–5 (general information), Table 12–6 (specimen collection), and Table 12–7 (identification profile).

Nongonococcal urethritis Nongonococcal urethritis, caused by *Chlamydia trachomatis* and *Ureaplasma urealyticum,* has been named nonspecific urethritis and postgonococcal urethritis because previously no specific agent could be isolated and the disease occurred even after adequate treatment for gonorrhea. Bowie and Holmes recommended using semiquantitative urethral Gram stained smear to define urethritis as ≥ four polymorphonuclear leukocytes in five fields under oil-immersion lens.[24] Most diagnoses are made clinically or from specimens cultured by reference and commercial laboratories,[25] since handling tissue culture is costly. Fortunately, recent developments provide some easy to adopt preliminary screening procedures, such as examination of a direct smear by direct fluorescent antibody test (DFAT)[26,27] and detection of chlamydial antigen by enzyme immunoassay (EIA)[27,28] without culturing except for further work-up in some cases.

The two known species of *Chlamydia* are *C. trachomatis* and *C. psittaci*. *C.*

Table 12–5 Laboratory diagnosis of STD—*Ureaplasma* and *Chlamydia* infection (general information)

Biologic characteristics
  Ureaplasma
  - Member of *Mycoplasma*, characterized by use of urea, hence named *Ureaplasma*. Lacks cell wall, hence resistant to penicillin. Minute colonies with "fried egg" appearance visible only under microscopic examination.

  Chlamydia
  - Obligate intracellular organism, appears as cytoplasmic inclusion body (elementary body 0.3 μm, reticulate body 1.0 μm) in mammalian cells.
  - Heat labile, slow grower, developmental cycle 72 hours at 35°C.
  - Susceptible to tetracycline, erythromycin, penicillin, chloramphenicol,[a] and toxin component in Dacron and cotton swabs.

Specimen collection and transport (see Table 12–6)
Identification profile
  Ureaplasma
  - Growth in U broth and U agar.[b]
  - Optimal pH for growth—6.3. Very sensitive to pH change.
  - Growth temperature—37°C.
  - Microscopic "fried egg" colonies appear in U agar/New York City agar in two to four days aerobically.
  - Strong urease producer, giving a (+) urea test.

  Chlamydia
  - (see Table 12–7)
  - Cell culture stained with monoclonal antibody, immunofluorescent test, iodine/Giemsa stain
    Immunotypes—A, B, Ba, C-K, L_1-L_3 (LGV: L_1-L_3); (NGU and ocular infections: D-K)
    Serologic tests[c]
    Complement fixation (group antigen)—titer $\geq$1:16
    ELISA (group antigen) titer $\geq$1:16
    Microimmunofluorescence (MIF) (pooled specific antigens) L_1/L_2, C/J, E/D, F/G, K/L_3 with nonspecific conjugates IgG, IgM, IgA.

[a]Inhibitory in cell culture. LGV, Lymphogranuloma venereum.
[b]Kenny GE. Mycoplasmas. In: Lennette EH, Balows A, Hausler WJ Jr, Shadomy HJ, eds. Manual of Clinical Microbiology, 4th ed. ASM, 1985;407–411.
[c]Non-LGV : *C. trachomatis*—fourfold rise in titer/seroconversion.
  LGV : *C. trachomatis*—single high titer $\geq$1:512 usually indicates active infection.

trachomatis TWAR strain, related to respiratory infection, and *C. psittaci*, the causative agent of psittacosis, will not be presented here. *Chlamydia* culture has been the most definitive procedure to diagnose NGU by *Chlamydia*,[25] especially with the aid of monoclonal antibody.[29] *Chlamydia* requires living cells to undergo its developmental cycle, which starts when the infectious elementary body (EB, 0.3μm) attaches to and then penetrates the host cell, followed by simple fission to form numerous reticular bodies (RB, 1.0 μm), maturation of reticulate bodies to matured EB, and release of EB from the host cell, thus completing the developmental cycle. These two morphologic forms—EB and RB—make up the cytoplasmic inclusion body. The complete developmental cycle requires 72 hours;

Table 12–6 Laboratory diagnosis of STD—*Ureaplasma* and *Chlamydia* infection (specimen collection)

Agent	Infection	Site	Preparation	Collection	Transport Media
Chlamydia trachomatis (D-K)	NGU	Endourethra	Compress urethra to let secretion flow down	Scrape with Ca alginate[a] minitip culturette 4 cm from the meatus	2 sucrose phosphate transport medium (2SP)[b] kept cold in wet ice for culture Transport medium for Ag test
	Urinary tract	Urine	Direct smear Clean catch	Scrape with minitip Sterile container for antigen test or for culture	Fix in acetone for antigen test
		Semen	Unsatisfactory for culture		
	Proctitis	Rectum	Insert anoscope	Scrape inflamed mucosa with Ca alginate swab	Same as above
	Epididymitis	Epididymis	Use local anesthesia[c]	Aspirate with sterile saline	
(L$_1$-L$_3$)	LGV	Endourethra Perianal node	See above Aspirate through normal skin	Same as above	Same as above
Ureaplasma urealyticum	NGU	Rectum See NGU above	See NGU above	See NGU above	Direct inoculation onto Neigen-Jembac with New York City medium/U medium

[a]Rotate and withdraw, express material into transport medium and discard swab; Dacron and cotton swab inhibitory.
[b]2SP (68.46 g sucrose, 2.088 g K$_2$HPO$_4$, 1.088 g Na$_2$HPO$_4$. Dist H$_2$O to 1000 ml. Adjust pH to 7.0 and autoclave; add bovine serum 5%, streptomycin 50 µg/ml, vancomycin 100 µg/ml, nystatin 25 U/ml). If delayed, store specimen at −70°C.
[c]Usually performed by a urologist.

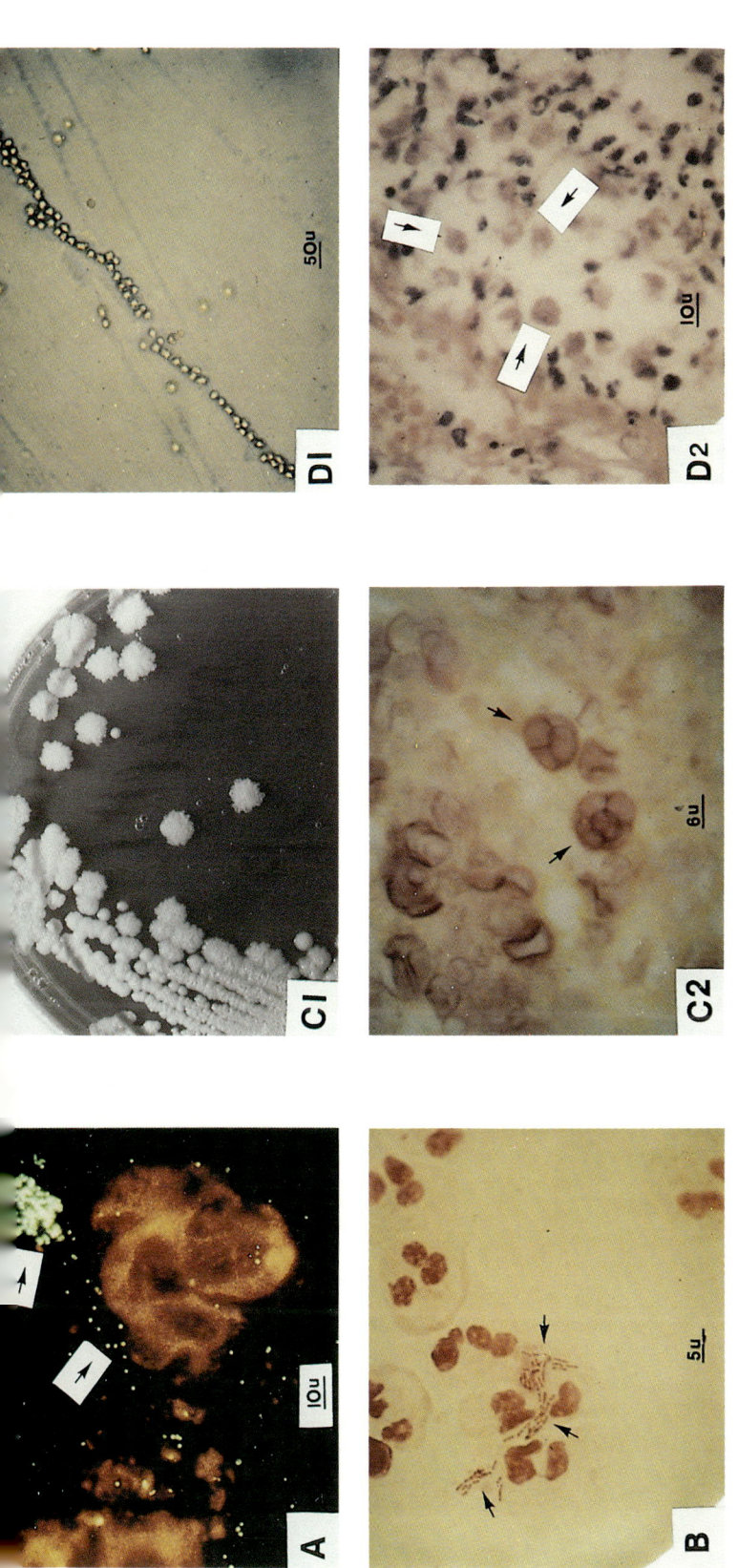

Plate I Types of Infectious Agents. **(A)** Chlamydia trachomatis. A stained touch preparation of a genital lesion from a homosexual man with AIDS showing numerous tiny green elementary bodies of C. trachomatis, some in clusters, some singly on the surface of epithelial cells (stained red), and some free in the background. (Indirect fluorescent test with anti-Chlamydia trachomatis monoclonal antibody) (500 ×). (Courtesy Difco Inc.) **(B)** Hemophilus ducreyi. A stained touch preparation of the aspirate from a bubo lesion of a homosexual man with chancroid showing gram-negative coccobacilli in a characteristic "school of fish" and cluster arrangement (Gram's stain) (500 ×). (Courtesy Professor E. Bottone) **(C1)** Prototheca wickerhamii. A Sabouraud agar plate showing numerous rough colonies and a tiny smooth colony of a unicellular achlorophylic algaelike organism. The organism was isolated from the autopsy material of the brain and CSF of a patient who died of AIDS (six-day old culture incubated at 37°C). (Courtesy Dr. Zigmund Kaminski,[123] Chapter 12) **(C2)** Prototheca wickerhamii. Stained smear from an olecranal lesion showing the typical spherical structures with multiple fissions from the lesion of the olecranon bursa. (Gram's smear) (500 ×). (Courtesy Dr. G. R. Healy) **(D1)** Acanthamoeba. Culture of Acanthamoeba on 1.5% nonnutrient agar showing numerous cysts arranged linearly. Streaked line of their motility is visible (Low-power objective). **(D2)** Acanthamoeba trophozoites (arrow) in lung histologic section of an AIDS patient (hematoxylin-eosin stain) (250 ×). (Courtesy Dr. C. A. Wiley,[122] Chapter 12)

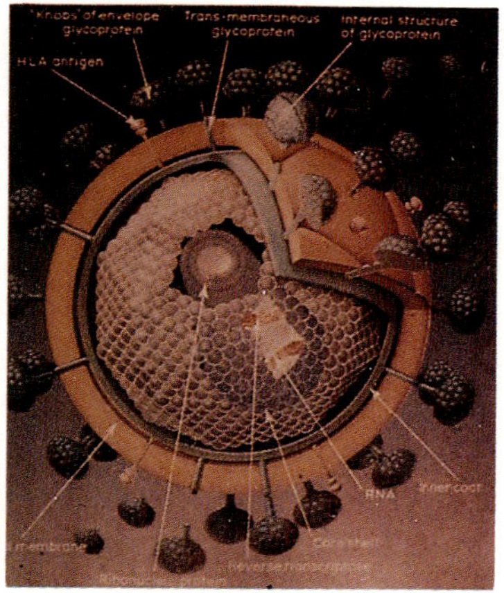

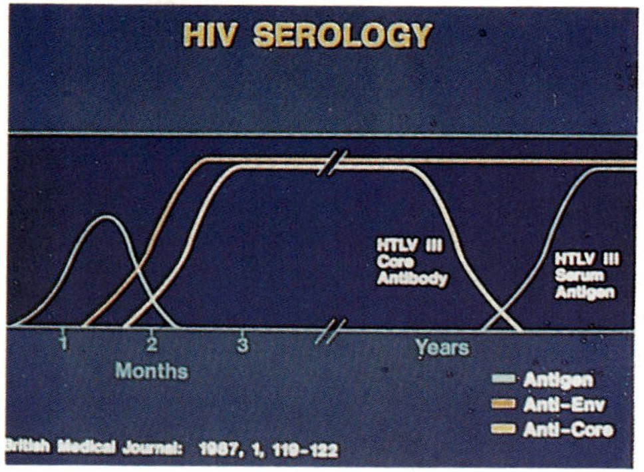

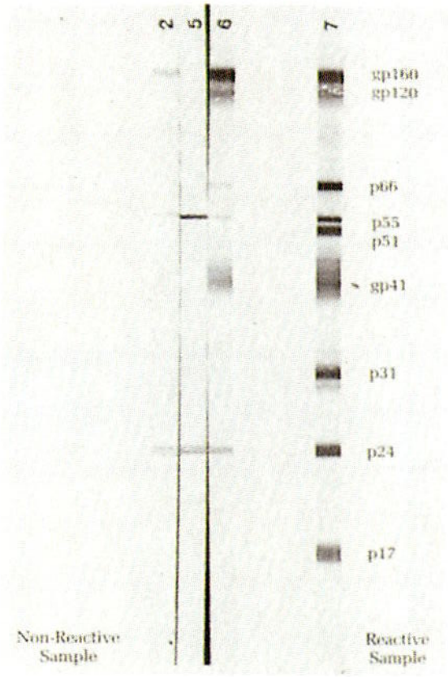

Plate II *HIV.* **(A)** *Schematic representation of the HIV showing HIV antigen, knobs of envelope glycoprotein, transmembranous glycoprotein, internal structure of glycoprotein, inner coat, RNA, core shell, reverse transcriptase, ribonucleic protein, and lipid membrane. (Courtesy Dr. Michael Koch,[42] Chapter 12)* **(B)** *Genomes of HIV and associated proteins and glycoproteins. (Courtesy Abbott Diagnostics)* **(C)** *HIV serology showing the rise and fall of the antigen titer, followed by the rise of antibody titers (antienvelope and anticore proteins) and reappearance of the antigen titer in the terminal stage of AIDS (Courtesy Abbott Diagnostics)* **(D)** *Western blot of positive serum by enzyme immunosorbent assay. The indeterminate strips are on the left (negative for p17 and p51), and the reactive strip, containing the specific pattern of p24, p31, gp41, and gp160 antigens is on the right. (Courtesy Dupont,[55] Chapter 12)*

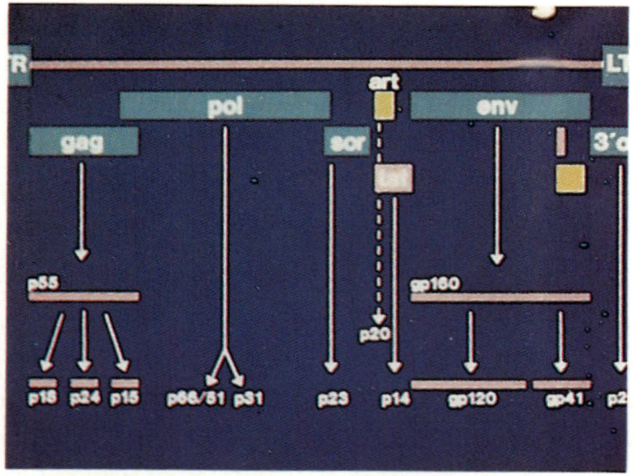

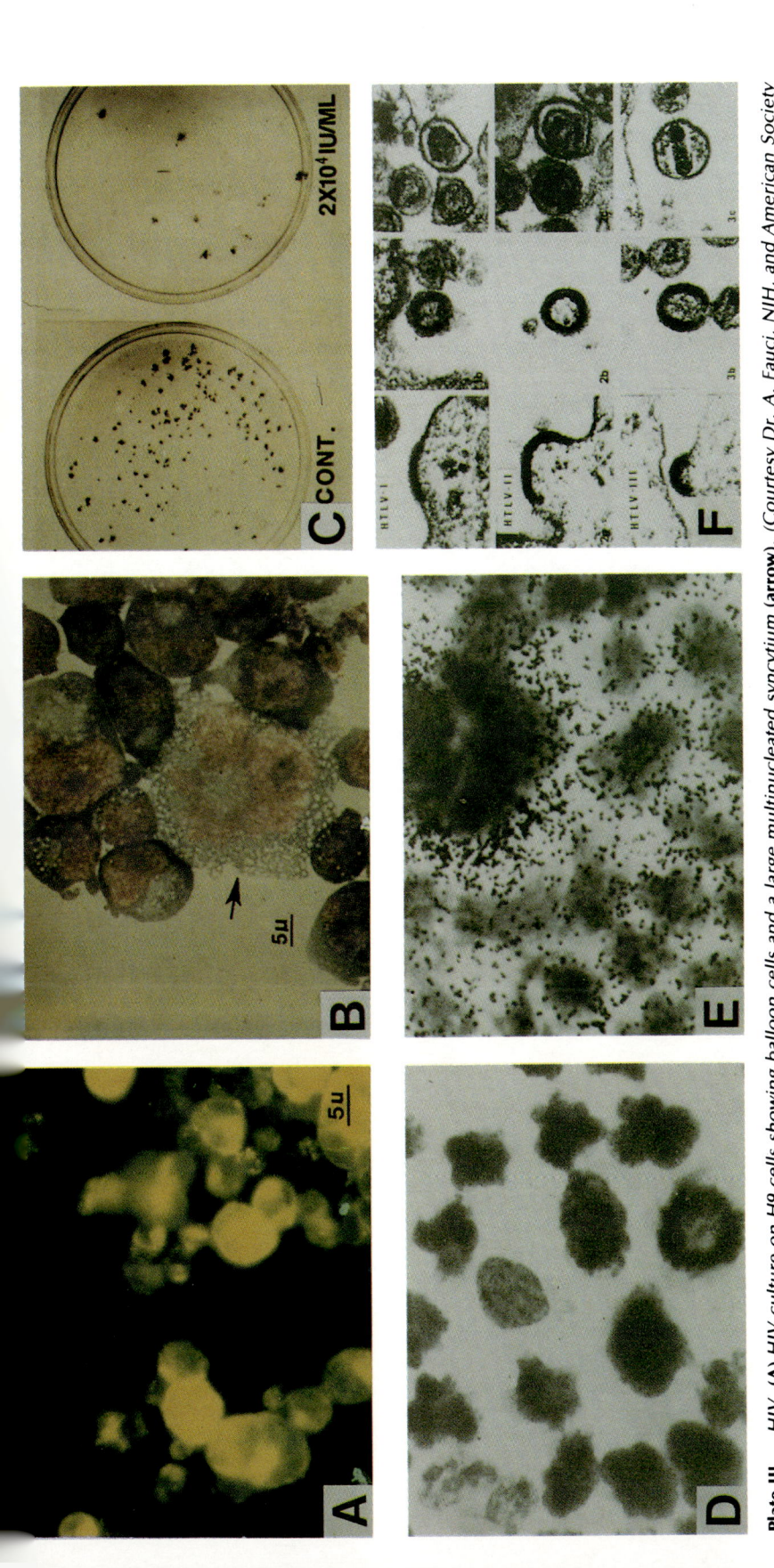

Plate III HIV. **(A)** HIV culture on H9 cells showing balloon cells and a large multinucleated syncytium (**arrow**). (Courtesy Dr. A. Fauci, NIH, and American Society for Microbiology, cover of ASM News, May 1987) **(B)** HIV culture on H9 cells showing fluorescent balloon cells and syncytium (indirect fluorescent test) (500 ×). (Courtesy Dr. D. Volsky) **(C)** Petri dish (control plate before irradiation) showing numerous plaques of HIV on MT2 cells on the left and reduction of plaques after irradiation on the right. (Courtesy Professor N. Yamamoto, University of Yamaguchi.[66] Chapter 12) **(D)** Uninfected H9 cells hybridized with HTLV-III probe. **(E)** H9/HTLV-IIIB cells, which are active viral producers, hybridized with HTLV-III probe. (Courtesy Flossie Wong-Staal, Ph.D., Chief, Molecular Genetics of Hematopoietic Cells Section, Laboratory of Tumor Cell Biology,[73] Chapter 12) **(F)** Electron micrographs of retroviruses (HTLV-I, HIV-1, and HTLV-II). (Courtesy Robert C. Gallo, M.D., Chief, Laboratory of Tumor Cell Biology,[48] Chapter 12)

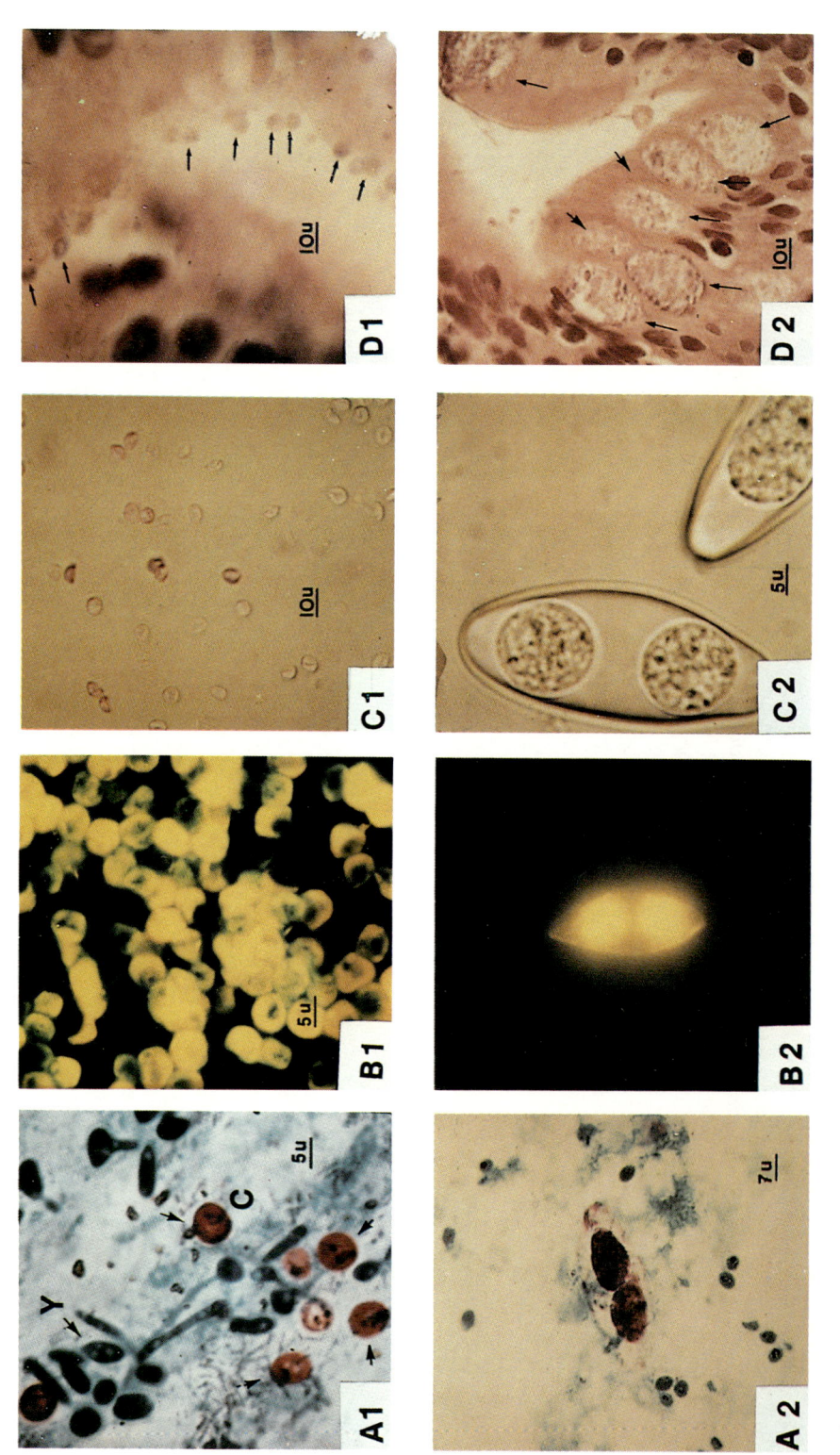

Plate IV

Plate IV *Comparison of Cryptosporidium and Isospora belli in various staining specimen preparations of AIDS patients.* **(A)** Modified Cold Kinyoun (MCK) stool preparations. **(A1)** Cryptosporidium sp. oocysts shown as acid-fast positive oval structures in red (C) and non-acid-fast yeasts in green (Y). (500 ×).[89] (Chapter 12) **(A2)** Isospora belli oocysts shown as large elliptical structures containing two acidfast positive (red) oval sporocysts and small oval, non-acid-fast green structures (yeasts) (500 ×). **(B)** Truant stained stool preparation (auramine-rhodamine). **(B1)** Cryptosporidium sp. oocysts appear as orange fluorescent oval structures (500 ×). **(B2)** Isospora belli oocysts appear as elliptical structures containing two fluorescent orange sporocysts (500 ×). **(C)** Sucrose flotation unstained stool preparation. **(C1)** Cryptosporidium sp. oocysts appear as tiny pink oval structures due to interaction between sucrose and optics (American Optic scope; low-power objective). **(C2)** Isospora belli oocysts. The one on the left shows two sporocysts, and the one on the right contains one sporoblast, at an immature stage (oil-immersion objective). **(D)** Histologic sections of duodenal biopsy (hematoxlin-eosin stain). **(D1)** Cryptosporidium sp. endogenous stages seen lining the microvilli (arrows) (500 ×). **(D2)** Isospora belli endogenous stages (arrows) appear in the cytoplasm of enterocytes (500 ×).

Plate V (See overleaf) *Comparative staining characteristics of Pneumocystis carinii (PC) and Cryptosporidium sp. (CR) in open lung biopsy from homosexual men with AIDS.* **(A)** Giemsa-Wright stained preparations (Hemacolor). **(A1)** PC cyst (C) containing eight sporozoites and numerous tiny trophozoites (T) in the background. Cyst wall is not stained and appears as a halo. **(A2)** Three CR oocysts (arrows), each containing four densely stained red spherical sporozoites within a macrophage.[156] (Chapter 12) **(B)** Gomori methenamine silver stained preparations (GMS). **(B1)** PC cysts stained black. **(B2)** CR oocysts failed to stain and appear as hollow circular structures. **(C)** MCK acid-fast stained preparations. **(C1)** PC cysts are non-acid-fast and invisible. **(C2)** CR oocysts are acid-fast and red (arrows). **(D)** Gram-Weigert stained preparations. **(D1)** PC cysts are stained purple (low-power objective). **(D2)** CR oocysts are stained purple, showing crescent-shaped sporozoite (oil-immersion lens). **(E)** Indirect fluorescent test with monoclonal antibody. **(E1)** PC shown as green dots representing the oocysts and trophozoites. (Courtesy Dr. J. A. Kovacs,[154] Chapter 12) **(E2)** CR shown as green spherical oocysts.

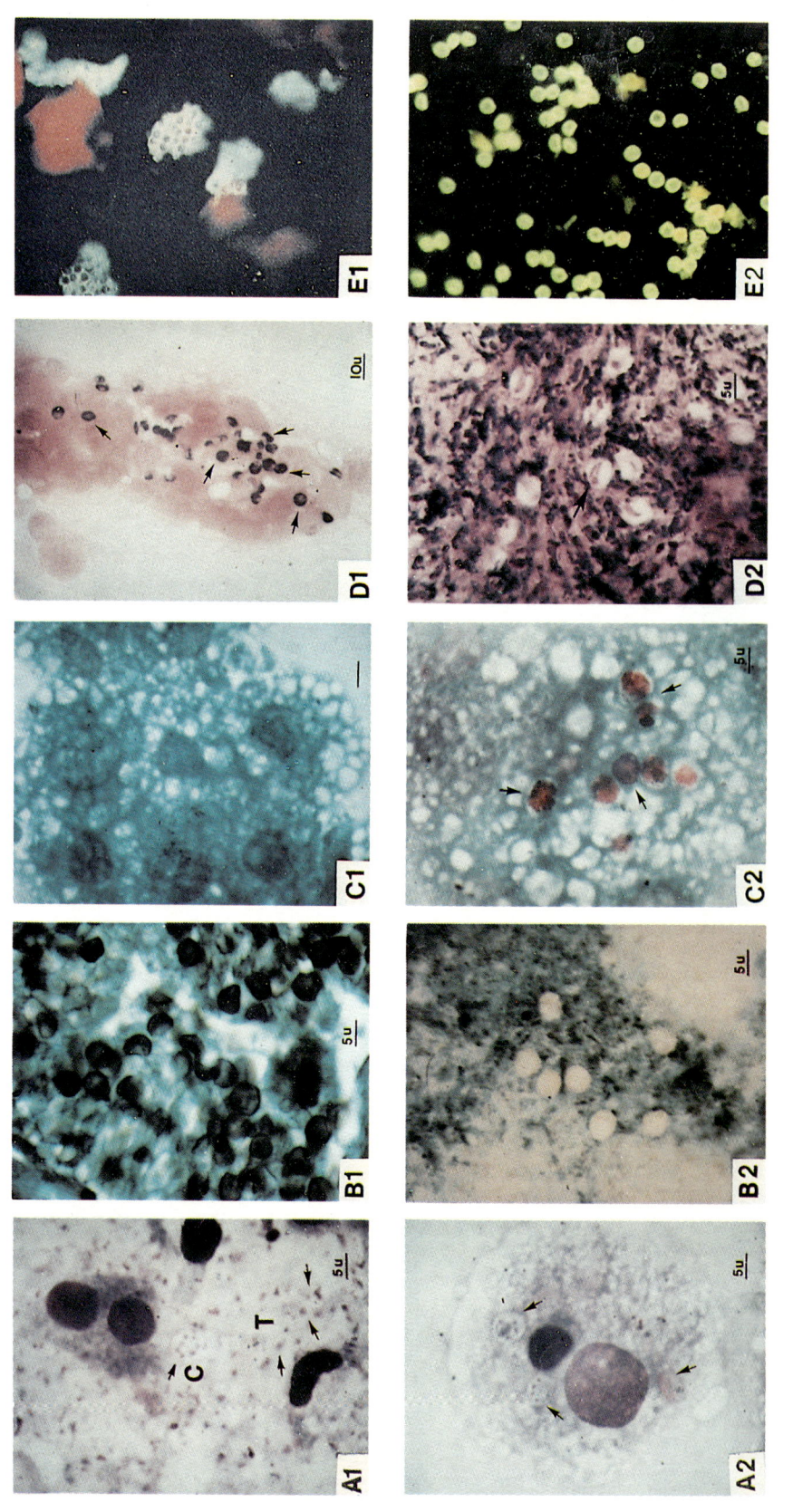

Plate V

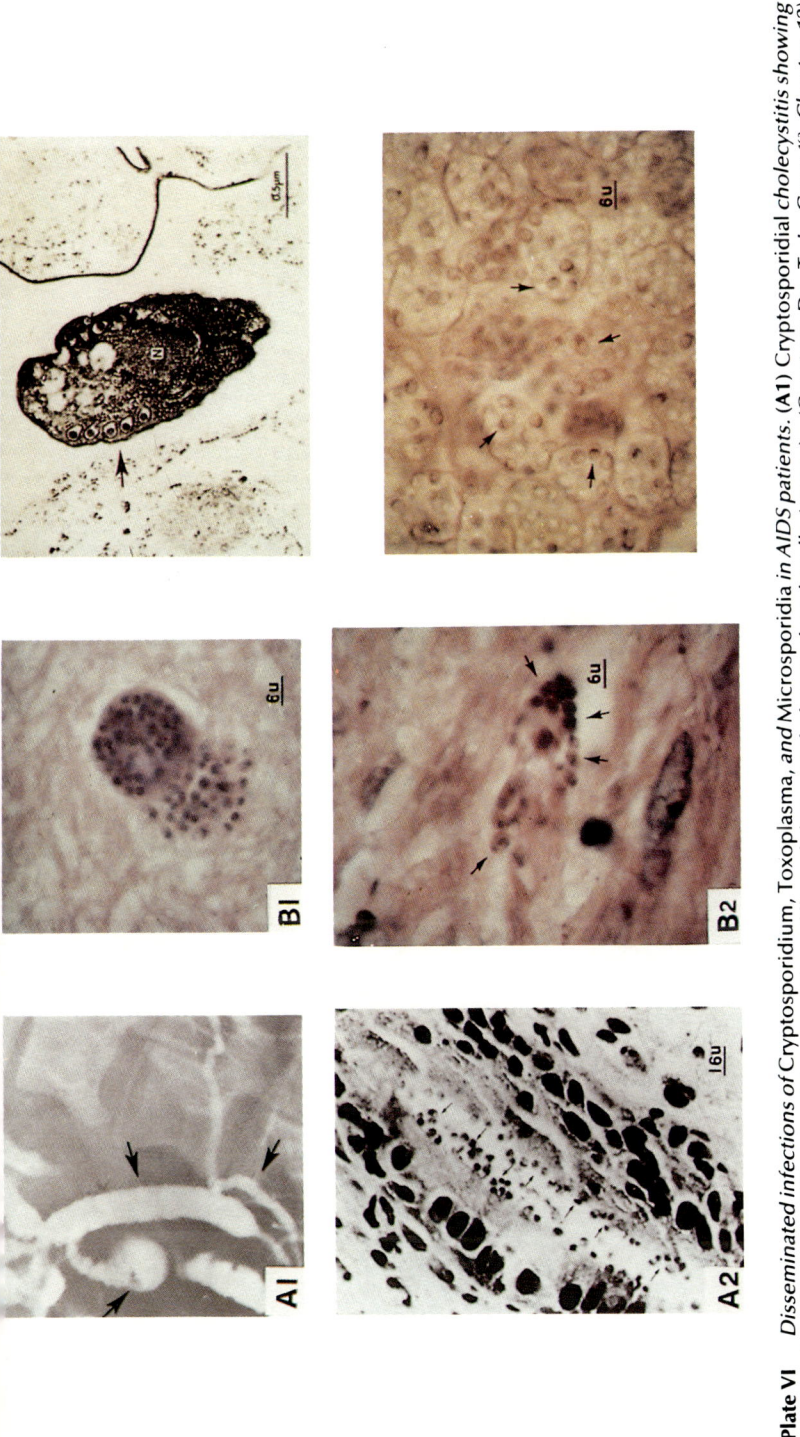

Plate VI *Disseminated infections of Cryptosporidium, Toxoplasma, and Microsporidia in AIDS patients.* **(A1)** *Cryptosporidial cholecystitis showing the small gallbladder, diffuse nodular intrabiliary filling defects, and shaggy ductal walls* (**arrows**). (Courtesy Dr. T. L. Gross,[163] Chapter 12) **(A2)** *Cryptosporidial hepatitis. Bile duct shown with numerous cryptosporidia* (**arrows**) *(hematoxylin-eosin stain) (480 ×).* (Courtesy Dr. D. G. Kahn,[162] Chapter 12) **(B1)** *Toxoplasma gondii cyst (liberating bradyzoites from a brain biopsy of an AIDS patient (hematoxylin-eosin stain) (500 ×).* **(B2)** *Toxoplasma gondii tachyzoites in the duodenum at autopsy (hematoxylin-eosin stain) (500 ×).* **(C1)** *Encephalitizoon cuniculi sporont containing a nucleus (N) and the cross-sections of the coiled polar tube (*) on each side of the posterior region of this parasite cell in the liver of a patient with AIDS (high-power electron microscope).* (Courtesy Dr. E. R. Schiff,[125] Chapter 12) **(C2)** *Pleistophora from a muscle biopsy showing clusters of spores surrounded by pansporoblastic membranes (hematoxylin-eosin stain) (1500 ×).* (Courtesy Dr. D. K. Ledford,[126] Chapter 12)

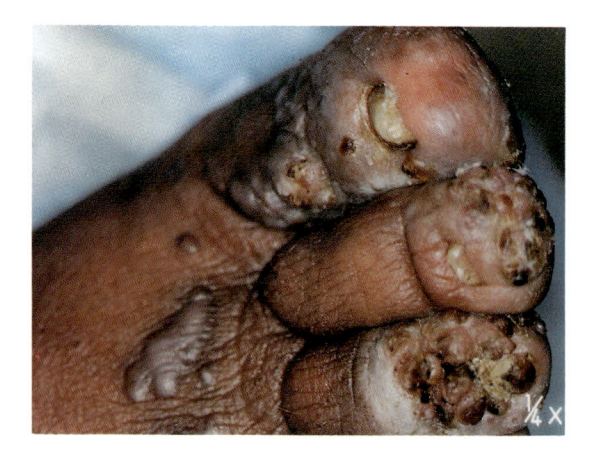

Plate VII *Violaceous nodules on the foot in classic Kaposi's sarcoma.*

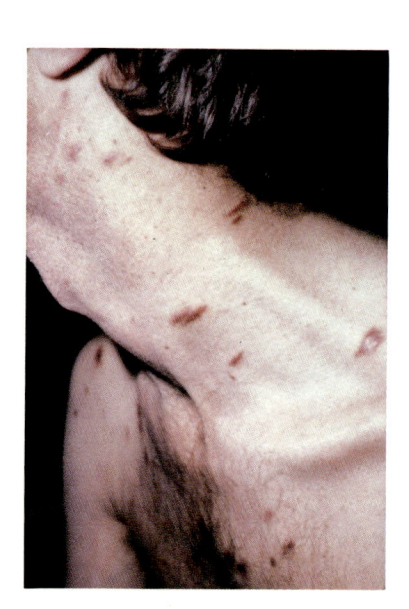

Plate VIII *Reddish purple oval papules in AIDS-associated Kaposi's sarcoma, following skin lines.*

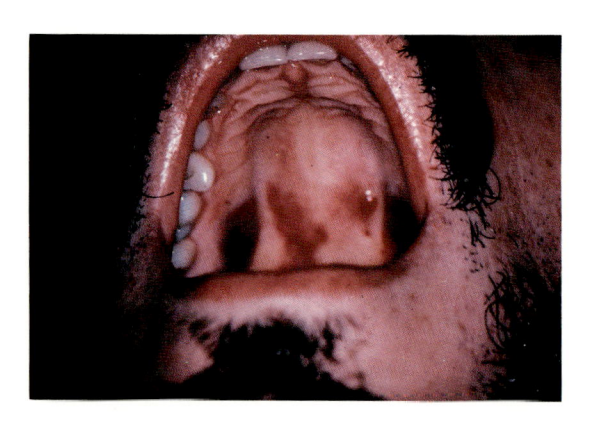

Plate IX *Reddish purple lesions in the oral cavity in AIDS-associated Kaposi's sarcoma.*

Table 12–7 Laboratory diagnosis of STD—Chlamydia infection (identification profile)

Specimens	
Transport for culture	Swabs, aspirates, scraping, pus, urine, biopsy material in transport medium (2SP) kept cold in wet ice/ice pack during transport for culture urine for antigen detection.
Transport for antigen	Direct smear: Direct immunofluorescent test (DFA). Roll swab on glass slide. Place a drop of acetone for fixative. Transport slide in slide container. EIA: place swab in transport medium containing preservative for the antigen, which remains stable at 4°C for 5–7 days.
Laboratory processing	
Pretreatment	If frozen, thaw quickly, agitating it in a 37°C H_2O bath. Tissue: Homogenize with antibiotic-supplemented cell culture medium or transport medium. Shake specimens with glass beads in transport medium to release elementary body before inoculation for culture. Sonication and filtration may improve the yield.[a]
Culture	
Cell cultures	McCoy cell, Hela 229, BHK 21 (C13) on coverslip/microtiter plate, pretreated with irradiation, IUdR, DEAE-D cytochalasin/cycloheximide to prevent cell replication.
Staining	To detect, intracytoplasmic *Chlamydia* inclusion.[25,26]

Methods	Direct Smear Preparation	Cell Culture (age, hr) Preparation	Staining Procedures (mins)	Sensitivity	Specificity
Fluorescent	Few seconds	18–40	30	Most	Most[14]
Giemsa		48–72	60	Moderate	Moderate
Iodine		48–72	15	Least	Least

Chlamydiazyme (Abbott Laboratories), IDEIA Chlamydia Test (Boots-Celltech Diagnostics Inc.).
[a]See Chapter 4.

however, the earliest time one can detect *Chlamydia* antigen is at approximately 48 hours by immunofluorescent test. A more rapid detection is available using monoclonal antibody against the major membrane protein of *C. trachomatis* in 18 hours by immunofluorescent test in microtiter culture plates.[26] Detection of inclusion by Giemsa stain followed by dark-field examination or glycogen by Jones iodine stain requires a longer turnaround time, from 48- to 72-hour-old cell culture.[25]

Contrary to the time-consuming culture technique, direct antigen test has slowly replaced culture as the preliminary diagnostic test, either by DFAT or EIA.

Nowadays a simple *Chlamydia* diagnostic kit (DFAT) provides the physician or other health care professional with a simple procedure to diagnose *Chlamydia* infection. The kit contains two types of swabs (one for males and one for females) to collect specimen, a slide attached to a slide container to smear the specimen, a small vial of acetone to fix the slide, and brief instructions for proper collection, handling, and transportation techniques. DFAT is easy to perform. Add anti-*Chlamydia* monoclonal antibody conjugated with isothiocyanate to the fixed slide. After 30 minutes of incubation at 37°C, wash the slide and coverslip for examination under a fluorescent scope with a 40X objective. Detection of EB as tiny green fluorescent dots free, in clusters, or on the surface of epithelial cells (stain red) is reported as positive (Plate IA). These reagents vary in sensitivity and specificity[27] according to manufacturer (e.g., Difco, Syva, Bartels, Ortho, and Organon).

EIA is the automated system that facilitates large-volume screening of specimens. Two methods are available: Chlamydiazyme (Abbott Laboratories) and IDEIA (Boots-Celltech Diagnostic, Inc.), which differ in principle and enzyme employment. Both require the collection of specimen in a special transport vial to preserve the antigen.

Chlamydiazyme is a *sandwich solid phase type* of assay. Add specimen to a specially treated bead in a microtiter plate at 37°C for 60 minutes. If *Chlamydia* is present, it will bind to the bead. Wash the bead of unbound antigen or other materials before adding polyclonal antibody to *Chlamydia*. After the second incubation at 37°C for 60 minutes, followed by washings, add a polyclonal antibody enzyme conjugate (goat-antirabbit-horseradish peroxidase) to the bead, which reacts with the antigen-antibody complex on the bead. Add O-phenylenediamine (OPD) containing hydrogen peroxide, the substrate for the horseradish peroxidase, resulting in a yellow-orange color due to enzyme reaction, which is stopped by adding 1N sulfuric acid after 30 minutes at 15° to 30°C. Absorbance is determined with a spectrophotometer. Positive and negative controls are provided to accompany each run. Overall test sensitivity is reported at 83.3%, and overall test specificity is 94.2%. One study stated that Chlamydiazyme is more sensitive but less specific than the direct smear test by DFAT (MicroTrak-Syva Co) but is better for detecting early infections.[28,29]

IDEIA *Chlamydia* test requires a 15-minute boiling of the specimen before it is added to a microplate coated with a monoclonal anti-*Chlamydia* antibody.

If *Chlamydia* is present, it will adsorb to the antibody during incubation. After excess unbound antigen is washed off, an enzyme-conjugated monoclonal antibody (alkaline phosphatase-anti-*Chlamydia* antibody) is added to each well to the "captured" antigen. Enzyme substrate is then added. This is followed by a second enzyme when the amplifier is added, producing a pink to red color. Color development is stopped by adding 3% weight by volume sulphuric acid. Color reaction is proportional to the quantity of chlamydial antigen initially bound in the well. Read absorbance using a spectrophotometer. Overall test sensitivity is reported at 92%, and overall test specificity is 98.4%.

Again, the success of laboratory diagnosis depends a great deal on knowing this organism's biologic properties to initiate proper collection, transport, and culture of clinical specimens. The pertinent information to those who have not handled laboratory requests for *Chlamydia* are summarized as follows: Table 12–5 for general information, Table 12–6 for specimen collection, and Table 12–7 for isolation techniques and identification profile. For instance, (1) Dacron swab is toxic to *Chlamydia*, and hence calgiswab is preferable; (2) because the organism is intracellular, vigorous scraping of the base of the lesion is needed to obtain inclusion-bearing cells; (3) to keep *Chlamydia* viable in the cellular components, tissue culture transport medium should contain serum (fetal calf/bovine) but not anti-*Chlamydia* agents such as tetracycline, erythromycin, or penicillin, which inhibit the agent in cell culture; (4) preparation of the infected site to collect specimen plays a major role in obtaining good results (see Table 12–6); (5) *Chlamydia* are heat labile, and hence the transport medium is best kept cool in wet ice or ice pack before and during transport, or stored at $-70°C$ if delay exceeds 24 hours; (6) before inoculation of monolayer cell culture, the cytoplasmic inclusion bodies must be released from the host cell by shaking the specimen with glass beads (commercially available in the transport medium vial) or by sonication and filtration (see Chapter 4); (7) inoculation of the monolayer followed by one-hour centrifugation at 33° to 35°C is necessary to concentrate the EB onto the small coverslip monolayer at the bottom of the 1 dram vial to enhance attachment and penetration; (8) a monolayer (McCoy, HeLa, BHK) pretreated with irradiation, cycloheximide, or cytochalasin will inhibit host cell metabolism and prime the cell to accept the EB more readily (see Table 12–7); (9) demonstration of *Chlamydia* in cell culture is by various stains depending on the age of the cell culture (see Table 12–7)[25,26]; (10) with the performance of any enzyme assay, specific optimal temperature for incubation must be maintained during the test, and reagents must be added accurately, with little deviation from specified time.

The microimmunofluorescent (MFI) test with monospecific antigens to detect antibody in serum[30] has proved more sensitive than complement fixation or enzyme-linked immunosorbent assay (ELISA) with group antigens. However, serologic testing has limited value in diagnosis of chlamydial infection except, perhaps, in invasive infection such as LGV. Concurrent gonorrhea, herpes, and syphilis in homosexual men with NGU is common, and hence laboratory tests to cover these agents are important.

Lymphogranuloma venereum. Lymphogranuloma venereum (LGV) is an STD caused by *C. trachomatis* L_1, L_2, L_3 and characterized by primary, painless, superficial ulcerative lesions at the site of inoculation, which may develop into secondary regional lymphadenopathy with fluctuant tender buboes involving the inguinal and sometimes femoral nodes.[31,32] The immunotypes L_1, L_2, and L_3 of *C. trachomatis* are similar to immunotypes A-K causing NGU described above, except that they can infect mucosal surfaces as well as being more invasive, causing systemic and destructive lesions. Ulcerative proctitis associated with mucopurulent discharge and perianal node involvement is increasingly seen in homosexual men. Oral infections without genital involvement have also been reported.[33] The laboratory diagnosis is essentially the same as for *C. trachomatis*, described above. The recovery rate of isolation of the agent depends on the methods used and the site of inoculum. Bubo biopsy/pus gives the following rate of detection: 98% in mouse brain, 78% in yolk sac, and only 24% to 30% in cell cultures.[31] Serologic tests for *Chlamydia* infection have been performed with group antigen with the complement fixation test. Because most patients visiting venereal disease clinics have titers of $\geq$ 1:16, elevated titer of $\geq$ 1:64 is usually regarded as the baseline for significant findings. To be more specific, the MIF test using antigen of specific immunotypes can be performed, but it is more time consuming. The MIF gives 4 to 15 times higher titers in LGV than in NGU caused by non-LGV *Chlamydia* strains. Proctitis caused by LGV may result in titers as high as 1:16,384.[33] False-positive tests may also be seen in non-LGV idiopathic epididymitis.

Ureaplasma urealyticum. *Ureaplasma urealyticum* is a *Mycoplasma* that grows well on New York City medium used to isolate gonococci and also in U broth and agar (see Tables 12–5 and 12–6). It was once called T strain *Mycoplasma* due to its characteristic tiny colonies when examined under bright-light microscopy. The organism is characterized by its use of urea, which explains the name *U. urealyticum*. There are at least 14 serotypes of *U. urealyticum*. Case-control studies indicate that urethral colonization is common in men without urethritis and is strongly correlated with the total number of female sex partners involved, while other studies suggest that some serotypes may play a pathogenic role in asymptomatic pyuria or urethritis.[31]

Syphilis

Syphilis is caused by *Treponema pallidum*. In the homosexual population, the chancres occur as painless indurated lesions usually found in the anal canal, oropharynx, lip, and external genitalia. Syphilis is frequently found concomitant with other STDs, especially hepatitis B in proctitis.[34] A 1987 report of four cases of neurosyphilis with HIV infection in one institution within 18 months may alert clinicians that "neurosyphilis may be an early infectious complication, or even the presenting one, in patients who subsequently have AIDS."[35] Laboratory tests to diagnose early infection for proper treatment of this treatable infection are crucial. The incidence of syphilis has decreased slightly since the encouragement of safe sex during the AIDS epidemic. Unfortunately, false negative results do occur.

Only two diagnostic methods are available: (1) demonstration of the spirochete by direct dark-field examination from the chancre/silver-stained tissue smear from an organ and (2) serologic tests. Culture of the organism is not available.

Direct Dark-Field Examination. A positive dark-field examination is the most definitive test, but it must be performed before treatment from a *primary* lesion. This lesion should be free of ointment or material that will interfere with the examination of the organism under the dark-field microscope. Remove surface contaminants with a sterile saline sponge. Place a coverslip over the lesion while it is being squeezed to allow serosanguineous fluid deep down in the lesion (and not blood) to be collected on the coverslip. If blood appears, remove it and repeat the collection. Examine the wet preparation immediately for thin, spiral spirochetes with tight coils. Nontreponemal spirochetes from the mouth, lip, or anal canal may present a problem in interpretation, and thus dark-field examinations should not be performed from these sites.

Serologic Tests. There are two groups of serologic tests. The nonspecific nontreponemal tests for presumptive screening test and for monitoring treatment responses include the reagin tests (Venereal Disease Research Laboratory [VDRL] and rapid plasma reagin [RPR]).[13] The specific treponemal tests microhemagglutination *T. pallidum* (MHA-TP), fluorescent *T. pallidum* absorption test (FTA-ABS), ELISA using treponemal antigen, and Nichols strain are for confirmation. Any titer is significant in the nontreponemal tests but must be confirmed by the treponemal tests to eliminate biologic false-positive results. Positive titers can be obtained between one and two weeks after the appearance of the chancre; MHA-TP detects a higher percentage of late syphilis, while FTA-ABS tends to give more positive tests in early syphilis. The FTA-ABS test may give false interpretation with autoimmune disease and Lyme disease. Apparently, this has not been reported in patients with HIV infection.[34] It is not recommended for use on spinal fluid. The VDRL and RPR are useful tests to monitor treatment with a slow disappearance of the titer, while treponemal tests remain positive for life.

Chancroid

The laboratory request for *Hemophilus ducreyi*, which causes chancroid, is extremely rare because of the lack of satisfactory clinical laboratory diagnostic procedures. Most diagnoses are made by clinical observation or by positive direct smear showing gram-negative coccobacilli arranged in chains, usually referred to as "school of fish," or clusters (see Plate IB). Recent new interest in the use of selective cultural medium with improved transport conditions may reverse the above condition. Laboratory diagnosis depends on appropriate specimen collection, transport, and growth conditions (Table 12–8). Chancroid (soft chancre) is characterized by the presence of single or multiple superficial, nonindurated, painful ulcers with bubo formation in the anogenital area. Approximately 50% of patients present with fluctuant unilateral inguinal lymphadenopathy. To avoid fistulae formation, aspirate the bubo for laboratory diagnosis through healthy

Table 12–8 Laboratory diagnosis of STD—Chancroid and granuloma inguinale

Causative Agent	Hemophilus ducreyi	Calymmatobacterium granulomatis
Infection	Chancroid (soft chancre)	Granuloma inguinale (donovanosis)
Infected site	Soft ulcerated lesion in anogenital area; bubo (fluctuant lymph node)	Ulcer at anus/perianal skin
Specimen collection	Scrape base of ulcer with cotton swab	Scrape base of ulcer with cotton swab
Direct smear	Gram: gram-negative coccobacilli in chain/intracellular (Plate IB)	Giemsa-capsulated bipolar bacilli in large cystic vacuole within macrophage
Direct transport cultural system	Chocolate agar/rabbit blood agar with vancomycin Transport in candle jar with moist paper towel to provide CO_2 and humidity	Embryonic egg by yolk sac route
Incubation	33° to 35°C	33° to 35°C
Identification profile	Colonies—small nonmucoid, translucent, can be pushed intact across the agar surface Oxidase, nitrate reduction, porphyrin test, alkaline phosphatase (+) Catalase, indole (−)	Death of embryo Giemsa smear shows capsulated, bipolar stained bacilli

adjacent normal skin. The organism thrives better in the presence of 3% to 5% CO_2 with 100% humidity; therefore, inoculate the specimen directly onto vancomycin (3%)-supplemented chocolate agar or rabbit-blood (5% defibrinated) agar and transport it in a candle jar (3% to 10% CO_2) with moist paper towel to provide 100% humidity. Incubate the culture at a lower temperature (33° to 35°C) for 48 hours before examination for the characteristic growth. Small, nonmucoid, gray, translucent colonies that can be pushed intact across the agar surface may appear in two to four days. The organism is identified by positive reactions in the oxidase, nitrate reduction, porphyrin, and alkaline phosphatase tests and negative reactions in the catalase and indole tests. An experimental EIA to detect serum IgG antibodies showed variable rates of sensitivity in different geographic areas. This may require a broader cross-reacting antigen for the test.[36]

Granuloma Inguinale

Granuloma inguinale, caused by *Calymmatobacterium granulomatis,* is another rare laboratory diagnostic request because of the lack of satisfactory cultural medium. The diagnosis is usually made clinically by direct Wright stained smear preparation of the inguinal/anal lesion, revealing large mononuclear cells containing capsulated rods called Donovan's bodies. The lesions may vary from irregular, nodular, indurated, sharply demarcated lesions with seropurulent foul-smelling discharge to hypertrophic necrotic lesions with tumorlike masses. Direct smear from tissue scraping of the lesions or by sections of a biopsy is the usual diagnostic procedure because the only culture technique available is by embryonic egg inoculation (see Table 12–8).

Parasitic Infections

Trichomoniasis

Trichomoniasis, caused by *Trichomonas vaginalis,* is usually asymptomatic in males but symptomatic in females. The trophozoite (no cyst stage has been reported) can be detected in urine or prostatic fluid. In the wet preparation of specimen, one can recognize the organism by the movement of its undulating membrane when examined under the low-power objective of light microscopy. The yield is higher in culture (modified Hollander medium) after incubation at 37°C overnight.

Parasitic Infestations

Sexually transmitted parasitic diseases are usually referred to as "minor" STDs. They include pediculosis and scabies.

Pediculosis (phthiriasis). The causative agent of pediculosis is *Phthirus pubis.* A contagious ectoparasitic infestation, it is caused by three types of lice: *Pediculus humanus* var. *capitis* (head louse), *P. humanus* var. *corporis* (body louse), and *Phthirus pubis* (pubic/crab louse). Only the pubic louse is transmitted sexually, through coitus or other intimate contact. Laboratory diagnosis has been detailed.[37]

Scabies. Scabies is an ectoparasitic infestation caused by *Sarcoptes scabieri,* a mite marked by characteristic pruritic skin lesions caused when the female mite excavates under the skin and forms serpiginous tunnels. Laboratory diagnosis has been detailed.[37]

Fungal Infections: Candidiasis

Candidiasis is caused by *Candida albicans.* Laboratory diagnosis is based on direct smear showing the oval budding yeasts with or without pseudohypha, which appear as white colonies with a yeast odor on Sabouraud dextrose agar and mycosel agar. *Candida* species can be identified by germ tube and various fermentation and assimilation tests.[13]

Viral Infections

The causative agents of viral infections are listed in Table 12–1.

Laboratory Diagnosis: Overview

Of all the viral genital infections, AIDS is the most devastating, with extremely high morbidity and mortality demanding immediate and urgent control measures to curb its worldwide distribution. A condensed general information of the diagnostic virologic work-up is listed in Table 12–9. Because of the AIDS epidemic, tremendous advances have been made in rapid and large-scale screening for viral agents, not only HIV but also opportunistic viruses. These are enzyme immunoassay (EIA), radioimmunoassay (RIA), immunoblotting assay (Western blot [WB]), and immunofluorescence (IF) using monoclonal antibody for specific virus. Last but not least is the rapid application of gene probes (DNA/RNA) in recombinant DNA and hybridization technologies in AIDS-associated diagnoses and research in virology to diagnose herpes simplex virus (HSV), cytomegalovirus (CMV), Epstein-Barr virus, (EBV), and human immunodeficiency virus (HIV): HIV-1 (Dupont) and HIV-2 (genetic system—Seattle). More of this is presented in the following sections.

An overview of virologic work-up in general, such as the biologic properties and growth cycle of viruses, procedures for direct demonstration of viral particles, isolation of viruses by tissue cultures, and various serologic tests to detect viral antigen and antibody are shown in Table 12–9. Specimen collection and transport are shown in Table 12–10, and the identification profile of each virus in STDs is briefly presented in Table 12–11. Plate II illustrates the schematic structure, genomes, serology, and Western blot (WB) of HIV, and Plate III shows the demonstration of HIV by electron microscopy, cell culture, IFA, plaque assay, and in situ hybridization.

AIDS

Human immunodeficiency virus (HIV), which causes AIDS, is an RNA retrovirus. It was discovered independently by Montagnier from the Institute of Pasteur[38] and Gallo from the National Cancer Institute.[39] HIV is a member of the nontransforming retrovirus group, formerly referred to as human T cell lymphotropic virus (HTLV-III)[39]/lymphadenopathy virus (LAV)[38] after the virus was repeatedly isolated from the blood of AIDS patients. Subsequent virus isolates are the AIDS-associated retrovirus (ARV), reported by Levy et al. in San Francisco[40] and Feorina et al. at CDC[41]; the Cambridge LAV (C-LAV) by Karpas et al. from the University of Cambridge, England[42]; and the LAV/NI from Volksy et al. in Nebraska.[43] All these viruses are reported isolates of HIV-1 when cocultivation technique was successful. During the last four years, pathogenesis of HIV has been widely investigated,[44] and a continuous vigorous attempt to curb this epidemic is of global importance. Other cofactors postulated to be involved in AIDS are discussed in Chapter 29.

Table 12–9 Laboratory diagnosis of viral infections—STDs and OIs (general information)[a]

Biologic properties
  DNA/RNA viruses, obligate parasites depending on eukaryotic cell growth.
  Heat labile, slow grower (exception—herpes simplex grows within 24 to 48 hours).
  Resistant to antibiotics, antiviral agents—acyclovir, arabinoside A, AZT.
  Multiplication depends on replication, appears as cytoplasmic/intranuclear inclusion bodies and other cytopathogenic effect (CPE).
  Growth: Tissue culture at 35°C, similar to *Chlamydia*.
  Growth cycle—viral particle: adsorption–penetration–replications = 48 hours–20 days or attachment, penetration-reverse transcription–replication–budding (retroviruses).
Specimen collection and transport (see Table 12–10)
Identification profile (see Table 12–11)
Direct smear preparation (see Table 12–11)
  Tzanck: alcohol-fixed, multinucleated giant cells with inclusions.
  Immunofluorescence (IFA): air dry, detects viral antigen as green fluorescent particles with monoclonal antibodies (HIV-1, HIV-1 p24, HTLV-I, CMV, EBV, HSV).
  Immunoperoxidase (IP): air dry, detect viral antigen as black grains.
  In situ hybridization: mononuclear cell prep. hybridized with a ^{35}S labeled HIV-specific RNA probe and exposed to autoradiography—intranuclear and intracytoplasmic black grains.
  Electron microscopy (EM): Fix in 2% to 4% phosphotungstic acid—detect virus particle in electron micrograph.
  Immuno electron microscopy (IEM): Viral antibodies present viral particles in clumps.
Tissue culture (TC)
  Primary monkey kidney (PMK), HeLa, rabbit kidney (RK), human embryonic lung fibroblast (HELF), human embryonic kidney, human amnion cells HEp-2 cells; immortal permissive cell lines such as H9 cells, Molt 4, MT2, MT4, CEM, CR3, and primary cocultivation of mononuclear cells etc. for HIV.
Serologic tests (see Table 12–11)
  Complement fixation, neutralization, hemagglutination inhibition (HI), immune adherence, passive hemagglutination (PHA) tests.
  ELISA (EIA): to detect Ab or Ag.
  Western blot: to detect Ab for HIV-1 and HIV-2.
  IFA: to detect Ag for HIV-1 and HIV-2;
    : to detect Ab for EBV.[a]
  Recombinant technology: Recombinant Ag (gp120, gp41) to detect HIV Ab.
  Nucleic acid probe (radioactive/non-radioactive): to detect DNA/RNA for HIV-1/HIV-2.
  Radioimmunoassay (RIA): to detect Ag for HIV, HBsAg, HAV.

[a]EBV antigens: EB-VCA, Epstein-Barr viral capsid antigen; EBNA, Epstein-Barr nucleoantigen; EA-R, restricted early antigen; EA-D, diffuse early antigen; HIV-1 and HIV-2, human immunodeficiency virus type 1 & type 2; CMV, cytomegalovirus; HSV-1 and HSV-2, herpes simplex virus type 1, type 2; HBVsAg, hepatitis B virus surface antigen; HBVcAg, hepatitis B virus core antigen; HAV, hepatitis A virus. Manufacturers: Abbott Diagnostics, Dupont, Electron Nucleonics, Gull, Wampole Inc.
AZT: azidothymidine.
Ag: antigen.

Table 12-10 Laboratory diagnosis of viral infections—STDs and OIs (specimen collection and transport)

Viruses	Respiratory	Rectal–Genital–Urinary	Blood/Fluid	Other Biopsy	Collection and Transport[b]
HIV-1	Sputum, bronchoalveolar lavage (BAL), lung tissue	Semen, urine, vaginal secretion, tissue (placenta, rectal, renal)	Blood/fluid, serum	Brain, LN, cornea	Transport medium (BSS[a] with 0.5% gelatin/calf serum. Keep cold in wet ice; if delay in processing, store at −70°C and not at −20°C.
HIV-2			Blood/fluid		
Hepatitis A/B virus			Serum	Liver	Same as above
Non-A, Non-B virus			Serum		Same as above
HSV-1 and HSV-2	Throat swab, mouth washing, BAL, lung biopsy	Same as above	Serum, buffy coat		Same as above, vesicle
CMV	Same as above	Same as above	Buffy coat	Kidney, salivary gland, GI tract, CSF, retina, pericardium, myocardium	Same as above
Adenovirus	Same as above, bronchial wash, lung biopsy	Same as above		Colon contents	Same as above
Varicella zoster			Serum, vesicular fluid	Vesicular lesion	Same as above
EBV	Same as above		Serum	LN, CNS	Same as above
Pox virus				Genital wart	
Papilloma virus				Anal wart	

[a] Paired sera (acute phase—not later than three days after onset, convalescent phase two to three weeks later).
[b] For culture.
LN, Lymph node.

Table 12–11 Laboratory diagnosis of STDs—Nondiarrheal viral infections (identification profile[a])

Viruses	Direct Smear Examination	Tissue Culture	Serology	Comment
Retrovirus HIV-1	EM: 100–120 nm cube, free/budding from host cell membrane, cylindrical structure present	Primary cocultivation, with mononuclear cells/ with immortal cell lines: H9, CR10, CEM Detects HIV by RT/IFA/ EIA/EM/in situ hybridization	Serum/plasma HIV-1 Ab (EIA+)[a] confirmed by (WB+) (protein bands p24, p31, and either gp41/gp160 or by RIP HIV Ag (EIA +)	Serologic evidence of previous exposure to HIV or current infection or Early exposure to HIV/at terminal infection
HIV-2	Identify HIV-2 DNA by HIV-2 specific DNA probe with DNA amplification by polymerase chain reaction technique	Same as above	HIV-1 Ab (EIA −)[a] WB for HIV-1 (indeterm)[a] WB for HIV-2(+) gag(p26), pol(p34) and env gp(140) present	HIV-2 infection
Herpesviruses HSV-1 and -2 Nonspecific type	EM: 150 nm enveloped particle Tzanck direct smear Hemacolor stain (™<1 minute)	Primary cell cults/cell lines Primary rabbit kidney cells, human amnion cells, human diploid fibroblast, HeLa	Complement fixation test, IFA test Latex aggl. test Immunoperoxidase test EIA test for Ag detection	Fourfold rise in titers; acute/reactivation infection Most of these tests are not sensitive for diagnosis in

Table 12–11 (continued)

Viruses	Direct Smear Examination	Tissue Culture	Serology	Comment
	Intranuclear (IN) Inclusion bodies (IB) Immunoperoxidase test (IP) (2 hours): rust color (IN, IB) IFA test (2 hours) with monoclonal antibodies HSV-1 and HSV-2 Nonradioactive NA probe applied to direct smear, paraffin tissue section/cells in transport medium	Vero cells, etc. CPE: rounding up of cells, eosinophilic, intranuclear inclusions in human amnion cells within 2–3 days (Cowdry type A) inclusions Large ground glass nucleus (early), eosinophilic IN inclusion (late) Test for viral Ag (IFA/IP) Typing: Type 1 Type 2 EE-CAM pock pock (Tiny) (Large) CCS-chick cell (−) (+) G pig cell (+) (+) BVDU + (−) (+) − (+) (+) BA-FA (+) or (+) (specific)		AIDS patients Primary rabbit kidney cells, human amnion cells, human diploid fibroblast, Vero cells, etc.

Virus	Morphology/Detection	Propagation	Serologic tests/Markers	Clinical significance
Hepatitis viruses				
Hepatitis A virus (HAV) (Enterovirus 72?)	EM: 27–32 nm cube	Propagation is difficult, low sensitivity. A new replicating virus, that grows out in three days, can be used to test for neutralizing anti-HAV	EIA, RIA HAV Ab (+) Anti HAV − IgM(+) Total anti-HAV-IgG(+)	Incubation period Acute infection Recovery period
HBV (Dane particle)	EM: 42 nm double enveloped particle HBsAg—surface antigen, HBcAg—core antigen, HBeAg—e antigen Detects by IFA/IP/EM/ nonradiometric synthetic NA probe	Not available	EIA/RIA/LA/NA probe Six serologic markers: HBeAg, HBsAg, anti-HBc total anti-HBc, anti-HBe, & anti-HBs HBsAg, HBeAg (+) HBsAg, HBeAg, anti-HBc-IgM, and total anti-HBc(+) Anti-HBc-IgM, total anti-HBc, and anti-HBe(+) HBsAg, total HBc (+) and HBeAg, anti-HBc-IgM anti-HBe (+/−) Above tests all (−)	Incubation period Acute phase Convalescent phase Chronic infection
Hepatitis Non-A, Non-B virus (NANBV)	IEM: 27 nm virus particle inside hepatocyte	Not available		Diagnosed by exclusion[a] Liver biopsy-bridging nucleus necrosis and abnormal AAL after transfusion
Hepatitis D (HDV)	35 nm double-shelled virus particle HDV Ag in liver	Not available	RIA, EIA Anti-delta agent $<10^2$ $>10^2$ Anti-D-IgM, HBsAg, anti-HBc-IgM, HBeAg(+)	Acute infection Chronic infection Acute HBV and acute HDV coinfections

Table 12-11 (continued)

Viruses	Direct Smear Examination	Tissue Culture	Serology	Comment
Poxvirus	300 nm × 200 nm × 100 nm brick-shaped particle. Hematoxylin-eosin molluscum body—eosinophilic hyaline spherical mass in cells of stratum malpighii of the epidermis Giemsa-stained preparation—large characteristic cytoplasmic inclusion body of the lesion			Diagnostic of *Molluscum contagiosum*
Papilloma virus	45–55 nm Hematoxylin-eosin section—acanthosis and papillomatosis Basophilic intranuclear inclusion bodies		Ag test—IP	Diagnostic of *Condyloma acuminatum*

[a]HIV-2 gene probe (Genetic Systems Corporation, Seattle). (+) reactive, (−) nonreactive, (indeterminate) insufficient number of bands/specific types of bands missing.
HIV-1: antibody, antigen test (EIA), WB and non-radioactive synthetic NA probe (Dupont); antibody, antigen tests (Abbott); antibody (Nucleo Electronic).
HSV: Auszyme II (Abbott Laboratories), Cordia H (Cordis Corp, Miami, Fla), Organon's Hepanostika (Europe).
Ag, antigen; Ab, antibody; EM, electron microscopy; IP, immunoperoxidase test; IFA, indirect fluorescent test; PMK, primary monkey kidney; CPE, cytopathic effect; EE, embryonic egg; CF, complement fixation test; IaD, immune adherence test; IB, inclusion body; CAM, chorioallantoic membrane; BVDU, E-5-(2bromovinyl)-2-deoxyuridine; BA-FA, biotin-aridin fluorescent antibody test; RIA, radioimmunoassay; EIA, enzyme immunoassay; IgG, immunoglobulin G; IgM, immunoglobulin M; PHA, passive hemagglutination; CCS, cell culture selection; IN, intranuclear; G. pig, guinea pig.

Although HIV has been isolated from patients with AIDS and AIDS-related complex (ARC), diagnosis of AIDS is based mostly on clinical presentation[45] and detection of HIV antibody by EIA, which is the accepted standard test worldwide.[2,52] Recently, HIV antigen detection[3] has been introduced, and it has been shown that patients in high-risk groups demonstrate antigen in the blood one to two years before the antibody is detected. Although still a research tool and not approved for standard screening of blood donors, HIV antigen testing is important in closing the diagnostic "window" between infection and antibody production. Isolation of HIV in culture is still in its infancy,[38–43,46–51] and only research centers and some large medical centers do it routinely for several reasons: (1) fear of the virus among laboratory personnel; (2) problem of confidentiality; (3) physical set-up, requiring a biosafety cabinet to process specimens with possible presence of HIV; (4) lack of persons trained to perform not only the tissue culture but to detect the virus by reverse transcriptase,[46,49] cocultivation,[38–43,50] electron microscopy,[38,39] RIA,[46] and immunoprecipitation[48]; and (5) cost. Recent advances, such as the indirect immunofluorescent test[41,43,52] and antigen capture assay (EIA)[46,53] are less cumbersome and less time consuming to set up and may pave the way for more clinical virology laboratories to offer this type of service to patients.

Currently, diagnosis of HIV infection (primarily of HIV-1, with only one documented case of HIV-2 in the United States)[54] can be established by a combination of the following procedures (see Tables 12–9 to 12–11 and Plates II and III).

HIV Serology. Serologic tests currently available for HIV are the antibody test by EIA[2] confirmed by Western blot[2,52,55] and the antigen capture assay[3,53] for earlier diagnosis, used in research. There are two strains of HIV, designated HIV-1 and HIV-2. HIV-1 is associated with the AIDS testing in the United States, and HIV-2 is associated with AIDS in east Africa and Europe. In 1988, the first documented case of HIV-2 infection in the United States was detected in a woman visiting New Jersey from West Africa.[54] Her serum, when tested for HIV antibody with HIV-1 antigen, was negative with an indeterminate Western blot but positive when a DNA amplification technique for HIV-2 was used.[54]

In 1983, Gallo et al. demonstrated that over 90% of AIDS and ARC patients were seropositive for antibodies to HIV from 1000 sera tested.[39] One year later, the Volksy and Sonnabend group reported that 100% of homosexual and bisexual individuals with AIDS or ARC from Greenwich Village, New York City, had HIV antibody (69% with lymphadenopathy syndrome (LAS), 31% asymptomatic). No heterosexual individuals tested positive at the beginning of the AIDS epidemic.[43] Current studies conducted in the United States on various segments of the population are now providing data on the incidence of HIV infection in the general population: hospital inpatients, 0.37%; hospital outpatients, 0.18%; Massachusetts infants, 0.23%; California women (premarital), 0.53%; California STD clinic, 0.67%; military applicants (total), 0.15%; and military applicants (> 26 years), 0.41%. A conservative assumption of the rate of HIV infection in the United States would be 0.15%.[56] Since these figures were based on antibody test alone, the true incidence may be much higher if antigen capture assay is included to detect early cases of AIDS.

Antibody Test

EIA[2,57] is the widely used mandatory procedure for blood screening for HIV-1 antibody in blood banks across the United States. Confirmatory tests are Western blotting, IFA, and radioprecipitation (RIP) assay.

Briefly, EIA (ELISA) is a *solid phase sandwich type enzyme immunoassay* in which the solid phase (polystyrene bead/well of microtiter plate) is coated with the HIV antigen (HIV propagated in T lymphocyte cell line H9/HTLV III_B) and is disrupted and inactivated with detergent and sonication before coating the solid phase. The patient's diluted specimen (serum/plasma) is added to the antigen for incubation in a $40° \pm 2°C$ water bath for one hour. Three known positive and two known negative sera are assayed for each run. HIV antibody IgG will bind to the solid phase. After washing off excess unbound antibody, goat antibody to human IgG conjugated with horseradish peroxidase (antihuman IgG:HRPO) is added for another hour of incubation at $40° \pm 2°C$. After washing off the beads/microtiter plate to remove unbound conjugate, the substrate O-phenylenediamine (OPD) solution containing hydrogen peroxide is added, and after 30 minutes of incubation at room temperature in the dark, a yellow-orange color develops in proportion to the amount of antibody to HIV, which is bound to the bead/microtiter well and is determined in the spectrophotometer with a substrate blank set at 492 nm. it is important to use a nonhemolyzed specimen to avoid getting inconsistent test results.

Samples considered positive after testing should be retested to establish whether they are repeatably reactive (e.g., Abbott Laboratories, Dupont, Genetic systems, ENI). All repeated reactive sera should be further confirmed with Western blot,[55,57] IFA,[59] or RIP.[57]

Western Blot

All sera proved to be reactive by duplicate test with EIA should be further documented with Western blot (immunoblot).[55,57] In this test, lysates of HIV producer cell clones are subjected to electrophoresis under reducing conditions on preparative sodium dodecyl sulfate (SDS)–polyacrylamide slab gels and electroblotted to nitrocellulose sheets. The sheets are cut into strips to be used for the Western blot assay. Currently, these strips are available commercially [HTLV-III immunoblot kit, Bio-Rad Laboratories, Richmond, CA; Biotech/Dupont HIV Western Blot kit (approved by FDA), Wilmington, DE]. Each strip, placed in a reaction tray (trough), is added to 0.5 ml human serum (1:100) to be tested. After incubation for one hour at room temperature with gentle agitation on a rotator, the strip is washed thoroughly with PBS, pH 7.4, supplemented with 10% Tween 80. Development process is of two types: chemical incubation (biotin-avidin test) and plates to reveal radioactivity strip (RIA). The former is more commonly used in laboratories, and thus the latter will not be discussed here.

Visualization of the specifically bound human immunoglobulins to HIV proteins is performed using a goat-antihuman immunoglobulin biotin conjugate, and avidin-horseradish peroxidase conjugate, with 4-chloro-1-naphthol as substrate. Bands visible on the strip represent different HIV proteins (see Plate IID). Biotech/Dupont uses a biotin-avidin system to enhance signal amplification. A conjugate of biotin-labeled goat anti-IgG binds readily to antigen-antibody complexes on the strip, and a Biotech/Dupont horseradish peroxidase-avidin (HRP-avidin) conjugate with its exceptionally high affinity for biotin tags these complexes. In most cases HIV seropositivity is defined by the presence of at least anti-p24 and anti-gp41. Recently, in the Food and Drug Administration (FDA)-approved Dupont strip, a showing of p24, p31, and either gp41 or gp160 is regarded as reactive. Most blots with positive results will have other virus-specific bands present; including p17, p51, p66, and gp120, while a lack of p31 in a *low-risk person* is read as indeterminate. Indeterminate samples are retested, and follow-up samples should be requested to check for validity.[55] No bands present is regarded as negative. Reactive strip, nondeterminative strip, and nonreactive strip are shown in Plate IID. Strips containing HIV IgG or IgM for WB are available commercially from Dupont. WB with recombinant derived p41 had been reported.[60] To replace the time-consuming Western blot assay, immunofluorescent test using HIV infected cells proves to give 100% correlation to Western blot.[59] More of this is presented in the discussion on cell culture below.

Because of the lack of control standard reagent for various laboratories to use, small discrepancies of serologic testings for HIV vary from laboratory to laboratory. CDC urges that "quality laboratory testing for HIV antibody is a critically important element for surveillance and detection of HIV infection. The laboratory testing process requires quality assurance for (1) collection, labelling and transport of specimens; (2) laboratory reagents and procedures; (3) interpretation of analytical results; and (4) communication from the laboratory scientist to the clinician and then to the person being tested."[55,57,58]

RIP is one of the standard assays used to confirm the presence of HIV antibodies to various proteins. HIV is grown in cell culture in the presence of a radioactive label, purified, and disrupted. Test serum is added to the material, isolated by precipitation, washed, resolved electrophoretically, and developed to show the radioactive pattern. A control is set up from uninoculated cell culture[57] (see Chapter 13).

Antigen Test

Another development is the antigen capture assay. One report showed that AIDS was diagnosed in one patient three months after HIV-Ag was first detected in serum and six months after seroconversion. Antigenaemia had been shown to be accompanied by the disappearance of IgG antibody reactivity to the major HIV core protein p24[3,53] (Plate IIC) indicating that HIV-Ag appears early and transiently in primary HIV infection. Antibody production follows, after which HIV-Ag may disappear. Its persistence or reappearance seems to correlate with clinical, immunologic, and neurologic deterioration.[3]

For screening, use the *solid phase sandwich technique* similar to EIA, described above for the HIV-ab test. Add polystyrene beads/wells coated with *HIV antibody* to undiluted serum or plasma. After an overnight incubation (16-20 hrs) at room temperature, wash off excess unbound antigen and add rabbit anti-HIV-IgG. Follow this with a four-hour incubation at 40°C; after removing excess antibody, add goat anti-rabbit antibody conjugated with peroxidase. After two hours of incubation at 40°C, wash the plate. Add substrate OPD, as with the *HIV antibody test* described above. After 30 minutes of incubation at room temperature in the dark, stop the reaction by 1N H_2SO_4. Read the absorbance at 492 nm with the dual wavelength spectrophotometer. The presence or absence of HIV antigen(s) is determined by relating the absorbance of the specimen to a cut-off value. The cut-off value is the absorbance of the negative control mean plus the factor 0.050. Specimens with absorbance values greater than or equal to the cut-off value are considered reactive for HIV antigen(s). Specimens with absorbance values less than the cut-off value are considered nonreactive for HIV antigen(s) by the criteria of the test. For the test to be valid, the difference between the means of the positive and negative controls (P-N) should be 0.400 or greater. If not, the technique may be suspect and the run must be repeated. If the P-N is consistently low, deterioration of reagents may exist.

Similarly, HIV antigen from tissue culture fluid can likewise be checked, except that the culture fluid must be inactivated by 5% Triton 100× before testing. Three negative and two positive controls must be assayed with each run, plus an additional three-cell culture control from uninfected cell culture. Comparative study with reverse transcriptase (RT) activity shows that it is 100 times more sensitive than RT and is less time consuming. A shorter test requiring only five hours has been shown to be compatible with the result of the long method except that the reactive result is less intense (Dupont).

Preliminary study of cerebrospinal fluid (CSF) HIV antibody was carried out at St. Vincent's Hospital and Medical Center of New York on 87 patients with neurologic symptoms. Findings revealed that 72 of 87 (83%) were positive for HIV antibody. Antigen and antibody assays were conducted on 47 patients. Of these, 15% had both antigen and antibody present, 68% had only antibody, and 17% were negative for both. HIV antibody was present in all cases but one of cerebral OI, and in all cases of neoplasm, HIV encephalitis, and myelitis. HIV antigen, however, was present in none of the neoplasms but in approximately one-third of the other groups.[61]

To study the time occurrence of specific markers following infection, one can use CIA-RA technology (Abbott Laboratories). CIA-RA (Abbott Laboratories) is a competitive immunoassay employing as antigen recombinant-DNA-produced HIV proteins. Antibodies from the patient sample compete for binding to the selected antigen coated on the beads with a standardized preparation of purified polyclonal human anti-HIV IgG labeled with horseradish peroxidase.

The antigen employed is recombinant-DNA (rDNA)envelope/core to determine the sequential appearance of these antibodies in AIDS/ARC and asymptomatic homosexual men (Abbott Laboratories).[53,60] Polystyrene beads are coated with purified human anti-HIV IgG and mixed with purified rDNA envelope (entire gp41, a small portion of gp120)/core protein (p15, p17 adjacent to p24) expressed in *Escherichia coli*. Each antigen is coated on a separate bead so that antibodies to core or envelop can be detected specifically. Briefly, 50µl of patient serum with 20 µl of diluent and 200 µl of antibody to envelop or core conjugated with horseradish peroxidase are added to the rDNA envelope- or core antigen-coated bead. Incubate it at room temperature. Wash the bead three times with distilled water and transfer it into an assay tube. Add 300 µl of freshly prepared o-phenylenediamine and incubate it for 30 minutes at room temperature. Stop color development by adding 1 ml molar sulphuric acid. Measure absorbance at 492 nm in a Quantum dual-wavelength spectrophotometer. A result is positive when the optical density is lower than the calculated cut-off value. This value is the absorbance of the mean of two positive controls plus the mean of two negative controls divided by two.[53] In one study, the presence of HIV anticore (anti-p24) and anti-envelope antibodies (anti-gp41) were assessed by both Western blot and CIA-RA. All positive samples were CIA-RA-envelope-antibody positive, while in 5 of 69 positive samples (7.2%) with Western blot were negative.[60] The apparent sequence of markers in ARC/AIDS patients is HIV Ag, antibody to envelope, followed by antibody to core (Plate IIC).[53]

Direct Demonstration of HIV. Direct demonstration of HIV from lesion/cell cultures can be performed with electron microscopy or the recent advances of using in situ hybridization, described below. For electron microscopy, fix clinical specimens in 1% glutaldehyde and process by the standard procedure for virology. The virus is an RNA retrovirus with 100 to 120 nm spherical virion containing the characteristic cylindric structure. The virus is either free or seen budding from the host cell (Plate IIIF).

HIV Culture. HIV has been isolated from blood, CSF, brain tissue, lymph node, tears, urine, semen, vaginal secretion, breast milk, alveolar fluid, synovial fluid,[58] placenta,[62] and even retina.[63] The growth medium used is RPRI 1640 (Roswell Park Memorial Institute) supplemented with glutamine, activated fetal calf serum, streptomycin, penicillin, and fungizone. A P-3 level type of biologic safety cabinet (ducted out) is required to handle a large volume of infective materials, and protective clothing with gloves and masks are needed for laboratory workers to avoid self-contamination. Sodium hypochlorite (bleach), 1:5 dilution, is effective in inactivating the virus[64] in case of spill in laboratory work.[58]

HIV causes cytopathic effects in the target cells, causing the cells to balloon out and form syncytium (multinucleated giant cell with multiple nuclei arranged in a characteristic ring formation) (Plate IIIA). One of the hallmarks of HIV infection is the depletion of T4 cells due to cell death from the cytolytic effect of HIV seen in primary cell culture from patients with AIDS/ARC.

Two methods of culturing HIV have been used with success. One is the cocultivation technique[39,47,51] which involves feeding the cell culture depleted of T cells with immortal cell lines, which are highly susceptible to and permissive for cytopathic variants of HIV.[43,65–68] The detection of HIV in cell culture can be achieved by (1) the presence of reverse transcriptase activity,[46,48,49,69] (2) antigen capture assay of culture fluid,[46,52,69] (3) immunofluorescence of infected cells[39,40,59,67] with known positive HIV serum from patients with AIDS/ARC (Plate IIIA) or monoclonal antibody to HIV core protein p24 (Dupont), (4) electron microscopy (Plate IIIF), (5) plaque assay of viral particle[69] (Plate IIIC), and (6) in situ hybridization (Plate IIID and E).

The cocultivation technique involves the preparation of two types of lymphocytes, one from a normal individual free of HIV antibody/antigen and HSV and the other from a patient suspected of having AIDS/ARC.[39,46,50,51] The peripheral blood can be collected in a vacutainer tube containing heparin. Approximately 200 ml of heparinized blood or plasma will yield approximately 2 to 6 $\times 10^8$ lymphocytes by the Ficoll-Hypaque gradient centrifugation, a lymphocyte separation medium (LSM). Centrifugation of LSM and blood mixture at 400 $\times$ gravity for 20 minutes will separate the mixture into four different layers (top layer, plasma and platelets; interface, mononuclear leukocytes; layer below interface, LSM; bottom layer, red blood cells [RBCs] and granulocyte deposit). The mononuclear leukocytes are removed from the interface, and after a washing with PBS pH 7.4, the cell pellet is suspended in growth medium (RPMI 1640, 20% inactivated fetal bovine serum, and 0.29 mg of glutamine/ml) containing phytohemagglutinin P (PHA-P, 0.1%) and incubated at 37°C in a 5% CO_2 atmosphere. PHA-P stimulates T cells to express T4 receptor sites, which HIV recognizes before infecting the cells. A final concentration of approximately 2 $\times 10^7$ cells/ml can be obtained within two to three days incubation. Approximately 0.5 ml of this cell culture can be added to lymphocyte culture from an AIDS patient.

The lymphocytes from AIDS/ARC patients are prepared as above, except the cell pellet is suspended in a growth medium without PHA: it contains interleukin-2 (IL-2), which stimulates growth of T4 cells; DEAE, which enhances infection of T4 by HIV, and antihuman interferon A, which counteracts activity of interferon. Cell cultures are checked for growth by performing the viable count with 0.4% trypan blue (0.1 ml culture fluid in 0.1 ml trypan blue). Viable cells are colorless, while dead cells stain blue. This is performed twice a week, and cell cultures are readjusted with fresh medium to give 1 $\times$ 10^5/ml.[51] Multinucleated giant cells (syncytium) shown with multiple nuclei in a characteristic ring formation (Plate IIIB) are visible in six- to 14-day-old cultures but not in giant cells in uninfected cells.[47,51] Cultures are observed for one month before being classified as negative. Detection of HIV can be carried out with IFA, RT, antigen capture assay, and electron microscopy.

The other method of culturing HIV is to use immortal cell lines. In 1984, Popovic found a cell line HT, a neoplastic aneuploid T cell line derived from an adult with lymphoid leukemia that is highly susceptible to and permissive for cytopathic effects of HIV. It can grow permanently after infection with the virus, and this immortalized T cell population with its clones (e.g., H9) have been used in the isolation and continuous high-level production of HIV from patients with AIDS and ARC.[47] Other cell lines isolated are (1) CCRF-CEM T cell line, developed from EBV-transformed B lymphoblastoid cell lines by Montagnier[65]; (2) Molt 4,[39,66] (3) CEM/LAV-NR2, a constitutive HIV producer line from CEM that does not require frequent "feeding" with uninfected CEM cells and is 100% viable, 100% positive for LAV antigens and very suitable for IFA studies[43]; (4) CR-10, another clone of CEM isolated by the Volksy group that is easy to use for IFA[67]; (5) MT2 and MT4 cell lines, which carry HTLV-1 but strongly express OKT4 surface antigens, were established from cord blood lymphocytes that had been cocultured with leukemic cells from patients with adult T cell leukemia[70]; and (6) C3, a clone from CEM, another immortal cell that grows rapidly and can generate high yield of HIV within a short time.[68] The advantage of these cell lines, especially CR10, is the easy attainment of cells for IFA or high yield of HIV for other assays, while MT-2 has the ability to attach to the plastic surface of the petri plate. This facilitates the use of these cells for plaque assay of HIV[70,71] (Plate IIIC).

Detection of HIV in cell culture can be carried out with RT, antigen assay, IFA, electron microscopy, plaque assay, and in situ hybridization.

1. *Reverse transcriptase (RT)*. RT is an enzyme that catalyzes transcription of its genetic code from its RNA genome to double-stranded DNA in all retroviruses. During transcription, the tritium-labeled thymidine is incorporated into the DNA. The DNA is trapped on the filter, and the labeled unincorporated thymidine washes through. Thus the level of DNA with tritium-labeled thymidine (radioactivity) indicates RT activity. Values of 10,000 to 40,000 cpm/0.4 ml suggests the presence of HIV in the specimen.[51]

2. *Immunofluorescence (IFA)*. RT assay is time consuming and not specific for HIV, since it is present in all retrovirus cultures. It has been compared with Western blot to detect HIV antibodies as a confirmatory test with good results.[59] Also, it has been used by various investigators to detect HIV in the cell cultures described above. We have been very successful in using CR-10 (courtesy Dr. D. Volksy) for IFA, since these lytic-resistant cells give a high yield of HIV more rapidly than H9. Cells from a five- to ten-day-old culture are washed with phosphate-buffered saline (PBS), pH 7.4, and resuspended in the same buffer at concentration 10^6/ml. With a micropipette tip, 10 μl cell suspension is spotted on a 12-well slide, air dried, and fixed in ice-cold acetone at $-20°C$ for 15 minutes. Slides can be stored at $-20°C$ until use. An equal volume of PBS-diluted patient serum is applied to cells and incubated for 30 minutes at 37°C. The goat fluorescein-conjugated antiserum to human immunoglobulin G is diluted and applied to the fixed cells for 30 minutes at room temperature. Slides are then washed extensively before microscopic examinations under EPI fluorescent scope. The infected cells are visible with bright green fluorescence (Plate IIIA), while the

uninfected cells are negative in this assay. Anticomplementary immunofluorescence has also been used to detect HIV antigen and antibody.[72] Monoclonal antibodies for gp120, p24, and p17 are available commercially (Dupont).

3. *Electron microscopy (EM)*. Viral particles are demonstrated by standard electron microscopy procedure.

4. *Plaque assay (PA)*. Quantitation of HIV by plaque-forming assay was developed by Harada and Yamamoto.[70] HTLV-I positive MT4 cell in suspension culture (150×10^4/ml) is chemically adhered to the poly-L-lysine-treated petri plate to serve as the monolayer. The monolayer is then seeded with HIV-infected cells (Molt-4/HTLV-III, H9/HTLV-III, or CEM/LAV). After one hour of incubation at 22°C, the plate is washed twice to remove unbound cells and is then overlaid with agarose-containing nutritional medium (RMPI 1640 medium, 10% heat inactivated fetal calf serum, 100 IU/ml penicillin, 100 μg/ml streptomycin, 0.6% agarose [Sea Plaque Agarose, Marine Colloid Corp., Rockland, ME]). The plate is incubated at 37°C with 5% CO_2 for three days before it is overlaid with agarose again. Plaques are visible after five to six days of incubation. The plaques can be sustained with a staining mixture containing 0.5 mg of 3,3'-diaminobenzidine tetrahydrochloride per ml and 0.02% H_2O_2 in PBS (Plate IIIC).[70,71]

5. *Nucleic acid probe*. The complementary structure of DNA offers a sensitive, specific means to detect viral genes and transcripts. The double-stranded structure of DNA allows the two strands to fit together through the pairing of complementary bases: adenine pairs with thymidine or uracil, in the case of RNA, and guanine pairs with cytosine. Molecular cloning technology leads to the isolation of complementary DNA (cDNA) and genomic DNA for numerous peptides, proteins, and enzymes. DNA sequences thus generated can then be used to make DNA or RNA probes for assessing the role of their respective mRNA in various functions in tissues. For instance, the viral RNA and mRNA that serve as an intermediary for coding HIV proteins can form sequence-specific, complementary, double-stranded structures with DNA. As a result, either RNA or DNA molecules can be labeled with radioactivity, a hapten, or an enzyme and used as probes to seek out complementary partners. Dupont now offers prelabeled radiometric probes, and hybridization (pairing of complementary pairs) of prelabeled [^{35}S]-RNA (Dupont NEP-200) and [^{35}S]-DNA (Dupont NEP-201) probes is less time consuming for in situ hybridization of HIV. Both are ready to be used directly in a hybridization reaction. The advantage of this new research tool is that it allows detection of the presence of HIV RNA/DNA directly from a tissue sample, such as lymph node, peripheral blood, or infected cell cultures from patients with AIDS.[73] The procedure consists of the following steps: cell sample preparation, cell fixation, prehybridization treatment, hybridization, and detection.[73] For each sample hybridized with HIV probe or control probe, analysis of 4 to 10×10^5 cells is carried out.[73] This [^{35}S]-RNA probe can detect 86% of the lymph node and 50% of the peripheral blood samples examined. However, the labeled cells were observed at very low frequency (0.01% of total mononuclear cells) and expressed viral RNA at relatively low abundance (20 to

300 copies per cell). The lymph node hyperplasia observed in HIV-associated lymphadenopathy is not directly due to proliferation of HIV-infected lymphocytes.[73]

RNA probes can be used in all hybridization protocols. For Northerns, Southerns, and dot blot experiments, the DNA probe may be preferable because the LTR region of the genome, which can cause cross-hybridization with human DNA, is not a targeted site. Compared with many nonradiometric probes, radiometric probes are compatible with staining. Also, they are more sensitive and require fewer steps.

The latest probe development is the enzyme-labeled synthetic nucleic acid nonradioactive probe (HIV SNAP probe kit, Dupont). Dupont's DNA probes consist of enzyme-conjugated single-stranded synthetic oligonucleotides 20 to 26 bases long that hybridize to a unique sequence of a designated DNA target. In this nonradiometric detection system, the enzyme, alkaline phosphatase, is covalently linked directly to the C5 position of a thymidine base through a 21-atom spacer arm. After hybridization, the enzyme is fully active and does not affect the sensitivity or efficiency of probe hybridization. The probes hybridize rapidly and specifically to the designated targets. They do not cross-react with nonspecific targets, and there is no nonspecific binding to filter material. Sensitivities equal to autoradiography with an overnight exposure are achieved in four hours or less. Limits of detection are in the range of 10 million copies of DNA. Higher levels of target are visualized in several minutes.

The enzyme-labeled DNA probes are supplied in lyophilized form and do not require denaturation before use. Hybridization is performed in 15 to 30 minutes. The probes are detected directly after hybridization by adding a substrate to form a colored precipitate. Each vial contains 1 µg of DNA probe, or sufficient material to hybridize more than 300 samples.

The DNA probes can detect dormant HIV genome in the absence of proliferation of the virus and can be used in all classic hybridization methods: Dot/Slot blots, Northerns, Southerns, and in situ hybridizations. As with other probes, color-developed SNAP probes hybridized to membrane-immobilized nucleic acids can be stripped and the sample rehybridized with another probe (Dupont NEP-001).

Currently, this probe kit has detected all variants of HIV tested to date, except for Zaire strains, and has reduced sensitivity to a Haitian strain.

Herpes Viruses

The members of the herpesvirus group are represented by DNA-containing enveloped viruses that include HSV-1, HSV-2, nonspecific HSV, CMV, varicella zoster virus (VZV), EBV, and the latest discovery—herpesvirus type 6 (HHV6). All are characterized by primary infections that become latent and may reactivate. Of these, HSV and CMV are well recognized as STDs in homosexual and bisexual men. There is growing indication of CMV in gastrointestinal infection causing diarrhea, which will be discussed below under STDs associated with diarrhea. VZV, EBV and HHV6 will be discussed under OIs in Homosexual Men with AIDS.

Laboratory Diagnosis: Overview. Most laboratories can do direct examination of a smear from a vesicle (Tzanck smear) stained with Giemsa/Hemacolor to search for multinucleated giant cells or, rarely, embedded for ultrathin sectioning by electron microscopy.[13] Rapid methods available are IFA, IP with monoclonal antibodies, and in situ hybridization. Some laboratories can do tissue cultures in various cell lines such as human embryonic lung, foreskin, rabbit kidney, monkey kidney, or human embryonic kidney and serologic tests such as complement fixation (CF), ELISA, or RIA to detect either viral antigens or antibodies. Ready-to-use transport media and tissue culture monolayers on coverslip/paddle are available commercially for HSV. Simple detection tests, such as an immunoperoxidase test, which can be read with light microscopy without a special instrument, is available for HSV and CMV, and thus microbiology or pathology laboratories can extend their coverage to these frequently encountered STDs routinely. Monoclonal antibodies are available for CMV late and early nuclear protein, all the EBV antigens, and HSV. The recently developed NA probe also has extended to radiometric CMV (DNA ^{32}P labeled probe) and nonradioactive enzyme-labeled synthetic nucleic acid probes (ENZO Biochem, Inc., and Dupont) for HSV. Again, successful virologic work depends on knowing the properties of the agent, as shown in Table 12–9. Precautions for specimen collection and transport are shown in Table 12–10; methods of identification are shown in Table 12–11.

HSV Infection. The causative agent of HSV is HSV-1 and -2 and HSV nonspecific. Diagnosis of a herpes infection is frequently made clinically by the characteristic vesicles on the mucous membrane. However, diagnosis is difficult in the case of rectal herpes, even by protoscopic examination.[74] In general, diagnostic procedures involve direct demonstration of agent (antigen/DNA) in smear, virus culture, and viral serology. These procedures are discussed below.

To prepare a satisfactory Tzanck smear, use young vesicle. With a sterile scalpel, unroof the vesicle and scrape the edge of the lesion vigorously to attain cellular components onto the slide, followed by immediate alcohol fixation (95% ethanol). The preparation can be stained by Giemsa-Wright's Hemacolor (Harleco Co.) in less than one minute, while immunoperoxidase (IP) and IFA with monoclonal antibodies both require two hours to demonstrate the multinucleated giant cell with intranuclear and intracytoplasmic inclusions. Unfortunately, the Tzanck smear is a very insensitive and nonspecific test because (1) the result depends greatly on the age of the vesicles, (2) similar findings are shown by all members of the HSV groups, and (3) unless monoclonal antibody is used,[75] it is difficult to detect specific viral antigen accurately from direct scraping, especially in cases of low infectivity.

The ELISA test (Dupont Herpes ELISA) can detect the presence of HSV in four hours.

As in HIV, nonradiometric, enzyme-labeled, oligonucleotide DNA probes are available to detect viral DNA sequences from HSV-1, HSV-2 and herpes nontype-specific sequence (SNAP herpes simplex virus probes, Dupont; viral DNA probe, ENZO Biochem, Inc.). They can be used with intact, fixed cells on microscope slides to detect the presence of HSV DNA in the cells. Intact cells, fixed on a microscope slide, are treated to destroy endogenous enzymes, denature the DNA, and allow for permeation of the probe into the cell. During hybridization, the DNA of the SNAP probe forms a specific Watson-Crick duplex with its viral DNA complement. If HSV is not present, no such duplex is formed. Washing removes excess, unreacted probe. The DNA oligonucleotide probe is covalently linked to alkaline phosphatase. Incubation of the hybridized sample with NBT and BCIP substrates results in deposition of blue color at the location of the viral nucleic acid. In the ENZO method, avidin-biotinylated horseradish peroxidase complex, the chromogen-substrate solution (freshly made), and fast-green counterstain were used, giving the cell with HSV DNA its characteristic red nuclear staining. A comparative study of this method to culture revealed HSV was isolated from 81% of vesicular lesions, 76% of pustules, and 67% of ulcers, while HSV DNA was detected in 77%, 76%, and 55% of lesions in these stages, respectively. The major drawback was the adequacy of the sample, and sensitivity dropped to 57% if samples with <20 cells were evaluated.[76] Also, it is not type specific. The advantage of nonradiometric hybridization is the absence of handling and disposal of radioactive materials.

Tissue culture, however, remains the most reliable method, and human foreskin fibroblast[76,77] appears to produce a high yield of positive findings. Furthermore, a ready-to-use commercial culture set (Immulok) can meet the demand even in small laboratories. Confirmation of positive cytopathic effect (CPE) can be carried out with IFA or immunoperoxidase test. With the fluorescent antibody technique with biotin-linked HSV (HSV-FA) antibody, characterized by high affinity of binding to avidin-fluorescein conjugate, even in cases of low infectivity, the final diagnostic report of a specimen can be reduced to 26 hours.[76,77]

Two strains of type 1 have been recovered from CSF[78] and type 2 from encephalitis in homosexual men with persistent lymphadenopathy.[79] Several techniques have been used to type isolates, such as selective cell culture system [E-5-(2 bromovinyl)-2 deoxyuridine (BVDU) assay] and monoclonal antibody.

Of the serologic diagnostic tests available, IFA is the most commonly used. With the use of HSV pooled antigen, a conversion from a negative to a positive titer of IgG of at least 1:10 is regarded as significant, especially in asymptomatic carriers. High titers ranging from 1:100 to 1:400 are usually seen in active infection. IgM indicates current infection. A recently developed rapid method is the latex agglutination test, producing a result comparable with the CF test. However, the titer is two to four doubling dilutions higher than CF titers. Prozone reaction may occur, necessitating adding higher diluted sera for the test in some patients.[77]

CMV is a DNA virus that has been demonstrated in urine, blood, upper respiratory tract, gastrointestinal tract, semen, and biopsy materials such as lung, spleen, liver, cornea, and brain in disseminated infections in patients with AIDS.[80] It is included here as an STD since high incidence has been noted in homosexual men and heterosexual patients who visited venereal disease clinics. Although it is an important OI, it is presented in Table 12–14 under OIs in AIDS. Laboratory diagnosis is established by demonstration of the virus in infected cells, cell culture, and serologic tests. Direct demonstration can be accomplished by Tzanck smear stained with Hemacolor, IFA, and tissue section by electron microscope, hematoxylin-eosin stain, and DNA probe. DNA probes have been used successfully to detect the presence of CMV in clinical samples such as urine and peripheral blood mononuclear cells. Dupont CMV Nick Translation kit involves the following four simple steps to detect CMV genome in tissue:

1. Sample immobilization. Samples are treated to release and denature nucleic acids. With a vacuum manifold, multiple samples can be conveniently immobilized on nylon or nitrocellulose membrane filters.
2. Nick translation of probe. The kit provides all the reagents necessary to label the purified DNA fragment to high-specific activity with ^{32}P. The labeled fragment is then purified using NENSORB 20 cartridges, provided in the kit.
3. Hybridization. Purified ^{32}P-labeled probe is added to membranes carrying target DNA and incubated at 70°C for 3.5 to 20 hours. This allows probe sequences to form hybrids with complementary target sequences on the membrane filter. Following hybridization, the membrane filters are washed to remove excess unhybridized probe.
4. Detection. Washed membrane filters are placed against x-ray film and exposed at $-70°C$ in the presence of CRONEX intensifying screens. A positive signal on the x-ray film indicates that the DNA probe is detecting complementary sequences that were present in the original sample.

Human embryonic lung and human foreskin cell cultures have been successful in isolating the virus, which is a slow grower, requiring four days to four weeks to show cytopathic effect (CPE) shown as clusters of large, pleomorphic cells or round refractile cells. On hematoxylin-eosin-stained preparation, large, acidophilic, intranuclear inclusion bodies surrounded by halos in large balloon-like cells can be seen in urine, semen, and tissue. The incidence of positive culture is much higher in semen than in urine, which may give false negative results (see Table 12–14).

Acute infection can be determined by a fourfold rise in antibody titer by CF, IHA, or ELISA tests. Tests for IgM antibody have been developed using ELISA techniques. Using the IFA technique, various modifications have been reported to improve detection of IgM-CMV antibody, such as the use of isolated fibroblast nuclei at early stages of viral reproduction to avoid the nonspecific fluorescence associated with the presence of IgG-F$_c$ receptors in the cytoplasm of infected cells. A rise in IgM antibody titers may be seen in recurrent as well as initial infections but may not be a reliable marker for active CMV infection in some populations, such as AIDS patients. Determination of IgG to CMV early antigens with monoclonal antibody frequently has been associated with recent or active infections. The level declines after virus excretion ceases, while IgG induced by late CMV antigens, which develop during a primary infection, usually persist for life.[81] Again, serology is not too helpful in AIDS patients for diagnosis.

Viral Hepatitis

The causative agents of viral hepatitis are hepatitis A (HAV), hepatitis B (HBV), hepatitis non-A, non-B virus (NANBV), and hepatitis D (HDV). HAV is an RNA virus and is the only hepatitis virus that has been cultured successfully.[82] Current diagnostic tests are EIA and RIA instead of immune adherence tests with IgM.

HBV is a DNA virus and can be diagnosed by various immunologic tests, including EIA, RIA, latex agglutination, and nonradiometric enzyme-labeled synthetic nucleic acid probe (SNAP Probe) for HB_s and HB_c. Various antigens and antibodies (hepatitis B surface antigen, HBsAg; hepatitis Be antigen, HBeAg; antihepatitis core antibody, anti-HBc) in serum have been used to diagnose infection (see Table 12–11). HBsAg has been demonstrated in rectal mucosal lesions from asymptomatic patients and in needle biopsy of liver in homosexual men by immunoperoxidase.

The nucleic acid genome of NANBV is unknown. There are at least two distinct viral agents of NANA, with different modes of transmission. The post-transfusion type of transmission is similar to HBV. The other agent is ET-NANB, which is transmitted by the fecal-oral route. This form of infection occurs as a result of inadequate sewage disposal.[83] The infection is diagnosed mostly by exclusion when tests for HAV and HBV and other causes for hepatitis are negative in transfusion cases. Liver biopsy may demonstrate bridging necrosis accompanied by abnormal alanine aminotransferase.

HDV is also called the delta agent and is believed to be a defective virus that replicates only in HBV-infected cells. HIV and HDV in homosexual men has been reported.[84] An RIA kit to detect antibody in serum is available to diagnose hepatitis D infection in lieu of liver biopsy.

Molluscum Contagiosum

Molluscum contagiosum, caused by pox virus, is a benign viral infection of the skin and mucous membranes. Sexually transmitted cases with lesions in the genital and perianal areas are increasingly reported, especially occurring around the pubic hairs, lower abdomen, and anal areas in homosexual men. Punched biopsy of the infected areas shows that the basal layer appears unaffected, but the cells of the stratum malpighii of the epidermis become filled with an eosinophilic hyaline spherical mass, known as the molluscum body, which appears to be pushing the nucleus to the cell periphery. The molluscum body consists of a large mass of DNA virus "clear bodies" and cellular debris in a gelatin matrix. The white caseous material from the lesion can be squeezed on a slide to reveal these inclusions (see Table 12–11).

Condyloma Acuminatum

Condyloma acuminatum is a STD caused by a human papilloma virus (HPV) that has never been grown in culture. It is commonly referred to as venereal or anal wart. Electron microscopy reveals the virus particles as unenveloped, 45 to 55 nm in diameter, with icosahedral symmetry. The virus has a double-stranded circular DNA genome. Virus extract from warts obtained from restriction enzyme analysis and DNA hybridization techniques are used to detect specific viral DNA sequences. Three methods are available: Southern blot hybridization, in situ filter hybridization, and in situ tissue section typing. The positive rates for the detection of HPV DNA in condyloma, 82% by Southern blot hybridization, 62% by in situ filter hybridization, and 72% by in situ tissue hybridization, indicate that there are various species of HPV. HPV-1, -2, and -4 are associated with common and plantar warts, while HPV-3 and -5 are found in plane warts and the lesions of epidermodysplasia verruciformis. HPV types 16 and 18 are strongly associated with cancer of the cervix, and types 6 and 11 are linked with condylomata acuminata.[85,86] The clinical diagnosis can be confirmed by biopsy, which reveals hypertrophic papillae with normal epiderm covering in histologic sections, nuclear basophilic inclusions in some epithelial cells by light microscopy, and detection of papilloma antigen by immunoperoxidase test (see Table 12–11).

SEXUALLY TRANSMITTED DISEASES ASSOCIATED WITH DIARRHEA

In 1976, diarrhea in homosexual men was called the "gay bowel syndrome." This was a misnomer because bacterial cultures and parasitic examinations were positive for multiple pathogens (*Shigella, Campylobacter, Entamoeba histolytica,* and *Giardia lamblia*), usually singly but sometimes concurrently. It became clear that full coverage of bacterial enteric pathogens and parasites from stool specimens, as well as agents of venereal disease from known or suspected homosexual patients, was needed. At present, the list of such infectious agents continues to increase, as shown in Table 12–1.

Most of the organisms are well-established agents that cause infectious diarrhea. The new members among the STDs are *N. gonorrhoeae*, HSV, and *Chlamydia*. Among AIDS patients with diarrhea we have learned to look for CMV, *Mycobacterium avium-intracellularis* (MAI), *Cryptosporidium* species, *Isospora belli*, and *Microsporidia*.

Bacterial Infections

Fresh stool specimens sent in sterile containers are preferable to rectal swab for bacterial cultures. These should be collected before antimicrobial treatment is started. Direct smear and cultural media for primary isolation are listed in Table 12–12. All media are incubated at 35°C, except with *Campylobacter* species. Campyl-BAP plates are inoculated in duplicate: One is incubated at 35°C and the other at 42°C, both in the presence of 10% CO_2. The cultures are not examined until after 48 hours of incubation, which should ensure higher yields of positive cultures. *C. jejuni* thrives better at 42°C, while *C. intestinalis* fails to grow at 42°C. Studies conducted in homosexual men indicated that *Campylobacter*-like organisms, now identified as *C. cinadei* and *C. fennelliae*, are prevalent in symptomatic gay men with proctitis and bacteremia, although they are rare in AIDS patients. These organisms required anoscopically-obtained rectal swab in additional cultural media such as Campy-Thio enrichment (BBL), Skirrow's selective blood agar, and Fennell's blood agar.[87,88]

Parasitic Infections

Since cryptosporidiosis was presented as far back as the first edition, there is a great need for clinical laboratories to learn how to identify the parasite. Also, the latest CDC guideline stated that chronic diarrhea due to *I. belli* will be regarded as indicating an AIDS-associated infection.

Laboratory Diagnosis: Overview

The success of diagnosing parasitic infection depends a great deal on the quality of the specimens received for examination and the types of tests requested (Tables 12–12 and 12–13). The ideal specimen will be one that is freshly passed and contains no interfering substances such as antibiotics, laxatives, and so on. Multiple specimens should be submitted because ameba are extruded periodically in the stool: Three specimens collected on three consecutive days is preferred to three specimens submitted for examination on the same day. Purged specimens are more satisfactory than formed stool for trophozoite detection if the patient does not have diarrhea. The most commonly used laxative for purging is Fleet's phosphosoda, which is given to the patient after overnight fasting. The first specimen is usually formed and can be used for enteric bacterial culture, and the subsequent liquid specimens are more satisfactory for parasitic examination. Cholecystokinin injection, which causes the gallbladder to contract, may enhance recovery of *Giardia* trophozoites from this site, especially with the use of Enterotest. Sigmoidoscopy or colonoscopy may aid in obtaining optimal (biopsy) specimens of visible lesion in the colon.

The specimen is best examined when fresh to check for motile trophozoites or larva, which will be lacking if the specimen is submitted in formalin or other preservative. The two procedures routinely used are direct preparation and concentration preparation. Both preparations are examined unstained and stained.

1. *Unstained preparation.* Unstained smear is prepared with saline or sucrose directly with the fecal specimens. Saline preparation is good to look for motile

Table 12–12 Laboratory diagnosis of STDs associated with diarrhea (general information)

Agent	Specimen	Collection	Smear Preparation	Processing
Bacteria	Stool	Before treatment	Gram: *Campylobacter*[a]	Standard cultural procedure
	Rectal swab[c]	Sterile container	Dark-field: *Campylobacter*	Modified special media for *Campylobacter*[b]
			Kinyoun: MAI	Thio enrichment broth
			Methylene blue for fecal leukocytes	Skirrow's selective blood agar
				Fennell's selective blood agar (37°C and 5% CO_2)
Parasites	Stool	Same as above	Three-step stool examination	Standard formalin ether concentration
	Duodenal aspirate		Iodine: *Entamoeba histolytica*	Sucrose flotation
			MCK: *Cryptosporidium* and *Isospora*	Culture for *E. histolytica*
			Sucrose: Same as above	
			EM: *Microsporidia*	
Viruses	Intestinal biopsy	See Table 12–10	Hematoxylin-eosin	None found in stool
	Intestinal		EM preparation	Look for viral inclusion bodies
				Look for viral particles
				Culture with stool filtrate

MAI—*Mycobacterium-avium intracellulare*.
[a] Stain with Kopeloff modified Gram's stain.
[b] *Campylobacter cinadei, C. fennelliae*
[c] Use anoscopically collected rectal swab in proctitis.

Table 12-13 Laboratory diagnosis of diarrhea-associated STDs—Parasites (identification profile)

Parasite	Specimen	Collection/ Diluent	Stages to Be Detected		Antigen/Antibody
Entamoeba histolytica	Fresh stool[a] Liquid/formed/ purged stool[b]	Sterile container	Iodine and trichrome smears	Cyst 10 to 20 μm spherical, one to four nuclei, uniform peripheral chromatin, diffuse glycogen	Culture Trophozoites/ cyst for zymodemes (pathogenic zymodemes II and XI)
			Trophozoite 10 to 60 μm irregular, fingerlike pseudopods		
	Rectal biopsy Liver aspirate Bile, duodenal aspirate	0.5 ml saline	Rapid motility Ingested RBCs, one nucleus		CIE/LA for Ag
Isospora belli See Chapter 10	Fresh stool Liquid/purged stool	Sterile container 0.5 ml saline	Tissue Asexual stages (meronts, sporont, in lamina propria)	Stool Sexual stage Oocyst— ellipsoidal, (25 to 30 μm) 2 spherical sporocysts (12 to 14 μm)	Not available
	Biopsy		See Plate IVA2 to D2		

Table 12–13 (continued)

Parasite	Specimen	Collection/Diluent	Stages to Be Detected		Antigen/Antibody
Cryptosporidium spp.	Fresh stool Duodenal aspirate Small bowel biopsy, bile, sputum, eosophageal swab	Sterile container 0.5 ml saline and formalin for pathology laboratory	Tissue Asexual stages meronts, sporonts, 2–3 μm, lining-brushed border of enterocytes or respiratory epithelium	Stool Sexual stage oocyst-oval-spherical; 4 to 5 μm Acid-fast (red) Iodine stain (colorless) Sucrose flotation (pink) DFA/IFA (green fluorescence)	IFA/ELISA
			See Plates IV A1 to D2, V A2 to E2, and VI A1 and A2		
Giardia lamblia	Fresh stool Duodenal aspirate	Sterile container Same as above	Trophozoite 10 to 20 μm, pear shaped, four pairs flagella	Cyst 8 to 19 μm Pear shaped, four nuclei	CIE for antigen

[a] Delayed in examination (one hour). Collect with preservative-polyvinyl alcohol (PVA), 3:1 pt stool/MIF kit (Marion Scientific). IFA, indirect fluorescent antibody; DFA, direct fluorescent antibody; LA, latex agglutination.
[b] Fleets phosphosoda for laxative after an overnight fasting. Use first specimen for culture and second, more liquid one during purging for ova and parasite examination.

trophozoites of *Entamoeba histolytica* or larva such as the rhabditiform larva and even the filariform larva of *Strongyloides stercoralis,* especially in immunocompromised patients such as AIDS patients.

Sucrose flotation has been most useful in identifying the coccidial oocysts. A drop of sucrose solution is added to one drop of stool filtrate on a slide with a coverslip. Allow ten minutes for the oocysts to float to the bottom of the coverslip. With careful focussing immediately below the coverslip, oocysts are easily detected. This works well in a busy clinical laboratory and can replace the time-consuming centrifugation procedure.[91] Due to the sucrose and optics in American Optic scope, the oocysts appear pink while yeasts will be colorless. However, it is not specific for *Cryptosporidium* and *I. belli* oocysts, since all coccidial oocysts can give this pink hue.

2. *Stained preparation* (Plate IV). Several staining methods are widely used to identify parasites. Iodine preparation will aid in identifying nuclei characteristics of amebic cysts or in differentiating cryptosporidial oocysts from yeasts. The yeast will stain brown, while cryptosporidia will be colorless with a greenish glassy hue.

Modified Cold Kinyoun (MCK) is an excellent screening procedure to identify the coccidial oocysts (*Cryptosporidium* and *Isospora*) (Plate IV), which are acid fast, and can also serve as a permanent record for future reference. Furthermore, automation is available—MIDAS II (EM diagnostics), which is used for Gram smear, can be programmed to stain a total of 20 slides in 10 minutes. The automation includes fixation of the fecal smear by methanol, staining by carbol fuchsin, washing, decolorization with acid alcohol, counterstaining with light green/methylene blue, washing, and drying.

Truant's stain (auramine-rhodamine), normally used to detect acid-fast bacilli, can also be applied to stain coccidial oocysts, which exhibit yellowish fluorescence. Those not exhibiting fluorescence will be invisible[89-91] (Plate IV B1, B2)

Both direct[92] and indirect fluorescent antibody tests[93-95] have been reported for detection of cryptosporidia oocysts. IFAT using monoclonal antibody[96] on stool smear has been used for screening specimen in a community outbreak of cryptosporidiosis (Meridian Inc.). The specificity and sensitivity are comparable to MCK and sucrose flotation (unpublished data). The advantage of IFAT is that one can screen the slide with less time. The disadvantages are that one cannot keep any permanent record of the slide, a fluorescent scope is required, and the reagent cost is less cost effective than acid-fast staining. Briefly, the stool filtrate placed on a slide is added to anticryptosporidial monoclonal antibody. After 30 minutes of incubation at 22°C, the slide is washed with PBS pH 7.4 to wash off excess antibody before the goat antihuman gamma globulin conjugated with isothiocyanate is added for the second incubation period of 30 minutes. The slide is thoroughly washed with PBS and is coverslipped with buffered glycerin to be examined under the fluorescent scope. Positive and negative controls are included for each run. Cryptosporidial oocysts appear as green fluorescent spherical structures, while yeasts are invisible. The whole procedure requires approximately 90 minutes (Plate V E2).

Because parasites may not be present in great numbers, stools must be concentrated for repeat smear examinations before being regarded as negative. Two methods in vogue are the formalin-acetate and the sucrose flotation.

1. *Formalin-acetate.* The conventional procedure of formalin-acetate has been used to concentrate stool specimens for most ova and parasites.[13]

2. *Sucrose flotation.* The modified sucrose flotation method is more satisfactory for coccidial oocysts (*I. belli* and *Cryptosporidium* species), especially with liquid stool devoid of fecal material. The sugar flotation procedure involves the use of sucrose[91] consisting of sucrose 500 g, water 320 ml, and phenol 6.5 g. After the stool is filtered through three pieces of gauze to get rid of clumps of fecal material, approximately 2 to 3 ml of filtrate is placed at the bottom of a 15 ml conical screw-capped tube. Approximately 8 ml of the sucrose solution is added to the filtrate. With a few wooden applicators, the contents are mixed well, avoiding the creation of any bubbles. The remainder of the tube is filled with sucrose solution to the top, and then the tube is recapped. (The tube is centrifuged at 500 × g [1000 rpm] for 15 minutes. A small aliquot from the top will be transferred to a glass slide. A coverslip is placed on the specimen and examined under the low-power bright-field objective, high-power objective, and oil-immersion lens for coccidial oocysts. The oocysts appear pink when examined with the American Optic microscope[89-91] (Plate IVC1 and C2). The sucrose solution can cause indentation of the oocysts, leading to their rupture and disappearance, so the preparation is best examined within 10 to 15 minutes. Atypical oocysts detected by this method have been reported. They may represent strain variations of *C. parvum* or a different species.[97] A more rapid method is to prepare fecal preparation with a drop of sucrose, as mentioned above.[91]

Serologic methods are IFA[98] and ELISA[99] using fecal cryptosporidial oocysts as the antigen or section from infected tissue. Infected tissue was first used by Tzipori but is not too practical to use in diagnostic clinical laboratories.

Amebiasis

Entamoeba histolytica is characterized by two stages, the trophozoite and the cyst. The former is best detected in liquid stool. The trophozoite is detected by rapid motility of the fingerlike pseudopods and sometimes the presence of ingested erythrocytes, indicating active infection, while the cyst is usually present in formed stool and may indicate chronic infection or a carrier. They are frequently mistaken for leukocytes; therefore, trichrome permanent smear is required for definitive identification (see Table 12–13). Sargeaunt et al. have used the electrophoretic mobility patterns of four enzymes from trophozoite culture of *E. histolytica*[100] to determine the zymodeme of the amebic populations. They concluded that the pathogenic strains are represented by zymodemes II and XI, while none of the isolates from homosexual men were considered pathogenic. The significance of this observation awaits documentation. For extra-intestinal amebiasis, a number of serologic tests are available. The ELISA test has been reported as more sensitive than the counterimmunoelectrophoresis in detecting amebic antibody.[13]

Isosporiasis

I. belli is usually rare in temperate countries and is endemic in the tropics. The formalin-acetate method of concentration is not too successful in concentrating this coccidial oocyst, but sucrose flotation proves useful. *I. belli* is oval, measuring 30 × 33 μm. In fresh stool specimen, the stage detected is the sporoblast, consisting of a mass of granules (Plate IVC2). After the parasite is exposed to the environment, sporulation takes place and two sporocysts are formed, each of which contains four banana-shaped sporozoites (Plate IVC2). The staining reactions are the same as those for cryptosporidia, since it is acid-fast with MCK (Plate IVA2) and Truant's stain (Plate IVB2) and appears pink in sucrose flotation (Plate IVC2). In tissue section of the intestinal tract, endogenous stages are located in the host cytoplasm (Plate IVD2), unlike cryptosporidia, which is found attached to the microvilli of the enterocytes (Plate IVD1). Since sporulation does not take place until the oocyst is outside the host, an epidemic by this parasite is rare[105-108] (see Table 12–13). (See Chapter 8 on Cryptosporidiosis, Isosporiasis, and Microsporidiosis.)

Cryptosporidiosis

This disease used to be diagnosed by small bowel biopsy (Plate IVD1), but for the past six years, stool examination has been the standard procedure. The three-step stool examination we have used since 1981 is easy to adapt in most clinical parasitology laboratories by incorporating acid-fast and sucrose flotation methods to the routine standard method of iodine preparation to detect this minute parasite, as described above[89-91] (Plate IVA1 to C1). In AIDS-related cryptosporidiosis, the patient usually suffers persistent diarrhea resistant to drug treatment. Hyperimmune bovine colostrum from cow infected with bacteria[101] and, more specific, with cryptosporidia[102,103] has been reported. Four cases of chronic cryptosporidiosis responding to hyperimmune colostrum from cow infected with cryptosporidia containing a high level of immunoglobulins within three to four days is most encouraging.[102,103] A double-blind study is currently set up at St. Vincent's Hospital and Medical Center in collaboration with the Vaccine Center, University of Maryland. Another treatment regimen, with transfer factor, has shown some response.[104] However, nonimmunocompromised individuals usually have self-limited infection lasting one to two weeks. More of this is discussed in Chapter 8.

Microsporidiosis

Microsporidia is another newly recognized protozoan causing diarrhea in AIDS.[109] However, it has not been detected in stool specimen, and hence it may not be transmitted sexually.

Giardiasis

Giardia lamblia is a flagellate that is easy to detect from stool specimen or duodenal aspirates by its characteristic features (see Table 12–13). The enterotest is superior to stool examinations in some cases and easier to do than duodenal aspiration. A thread with a wax button at the end is swallowed by the patient after overnight fasting. After one hour, the thread is pulled from the stomach and examined for *Giardia*. It is presently the test of choice in suspected giardiasis if the stool is negative. Improved detection of the parasite has been shown when cholecystokinin injection is given before the string is retrieved. Recent reports show that counter-immuno-electrophoresis (CIE) of the stool filtrate is a promising diagnostic test.

Enterobiasis

Enterobius is a pinworm that causes intense itching in the perianal area. The standard procedure is to take an adhesive-tape swab of the perianal area first thing in the morning, before taking a bath or having a bowel movement, or in the evening before retiring. The egg is flattened on one side and may contain motile larva. The female worm may contain hundreds of eggs.

Endolimax and Blastocystis Infections

Endolimax nana is an amoeba (trophozoite 6 × 10 μm, cyst 5 × 10 μm) usually regarded as a commensal when detected in stool examination. *Blastocystis hominis* trophozoite and cyst are frequently seen in the stool of homosexual men with or without AIDS. Large numbers found in symptomatic patients may be significant, requiring treatment.

OPPORTUNISTIC INFECTIONS IN HOMOSEXUAL MEN WITH AIDS

The laboratory diagnosis of OIs seen in patients with AIDS is outlined in Table 12–14. The list continues to increase as the epidemic spreads worldwide.[109,110] (See Table 12–15.)

Laboratory Diagnosis: Overview

Pneumocystis carinii still ranks as the most common OI in the AIDS population and has been used as the index for individuals to qualify for azidothymidine (AZT) treatment programs. More disseminated infections are noted in agents such as *Cryptococcus neoformans*,[111,112] *Histoplasma capsulatum*,[113,114] *Coccidioides immitis*,[115] *Sporotrix schenckii*,[116] *Mycobacterium kansasii*,[117] *Herpes zoster*,[118] and even *P. carinii*.[119] Other OIs not encountered, or unknown, when the

Table 12–14 Laboratory diagnosis of OIs in AIDS (Identification profile)[a]

Infection	Agent	Clinical Specimens	Identification Profile	Serology
Parasites				
Pneumocystis carinii pneumonia (PCP)	Pneumocystis carinii	Lung biopsy Bronchoalveolar lavage (BAL) Induced sputum	Touched preparation Cyst and Trophozoites Hemacolor <1 min*, IFA (monoclonal Ab) 1 hr Cyst only Gram Weigert—15 mins Toluidine blue—30 mins Histologic sections H & E—foamy material GMS—Cyst stains black (see Plate V)	None reliable (Ag test—CIE,LA) (Ab test—IFA,EIA)
Disseminated infection		Same as above plus epicardium, endocardium, liver, pancreas, kidney, adrenal, thyroid, eyes		
Toxoplasmosis: CNS, pulmonary, disseminated infection	Toxoplasma gondii	Lung biopsy, brain biopsy, CSF, GI tract	Touch preparation Hemacolor Tachyzoite—crescent shaped, stains purple IFA Histologic section Necrosis showing tachyzoite, and tissue cyst (100 μm) with bradyzoites (see Plate VI B1 and B2) Mouse inoculation—IP/SC 7 to 14 days (+)	IFA—4× rise in titer IgG—>1:10,000 IgM—>1:100 IHA—4× rise in titer IgG—>1:1000 Sabin dye test >1:1000 Elisa >1:1000 Serology not reliable in AIDS patients
Cryptosporidiosis: intestinal, pulmonary, hepatic, biliary		Stool, bile Biopsy: intestinal, rectal, lung,	Cryptosporidium vs P. carinii Oocyst Cyst Size 4–5 μm 5 to 6 μm Shape Spherical Spherical	IFA, Elisa—fourfold rise in titer

Table 12–14 (continued)

Infection	Agent	Clinical Specimens	Identification Profile	Serology
disseminated infection		liver, gallbladder, etc.	Hemacolor — Purple Gram-Weigert — Purple GMS — Black MCK — Unstained IFA/DFA — Acid-fast (red) Green fluorescence (see Plates V, VI A1-2) Non-acid-fast	
Acanthamoebic infection, CNS, pulmonary	*Acanthamoeba* spp.	CSF, biopsy: brain, lung, skin nodule	Touch preparation Hemacolor — purple troph./cyst Trichrome — cytoplasm (green); karyosome (red) Calcofluor white — trophozoite (orange); cyst wall (green) Culture 22°C and 35°C 1.5% nonnutrient agar overlay with *E. coli*	IFA CIE
Microsporidiosis	Microsporidia (*Enterocytozoon bieneusi*) (*E. cuniculi*, *Pleistophora* sp.)	Endoscopy biopsy (duodenum)	*Plasmodia* with uninucleate to multinucleated stages, free parasite ranges 2 to 9 μm Giemsa stained prep. — hyaline pale-blue cytoplasm, reddish-purple nuclei. Some strains are acid-fast.	IFA

Fungi

Candidiasis	*Candida* sp.	Sputum, blood, etc.	Direct smear and culture to show budding yeasts and pseudohyphae	Not available
Trichosporoniasis	*Trichosporon beigelli*	Urine, blood, lung bx	Direct smear and culture to show arthrospores and blastospores	Same as above
Cryptococcosis	*Cryptococcus neoformans*	CSF, blood, bone marrow, urine, sputum, BAL, brain, lung biopsies	India ink preparation capsulated spherical budding yeast Capsules vary in size due to strain variation Culture—mucoid, white colonies on Sabouraud agar/blood agar plates	Antigen test (LA) Titer 1:1 to >1:10^6 Antibody test seldom can detect early enough to be +
Cunninghamella infection	*Cunninghamella berthiolate*	Wound swab	Wide nonseptate hyphae, sporangiophore, ending in a vesicle Sporangiophore bear multiple sporangiola (conidia) Culture—fluffy colony on Sabouraud agar plate	None available
Aspergillosis	*Aspergillus fumigatus*	Buffy coat, bone marrow, biopsy/autopsy—brain, lung, intestinal tissue, adrenal, kidney	Septate hyphae Vesicle-shaped conidiophore bearing conidia	Immunoprecipitin

Table 12–14 (continued)

Infection	Agent	Clinical Specimens	Identification Profile	Serology
Alternaria infection	*Alternia alternata*	Nasal biopsy	Septate hyphae Conidia at the apices of conidiophore, taper toward the distal ends, characteristic horizontal and vertical septa	
Virus				
CMV infection (Enteritis, colitis, eosophagitis, gastritis, hepatitis, chorioretinitis, pneumonia, encephalopathy, disseminated infection)	CMV 150 nm cube	Sputum, BAL, buffy coat, urine, CSF, stool, biopsy (kidney, brain, pericardium, myocardium, etc.)	H&E "owl eye" (Cowdry type A) single, large, eosinophilic intranuclear inclusion surrounded by a halo in susceptible cells Fibroblast culture—supports replication, enhances infectivity by centrifugation into cell CPE: 2 to 3 days to 2 to 3 weeks, perinuclear in enlarged infected cells (cytomegaly) (Cowdry type A) single, large, eosinophilic intranuclear inclusions surrounded by a halo in susceptible cells	Anticomplement fluorescent test 4× rise in titer Both false + and − results seen in immunocompromised patients
Varicella-Zoster	(V-Z) virus EM: 150 nm cube with envelope	Direct smear Vesicle: IFA/IP for inclusions	Diploid human cell lines or primary human cell cultures—WI-38 diploid fibroblasts and human embryonic kidney cells	In situ hybridization for Ag

EBV infection (Infectious mononucleosis, Burkitt lymphoma, nasopharyngeal carcinoma)	EBV EM: 150 nm cube Specific antigens: Viral capsid Ag (VCA) Early Ag-diffuse (EA-D) Early Ag-restricted (EA-R) Nuclear Ag (NA)	Biopsy	CPE: small foci of rounded and swollen refractile cells in 5 to 7 days or longer. It differs from CMV by having CPE in epithelial cells Identification: IFA, dot blot hybridization DNA hybridization (molecular cloned EBV-DNA probe)	Heterophile test CF/EIA/IFA/Indirect anticomplementary IFA Infectious mononucleosis Heterophile test (+) Early EBV infection VCA-IgG, IgM(+), EA-D(+) Late EBV infection VCA-IgG, EBNA(+) Chronic EBV infection VCA-IgG ≥ 1:5120 EA (D/R) ≥ 1:640 EBNA (−1 low)
PML infection	Parvovirus JC	Brain biopsy Bone marrow	IFA	IFA Serum 4× rise in titer CSF and serum

CF, complement fixation test; H&E, hematoxylin-eosin preparation; GMS, Gomori methenamine silver; DFA, direct fluorescent antibody test; IFA, indirect fluorescent antibody test; IHA, indirect hemagglutination test; LA, latex agglutination test; MCK, modified cold Kinyoun stain; Hemacolor-Giemsa-wright; PML, progressive multifocal leukoencephalopathy; IP, intraperitoneal inoculation; SC, subcutaneous inoculation; EIA, enzyme immunoassay; EBV infection includes infectious mononucleosis, Burkitt lymphoma, and nasopharyngeal carcinoma.

Table 12–15 Total frequency of OI diagnosis among AIDS patients in New York State as of Feb. 13, 1988[186]

Diagnosis	Number	%
P. carinii pneumonia	9112	65.7
Kaposi's sarcoma	2341	16.9
Esophageal candidiasis	1151	8.3
Cryptococcosis	979	7.1
MAI	577	4.2
CMV	537	3.9
Toxoplasmosis of the brain	343	2.5
Cryptosporidiosis	310	2.2
Chronic mucocutaneous herpes	280	2.0
Lymphoid interstitial pneumonia	143	1.0
Immunoblastic lymphoma	94	0.7
Atypical mycobacteria	88	0.6
Primary lymphoma of the brain	78	0.6
Progressive multifocal leukoencephalopathy	67	0.5
HIV wasting	62	0.5
Bacterial infections	61	0.4
M. tuberculosis[a]	55	0.4
Burkitt's lymphoma	44	0.3
HIV encephalopathy	41	0.3
Candidiasis of the lungs	33	0.2
Histoplasmosis	32	0.2
Salmonella septicemia	22	0.2
CMV retinitis	16	0.1
Isosporiasis	13	0.1
Coccidioidomycosis	1	<0.1

[a]Tuberculosis data from New York City is not included.

first edition of this book was published include CNS infections caused by *Listeria monocytogenes*,[120] *Acanthamoeba polyphaga*,[121,122] and *Prototheca wickerhamii*[123]; and persistent diarrhea caused by a newly recognized protozoan called *Microsporidia*,[124–127a] which also involves the liver[125] and muscles.[126] The intestinal spirochetes[128] and the "nonpathogenic amoeba"[129] may be regarded as OI in some patients when they are present in an unusually heavy load. Another rare parasite reported is *Strongyloides*.[130] Blood-borne parasites such as malaria in patients with positive HIV serology have been reported. There is speculation that *Plasmodia*, causing stickiness of the blood, may have caused false-positive HIV serology.[131] Rectal leishmaniasis is another rare infection reported in homosexual men with AIDS.[132] Disseminated bacterial infections are well represented by MAI,[133,134] *Mycobacterium tuberculosis*,[135–137] and *Campylobacter* sp.[138] Other rare infections are the spinal cord abscess caused by *M. tuberculosis*,[139] lung abscesses caused by *Corynebacterium pseudodiphtheriticum*,[140] *C. equi* (Rhodococcus),[141] *Hemophilus parainfluenzae* prostatitis,[142] and botryomycosis.[143] The most exciting report is the association of a gram-negative coccobacillus to disseminated skin nodules in epithelioid angiomatosis[144] and epithelioid angiomatosislike infection. Cat-scratch disease bacillus is given to this gram-negative bacillus.[145-146] Others have indicated *Bartonella* is the most likely agent (Dr. C. J. Cockerell, personal communication).

Advancements in methodologies include rapid recovery of MAI, *M. tuberculosis,* and *Histoplasma capsulatum* by automatic Bactec blood culture system,[147] and Dupont isolator, another new collecting system for blood and bone marrow[148-149]; ultra-nebulizer to induce sputum for the detection of PCP[149,150] and HIV antigen[151] in lieu of added methodology for invasive procedures such as open lung biopsy and bronchoalveolar lavage.[152] Rapid identification of *Mycobacteria* by gene probe, which requires only a few hours from colonies or from positive Bactec 13A blood cult or Bactec 12A bone marrow culture vials (Johnson Laboratories)[153,154] versus the standard procedure of several weeks by biochemical tests,[153,154] and automated instruments for staining a maximum of 20 slides for acid-fast and Gram's stain, have been remarkable.[155] Recent advances in diagnosing cryptosporidiosis are the immunofluorescent test to detect fecal oocysts in stool specimens[95-98]; and serologic tests are IFA and ELISA, using fecal oocysts as antigen,[98,99] as mentioned above. Advanced technology in virology includes antigen capture assay, nucleic acid hybridization (DNA and RNA probes), application of cocultivation technique, and discovery of immortal cell lines for the isolation of HIV from clinical specimens. Calcofluor white fluorescent stain for fungi and *Acanthamoeba*,[154] caffeine culture and medium[155] to identify *Cryptococcus neoformans* by the brown colonies, and Warthin Starry stain[145] to identify cat-scratch disease bacilli are recent rapid staining procedures. These are some of the recent developments in clinical microbiology for the laboratory diagnosis of STDs and OIs in AIDS.

Parasitic Infections

Pneumocystis Pneumonia

P. carinii pneumonia heads the list of OIs in AIDS patients (see Table 12–15). Extrapulmonary infections have included eye and ear, and disseminated infections have involved lung, epicardium, endocardium, jejunal mucosa, colonic serosa, omentum, mesentery, appendices epiploicase, liver, pancreas, kidneys, right ureteral mucosa, adrenals, thyroid, and bone marrow.[156-160] Open lung biopsy used to be the standard procedure for detecting *P. carinii*. For the past few years it has been replaced by bronchoalveolar lavage and transbronchial aspirate with or without biopsy.[152] Recently, less invasive procedures such as induced sputum have been used.[149,150] A recent report indicated improved detection of *P. carinii* in sputum with use of monoclonal antibodies.[159] Our current procedures are bronchoalveolar lavage and transbronchial aspirate with or without biopsy. Positive specimens average one to six a week, with a high percentage showing numerous trophozoites and rare cysts. Rarely, open lung biopsy is received, especially in pediatric patients when the other methods give negative results. We are in the process of adopting the induced sputum using the ultra-nebulizer, an instrument to obtain satisfactory induced sputum. These procedures are described briefly as follows.

(1) *Open lung biopsy.* A minute piece of biopsy is submitted on a piece of sterile gauze slightly wet with a few drops of nonantimicrobial saline and is transported to the laboratory in a sterile plastic container. Touch preparations are made by touching the cut surface of the biopsy on a sterile glass slide in four to six spots, without smearing them, to preserve the cellular architecture. Rapid diagnosis can be stained with Hemacolor (Giemsa-wright stain) in less than one minute. The cysts, spherical structures measuring 4 to 6 μm, can be detected by the halo representing the unstained cyst wall and the internal crescent-shaped sporozoites varying from 1 to 8. Cell-free trophozoites are usually seen in clusters with some cysts embedded in them (Plate VA1).[159] Other stains used to demonstrate cysts only are toluidine blue (cyst wall stains blue), Gomori methenamine silver stain (cyst wall stains black) (Plate VB1), and Gram-Weigert (cysts stain purple) (Plate VD1). All the latter stains are more time consuming, 20 minutes or more, except for a short-cut Gomori silver stain that takes 15 minutes. The latest development is the monoclonal antibody in the immunofluorescent test, which stains both cysts and trophozoites[158,159] (Plate VE1). It is important to include stain that demonstrates the trophozoites, since they are frequently seen in clusters in patients with full-blown *P. carinii* infection.

(2) *Cryptosporidium* should also be checked when lung specimens are submitted for *P. carinii* testing. The comparison of these two parasites is shown in Plate V. Recently, a sputum sent for *Mycobacteria* showed moderate cryptosporidial oocysts in a patient who had no diarrhea. Examination of the stool did reveal rare oocysts, and a few days later the patient did develop liquid diarrhea. Unfortunately, no stool examination was performed before the sputum was detected positive; however, the sequence of events may indicate that the portal of entry of the oocysts is through inhalation, and the patient may have swallowed the organisms into the intestinal tract, thus leading to diarrhea in this case.

Cryptosporidiosis

Cryptosporidium species have been reported as common causes of diarrhea in patients with AIDS, as described above.[89,90] Look for them in other patients with diarrhea, whether they are immunocompromised or not. Search for *Cryptosporidium* as well when lung specimens are submitted for *P. carinii*. Giemsa and hematoxylin-eosin stains will not be helpful in differentiating the two in lung tissue because of their similar size and shape (5 to 6 μm). Differential staining procedures may help, such as MCK, which shows the oocysts red (acid-fast +) (Plate VC2).[161] They are not stained in the Gomori silver stain (Plate VB2), while in Gram-Weigert's stain they stain purple showing crescent-shaped sporozoites (Plate VD2). On the other hand, *P. carinii* is acid-fast negative (not red) and will not be visible but appear faintly green or blue as the counterstain background

(Plate VC1), the same color as the counterstain (light green or blue), but positive (black) in the Gomori silver stain (Plate VB1) and purple in Gram-Weigert's smear (Plate VD1). Furthermore, *Pneumocystis* is in the interstitium as well as in the alveoli, while *Cryptosporidium* lines the alveoli and is not detected in the cytoplasm of host cells when examined under light microscopy (Plate IVD1 and D2).

Disseminated cryptosporidiosis involving the intestinal tract, including the gallbladder,[162] common bile duct (Plate VIA1),[163] and liver[162] (Plate VIA2), has been reported. There was a case of esophagitis in an immunocompetent child.[164] Stool examination should be performed concurrently because cryptosporidiosis is primarily an enteritis.[90,165] IFA testing using fecal cryptosporidial oocyst as the antigen to detect specific cryptosporidial IgG, IgM and IgA in AIDS and non-AIDS individuals revealed a low level or no IgM and IgA in AIDS individuals.[98] Although cryptosporidiosis is both a cell- and humoral-mediated immunity, the mucosal immunoglobulin may also play an important role, since some patients with persistent cryptosporidiosis responded well to hyperimmune colostrum from cow infected with *Cryptosporidium*.[102,103]

Toxoplasmosis

The unusual feature of toxoplasmosis in homosexuals with AIDS is the high incidence of CNS toxoplasmosis. Although serologic tests are the standard diagnostic procedures, they are not reliable in documenting CNS toxoplasmosis in AIDS patients, even with the use of the IgM-IFA test. Cerebrospinal fluid (CSF) in one case revealed a fourfold increase in titer when the serum did not. Brain biopsy may be necessary to establish the diagnosis by hematoxylin-eosin stain (Plate VIB1) or by rapid Hemacolor stain. Toxoplasma is periodic acid Schiff (PAS) + and Gomori methenamine silver (GMS) +, and the antigen is detectable by IP.[166] One report of isolation of *T. gondii* in tissue culture from blood is of interest.[167]

Acanthamoeba Meningoencephalitis and Skin Nodules

Two cases of acanthamoebic infections have been reported in AIDS patients.[121,122] The organism was mistaken for macrophage in the skin nodules and was identified in the brain when the patient died of acanthamoebic encephalitis.[122] The other case involved only the brain (Plate ID2). The organism is easily cultured in 1.5% nonnutrient agar supplied with gram-negative bacilli (*Escherichia coli/ Enterobacter* sp.) as food. Two plates can be set up, one incubated at 22°C and the other at 37°C. The pathogenic strain of *Acanthamoeba polyphaga* or *A. castellanii* grows better at 37°C. Trophozoites will be visible within one to three days and will form cysts after three days when food is depleted. They tend to grow in a straight line because they are very motile (Plate ID1).[168–170]

Microsporidiosis

This protozoan is another newly recognized opportunistic agent detected in AIDS patients with diarrhea. There are four genera—*Nosema cuniculi, Encephalitozoon* sp., *Enterocytozoon,* and *Pleistophora*. They usually infect insects, fish, and mammals. The clinical manifestations in individuals with AIDS include gastroenteritis, myositis, and hepatitis. The infective stage is the spore, varying from 1.5 to 4 μm oval structures. They stain poorly with hematoxylin-eosin stain (Plate VIC2) and variably in Gram and Ziehl-Neelsen stains.[124-127] All diagnoses are made with biopsies, and none are detected in stool specimen. Because of size and morphology resembling bacilli, this protozoan is difficult to detect in fecal smear. (This is further discussed in Chapter 8.)

Fungal Opportunistic Infections

Yeasts

The most common opportunistic fungal infections are those caused by yeasts (*Candida* sp., *Cryptococcus neoformans, Trichosporon* sp.). Candidiasis should be diagnosed by smear and culture from scraping, biopsy, blood, and bone marrow. *Candida* sp. (*C. albicans, C. parapsilopsis, C. tropicalis*) can be recognized as white, dull, colonies with a yeastlike odor. They are characterized by budding oval yeast cells with pseudohyphae. Speciation is based on carbohydrate fermentation and assimilation.[13]

Candida infections are marked by oroesophageal lesions that are persistent (8.3% of OIs in AIDS, see Table 12–15).[183] Revised CDC guidelines state that candidiasis indicative of AIDS infection requires diagnosis by gross inspection by endoscopy/autopsy or by microscopy (histology/cytology) on a specimen obtained directly from the tissues affected (including scrapings from the mucosal surface), not from a culture.[45]

Disseminated fatal *Trichosporon* infection has been reported in immunocompromised host.[171] It produces yeastlike colonies on Sabouraud agar plate. Microscopically, it is recognized by its budding yeast cells, hyphae, pseudohyphae, rectangular arthrospores, and blastoconidia.

Cryptococcus meningitis in AIDS has been seen frequently (7.1%; see Table 12–15).[183] It is identified by its spherical yeast cells with a polysaccharide capsule easily exhibited as a halo in India ink preparation and mucoid, white, yeastlike colonies on Sabouraud or blood agar plate. Capsule size varies and is noted in isolates in our hospital even in the pre-AIDS period. Although it has been associated with immunocompromised hosts, such as those with Hodgkin's disease and leukemia in bygone years,[111,112] it has become a frequent finding in disseminated infection in AIDS individuals. It has been isolated not only from CSF and brain tissue but also from bone marrow, blood cultures, and bronchoalveolar lavage requested for *P. carinii*. The large capsule is easily delineated as a halo around the budding yeasts when the specimen is stained with MCK for an acid-fast organism (unpublished data). One striking feature of AIDS-associated cryptococcus infection is the extremely high titer of crytococcus antigen, in the range of 1 to 2 million. Although antigen titer is frequently used to monitor treatment in the pre-AIDS period, it is extremely time consuming and costly to monitor sera/CSF specimens from AIDS patients, since the extremely high titer of antigen decreases slowly or not at all.

Molds

Compared with opportunistic yeast infections, the filamentous fungi represented by the dimorphic fungi (*Histoplasma capsulatum*,[113,114] *Blastomyces* sp., *Coccidioides immitis*,[115] *Sporotrichum schenckii*),[116] members of the *Mucorales* (*Pseudallescheria* sp. and *Cunninghamella* sp.[172]), *Aspergillus* sp. and *Alternaria* sp.[173] are less frequent.

Disseminated histoplasmosis with skin lesions on the face, arms, and hands indicates reactivation of previous exposure.[113,114] Oval structure 1 to 2 μm can be demonstrated easily from bone marrow preparation and bone marrow culture in Bactec blood culture vial in a week at 37°C. We encountered three cases within one week. One case caused some confusion in identification because the original organism detected in biopsy was a large oval structure (10 to 15 μm) resembling *Paracoccidiodes* sp. Definitive identification was possible when the culture revealed numerous tuberculate spores typical of *Histoplasma capsulatum*.

Cunninghamella bertholletiae, one member of the *Mucorales*, is rarely isolated even in immunocompromised hosts. It is characterized by sporangiophore, vesicle, and sporangiola (conidia). It grows rapidly, similar to *Mucor*, and the hyphae are broad and nonseptate. Only one case has been reported in an AIDS patient, involving a leg lesion.[172]

Bacterial Infections

Besides the usual gram-negative enteric bacilli, *Staphylococcus aureus* and *Streptococcus pneumoniae*, the unusual emergence of Mycobacteria is unique, especially disseminated mycobacteriosis by MAI and unusual increased incidence of *M. tuberculosis*. Recent reports of cat-scratch disease bacillus in relation to epithelioid angiomatosis nodules is of great interest.[144–146,174]

Mycobacteria

MAI is frequently isolated as a colonizing organism but was seldom found invading, until the AIDS epidemic.[110,134] Since the first edition, *M. tuberculosis* has also been included as an increasingly important OI with AIDS.[135–137] At St. Vincent's, we have isolated 100 MAI and 75 *M. tuberculosis* cases in one year. MAI has been isolated from bone marrow, spleen, liver, lung, stool, intestinal biopsies, and brain biopsy. The primary site of infection is unknown. Usually it is detected in the stool requested for cryptosporidiosis before the clinician suspects it. Growth of MAI and *M. tuberculosis* may be slow (six weeks) or rapid (one week) in rare instances. Developments of the last two years showed that the organism can be detected directly from sputum or positive culture can be identified within a few hours by generic probe (GEN-PROBE, Inc.). Since the probe can detect both dead and viable organisms, the probe to detect the organism from sputum directly has been recalled for further investigation. Mycobacterial probe employs the principle of nucleic acid hybridization to confirm the identification of *M. avium* and *M. intracellulare*, which are difficult to differentiate by biochemical profile isolated in culture from clinical specimens. The kit contains ^{125}I-labeled cDNA probe that is homologous to ribosomal RNA sequences unique to the tuberculosis complex. The other probes are those which identify *M. avium* and *M. intracellulare* even in mixed cultures. Using "insolution" hybridization and "ribosomal RNA detection," it is possible to identify positive samples within two hours instead of weeks or months. Blood or bone marrow cultures in Bactec vials (13A and 12A) and Dupont Isolator can likewise be identified within 2 hours.[153,154]

Cat-Scratch Disease Bacillus

This bacillus is a gram-negative coccobacillus that is very faintly stained by Gram smear unless modified Gram stain (Kopeloff stain) is used. The organism has recently been associated with AIDS patients with disseminated pedunculated skin nodules over the face, trunk, and extremities in epithelioid angiomatosis. We encountered one case, a homeless black male who denies drug abuse or homosexuality. His mother is a prostitute. A smear from a young lesion showed numerous minute gram-negative coccobacilli. The biopsy from one of these lesions showed bacilli resembling cat-scratch disease bacilli under electron microscopy (Figure 12–2). The organism does not need blood to grow, and the optimal temperature for growth is 30°C. Diphasic brain-heart infusion agar is the medium of choice. The organism requires ten days to grow. The colonies are invisible to the naked eye and require observation under the stereoscope.[144,145,174] The growth in diphasic medium resembles a haystack (Colonel DJ, Wear AFIP, personal communication). Compared with *Bartonella*, it does not require blood for growth, and it has a single flagellum shown by transmission electron microscopy. More investigation is underway.

Algal Infection

Prototheca Wickerhamii

This algae was detected in the CSF of an AIDS patient. The organism is the first such case diagnosed in meningitis. The colonies resemble yeast on Sabouraud agar. Both smooth and rough colonies appear in this patient's culture. The characteristic structure is the multiple fission form. Identification is by assimilation and IFA tests (Plate IC1 and C2).[123]

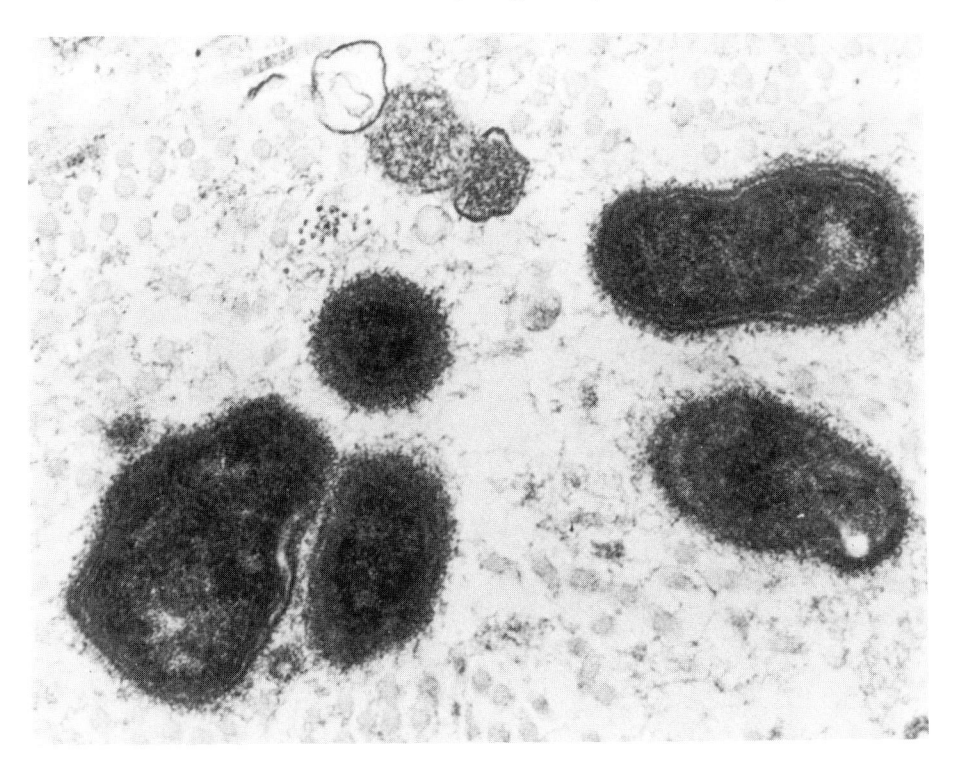

FIGURE 12–2 *Possible cat-scratch disease bacillus from biopsy of skin nodules of an AIDS patient viewed on Siemens Elmskop 1 electron microscope. (Courtesy Drs. Dorthea Zucker-Franklin, Department of Medicine, and Clay J. Cockerell, Department of Dermatology, New York University Medical Center, New York, N.Y.)*

Viral Infections

Progressive Multifocal Leukoencephalopathy

In the first edition, cases of AIDS-associated progressive multifocal leukoencephalopathy (PML) were rarely reported.[175–179] One report showed the incidence was as high as 3.8% of patients with AIDS.[176] A historical event 30 years ago[177] has progressed to an increasing understanding of the causative agent—Papovo virus (JC virus), which had been shown to be a harmless passenger, producing no disease except in immunocompromised hosts. Now it is clear that, like other opportunists, PML is another reactivation infection. Although standard procedure is to demonstrate the agent by IFA, electron microscope, or culture, recent development using DNA hybridization and immunocytochemical studies have been successful in demonstrating the organism in CNS[175–179] and, more recently, in B lymphocytes in the bone marrow and spleen of AIDS patients.[179] It is by this route that JC virus reaches the brain.[179]

Adenoviral Infection

Genital infections by adenovirus have been uncommon. A cluster of infections caused by adenovirus 19 in the genital tract of men and women has been associated with an outbreak of eye infection. Adenoviruses of especially high serotypes, such as 34 and 35, have been isolated from AIDS patients. Their role in causing disease in these patients is unclear.[180]

Varicella Zoster Infection

Herpes zoster has been documented as both a dermatomal and a disseminated disease in AIDS patients, occurring in 10% and 6% of patients, respectively, in one series.[181]

EBV Infections

EBV is ubiquitous in humans, and it is estimated that > 80% of the U.S. population carries some form of antibody to it. EBV is associated with acute infectious mononucleosis, Burkitt's lymphoma, the X-linked lymphoproliferative syndrome, nasopharyngeal carcinoma, and chronic mononucleosis syndrome characterized by fatigue.[182-184] It has been suggested that infection with EBV is an important cofactor in conditions leading to the development of AIDS and that HIV infection itself may reactivate latent EBV, thereby resulting in increased titers of antibodies to this herpesvirus.[183] EBV has been demonstrated in saliva and peripheral blood in low numbers. Isolation of virus in B lymphocytes is time consuming. IFA is used to detect antibodies to four antigens (viral capsid, VCA; early antigen EA [diffuse/restricted]; Epstein-Barr nuclear antigen [EBNA], a more specific test than Paul-Bunnel heterophile test). Patient (1) is susceptible if anti-VCA is absent (<1:10), (2) has a primary EBV infection if anti-VCA is present and anti-EBNA is absent, and (3) is immune due to past infection if both anti-VCA and EBNA are present.

Herpesvirus 6 (HHV-6)

A newly discovered herpesvirus, HHV6[182] is a large, enveloped particle whose inner core contains a double-stranded DNA genome of ~165,000 kilobase pairs long. Unlike EBV, it lyses but does not transform B lymphocytes. It can be propagated in a T-cell line called HSB-2. Anticomplement immunofluorescence assay of sera from HIV-seropositive homosexual men with lymphadenopathy, HIV-seronegative homosexual men, and homosexual men with AIDS shows a lack of correlation between human HHV-6 infection and the course of AIDS infection.[186]

REFERENCES

1. Coffin J, Haase A, Levy JA, et al. What to call the AIDS virus? (Letter from the International Committee on the Taxonomy of Viruses.) Nature 1986;321:10.

2. Weiss SH, Goedert JJ, Sarngadharan MG, Bodner AJ, et al. The AIDS seroepidemiology collaborative working group, Gallo RC, Blattner WA. Screening test for HTLV-III (AIDS agent) antibodies. Specificity, sensitivity, and applications. JAMA 1985;253:221–225.
3. Goudsmit J, Paul DA, Lange JMA, et al. Expression of human immunodeficiency virus antigen (HIV-Ag) in serum and cerebrospinal fluid during acute and chronic infection. Lancet 1986;2:8500–8504.
4. AIDS Weekly Surveillance Report—United States AIDS Program, Center for Infectious Diseases, Centers for Disease Control, Dec. 5, 1988.
5. Peterman TZ, Curran JW. Sexual transmission of human immunodeficiency virus: Special communication. JAMA 1986;256:2222–2226.
6. Hayward WL, Curran JW. The epidemiology of AIDS in the U.S. Scientific American 1988;259, no.4:72–82.
7. Malief CJM, Goudsmit J. Transmission of lymphotropic retroviruses (HTLV-I and LAV/HTLV-III) by blood transfusion and blood products. Vox Sanguinis 1986; 50:1–11.
8. Centers for Disease Control. Update: Acquired immunodeficiency syndrome and human immunodeficiency virus infection among health-care workers. MMWR 1988;37:229–238.
9. Boffey PM. Worker is infected by AIDS virus in laboratory. *The New York Times*, Sept. 5, 1987.
10. Sullivan R. AIDS deaths in New York are showing new pattern. *The New York Times*, Oct. 22, 1987.
11. Eijrond BDP, Van Den Hoek JAR, Emsbroek JA, et al. Declining incidence of sexually transmitted diseases as a result of an AIDS-prevention campaign (Abstr. F85). Third International conference on AIDS, Washington, DC, June 8, 1987.
12. Handsfield HH, Sandstrom EG, Knapp JS, et al. Epidemiology of penicillinase-producing *Neisseria gonorrhoeae* infection. Analysis by auxotyping and serogrouping. N Engl J Med 1982;306:950.
13. Lennette EH, Balows A, Hausler WJ Jr, Shadomy HJ, eds. Manual of clinical microbiology, 4th ed. Washington, DC: American Society for Microbiology, 1985.
14. Faur YC, Weisburd MH, Wilson ME, et al. New York City medium for the simultaneous isolation of *Neisseria gonorrhoeae*, large colony mycoplasma and T-mycoplasma. Appl Microbiol 1974;27:1041.
15. Centers for Disease Control. Sexually transmitted diseases treatment guidelines. MMWR (suppl) 1982;31:33.
16. Lue YA, Heard L, McLean TI. Comparative evaluation of a modified Gonogen procedure and the Phadebact test for the identification of *N. gonorrhoeae* (Abstr. C-364). In: Abstracts of the 86th Annual Meeting for the American Society for Microbiology, New York: 1986.
17. Amuso P, Hester J, Frankel J. Comparison of coagglutination tests for the identification of *Neisseria gonorrhoeae* (Abstr. C363). In: Abstracts of the Annual Meeting for the American Society for Microbiology, New York: 1986.
18. Capozzi JM, Baron EJ, Tyburski MB, Berman M. Comparison of three commercially produced rapid methods and conventional biochemicals for identification of *Neisseria* species (Abstr. C-360). In: Abstracts of the 86th Annual Meeting for the American Society for Microbiology, New York: 1986.
19. Farano P, Filipczak, Bondi J, et al. Comparison of the Gonocheck II with a new 1-hour innovative diagnostic system procedure for the identification of gram negative bacteria isolated on Thayer-Martin medium (Abstr. C-357). In: Abstracts of

the 86th Annual Meeting for the American Society for Microbiology, New York: 1986.
20. Armstrong A, Miller T. Detection of *Neisseria gonorrhoeae* L-forms with gonozyme (Abstr. C-23). In: Abstracts of the Annual Meeting for the American Society for Microbiology, New York: 1983.
21. Janda WM, Morello JA, Lerner SA, et al. Characteristics of pathogenic *Neisseria* spp. isolated from homosexual men. J Clin Microbiol 1983;17:85.
22. Judson FN, Ehret JM, Eickhoff TC. Anogenital infection with *Neisseria meningitidis* in homosexual men. J Infect 1978;137:458.
23. Carlson BL, Fiumara NJ, Kelly JR, McCormack WM. Isolation of *Neisseria meningitidis* from anogenital specimens from homosexual men. Sex Transm Dis 1980;7:71.
24. Bowie WR, Holmes KK. Non-gonococcal urethritis. Clin Microbiol Newsletter 1980;2:1.
25. Bird BR, Forrester FT. Laboratory diagnosis of *Chlamydia trachomatis* Infections. Atlanta: U.S. Department of Health and Human Services, Virology training branch, October 1981.
26. Stamm WE, Tam M, Koester M, et al. Detection of *Chlamydia trachomatis* inclusions in McCoy cell cultures with fluorescent-conjugated monoclonal antibodies. J Clin Microbiol 1983;17:666.
27. Judson FN, Ehret JM, Moore DF. Comparison of Ortho and Syva direct fluorescent antibody tests with culture for detection of *Chlamydia trachomatis* (Abstr. C-17). In: Abstracts of the 86th Annual Meeting of American Society for Microbiology, New York: 1986.
28. Josephson SL, Kehl KS, Thomason JL, Williams JE. Comparison of Chlamydiazyme and MicroTrak in an obstetrical-gynecological population. (Abstr. C-12). In: Abstracts of the 86th Annual Meeting of American Society for Microbiology, New York: 1986.
29. Vincelette J, Couturier B, Lefebvre J, et al. Comparative evaluation of direct immunofluorescence (Microtrak), enzyme immunoassay (Chlamydiazyme) and culture for diagnosis of *Chlamydia trachomatis* genital infections (Abstr. C-15). In: Abstracts of the 86th Annual Meeting of the American Society for Microbiology, New York: 1986.
30. Wang SP, Grayston JT, Alexander ER, Holmes KK. A simplified microimmunofluorescent test with trachoma-lymphogranuloma venereum (*Chlamydia trachomatis*) antigens for use as a screening test for antibody. J Clin Microbiol 1975;1:250.
31. Bowie WR. Urethritis in males. In: Holmes KK, Mardh P, Sparling PF, Wiesner PJ, eds. Sexually transmitted diseases. New York: McGraw-Hill, 1984;281–291.
32. Perine PL, Osoba AO. Lymphogranuloma venereum. In: Holmes KK, Mardh P, Sparling PF, Wiesner PJ, eds. Sexually transmitted diseases. New York: McGraw-Hill, 1986:281–291.
33. Bolan RK, Sands M, Schachter J, et al. *Lymphogranuloma venereum* and acute ulcerative proctitis. Am J Med 1982;72:703.
34. Bleeker A, Coutinho RA, Bakker-kok J, et al. Prevalence of syphilis and hepatitis B among homosexual men in two saunas in Amsterdam. Br J Vener Dis 1981;57:196.
35. Johns DR, Tierney M, Felsenstein F. Alteration in the natural history of neurosyphilis by concurrent infection with the human immunodeficiency virus. N Engl J Med 1987;316:1569–1572.

36. Museyi K, van Dyck E, Vervoort T, et al. Use of an enzyme immunoassay to detect serum IgG antibodies to *Haemophilus ducreyi*. J Infect Dis 1988;157:1039–1043.
37. Dohany AL, Burton JJS. Arthropods of medical importance. In Braude AI, ed. Medical microbiology and infectious diseases. Philadelphia: W.B. Saunders, 1981:196–210.
38. Barre-Sinoussi F, Chermann JC, Rey F, et al. Isolation of a T-lymphotropic retrovirus from a patient at risk for acquired immune deficiency syndrome (AIDS). Science 1983;220:868.
39. Gallo RC, Sarin PS, Gelmann EP, et al. Isolation of human T-cell leukemia virus in acquired immune deficiency syndrome (AIDS). Science 1983;220:865–867.
40. Levy JD, Hoffman SM, Kramer JA, et al. Isolation of lymphocytopathic retroviruses from San Francisco patients with AIDS. Science 1984;225:840–842.
41. Feorina PM, Kalyanaraman VS, Haverkos HW, et al. Lymphadenopathy associated virus infection of a blood donor-recipient pair with acquired immunodeficiency syndrome. Science 1984;225:69–72.
42. Koch Von MG. AIDS—Vom molekul zur Pandemie. Heidelberg: Spektrum Der Wissenschaft. 1987.
43. Casareale D, Dewhurat S, Sonnabend J, et al. Prevalence of AIDS-associated retrovirus and antibodies among male homosexuals at risk for AIDS in Greenwich Village. AIDS Research 1984/5;11:407–421.
44. Ho DD, Pomerantz RJ, Kaplan JC. Pathogenesis of infection with human immunodeficiency virus. N Engl J Med 1987;317:278–286.
45. AIDS Program. Center for Infectious Diseases, Centers for Disease Control. Revision of the CDC surveillance case definition for acquired immunodeficiency syndrome. MMWR Supplement 1987;36/1S:3S–15S.
46. Gupta P, Balachandran R, Grovit K, et al. Detection of human immunodeficiency virus by reverse transcriptase assay, antigen capture assay, and radioimmunoassay. J Clin Microbiol 1987;25:1122–1125.
47. Popovic M, Sarngadharan MG, Read E, Gallo RC. Detection, isolation, and continuous production of cytopathic retroviruses (HTLV-III) from patients with AIDS and pre-AIDS. Science 1984;224:497–500.
48. Gallo RC, Salahuddin SZ, Popovic M, et al. Frequent detection and isolation of cytopathic retroviruses (HTLV-III) from patients with AIDS and at risk for AIDS. Science 1984;224:500–503.
49. Sarngadharan MG, Alludeen HS, Gallo RC. Reverse transcriptase of RNA tumor viruses and animal cells. Methods Cancer Res 1976;12:3.
50. Schupbach J, Popovic Mikulas, Gilden RV, et al. Serological analysis of a subgroup of human T-lymphotropic retroviruses (HTLV-III) associated with AIDS. Science 1984;224:503–505.
51. Velleca WM, Palmer DF, Feorino PM. Isolation, culture and identification of human T-lymphotropic virus type III/lymphadenopathy-associated virus. Procedure guide (developmental), Centers for Disease Control, March 1986.
52. Gallo D, Diggs, JL, Shell GR, et al. Comparison of detection of antibody to the acquired immune deficiency syndrome virus by enzyme immunoassay, immunoflourescence and Western Blot methods. J Clin Microbiol 1987;23:1072–1077.
53. Allain J-P, Paul DA, Laurian Y, Senn D, and members of the AIDS-Haemophilia French study group. Serological markers in early stages of human immunodeficiency virus infection in haemophiliacs. Lancet 1986;2:1233–1236.
54. Centers for Disease Control. AIDS due to HIV-2—New Jersey. MMWR 1988;37:33–34.

55. Centers for Disease Control. Update: serologic testing for antibody to human immunodeficiency virus. MMWR 1988;36:833–844.
56. Abbott Diagnostics Educational Services. HIV Journal Articles: Serology. April 1987.
57. Weiss SH. Laboratory detection of human immunodeficiency virus. In: Wormser G, Stahl RE, Bottone EJ, eds. AIDS and other manifestations of HIV infection. Noyes Publications, 1987.
58. Centers for Disease Control. Recommendations for prevention of HIV transmission in health-care settings. MMWR Supplement 1987;36/2S:3S–18S.
59. Carlson JR, Yee J, Hinrichs SH, et al. Comparison of indirect immunofluorescence and western blot for detection of anti-human immunodeficiency virus antibodies. J Clin Microbiol 1987;25:494–497.
60. Hofbauer JM, Schulz TF, Hengster P, et al. Comparison of western blot (immunoblot) based on recombinant-derived p41 with conventional tests for serodiagnosis of human immunodeficiency virus infections. J Clin Microbiol 1988;26:116–120.
61. Ma P, McCaffrey M, Masdeu J. CSF HIV immunology in some neurologic syndromes of AIDS, No. 880329. Fourth International Conference on AIDS. Stockholm, Sweden, June 12–16, 1988.
62. Hill WC, Bolton V, Carlson JR. Isolation of acquired immunodeficiency syndrome virus from the placenta. Am J Obst Gynecol 1987;157:10–11.
63. Pomerantz RJ, Kuritzkes DR, De La Monte S, et al. Infection of the retina by human immunodeficiency virus type 1. N Engl J Med 1987;317:1643–1647.
64. Martin LS, McDougal JS, Loskoski SL. Disinfection and inactivation of the human T lymphotropic virus Type III/lymphadenopathy-associated virus. J Infect Dis 1985;152:400–403.
65. Montagnier L, Gruest J, Chamaret S, et al. Adaptation of lymphadenopathy associated virus (LAV) to replication in EBV-transformed B lymphoblastoid cell lines. Science 1984;225:63–66.
66. Koyanagi Y, Harada S, Yamamoto N. Establishment of a high production system for AIDS retroviruses with a human T-leukemic cell line MOLT-4. Cancer Lett 1986;30:299–310.
67. Casareale D, Stevenson D, Sakai K, Volsky DJ. A human T-cell line resistant to cytopathic effects of the human immunodeficiency virus (HIV). Virology 1987;156:40–49.
68. Montefiori DC, Mitchell WM. Infection of the HTLV-II-bearing T cell line C3 with HTLV-III/LAV is highly permissive and lytic. Virology 1986;155:726–731.
69. Feorino P, Forrester B, Schable C, et al. Comparison of antigen assay and reverse transcriptase assay for detecting human immunodeficiency virus in culture. J Clin Microbiol 1987;25:2344–2346.
70. Harada S, Koyanagi Y, Yamamoto N. Infection of HTLV-III/LAV in HTLV-I-carrying cells, MT-2 and MT-4 and application in a plaque assay. Science 1985;229:563–566.
71. Matsui T, Nakashima H, Yoshiyama H, et al. Plaque staining assay for non-/weakly cytotoxic human immunodeficiency virus. J Clin Microbiol 1987;25:1305–1307.
72. Blumberg RS, Sandstrom EG, Paradis TJ, et al. Detection of human T-cell lymphotropic virus type III-related antigens and anti-human cell lymphotropic virus type III antibodies by anticomplementary immunofluorescence. J Clin Microbiol 1987;23:1072–1077.

73. Harper ME, Marselle LM, Gallo RC, Wong-Staal F. Detection of lymphocytes expressing human T-lymphotropic virus type III in lymph nodes and peripheral blood from infected individuals by in situ hybridization. Proc Natl Acad Sci USA 1986;83:772–776.
74. Moseley RC, Corey L, Benjamin D, et al. Comparison of viral isolation, direct immunofluorescence and indirect immunoperoxidase techniques for detection of genital herpes simplex virus infection. J Clin Microbiol 1981;13:93.
75. Nerukar LS, Jacob AJ, Madden DL, Sever JL. Detection of genital herpes simplex infections by a tissue culture-fluorescent-antibody technique with biotin-avidin. J Clin Microbiol 1983;17:149.
76. Langenberg A, Smith D, Brakel CL, et al. Dectection of herpes simplex virus DNA from genital lesions by *in situ* hybridization. J Clin Microbiol 1988;26:933–937.
77. DeGirolami PC, Dakos J, Eichelberger K, Biano S. Evaluation of a new latex agglutination method for detection of antibody to herpes simplex virus: Notes. J Clin Microbiol 1988;26:1024–1025.
78. Heller M, Dix RD, Baringer JR, et al. Herpetic proctitis and meningitis: recovery of two strains of herpes simplex virus type 1 from cerebrospinal fluid. J Infect Dis 1987;146:584–588.
79. Dix RD, Waitzman DM, Follansbee S, et al. Herpes simplex virus type 2 encephalitis in two homosexual men with persistent lymphadenopathy. Ann Neurol 1985;17:203–206.
80. Drew WL, Mintz L, Miner RC, et al. Prevalence of cytomegalovirus infection in homosexual men. J Infect Dis 1981;43:188.
81. Lentz EB, Dock NL, McMahon CA, et al. Detection of antibody to cytomegalovirus-induced early antigens and comparison with four serologic assays and presence of viruria in blood donors. J Clin Microbiol 1988;26:133–135.
82. Gauss P, Muller V, Fosner GG, Deinhardt F. Propagation of hepatitis A virus in human embryo fibroblasts. J Med Virol 1981;7:233.
83. Centers for Disease Control. Enterically transmitted non-A, non-B hepatitis—Mexico. MMWR 1987;36:597–601.
84. Solomon, RE, Kaslow RA, Phair JP, et al. Human immunodeficiency virus and hepatitis delta virus in homosexual men. Ann Intern Med 1988;108:51–54.
85. Zachow KR, Ostrow RS, Bender M, et al. Detection of human papillomavirus DNA in anogenital neoplasia. Nature 1982;300:771–773.
86. Caussy D, Orr W, Daya AD, et al. Evaluation of methods for detecting human papillomavirus deoxyribonucleotide sequences in clinical specimens. J Clin Microb 1988;26:236–243.
87. Blaser UJ, Berkowitz ED, LaForce FM, et al. Campylobacter enteritis: Clinical and epidemiologic features. Ann Intern Med 1979;91:179.
88. Fennell CL, Totten PA, Quinn TC, et al. Characterization of campylobacter-like organisms isolated from homosexual men. J Infect Dis 1984;149:58.
89. Ma P, Soave R. Three-step stool examination for cryptosporidiosis in 10 homosexual men with protracted watery diarrhea. J Infect Dis 1983;147:824–828.
90. Ma P. Cryptosporidiosis and immune enteropathy: A review. In: Remington JS, Swartz MN, eds. Current clinical topics in infectious diseases. New York: McGraw-Hill, 1987;8:99–153.
91. Ma P. Biology and diagnosis of *Cryptosporidium* sp. In: Actor P, Evangelista A, Poupard J, Hinks E, eds. Infections in the immunocompromised host. New York: Plenum Publishing Co., 1986;135–152.

92. Sterling CR, Arrowood MJ. Detection of *Cryptosporidium* sp. infections using a direct immunofluorescent assay. Pediatric Infect Dis 1986;5:S139–142.
93. Tsaihong J, Ma P. Identification of fecal cryptosporidial oocysts by comparing sucrose wet preparation, modified cold Kinyoun stain and indirect fluorescent test (Abstr. C85). In: Proceeding and Abstract of the 84th Annual Meeting of the American Society for Microbiology, Washington, D.C., 1984.
94. Casemore DP, Armstrong M, Sands RL. Laboratory diagnosis of cryptosporidiosis. J Clin Pathol 1985;38:1337–1341.
95. Stibbs HH, Ongerth JE. Immunofluorescence detection of *Cryptosporidium* oocysts in fecal smears. J Clin Microbiol 1986;24:517–521.
96. Garcia LS, Brewer TC, Bruckner DA. Fluorescence detection of *Cryptosporidium* oocysts in human fecal specimens by using monoclonal antibodies. J Clin Microbiol 1987;25:119–121.
97. Baxby D, Blundell N, Hart CA. Excretion of atypical oocysts by patients with cryptosporidiosis (letter). Lancet 1987;25:1:974.
98. Ma P, Tsaihong J. Immune response of AIDS and non-AIDS individuals to *Cryptosporidium* (session 72, Abstr. 833). In: 27th Interscience Conference on Antimicrobiol Agents and Chemotherapy, New York, Oct. 6, 1987.
99. Ungar BLP, Soave R, Fayer R, Nash TE. Enzyme immunoassay detection of immunoglobulin M and G antibodies to *Cryptosporidium* in immunocompetent and immunocompromised persons. J Infect Dis 1986;153:570–578.
100. Allason-Jones E, Mindel A, Sargeaunt P, Williams P. *Entamoeba histolytica* as a commensal intestinal parasite in homosexual men. N Engl J Med 1986;315:353–356.
101. Kotler DP. Preliminary observations of the effect of cow milk globulin upon intestinal cryptosporidiosis in AIDS. Third International Conference on AIDS. THP 148, Washington, D.C., 1987.
102. Tzipori S, Roberton D, Chapman C. Remission of diarrhoea due to cryptosporidiosis in an immunodeficient child treated with hyperimmune bovine colostrum. Br Med J 1986;293:1276–1277.
103. Tzipori S, Roberton D, Cooper DA, White L. Chronic cryptosporidial diarrhoea and hyperimmune cow colostrum. Lancet 1987;2:344.
104. Louie E, Borkowsky W, Klesius PH, et al. Treatment of cryptosporidiosis with oral bovine transfer factor. Clin Immunol Immunopath 1987;44:329–334.
105. Ma P, Kaufman DL. Symptomatic *Isospora belli* in two homosexual men (Abstr. 131). Paper presented at the 12th International Congress of Microbiology, Boston, 1982.
106. Ma P, Kaufman D, Montana J. *Isospora belli* diarrheal infection in three homosexual men. AIDS Res 1984;1:327–338.
107. DeHovitz JA, Pape JW, HBoncy M, Johnson WD. Clinical manifestations and therapy of *Isospora belli* infection in patients with the acquired immunodeficiency syndrome. N Engl J Med 1986;315:87–90.
108. Soave R, Warren J. *Cryptosporidium* and *Isospora belli* infections. J Infect Dis 1988;157:225–229.
109. Ma P. Protozoa and acquired immune deficiency syndrome (AIDS). ATCC Quartetly 1987;7:1,2,7.
110. Armstrong D. Opportunistic infections in the acquired immune deficiency syndrome. Semin Oncol (Suppl 3) 1987;14;40–47.

111. Pipard MJ, Dalgleish A, Bigson P, et al. Acquired immunodeficiency with disseminated cryptococcosis. Arch Dis Child 1986;61:289–291.
112. Witt D, McKay D, Schwam L, et al. Acquired immune deficiency syndrome presenting as bone marrow and mediastinal cryptococcosis. Am J Med 1987;82:149–150.
113. Dietrich P-Y, Pugin P, Regamey C, et al. Disseminated histoplasmosis and AIDS in Switzerland (letter). Lancet 1986;ii:752.
114. Mandell W, Goldberg DM, Neu HC. Histoplasmosis in patients with the acquired immune deficiency syndrome. Am J Med 1986;6:974–978.
115. Bronnimann DA, Adam RD, Galgiani JN, et al. Coccidioidomycosis in the acquired immunodeficiency syndrome. Ann Intern Med 1986;106:372–379.
116. Bibler MR, Luber HJ, Glueck HI, Estes SA. Disseminated sporotrichosis in a patient with HIV infection after treatment for acquired factor VIII inhibitor. JAMA 1986;256:3125–3126.
117. Sherer R, Sable R, Sonnenberg M, et al. Disseminated infection with *Mycobacterium kansasii* in the acquired immunodeficiency syndrome. Ann Intern Med 1986;105:710–712.
118. Mandal BK. *Herpes zoster* and the immunocompromised. J Infect 1987;14:1–5.
119. Grimes MM, LaPook JD, Bar MH, et al. Disseminated *Pneumocystis carinii* infection in a patient with acquired immunodeficiency syndrome. Hum Pathol 1987;18;307–308.
120. Gould IA, Belok LC, Handwerger S. *Listeria monocytogenes:* A rare cause of opportunistic infection in the acquired immunodeficiency syndrome (AIDS) and a new cause of meningitis in AIDS. A case report. AIDS Res 1986;3;231–234.
121. Gonzalez MM, Gould E, Dickinson G, et al. Acquired immunodeficiency syndrome associated with *Acanthamoeba* infection and other opportunistic organisms. Arch Pathol Lab Med 1986;110:749–751.
122. Wiley CA, Safrin RE, Davis CE, et al. Acanthamoeba meningoencephalitis in a patient with AIDS. J Infect Dis 1987;155:130–133.
123. Kaminski ZC, Kapila R, Kloser P. *Prototheca wickerhamii* meningitis in a patient with acquired immunodeficiency syndrome (Abstr. 1A.11). Pan American Congress for Infectious Diseases, San Juan, Puerto Rico, 1986.
124. Modigliani R, Bories C, Le Charpentier Y, et al. Diarrhoea and malabsorption in acquired immune deficiency syndrome: a study of four cases with special emphasis on opportunistic protozoan infestations. Gut 1985;26:179–187.
125. Terada S, Reddy KR, Jeffers LJ, Cali A. Microsporidan hepatitis in the acquired immunodeficiency syndrome. Ann Intern Med 1987;107:61–62.
126. Ledford DK, Overman MD, Gonzalvo A, et al. Microsporidiosis myositis in a patient with the acquired immunodeficiency syndrome. Ann Intern Med 1985;102:628–630.
127. Rijpstra AC, Canning EU, van Ketel RJ, et al. Use of light microscopy to diagnose small-intestinal microsporidiosis in patients with AIDS. J Infect Dis 1988;157:827–831.
127a. Shadduck JA. Human microsporidiosis and AIDS. Rev Infect Dis (in press).
128. Surawicz CM, Roberts PL, Rompalo A, et al. Intestinal spirochetosis in homosexual men. Am J Med 1987;82:587–592.
129. Peters CS, Sable R, Janda WM, et al. Prevalence of enteric parasites in homosexual patients attending an outpatient clinic. Clin Microbiol 1986;24:684–685.

130. Drabick JJ, Egan JE, Brown SL, et al. Dicroceliasis (lancet fluke disease) in an HIV seropositive man. JAMA 1988;259:567–568.
131. Volsky DJ, Wu YT, Stevenson M, et al. Antibodies to HTLV-III/LAV in Venezuelan patients with acute malarial infections. N Engl J Med 1986;314:647–648.
132. Rosenthal PJ, Chaisson RE, Hadley WK, et al. Rectal leishmaniasis in a patient with acquired immunodeficiency syndrome. Am J Med 1988;84:307–309.
133. Centers for Disease Control. Diagnosis and managmeent of mycobacterial infection and disease in persons with human immunodeficiency virus infection. Ann Intern Med 1987;106;254–256.
134. Young LS, Inderlied CB, Berlin OG, Gottlieb MS. Mycobacterial infections in AIDS patients with an emphasis on the *Mycobacterium avium complex*. Rev Infect Dis 1986;8:1024–1033.
135. Sunderam G, McDonald RJ, Maniatis T, et al. Tuberculosis as a manifestation of the acquired immunodeficiency syndrome (AIDS). JAMA 1986;256:362–366.
136. Saltzman BR, Motyl MR, Friedland GH, et al. *Mycobacterium tuberculosis* bacteremia in the acquired immunodeficiency syndrome. JAMA 1986;256:390–391.
137. Barnes PF, Arevalo C. Six cases of *Mycobacterium tuberculosis* bacteremia. J Infect Dis 1987;156:377–179.
138. Wheeler AP, Gregg CR. Campylobacter bacteremia, cholecystitis, and the acquired immunodeficiency syndrome (letter). Ann Intern Med 1986;105:804.
139. Doll DC, Yarbro JW. Mycobacterial spinal cord abscess with an ascending polyneuropathy (letter). Ann Intern Med 1987;106:333–334.
140. Andavolu RH, Jagadha V, Lue Y, Mclean T. Lung abscess involving *Corynebacterium pseudodiphtheriticum* in a patient with AIDS-related complex. NY State J Med 1986;86:594–596.
141. Samies JH, Hathaway BN, Echols RM, et al. Lung abscess due to *Corynebacterium equi*: Report of the first case—acquired immune deficiency syndrome. Am J Med 1986;80:685–688.
142. Clairmont GJ, Zon LI, Groopman JE. *Hemophilus parainfluenzae* prostatitis in a homosexual man with chronic lymphadenopathy syndrome and HTLV-III infection. Am J Med 1987;82:175–178.
143. Toth IR, Kazal HL. Botryomycosis in acquired immunodeficiency syndrome. Arch Pathol Lab Med 1987;111:246–249.
144. Cockerell CJ, Webster GF, Whitlow MA, Friedman-Kien AE. Epithelioid angiomatosis: Vascular disorder in patients with the acquired immunodeficiency syndrome or AIDS-related complex. Lancet 1987;ii:654–656.
145. Stoler MH, Bonfiglio TA, Steigbigel RT, Pereira M. An atypical subcutaneous infection associated with acquired immune deficiency syndrome. Am J Clin Pathol 1983;80:714–718.
146. Angritt P. Tuur SM, Macher AM, et al. AIDS case for diagnosis series, 1988. Military medicine. Military Medicine 1988;153:M25–M32.
147. Kiehn TE, Edwards FF, Brannon P, et al. Infections caused by *Mycobacterium avium complex* in immunocompromised patients: Diagnosis by blood culture and fecal examination, antimicrobial susceptibility tests and morphological and seroagglutination characteristics. J Clin Microbiol 1985;21:168–173.
148. Kiehn TE, Cammarata R. Laboratory diagnosis of mycobacterial infections in patients with acquired immunodeficiency syndrome. J Clin Microbiol 1986;24:708–711.

149. Luce JM. Sputum induction in the acquired immunodeficiency syndrome (editorial). Am Rev Resp Dis 1986;133:523–524.
150. Bigby TD, Margolskee D, Curtis JL, et al. The usefulness of induced sputum in the diagnosis of *Pneumocystis carinii* pneumonia in patients with the acquired immunodeficiency syndrome. Am Rev Resp Dis 1986;133:515–518.
151. Resnick L, Pitchenik AD, Fisher E, et al. Detection of HTLV-III/LAV-specific IgG and antigen in bronchoalveolar lavage fluid from two patients with lymphocytic interstitial pneumonitis associated with AIDS-related complex. Am J Med 1987; 82:553–556.
152. Gagliardi AM, Stover DE, Zaman MK. Endobronchial *Pneumocystis P. carinii* infection in a patient with the acquired immune deficiency syndrome. Chest 1987; 91:463–464.
153. Lutz B, Galliher K, Greenwood JR. Combined use of the Bactec 460 and fGenprobe DNA probes for rapid isolation and identification of *Mycobacterium tuberculosis* and *M. avium* complex. 88th Annual Meeting of the American Society for Microbiology, Abstract, Miami, Florida: 1988.
154. Marines HU, Osato MS, Font RL. The value of calcofluor white in the diagnosis of mycotic and Acanthamoeba infections of the eye and ocular adnexa. Ophthamology 1986;94:23–26.
155. Ma P, Tsaihong J. A rapid automatic multistaining for microbiology EM MIDAS® II (Abstr. 123). In: First Annual ASM Conference on Biotechnology, March 20, 1986.
156. Maher AM, Bardenstein DS, Zimmerman LE, et al. *Pneumocystis carinii* choroiditis in a male homosexual with AIDS and disseminated pulmonary and extrapulmonary *P. carinii* infection. N Engl J Med 1987;316:1092.
157. Heyman MR, Rasmussen P. *Pneumocystis carinii* involvement of the bone marrow in acquired immunodeficiency syndrome. Am J Clin Pathol 1987;87:780–783.
158. Linder E, Lundin L, Vorma H. Detection of *Pneumocystis carinii* in lung-derived samples using monoclonal antibodies to an 82 kDa parasite component. J Immunol Meth 1987;98:57–62.
159. Kovacs JA, Ng VL, Masur H, et al. Diagnosis of *Pneumocystis carinii* pneumonia: Improved detection in sputum with use of monoclonal antibodies. N Engl J Med 1988;318:589–593.
160. Walzer PD. Diagnosis of *Pneumocystis carinii* pneumonia. J Infect Dis 1988;157: 629–632.
161. Ma P, Villanueva TG, Kaufman D, Gillooly J. Respiratory cryptosporidiosis in the acquired immunodeficiency syndrome. JAMA 1984;252:298–1301.
162. Kahn DG, Garfinkle JM, Klonoff DC, et al. Cryptosporidial and cytomegaloviral hepatitis and cholecystitis. Arch Pathol Lab Med 1987;111:879–881.
163. Gross TL, Wheat J, Bartlett M, et al. AIDS and multiple system involvement with *Cryptosporidium*. Am J Gastroenterol 1986;81:456–458.
164. Harari MD, West B, Dwyer B. *Cryptosporidium* as cause of laryngotracheitis in an infant. Lancet 1986;1:1207.
165. Fayer R, Ungar BLP. *Cryptosporidium* spp. and cryptosporidiosis. Microbiol Rev 1986;50;458–483.
166. Jenkins KA, Remington JS. *Toxoplasma gondii* infection of the central nervous system use of the peroxidase-antiperoxidase method to demonstrate toxoplasma in formalin fixed, paraffin embedded tissue sections. Hum Pathol 1981;12:690.

167. Hofflin JM, Remington JS. Tissue culture isolation of *Toxoplasma* from blood of a patient with AIDS. Arch Intern Med 1985;145:925–926.
168. Ma P, Willaert E, Juechter KB, Stevens AR. A case of keratitis due to *Acanthamoeba* in New York, New York, and features of 10 cases. J Infect Dis 1981;143:662–667.
169. Ma P, Visvesvara GS, Martinez AJ, et al. Free-living amoebic infections. Seminar, session 238A, tape available. Annual Meeting of American Society for Microbiology. Atlanta, 1987.
170. Ma P, Visvesvara, GS, Martinez AJ, et al. Naegleria and acanthamoeba infections. A review (submitted for publication).
171. Walling DM, McGraw DJ, Merz WG, et al. Disseminated infection with *Trichosporon beigelii*. Rev Infect Dis 1987;9:1013–1019.
172. Mostaza JM, Barbado FJ, Fernandez-Martin J, et al. Cutaneo-articular mucomycosis (*Cunninghamella bertholletiae*) in a patient with acquried immunodeficiency syndrome (AIDS). Rev Infect Dis (in press).
173. Wiest PM, K Wiese, Jacobs MR, et al. Alternaria infection in a patient with acquired immunodeficiency syndrome: Case report and review of invasive alternaria infections. Rev Infect Dis 1987;9:799–803.
174. Le Boit P, Egbert B, Stoler MH, et al. Epithelioid angiomatosis-like vascular proliferation in patients with AIDS. Manifestations of cat scratch disease bacillus infection. Lancet 1988;8592:960–963.
175. Miller JR, Barrett RE, Britton CB, et al. Progressive multifocal leukoencephalopathy in a male homosexual with T-cell immune deficiency. N Engl J Med 1982;307;1436.
176. Aksamit AJ, Mourrain P, Sever JL, Major EO. Progressive multifocal leukoencephalopathy: Investigation of three cases using in situ hybridization with JC virus biotinylated DNA probe. Ann Neurol 1985;18:490–496.
177. Walker DL. Progressive multifocal leukoencephalopathy. In: Vinken PJ, Bruyn GW, Klawans HL, eds. Infections of the nervous system, part II. Handbook of clinical neurology, rev. Series 3, vol. 47. Amsterdam: North-Holland Publishing Co., 1978;307–309.
178. Aksamit AJ, Sever JL, Major EO. Progressive multifocal leukoencephalopathy: JC virus detection by in situ hybridization compared with immunohistochemistry. Neurology 1986;36:499–504.
179. Houff SA, Major EO, Katz DA, et al. Involvement of JC virus-infected mononuclear cells from the bone marrow and spleen in the pathogenesis of progressive multifocal leukoencephalopathy. N Engl J Med 1988;318:301–305.
180. Horwitz MS, Valderrama G, Korn R, Spigland I. Adenovirus isolates from the urines of AIDS patients: characterization of Group B recombinants. In: Acquired immune deficiency syndrome. Alan R. Liss, 1984:187–207.
181. Quinnan GV, Masure H, Rook AH, et al. Herpes virus infections in the acquired immunodeficiency syndrome. JAMA 1984;252:72.
182. Volsky DJ, Lai PK. B-cell abnormalitieis in AIDS: Role of HIV and Epstein-Barr virus. In: Wormser GP, Stahl RE, Bottone EJ, eds. AIDS and other manifestations of HIV infection. Park Ridge, NJ: Noyes, 1987;347–366.
183. Strauss SE. The chronic mononucleosis syndrome. J Infect Dis 1988;157:405–412.
184. Barnes DM. Mystery disease at Lake Tahoe challenges virologists and clinicians. Science 1986;234:541–542.

185. Lehman JS, Mikl J. AIDS epidemiology program. In AIDS surveillance monthly update, Bureau of Communicable Disease Control. New York State Department of Health. January 1988;18.
186. Spira TJ, Bozeman LH, Sanderlin KC, et al. Lack of correlation between human herpes virus-6 infection and the course of human immunodeficiency virus infection. Abstract 847. Program and Abstracts of the Twenty-Eighth Interscience Conference on Antimicrobial Agents and Chemotherapy. Los Angeles, 1988.

ADDITIONAL READING

1. What science knows about AIDS. Scientific American 1988;259, no.4:40–134.
2. Hoofnagle JH. Type D (delta) hepatitis. JAMA 1989;261(9):1321–1325.

PART IV

Infectious and Neoplastic Complications of AIDS

Chapter 13

The Etiologic Agent of AIDS

David W. Archibald

M. Essex

A T-lymphotropic virus has been established as the agent of acquired immunodeficiency syndrome (AIDS) and related pathologic conditions.[1-5] This cytopathic human retrovirus, tropic for the T4 subset of lymphocytes, had been termed human T lymphotropic virus type 3 (HTLV-3),[2,5] lymphadenopathy-associated virus (LAV),[1] and AIDS-related virus (ARV).[6] The term human immunodeficiency virus (HIV) has since been accepted. These different isolates have a high degree of cross-reactivity by both serologic and nucleic acid analysis, demonstrating that they are members of a new human retrovirus family.[7-10]

Other human retroviruses, HTLV-1, HTLV-2, and HIV-2, share features with HIV, including tropism for T lymphocytes, utilization of Mg^{++} in their reverse transcriptase, possession of a major core protein of approximately 24 kilodaltons (kd) molecular weight, and possession of a transactivating gene *(tat)* capable of regulating transcription. HIV-2 is a new agent that has been identified in both healthy and immunodeficient people in West Africa.[11-14] HIV-2 shares more common epitopes with the simian immunodeficiency virus (SIV) than the prototype HIV that infects people in the United States and Europe.

The first human retrovirus, HTLV-1, was reported by Gallo et al. in 1980.[15] This type C retrovirus was isolated from an American patient with mycosis fungoides. Various other similar viral isolates have since been discovered.[16] Infection with HTLV-1 has been associated with T cell malignancies, most especially the aggressive adult T cell leukemia/lymphoma (ATLL).[17,18]

HTLV-1 infects and transforms T lymphocytes in vitro[19] and is associated with an increased incidence of infectious diseases in hospitalized patients in Japan.[20] Another horizontally transmitted type C retrovirus, feline leukemia virus, causes both T cell malignancies and immunosuppression in cats.[21,22] These and other observations about the biology of AIDS and the characteristics of HTLV-1 gave rise to experiments to seek a related retrovirus as a possible etiologic

---

This work was supported in part by Grants DE08553 and NS26665 from the National Institutes of Health.

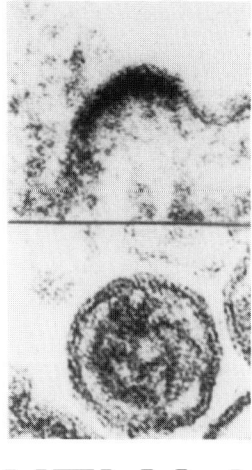

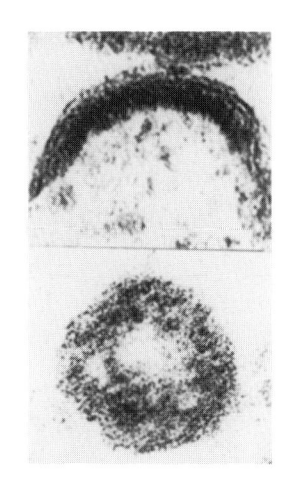

HTLV-1 **HTLV-2**

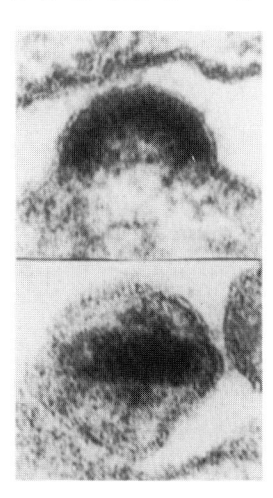

HIV-1

FIGURE 13–1 *Electron micrographs of HTLV-1, HTLV-2, and HIV-1 showing cell surface budding and individual particles. Photograph courtesy of R. Gallo.*

agent of AIDS. Partial cross-reactivity of HTLV-1 infected cells with the sera of some patients with AIDS further suggested the possibility of a relationship between an HTLV type of agent and AIDS.[23,24] Further investigation of the AIDS agent resulted in isolation of retroviral particles by researchers in France at the Pasteur Institute, which were termed LAV,[1] and by investigators in the United States at the National Cancer Institute, which were termed HTLV-3.[2–5]

Infection with HIV is detected by either the appearance of serum antibodies to virally related antigens or by viral recovery through culture of peripheral blood or other body fluids.[25-31] Since viral isolation is difficult and time consuming, large scale assays for infection depend on the demonstration of virus-specific antibodies. Most people infected with HIV will develop a circulating antibody response to viral antigens.[30,32,33] Documented seroconversion has been found to occur as early as 26 weeks following viral inoculation by an accidental needle stick[34] and may occur 1 to 2 weeks following an acute HIV infection. Because for the foreseeable future large-scale testing for HIV infection will depend on the detection of antibodies to viral proteins, knowledge of the viral antigens and the immune response to them is essential to interpret the course of infection with HIV. The immune response to these antigens is discussed below.

SEROLOGICALLY DETERMINED ANTIGENS

There are nine distinct functional regions in the HIV genome, eight of which have been shown to encode one or more serologically determined antigens. The first open reading frame encountered after the 5' long terminal repeat of the HIV genome is the *gag* gene, which encodes a polyprotein of approximately 55 kd. The *gag* precursor protein, p55, is found in large quantities in virus-infected cells and is present in lower amounts in extracellular virus.[3] The non-glycosylated 55 kd protein is cleaved into three proteins: p17, a myristylated protein at the amino terminus[35]; p24, the major viral core protein[35-38]; and p15, which is at the carboxy terminus of p55.[37,38] Both p17 and p24 are found in high concentrations in both infected cells and concentrated virus. P17, however, is not a strongly immunogenic antigen. A 38 kd protein is often detected in infected cells by sera that are reactive against p55 and p24. It is thought to be a p55 breakdown product.[35,38] The major core proteins of other T lymphotropic viruses are similar in size to p24 and exhibit some antigenic cross-reactivity. HTLV-1, HTLV-2, and HIV-2,[14,23,39,40] as well as retroviruses that infect nonhuman primates,[41-43] all have major core proteins of approximately 24 kd.

The second open reading frame in the HIV genome is the *pol* gene, which has the potential to code for a polyprotein of approximately 150 kd. Three serologically defined proteins, p64, p53, and p34, have been mapped to this region.[44,45] Proteins of 64 and 53 kd have been shown to determine the viral reverse transcriptase activity. Edman degradation of the first 17 amino acid residues of p64 and p53 resulted in a perfect translation of the predicted sequence of a segment of the nucleotide sequence of the *pol* gene.[44] Further, p64 and p53 were both precipitated by a monoclonal antibody that binds to an antigen containing the reverse transciptase activity.[44] Both p64 and p53 are highly immunogenic, and antibodies to these two proteins are found in essentially all infected persons regardless of their clinical status or risk group when assayed by Western blotting.[44-46] Antibodies to p64 and p53 should prove valuable as specific determinants of infection, especially in assays using electrotransfer, such as Western blotting. Finally, the *pol* gene product has also been shown to be an important target for cytotoxic T lymphocytes in vitro.[47]

A protein of approximately 34 kd, which is also highly immunogenic, is encoded by the 3' end of the *pol* gene. Radiosequence analysis of labeled p34 showed this protein to be a translation of the predicted sequence of the endonuclease segment of *pol*.[45] The endonuclease function may be needed for proviral DNA integration into the host cell chromosome. P34 is most easily detected by Western blotting but is also found by radioimmunoprecipitation (RIP).[45]

Unlike most other human, simian, mammalian, and avian retroviruses, HIV has additional open reading frames between the *pol* and *env* genes. An open reading frame *(vif)* whose 5' end overlaps with the 3' end of the *pol* gene codes for a protein of 23 kd that induces antibody production in some infected individuals.[48] *Vif* is therefore probably expressed in vivo. Whether p23 or *vif* has a role in viral pathogenesis is unknown. Deletions or nucleotide substitutions in *vif* have not affected the virus's cytopathic or replicative ability.[49,50] However, elimination of *vif* appears to impede virus transmission while maintaining control levels of viral mRNA and particle numbers. *Vif* may thus be involved in an unknown post-translational virus maturation step.[50] The protein is rich in the unusual amino acid tryptophan, which suggests that the structural constraints of this amino acid may have a role in its function.[7,48]

3' to the *vif* gene and immediately 5' to the envelope gene is an exon of a small open reading frame that contains a region necessary for stimulation of gene expression directed by the viral long terminal repeat.[51,52] This phenomenon, termed transactivation, is mediated by virus-specific transacting factors that stimulate increased viral gene expression. Transactivation in HTLV-1 and HTLV-2 is mediated by gene products encoded 3' to the *env* gene.[53,54] These nuclear proteins are encoded by a gene called *tat,* for transactivating transcriptional regulation. Analogous functional properties are found in the *tat* gene region of HIV, although the locations of *tat* in the genome differ between HTLV-1 and HIV.[55]

No protein product for *tat* has been found in purified HIV; however, the finding of this open reading frame in spliced mRNA[51] and the loss of transactivating ability of proviruses with the deletion of this reading frame suggest that the presumed HIV protein product is involved in transactivation.[56] Further, lymphoid and epithelial cells transfected with plasmids containing the *tat*3 region express a 14 kd protein that is recognized by the sera of some infected patients.[55] However, no homology exists between the potential product and the *tat* proteins of HTLV-1 and -2. *Tat*3 has a strongly basic domain rich in arginine and lysine residues, which may play a role in binding to nucleic acids.[51]

Another gene *(rev)* encoding a potential protein of approximately 116 amino acids has been shown to be necessary for posttranscriptional transactivation of *env* mRNA and *gag* mRNA and for viral replication. It is located in a region of the genome similar to *tat* but is in a different reading frame. Like *tat,* it is a highly basic protein.[57,58]

The sixth gene, designated *env,* is a large open reading frame that has the potential to encode for a polyprotein of 90 kd.[37,38,59] Because of its high degree of glycosylation, the *env* protein actually migrates as a glycoprotein of approximately 160 kd molecular weight in sodium dodecylsulfate polyacrylamide gel electrophoresis (SDS-PAGE). Gp160 is found in infected cells but not in purified virus preparations. Cleavage of gp160 results in the formation of gp120, the aminoterminus peplomer attachment protein, and gp41, the carboxy terminus transmembrane protein of the virus. Both proteins are found in both virus particles and infected cells.[38] Treatment of HIV-infected cells with tunicamycin, a glycosylation inhibitor, results in a new protein species of approximately 88 kd by RIP and SDS-PAGE.[59] Endoglycosidase H digestion of lentil-lectin-affinity purified gp160 and gp120 results in the appearance of an 88 kd band (the unglycosylated gp160) and a smaller broad band, presumably the incomplete digestion product of gp120.[59]

Gp120 is believed to be the viral antigen responsible for the tropism of the virus for the helper/inducer T cells and has been shown to be closely associated with the CD4 molecule in cross-linking experiments. When radiolabeled HIV was bound to CD4+ cells, which were then lysed, a viral glycoprotein of 120 kd coprecipitated with the CD4 molecule.[60] There are approximately 22 to 29 N-linked glycosylation sites in gp120,[61] which explains the high degree of glycosylation seen in this protein. The carbohydrate portion of the molecule may be important in the binding of gp120 to the cell receptor.[62] The most immunogenic HIV proteins are gp160 and gp120 when tested by assays based on equimolar amounts of undenatured antigen.[26,59,63] As assayed by RIP SDS-PAGE, the greatest proportion of patients with AIDS or ARC, healthy homosexuals and hemophiliacs, react to these proteins. These data are in accord with the findings that *env* genes of animal retroviruses encode the most immunogenic proteins as detected by the sera of infected animals.[64,65]

Gp41 is the transmembrane protein and the second product of gp160 cleavage. When antibodies to gp41 were detected with electrotransfer assays, this was considered the most sensitive diagnostic criterion of HIV infection in earlier studies.[4,66] Gp41 is not readily detected by RIP SDS-PAGE but, more commonly, with Western blotting. The protein consists of a hydrophobic membrane-spanning segment, hydrophilic anchor sequence, and an additional carboxy terminal stretch of 150 amino acids whose function is unknown.[67]

Analysis of nucleotide sequence and deduced amino acid sequences of five independently isolated HIVs has revealed that the envelope gene is the most variable viral gene,[61] with an estimated rate of 10^{-3} nucleotide substitutions per site per year.[68] Genetic variation of sequential virus isolates from the same persistently infected individuals has also been shown to be the greatest in the *env* gene.[68] Within the envelope gene, changes were most prevalent in the extracellular region. Predicted secondary protein structure and hydrophobicity revealed that these hypervariable regions are potential antigenic sites. There was marked conservation of other sites in the overall envelope. In five isolates studied, all 18 cysteine residues in the extracellular region were conserved,[61] suggesting that overall tertiary structure is maintained. Some of the conserved regions may also be possible antigenic sites. Rabbit antisera to amino acids 254 to 274 of a conserved region of gp120 demonstrated neutralization without affecting virus binding to CD4-positive cells. This may indicate a domain separate from binding that is necessary for HIV infectivity.[69] Similarly, Kowalski et al. developed a series of HIV *env* gene mutants that suggested that the ability of envelope glycoprotein to form syncytia depends on five separate processes. Envelope gene mutations that (1) decreased virus-receptor binding, (2) impaired virus lipid-cell membrane fusion, (3) affected anchorage of envelope protein in the membrane, (4) disrupted the association of gp120 and gp41, and (5) disturbed proteolytic processing of the precursor, were isolated to different domains in the gene.[70]

A molecular clone of HIV that has excisions spanning the carboxy terminus of the *env* gene and the *nef* gene gave rise to a replication-competent, noncytopathic virus. However, variants containing excision of only the *nef* gene produced cytopathic viruses.[71] Thus the carboxyterminus of *env* (gp41) appears to have a role in T cell killing.[71] Further synthesis of data on envelope functional

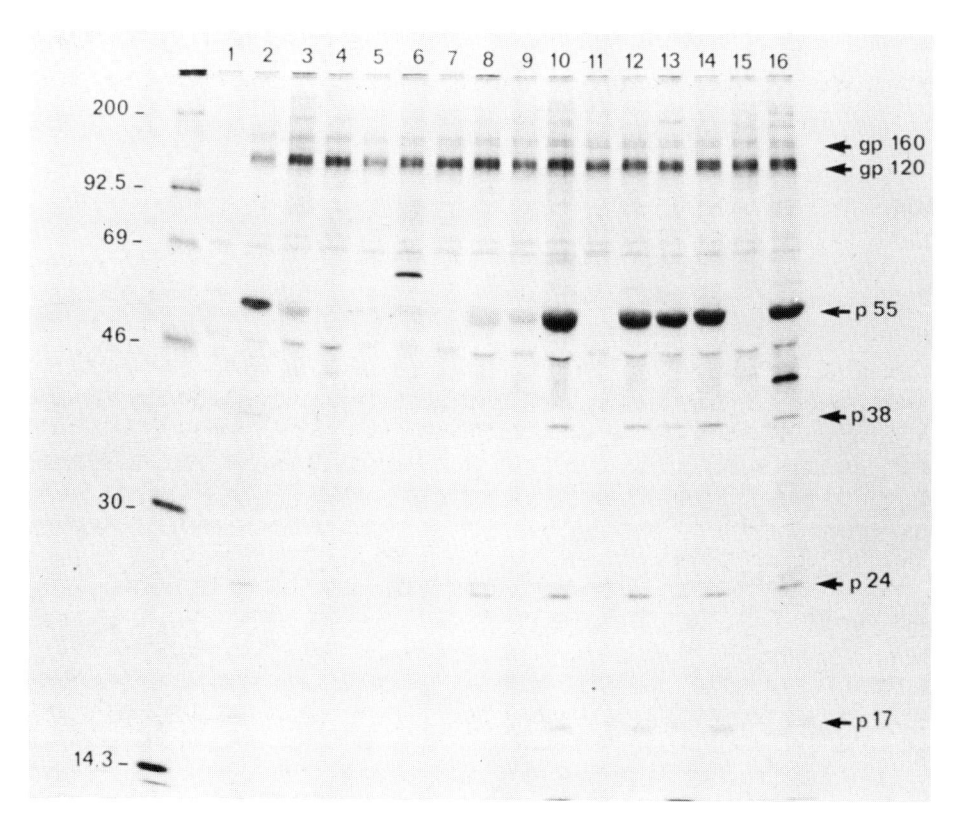

FIGURE 13–2 Radioimmunoprecipitation of ^{35}S-labelled HIV-1 infected cell lysates with sera from patients with AIDS and ARC (Lanes 2–10) demonstrating the major viral antigens.

domains, variable and conserved regions, neutralizing and blocking antibodies, patterns of glycosylation, and target sequences of cell-mediated immunity will be necessary to establish an HIV vaccine strategy.

The seventh gene, designated *nef* or p27,[7,72] has been shown to encode a myristilated protein found in infected cells. Myristilation may indicate that the protein has a function associated with the cellular membrane. Additionally, *nef* has been reported to show guanosine triphosphate (GTP) binding capacity, GTPase activity, and autophosphorylation ability.[73] *nef* migrates with a size of approximately 27 kd in SDS-PAGE. P27 was recognized by 37% of sera seropositive for other antigens as assayed by RIP SDS-PAGE and thus cannot be considered as immunogenic as the antigens encoded by the *env* genes.[72] As described previously, p27 is not absolutely necessary for viral replication or cytopathic effects but may be involved in the maintenance of latent infection.[71,73,74] Very recently, a gene product has been identified as encoded by the open-reading frame designated *vpu*.[75] A protein of about 16,000 kd, antibodies to this molecule are found in about a third of all HIV-1 infected individuals, but in more than 90% of those that became infected very recently. Thus far this is the only gene that is unique to HIV-1, not being present in HIV-2 or SIV. The final gene *vpr*, of unknown function, is located between *vif* and *tat*.

ANTIGENS DETECTED WITH IMMUNODIAGNOSTIC TESTS

Several tests are currently used to detect HIV exposure in patients and blood donors. All depend on the binding or nonbinding of virus-specific antibodies in the test serum to particular viral antigens. The enzyme-linked immunosorbent assay (ELISA),[3,5] Western blotting[3,5] or immunoblotting assay, RIP assay with SDS-PAGE (RIPA),[26,59] cytoplasmic immunofluorescence assay,[76] and membrane immunofluorescence assay[26,59] are used most often. The ELISA tests use concentrated virus as the source of antigen. The Western blotting and RIPA tests can use either concentrated virus or homogenate from infected cells as a source of antigen. The fluorescent assays require infected cells.

The different assays have advantages and disadvantages. Tests using only the proteins in extracellular virus, such as ELISA and Western blot, may lack sensitivity because some viral preparations lose glycoproteins and therefore contain little or no gp160 and gp120 and lesser amounts of gp41. The *gag* proteins, p24 and p17, are easily concentrated, but they are not as immunogenic as the glycoproteins.[26,59] The ELISA test is the least expensive and most easily performed, but it gives both false-positive results, due to a lack of specificity, and false-negative results, due to a failure to detect positive samples containing antibodies only to the viral glycoproteins.

Western blotting has been used as the standard confirmatory assay when a sample has tested positive by repeat ELISAs. However, unless a profile of antigens is detected, i.e. p17, p24, and gp41, the presence of a single faint band may be difficult to interpret. Intensity and migration patterns can vary greatly. Reactivity to the reverse transcriptase p53 and p64 proteins may actually be a more sensitive determination of infection than p24 or gp41.[44–46]

The membrane and cytoplasmic immunofluorescence tests work well in research laboratories and in selected reference laboratories but are time consuming and difficult because a constant source of viable cells must be maintained.

The most specific test is the RIPA assay because it shows a distinct profile to all HIV antigens. Because it is expensive and difficult to perform, it is unlikely to be available anywhere except in research laboratories at present.

Tests using procedures that allow detection of antibodies to all viral proteins show that some proteins are more immunogenic than others. In HIV the surface proteins encoded by the *env* gene are more antigenic in the infected individual than the proteins found in the virus core. Gp120 has been demonstrated to be associated with a T4 cell surface antigen that may be part of the virus receptor.[60] The antigens on the surface of the virus are usually the same antigens found on the surface of infected cells, and these are the antigens affected by neutralizing antibodies and cell-mediated responses.

In the RIPA assay, gp120 and gp160 are the most immunogenic of any of the viral antigens; antibodies are found in 97% to 100% of patients with AIDS or AIDS-related complex (ARC). Approximately half the sera of AIDS patients have detectable antibodies to p24.[26,63] Further, patients with AIDS have decreased titers of antibodies to p24 in accordance with disease progression. Antibodies to gp120 are present in essentially all patients with AIDS, even those with late-stage disease. These results suggest that gp120 may be more appropriate than p24 for screening if simple and cost-effective assays can be made available.[38]

Although most individuals infected with HIV develop a circulating antibody response, the disease progresses in the face of significant systemic titers. Naturally occurring, neutralizing antibodies have been identified,[69,77] but the titers are low and there are no major differences in rates or titers when healthy carriers are compared with patients with AIDS.

The finding of genomic variation, especially in the extracellular envelope gene, in regions of predictive antigenicity, supports the hypothesis of host immunologic pressure selecting for HIV variants.[61] Other lentiviruses, equine infectious anemia virus and visna virus, have progressive changes in the envelope genes that affect envelope antigenicity.[78,79] Nonetheless, antibodies are always present in an infected individual. Low titers of neutralizing antibody may be protective if present before live virus is encountered. There is precedent for this occurrence in infection with feline leukemia virus, wherein low serum neutralizing titers are associated with protection.[80] The complexity of chronic retroviral-induced disease and the failure to characterize fully the host response to the virus may account for the present paradox—failure of viral neutralization in the face of high serum virus-specific titers. The cell-mediated response is especially inadequately characterized.

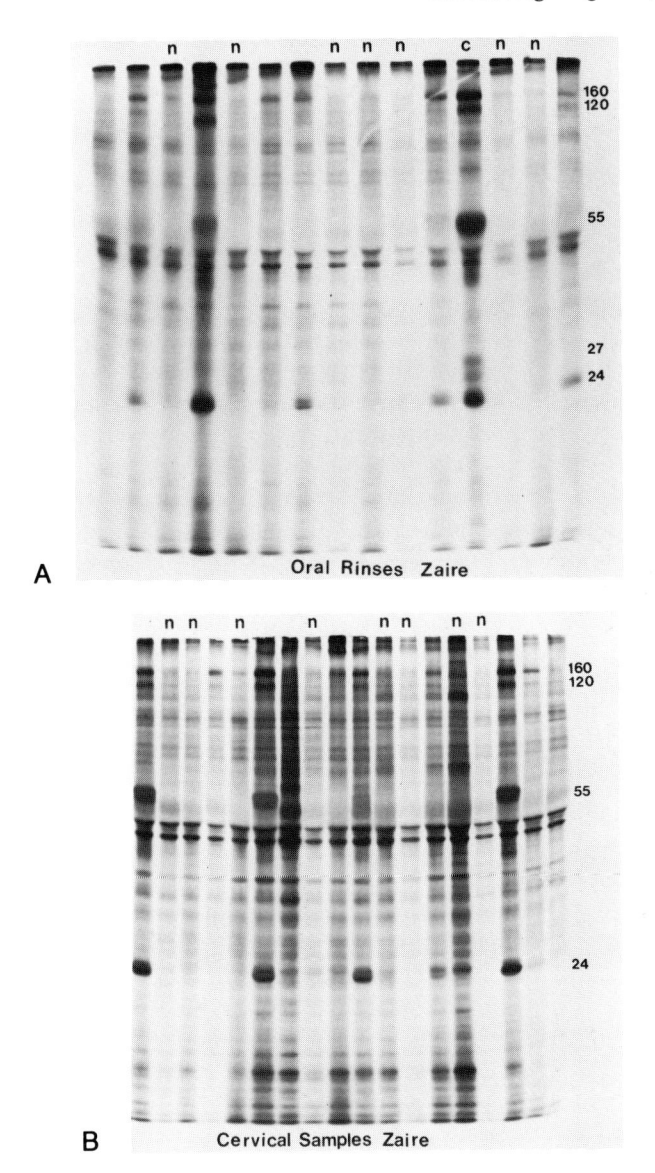

FIGURE 13-3 *Radioimmunoprecipitation of oral rinses (A) or cervical secretions (B) from female prostitutes in Zaire demonstrating the presence of secretory antibodies to viral antigens. Soluble cell lysates were prepared from Molt-HIV-infected cells. The cells were exposed to ^{35}S-cysteine, harvested, and lysed with RIPA buffer. The lysates were then reacted with anti-human IgA-coated-Protein-A beads that previously had been incubated with the rinse samples. Samples were from subjects as follows: lanes with no label show HIV-antibody positive women, lanes with label n show antibody negative women, and lanes with label c show a positive control sample.*

SECRETORY IMMUNE RESPONSE TO HIV

Mucosal surfaces exposed to body fluids in the oral cavity and reproductive tract represent potential sites for local immunization.[81–84] In certain viral infections, antibodies, especially of the IgA class, synthesized and secreted locally by mucosal plasma cells, are more effective in preventing reinfection than systemic circulating antibodies.[85,86]

Secretory immunoglobulin A (sIgA) is the major class of immunoglobulin bathing the body's mucosal surfaces; it is assumed to play a protective role as a first line of defense against invading virus particles. Tomasi proposed two mucosal defense mechanisms mediated by immunoglobulins.[87] In the first-line defenses, sIgA and possibly other locally synthesized immunoglobulins trap particles at the mucosal surfaces, inhibit adherence to the mucosa by coating the particle surface, neutralize the virus, and perhaps aid in the opsonization of the particle. The last mechanism must be mediated by immunoglobulins other than IgA. In the second-line defenses, serum-derived IgG neutralizes the virus, aids in opsonization, and forms immune complexes that fix complement, causing local inflammation, opsonization, and chemotaxis. This protective role has been well demonstrated in the upper respiratory tract, where virus-specific antibodies in secretions have been shown to correlate better with immunologic resistance than do antibodies in serum.[85] Oral immunization with live attenuated polio virus elicits antibodies in the nasopharyngeal fluid, gastrointestinal secretions, and serum.[86,87] Intravaginal immunization with inactivated polio vaccine has been shown to elicit IgA antibodies in the vagina within seven days, but it does not elicit an antibody response in the serum or nasopharynx.[88] Intramuscular immunization with polio vaccine results in an IgG response in genital tract secretions two or more weeks after immunization.[88] Cervical excretion of cytomegalovirus (CMV) has been shown to correlate with secretory antibody levels.[89] Thus local or systemic immunization may produce a cervical antibody response. Similar responses are found in other mucosal areas. Therefore, local immunization of mucosal areas such as the oral cavity or female genital tract could theoretically stimulate HIV-specific antibody production independent of circulating antibody.

We have demonstrated that antibodies to HIV are found in secretions of persons at risk for AIDS infection.[90–93] Parotid saliva,[92] whole saliva,[90–92] cervical secretions,[93] and, in individual cases, semen and milk contain these virus-specific antibodies. In parotid saliva and milk, the immune response to other antigens is attributable primarily to sIgA class antibodies. There is little serum transudate in either fluid, and sIgA comprises essentially all the immunoglobulins present. In the other secretory fluids, IgG class antibodies from serum may be involved in some of the humoral response, but locally synthesized sIgA is the most significant contributor.[94]

Essentially all seropositive individuals demonstrate antibodies in their secretions. As with serum antibody findings, antibodies found in secretions react most strongly to the *env* proteins. IgA antibodies to *gag* proteins p24, p38, and p55 are found in approximately 21% of whole saliva samples that contain antibodies to gp160 and gp120, 20% of positive parotid saliva samples, and 71% of positive cervical secretions when assayed by RIPA. Lower reactivity to *gag* antigens in secretions may reflect lower antibody concentrations in secretions rather than a difference in the systemic and secretory immune response.

Recently, we have demonstrated reactivity to *gag* and *pol* antigens in more than 50% of parotid samples from HIV-infected individuals by Western blotting using large sample volumes of affinity-purified parotid antibodies. However, limiting antibody dilution titres in parotid saliva to *env* antigens were between 1:300 and 1:30, whereas antibody titres to *gag* or *pol* antigens were usually only 1:3. Although weaker than the IgA response, we have also demonstrated a significant IgG antibody response to HIV antigens in the parotid samples of some infected individuals. This could be the result of a subclinical parotitis in some infected individuals, which would increase the number of IgG B cells in the glands (Trainin Z, Sun D, Essex M, Archibald D, unpublished data).

Diagnosis of HIV infection is extremely important, and not only to screen donated blood. Large-scale screenings of populations may be necessary for planning public health resource allocations. In other cases, certain individuals may

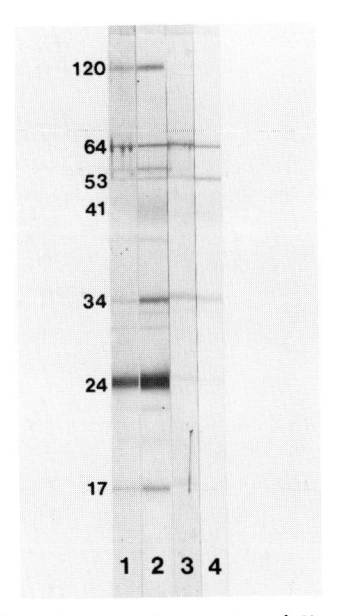

FIGURE 13–4 Western blot of serum (Lanes 1 and 2) and saliva (Lanes 3 and 4) from a patient with AIDS. Lanes 1 and 3 were incubated with an anti-human IgA serum. Lanes 2 and 4 with an anti-human IgG serum.

desire to know their HIV status without risking the release of the information. Collection of saliva is less expensive than collection of serum; therefore, a reliable HIV diagnostic kit that used saliva might be worthwhile for screening populations in Africa or other areas. Saliva collection also requires no trained medical personnel. In situations that might require antibody testing by persons unable to perform venipuncture, such as in a prison population, a saliva test would be useful. The demonstration that accurate Western blotting can be accomplished using saliva gives promise for such a test.[91]

Heterosexual transmission of HIV appears to be somewhat less common than homosexual transmission, and some factors in female genital secretions, such as locally secreted antibodies, may reduce transmissibility. Transmission from males to females may be lessened by neutralizing antibodies in the female genital tract that were elicited by inoculations of infected semen that did not cause infection. It is conceivable that these repeated virus challenges with small inocula could initiate local protective immunity. However, as yet, it is unclear what role, if any, antibodies in mucosal secretions play in the pathogenesis of HIV infection. The presence of mucosal antibodies may inhibit or diminish the infectivity of virus in secretions and therefore may be a highly desired end product of any vaccine. Research in the next few years should clarify the role of systemic and secretory humoral immunity to HIV, which will be important for better diagnosis, treatment, and prevention of HIV infection.

REFERENCES

1. Barré-Sinoussi F, Chermann JC, Rey F, et al. Isolation of a T-lymphotropic retrovirus from a patient at risk for acquired immunodeficiency syndrome (AIDS). Science 1983;220:868.
2. Popovic M, Sarngadharan MG, Read E, Gallo RC. Detection, isolation, and continuous production of cytopathic retroviruses (HTLV-III) from patients with AIDS and pre-AIDS. Science 1984;224:497.
3. Schupbach J, Popovic M, Gilden RV, et al. Serological analysis of a subgroup of human T-lymphotropic retroviruses (HTLV-III) associated with AIDS. Science 1984;224:503.
4. Sarngadharan MG, Popovic M, Bruch L, et al. Antibodies reactive with a human T-lymphotropic retrovirus (HTLV-III) in the serum of patients with AIDS. Science 1984;224:506.
5. Gallo RC, Salahuddin SZ, Popovic M, et al. Frequent detection and isolation of cytopathic retroviruses (HTLV-III) from patients with AIDS and at risk for AIDS. Science 1984;224:500.
6. Levy JA, Hoffman AD, Kramer SM, et al. Isolation of lymphocytopathic retroviruses from San Francisco patients with AIDS. Science 1984;225:840.
7. Ratner L, Haseltine W, Patarca R, et al. Complete nucleotide sequence of the AIDS virus, HTLV-III. Nature 1985;313:277.
8. Muesing MA, Smith DH, Cabradilla CD, et al. Nucleic acid structure and expression of the human AIDS/lymphadenopathy retrovirus. Nature 1985;313:450.

9. Sanchez-Pescador R, Power MD, Barr PJ, et al. Nucleotide sequence and expression of an AIDS-associated retrovirus (ARV-2). Science 1985;227:484.
10. Wain-Hobson S, Sonigo P, Danos O, et al. Nucleotide sequence of the AIDS virus, LAV. Cell 1985;40:9.
11. Barin F, M'Boup S, Denis F, et al. Serological evidence for a virus related to simian T-lymphotropic retrovirus III in residents of West Africa. Lancet 1985;2:1387.
12. Kanki PJ, Barin F, M'Boup S, et al. New human T lymphotropic retrovirus related to simian T-lymphotropic virus type 3. Science 1986;232:238.
13. Clavel F, Guetard D, Brun-Vezinet F, et al. Isolation of a new human retrovirus from West African patients with AIDS. Science 1986;233:343.
14. Clavel F. HIV-2, the West African AIDS virus. AIDS 1987;1:135.
15. Poiesz BJ, Ruscetti FW, Gazdar AF, et al. Detection and isolation of type C retrovirus particles from fresh and cultured lymphocytes of a patient with cutaneous T-cell lymphoma. Proc Natl Acad Sci USA 1980;77:7415.
16. Popovic M, Sarin PS, Robert-Guroff M, et al. Isolation and transmission of human retrovirus (human T-cell leukemia virus). Science 1983;219:856.
17. Kalyanaraman VS, Sarngadharan MG, Bunn PA, et al. Antibodies in human sera reactive against an internal structural protein of human T-cell lymphoma virus. Nature 1981;294:271.
18. Hinuma Y. Human leukemia virus associated with adult T-cell leukemia. Gan (Jap J Cancer Res) 1983;74:777.
19. Essex M. Adult T-cell leukemia-lymphoma; role of human retrovirus. J Natl Cancer Inst 1982;69:981.
20. Essex M, McLane MF, Tachibana N, et al. Seroepidemiology of HTLV in relation to immunosuppression and the acquired immunodeficiency syndrome. In: Gallo RC, Essex M, Gross L, eds. Human T-cell leukemia/lymphoma virus. Cold Spring Harbor, N.Y.: Cold Spring Harbor Press, 1984;355–362.
21. Hoover EA, Perryman LE, Kociba GJ. Early lesion in cats inoculated with feline leukemia virus. Cancer Res 1973;33:143.
22. Essex M, Hardy Jr W, Cotter S, et al. Naturally occurring persistent feline oncornavirus infections in the absence of disease. Infect Immun 1975;11:470.
23. Essex M, McLane MF, Lee T-H, et al. Antibodies to cell membrane antigens associated with human T-cell leukemia virus in patients with AIDS. Science 1983;220:859.
24. Gallo RC, Sarin PS, Gelmann EP, et al. Isolation of human T-cell leukemia virus in acquired immune deficiency syndrome (AIDS). Science 1983;220:865.
25. Groopman JE, Salahuddin SZ, Sarngadharan MG, et al. Virologic studies in a case of transfusion-associated AIDS. N Engl J Med 1984;311:1419.
26. Kitchen LW, Barin F, Sullivan JL, et al. Aetiology of AIDS—antibodies to human T-cell leukaemia virus (type III) in haemophiliacs. Nature 1984;312:367.
27. Geodert JJ, Sarngadharan MG, Biggar RJ, et al. Determinants of retrovirus (HTLV-III) antibody and immunodeficiency conditions in homosexual men. Lancet 1984;2:771.
28. Groopman JE, Sarngadharan MG, Salahuddin SZ, et al. Apparent transmission of human T-cell leukemia virus type III to a heterosexual woman with the acquired immunodeficiency syndrome. Ann Intern Med 1985;102:63.
29. Laurence J, Brun-Vezinet F, Schutzer SE, et al. Lymphadenopathy-associated viral antibody in AIDS. N Engl J Med 1984;311:1269.
30. Essex M, McLane MF, Kanki PJ, et al. Retroviruses associated with leukemia and ablative syndromes in animals and in human beings. Cancer Res 1985;45:4534s–4538s.

31. Kalyanaraman VS, Sarngadharan MG, Nakao Y, et al. Natural antibodies to the structural core proteins (p24) of the human T-cell leukemia (lymphoma) retrovirus found in sera of leukemia patients in Japan. Proc Natl Acad Sci USA 1982;79:1653.
32. Salahuddin SZ, Groopman JE, Markham PD, et al. HTLV-III in symptom-free seronegative persons. Lancet 1984;2:1418.
33. Sarngadharan MG, Popovic M, Bruch L, et al. Antibodies reactive with human T-lymphotropic retroviruses (HTLV-III) in the serum of patients with AIDS. Science 1984;224:506.
34. Stricof RL, Morse DL. HTLV-III/LAV seroconversion following deep intramuscular needlestick injury. N Engl J Med 1986;314:1115.
35. Veronese F, Copeland TD, Oroszlan S, et al. Biochemical and immunological analysis of human immunodeficiency virus gag gene products p17 and p24. J Virol 1988;62:795.
36. Veronese F, Sarngadharan MG, Rahman R, et al. Monoclonal antibodies specific for p24, the major core proteins of human T-cell leukemia virus type III. Proc Natl Acad Sci USA 1985;82:5199.
37. Robey GW, Safai B, Oroszlan S, et al. Characterization of envelope and core structural gene products of HTLV-III with sera from AIDS patients. Science 1985;228:593.
38. Essex M, Allan J, Kanki P, et al. Antigens of human T-lymphotropic virus type III/lymphadenopathy-associated virus. Ann Intern Med 1985;103:700.
39. Lee TH, Coligan JE, Homma T, et al. Human T-cell leukemia virus-associated membrane antigens: Identity of the major antigens recognized after virus infection. Proc Natl Acad Sci USA 1984;31:3856.
40. Biberfeld G, Brown F, Esparza J, et al. Meeting report: WHO Working Group on characterization of HIV-related retroviruses: criteria for characterization and proposal for a nomenclature system. AIDS 1987;1:189–190.
41. Kanki PJ, McLane MF, King NW Jr, et al. Serologic identification and characterization of a macaque T-lymphotropic retrovirus closely related to human T-lymphotropic retroviruses (HTLV) type III. Science 1985;228:1199.
42. Daniel MD, Letvin NL, King NW, et al. Isolation of T-cell tropic HTLV-III-like retrovirus from macaques. Science 1985;228:1201.
43. Kanki PJ, Kurth R, Becker W, et al. Antibodies to simian T-lymphotropic virus type III in African green monkeys and recognition of STLV-III viral proteins by AIDS and related sera. Lancet 1985;2:1330.
44. Veronese F, Copeland TD, Devico AL, et al. Characterization of highly immunogenic p66/p51 as the reverse transcriptase of HTLV-III/LAV. Science 1986;231:1289.
45. Allan JS, Coligan JE, Lee T-H, et al. Immunogenic nature of a Pol gene product of HTLV-III/LAV. Blood 1987;69:331.
46. Groopman JE, Chen FW, Hope JA, et al. Serological characterization of HTLV-III infection in AIDS and related disorders. J Infect Dis 1986;153:736.
47. Walker BD, Flexner C, Paradis TJ, et al. HIV-1 reverse transcriptase is a target for cytotoxic T lymphocytes in infected individuals. Science 1988;240:64.
48. Lee TH, Coligan JE, Allan JS, et al. A new HTLV-III/LAV protein encoded by a gene found in cytopathic retroviruses. Science 1986;231:1546.
49. Sodroski J, Goh WC, Rosen C. Replicative and cytopathic potential of HTLV-III/LAV with sor gene deletions. Science 1986;231:1549.
50. Fisher AG, Ensoli B, Ivanoff L, et al. The sor gene of HIV-1 is required for efficient virus transmission in vitro. Science 1987;237:888.

51. Arya SK, Guo C, Josephs SF, Wong-Staal F. Trans-activator gene of human T-lymphotropic virus type III (HTLV-III). Science 1985;229:69.
52. Sodroski J, Patarca R, Rosen C, et al. Localization of the trans-activating region of the genome of human T-cell lymphotropic virus type III. Science 1985;229:74.
53. Lee TH, Coligan JE, Sodroski JG, et al. Antigens encoded by the 3′ terminal region of human T-cell leukemia virus: evidence for a functional gene. Science 1984;226:57.
54. Slamon DJ, Shimothna K, Cline MJ, et al. Identification of the putative transforming protein of the human T-cell leukemia viruses HTLV-I and HTLV-II. Science 1984;226:61.
55. Rosen CA, Sodroski JG, Goh WC, et al. Post-transcriptional regulation accounts for the transactivation of the human T-lymphotropic virus type III. Nature 1986;319:559.
56. Goh WC, Rosen C, Sodroski J, et al. Identification of a protein encoded by the trans activator gene tat III of human T-cell lymphotropic retrovirus type III. J Virol 1986;59:181.
57. Sodroski J, Goh WC, Rosen C, et al. A second post-transcriptional trans-activator gene required for HTLV-III replication. Nature 1986;321:412.
58. Terwilliger E, Burghoff R, Sia R, et al. The art gene product of human immunodeficiency virus is required for replication. J Virol 1988;62:655.
59. Allan JS, Coligan JE, Barin F, et al. Major glycoprotein antigens that induce antibodies in AIDS patients are encoded by HTLV-III. Science 1985;228:1091.
60. McDougal JS, Kennedy MS, Sligh JM, et al. Binding of HTLV-III/LAV to T4+ cells by a complex of the 110K viral protein and the T4 molecule. Science 1986;231:382.
61. Starcich BR, Hahn BH, Shaw GM, et al. Identification and characterization of conserved and variable regions in the envelope gene of HTLV-III/LAV, the retrovirus of AIDS. Cell 1986;45:637.
62. Putney SD, Matthews TJ, Robey WG, et al. HTLV-III/LAV-neutralizing antibodies to an E. coli-produced fragment of the virus envelope. Science 1986;234:1392.
63. Barin F, McLane MF, Allan JS, et al. Virus envelope protein of HTLV-III represents major target antigen for antibodies in AIDS patients. Science 1985;228:1094.
64. Taniyama T, Holden HT. In vitro induction of T-lymphocyte-mediated cytotoxicity by infectious murine type c oncornaviruses. J Exp Med 1979;150:1367.
65. Flyer DC, Burakoff SJ, Faller DV. Cytotoxic T lymphocyte recognition of transfected cells expressing a cloned retroviral gene. Nature 1983;305:815.
66. Safai B, Sarngadharan MG, Groopman JE, et al. Seroepidemiological studies of human T-lymphotropic retrovirus type III in acquired immunodeficiency syndrome. Lancet 1984;2:1438.
67. Veronese F, deVico AL, Copeland TD, et al. Characterization of gp41 as the transmembrane protein coded by the HTLV-III/LAV envelope gene. Science 1985;229:1402.
68. Hahn BH, Shaw GM, Taylor ME, et al. Genetic variation in HTLV-III/LAV over time in patients with AIDS or at risk for AIDS. Science 1986;232:1548.
69. Ho DD, Kaplan JC, Rackauskas IE, Gurney ME. Second conserved domain of gp120 is important for HIV infectivity and antibody neutralization. Science 1988;239:1021.
70. Kowalski M, Potz J, Basiripour L, et al. Functional regions of the envelope glycoprotein of human immunodeficiency virus type I. Science 1987;237:1351.
71. Fisher AG, Ratner L, Mitsuya H, et al. Infectious mutants of HTLV-III with changes in the 3′ region and markedly reduced cytopathic effects. Science 1986;233:655.

72. Allan JS, Coligan JE, Lee TH, et al. A new HTLV-3/LAV encoded antigen detected by antibodies from AIDS patients. Science 1985;230:810.
73. Guy B, Kieny MP, Riviere Y, et al. HIV F/3 orf encodes a phosphorylated GTP-binding protein resembling an oncogene product. Nature 1987;330:266.
74. Terwilliger E, Sodroski JG, Rosen CA, Haseltine WA. Effects of mutations within the 3' orf open reading frame region of human T-cell lymphotropic virus type III (HTLV-III/LAV) on replication and cytopathogenicity. J Virol 1986;60:754.
75. Matsuda Z, Chou MJ, Matsuda M, et al. Human immunodeficiency virus type 1 has an additional coding sequence in the central region of the genome. Proc Natl Acad Sci USA 1988;85:6968.
76. Sandstrom EG, Schooley RT, Ho DD, et al. Detection of human anti-HTLV-III antibodies by indirect immunofluorescence using fixed cells. Transfusion 1985;25:308.
77. Robert-Guroff M, Brown M, Gallo RC. HTLV-III neutralizing antibodies in patients with AIDS and AIDS-related complex. Nature 1985;316:72.
78. Clements JE, Pedersen FS, Narayan O, Haseltine WA. Genomic changes associated with antigenic variation of visna virus during persistent infection. Proc Natl Acad Sci USA 1980;77:4454.
79. Salinovich O, Payne SL, Montelaro RC, et al. Rapid emergence of novel antigenic and genetic variants of equine infectious anemia virus during persistent infection. J Virol 1986;57:71.
80. Hardy WD, Hess PW, MacEwen EG, et al. Biology of feline leukemia virus in the natural environment. Cancer Res 1976;36:582.
81. Zagury D, Bernard J, Leibowitch J, et al. HTLV-III in cells cultured from semen of two patients with AIDS. Science 1984;226:459.
82. Ho DD, Schooley RT, Rota TR, et al. HTLV-III in the semen and blood of a healthy homosexual man. Science 1984;226:451.
83. Vogt MW, Craven DE, Crawford DF, et al. Isolation of HTLV-III/LAV from cervical secretions of women at risk for AIDS. Lancet 1986;1:525.
84. Wofsy CB, Cohen JB, Hauer LB, et al. Isolation of AIDS-associated retrovirus from genital secretions of women with antibodies to the virus. Lancet 1986;1:527.
85. Perkins JC, Tucker DN, Knopf HLS, et al. Evidence for protective effect of an inactivated rhinovirus vaccine administered by the nasal route. Am J Epidemiol 1969;90:319.
86. Ogra PL, Karzon DT, Righthand F, MacGillivary M. Immunoglobulin response in serum and secretions after immunization with live and inactivated polio vaccine and natural infection. New Engl J Med 1968;270:893.
87. Tomasi TB. The immune system of secretions. Englewood Cliffs, N.J.: Prentice-Hall, 1976;109–120.
88. Ogra PL, Ogra SS. Local antibody response to poliovaccine in the human female genital tract. J Immunol 1973;110:1307.
89. Waner JL, Hopkins DR, Weller TH, Allred EN. Cervical excretion of cytomegalovirus: correlation with secretory and humoral antibody. J Infect Dis 1973;136:805.
90. Archibald DW, Zon L, Groopman JE, et al. Antibodies to human T-lymphotrophic virus type III (HTLV-III) in saliva of acquired immunodeficiency syndrome (AIDS) patients and in persons at risk for AIDS. Blood 1986;67:831.
91. Archibald DW, Zon L, Groopman JE, et al. Salivary antibodies as a means of detecting human T cell lymphotropic virus type III/lymphadenopthy-associated virus infection. J Clin Microb 1986;24:873.

92. Archibald DW, Barr CE, Torosian JP, et al. Secretory IgA antibodies to human immunodeficiency virus in the parotid saliva of patients with AIDS and AIDS-related complex. J Infect Dis 1987;155:793.
93. Archibald DW, Witt DJ, Craven DE, et al. Antibodies to human immunodeficiency virus in cervical secretions from women at risk for AIDS. J Infect Dis 1987;156:240.
94. Tomasi TB. The immune system of secretions. Englewood Cliffs, N.J.: Prentice-Hall, 1976;6–12.
95. Trainin Z, Sun D, Essex M, Archibald D, unpublished data.

Chapter 14

Revision of the CDC Surveillance Case Definition for AIDS

Reported by Council of State and Territorial Epidemiologists; AIDS Program, Center for Infectious Diseases, CDC

INTRODUCTION

The following revised case definition for surveillance of acquired immunodeficiency syndrome (AIDS) was developed by CDC in collaboration with public health and clinical specialists. The Council of State and Territorial Epidemiologists (CSTE) has officially recommended adoption of the revised definition for national reporting of AIDS. The objectives of the revision are (a) to track more effectively the severe disabling morbidity associated with infection with human immunodeficiency virus (HIV) (including HIV-1 and HIV-2); (b) to simplify reporting of AIDS cases; (c) to increase the sensitivity and specificity of the definition through greater diagnostic application of laboratory evidence for HIV infection; and (d) to be consistent with current diagnostic practice, which in some cases includes presumptive, i.e., without confirmatory laboratory evidence, diagnosis of AIDS-indicative diseases (e.g., *Pneumocystis carinii* pneumonia, Kaposi's sarcoma).

The definition is organized into three sections that depend on the status of laboratory evidence of HIV infection (e.g., HIV antibody) (Figure 14–1). The major proposed changes apply to patients with laboratory evidence for HIV infection: (a) inclusion of HIV encephalopathy, HIV wasting syndrome, and a broader range of specific AIDS-indicative diseases (Section II.A); (b) inclusion of AIDS patients whose indicator diseases are diagnosed presumptively (Section II.B); and (c) elimination of exclusions due to other causes of immunodeficiency (Section I.A).

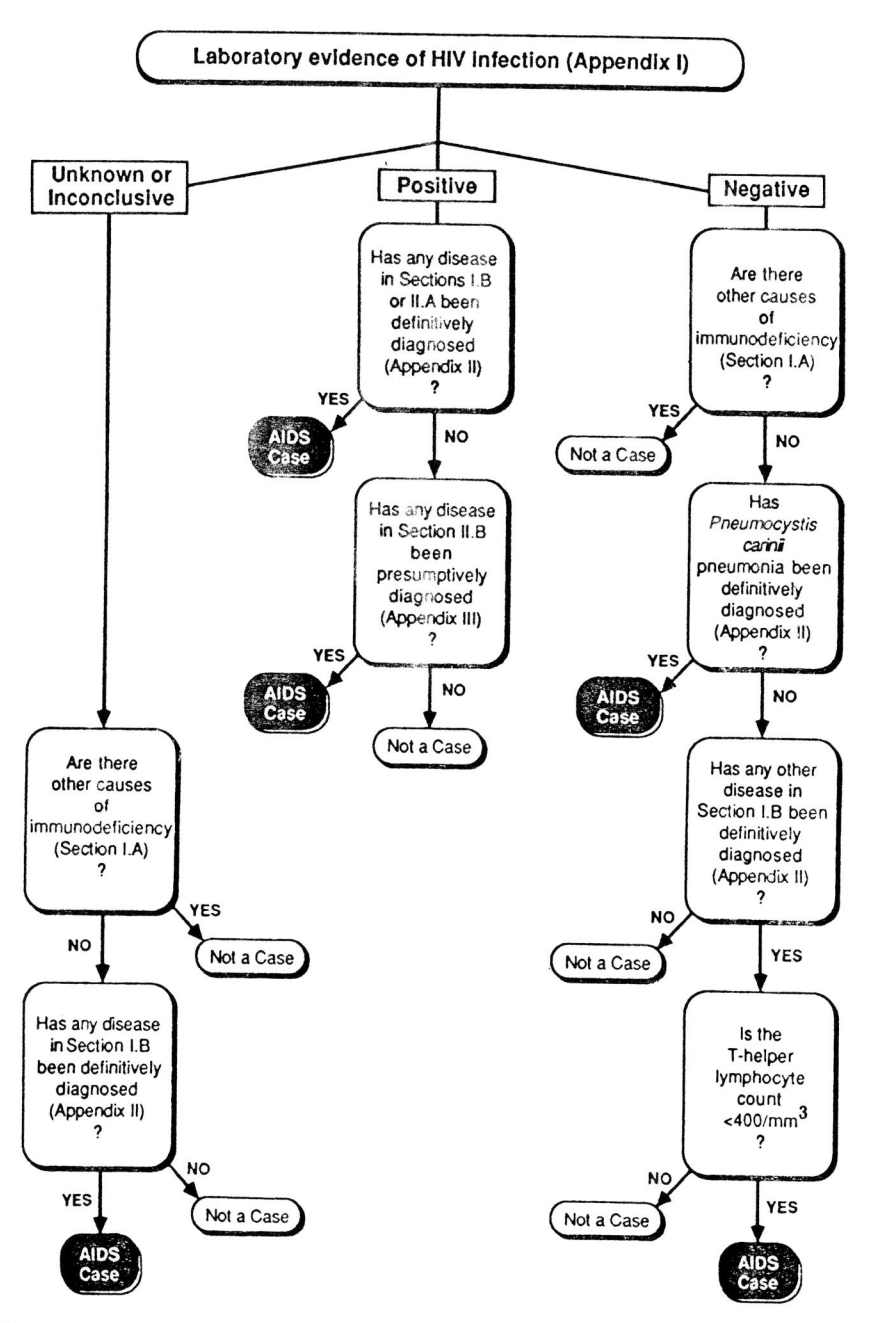

FIGURE 14–1 *Flow diagram for revised CDC case definition of AIDS, Sept. 1, 1987.*

Application of the definition for children differs from that for adults in two ways. First, multiple or recurrent serious bacterial infections and lymphoid interstitial pneumonia/pulmonary lymphoid hyperplasia are accepted as indicative of AIDS among children but not among adults. Second, for children <15 months of age whose mothers are thought to have had HIV infection during the child's perinatal period, the laboratory criteria for HIV infection are more stringent, since the presence of HIV antibody in the child is, by itself, insufficient evidence for HIV infection because of the persistence of passively acquired maternal antibodies <15 months after birth.

The new definition is effective immediately. State and local health departments are requested to apply the new definition henceforth to patients reported to them. The initiation of the actual reporting of cases that meet the new definition is targeted for September 1, 1987, when modified computer software and report forms should be in place to accommodate the changes. CSTE has recommended retrospective application of the revised definition to patients already reported to health departments. The new definition follows:

1987 REVISION OF CASE DEFINITION FOR AIDS FOR SURVEILLANCE PURPOSES

For national reporting, a case of AIDS is defined as an illness characterized by one or more of the following "indicator" diseases, depending on the status of laboratory evidence of HIV infection, as shown below.

I. Without Laboratory Evidence Regarding HIV Infection

If laboratory tests for HIV were not performed or gave inconclusive results (*See* Appendix 14–A) and the patient had no other cause of immunodeficiency listed in Section I.A below, then any disease listed in Section I.B indicates AIDS if it was diagnosed by a definitive method (*See* Appendix 14–B).

A. **Causes of immunodeficiency that disqualify diseases as indicators of AIDS in the absence of laboratory evidence for HIV infection**
   1. high-dose or long-term systemic corticosteroid therapy or other immunosuppressive/cytotoxic therapy ≤3 months before the onset of the indicator disease
   2. any of the following diseases diagnosed ≤3 months after diagnosis of the indicator disease: Hodgkin's disease, non-Hodgkin's lymphoma (other than primary brain lymphoma), lymphocytic leukemia, multiple myeloma, any other cancer of lymphoreticular or histiocytic tissue, or angioimmunoblastic lymphadenopathy
   3. a genetic (congenital) immunodeficiency syndrome or an acquired immunodeficiency syndrome atypical of HIV infection, such as one involving hypogammaglobulinemia

B. **Indicator diseases diagnosed definitively** (*See* Appendix 14–B)
   1. candidiasis of the esophagus, trachea, bronchi, or lungs
   2. cryptococcosis, extrapulmonary
   3. cryptosporidiosis with diarrhea persisting >1 month
   4. cytomegalovirus disease of an organ other than liver, spleen, or lymph nodes in a patient >1 month of age
   5. herpes simplex virus infection causing a mucocutaneous ulcer that persists longer than 1 month; or bronchitis, pneumonitis, or esophagitis for any duration affecting a patient >1 month of age
   6. Kaposi's sarcoma affecting a patient <60 years of age
   7. lymphoma of the brain (primary) affecting a patient <60 years of age
   8. lymphoid interstitial pneumonia and/or pulmonary lymphoid hyperplasia (LIP/PLH complex) affecting a child <13 years of age
   9. *Mycobacterium avium* complex or *M. kansasii* disease, disseminated (at a site other than or in addition to lungs, skin, or cervical or hilar lymph nodes)
   10. *Pneumocystis carinii* pneumonia
   11. progressive multifocal leukoencephalopathy
   12. toxoplasmosis of the brain affecting a patient >1 month of age

II. With Laboratory Evidence for HIV Infection

Regardless of the presence of other causes of immunodeficiency (I.A), in the presence of laboratory evidence for HIV infection (See Appendix 14–A), any disease listed above (I.B) or below (II.A or II.B) indicates a diagnosis of AIDS.

A. **Indicator diseases diagnosed definitively** (*See* Appendix 14–B)
   1. bacterial infections, multiple or recurrent (any combination of at least two within a 2-year period), of the following types affecting a child <13 years of age:
      septicemia, pneumonia, meningitis, bone or joint infection, or abscess of an internal organ or body cavity (excluding otitis media or superficial skin or mucosal abscesses), caused by *Haemophilus, Streptococcus* (including pneumococcus), or other pyogenic bacteria
   2. coccidioidomycosis, disseminated (at a site other than or in addition to lungs or cervical or hilar lymph nodes)
   3. HIV encephalopathy (also called "HIV dementia," "AIDS dementia," or "subacute encephalitis due to HIV") (*See* Appendix 14–B for description)
   4. histoplasmosis, disseminated (at a site other than or in addition to lungs or cervical or hilar lymph nodes)
   5. isosporiasis with diarrhea persisting >1 month
   6. Kaposi's sarcoma at any age
   7. lymphoma of the brain (primary) at any age

8. other non-Hodgkin's lymphoma of B-cell or unknown immunologic phenotype and the following histologic types:
   a. small noncleaved lymphoma (either Burkitt or non-Burkitt type) (See Appendix IV[a] for equivalent terms and numeric codes used in the *International Classification of Diseases,* Ninth Revision, Clinical Modification)
   b. immunoblastic sarcoma (equivalent to any of the following, although not necessarily all in combination: immunoblastic lymphoma, large-cell lymphoma, diffuse histiocytic lymphoma, diffuse undifferentiated lymphoma, or high-grade lymphoma) (See Appendix IV[a] for equivalent terms and numeric codes used in the *International Classification of Diseases,* Ninth Revision, Clinical Modification)

   Note: Lymphomas are not included here if they are of T-cell immunologic phenotype or their histologic type is not described or is described as "lymphocytic," "lymphoblastic," "small cleaved," or "plasmacytoid lymphocytic"

9. any mycobacterial disease caused by mycobacteria other than *M. tuberculosis,* disseminated (at a site other than or in addition to lungs, skin, or cervical or hilar lymph nodes)
10. disease caused by *M. tuberculosis,* extrapulmonary (involving at least one site outside the lungs, regardless of whether there is concurrent pulmonary involvement)
11. *Salmonella* (nontyphoid) septicemia, recurrent
12. HIV wasting syndrome (emaciation, "slim disease") (See Appendix 14–B for description)

B. **Indicator diseases diagnosed presumptively (by a method other than those in Appendix 14–B)**

   Note: Given the seriousness of diseases indicative of AIDS, it is generally important to diagnose them definitively, especially when therapy that would be used may have serious side effects or when definitive diagnosis is needed for eligibility for antiretroviral therapy. Nonetheless, in some situations, a patient's condition will not permit the performance of definitive tests. In other situations, accepted clinical practice may be to diagnose presumptively based on the presence of characteristic clinical and laboratory abnormalities. Guidelines for presumptive diagnoses are suggested in Appendix 14–C.

   1. candidiasis of the esophagus
   2. cytomegalovirus retinitis with loss of vision
   3. Kaposi's sarcoma

---

[a]Centers for Disease Control, Revision of the CDC surveillance case definition for AIDS. MMWR 1987;36:1S.

4. lymphoid interstitial pneumonia and/or pulmonary lymphoid hyperplasia (LIP/PLH complex) affecting a child <13 years of age
5. mycobacterial disease (acid-fast bacilli with species not identified by culture), disseminated (involving at least one site other than or in addition to lungs, skin, or cervical or hilar lymph nodes)
6. *Pneumocystis carinii* pneumonia
7. toxoplasmosis of the brain affecting a patient >1 month of age

III. With Laboratory Evidence Against HIV Infection

With laboratory test results negative for HIV infection (*See* Appendix 14–A), a diagnosis of AIDS for surveillance purposes is ruled out *unless:*
A. all the other causes of immunodeficiency listed above in Section I.A are excluded; AND
B. the patient has had either:
   1. *Pneumocystis carinii* pneumonia diagnosed by a definitive method (*See* Appendix 14–B); OR
   2. a. any of the other diseases indicative of AIDS listed above in Section I.B diagnosed by a definitive method (*See* Appendix 14–B); AND
      b. a T-helper/inducer (CD4) lymphocyte count <400/mm^3.

COMMENTARY

The surveillance of severe disease associated with HIV infection remains an essential, though not the only, indicator of the course of the HIV epidemic. The number of AIDS cases and the relative distribution of cases by demographic, geographic, and behavioral risk variables are the oldest indices of the epidemic, which began in 1981 and for which data are available retrospectively back to 1978. The original surveillance case definition, based on then-available knowledge, provided useful epidemiologic data on severe HIV disease.[1] To ensure a reasonable predictive value for underlying immunodeficiency caused by what was then an unknown agent, the indicators of AIDS in the old case definition were restricted to particular opportunistic diseases diagnosed by reliable methods in patients without specific known causes of immunodeficiency. After HIV was discovered to be the cause of AIDS, however, and highly sensitive and specific HIV-antibody tests became available, the spectrum of manifestations of HIV infection became better defined, and classification systems for HIV infection were developed.[2-5] It became apparent that some progressive, seriously disabling, and even fatal conditions (e.g., encephalopathy, wasting syndrome) affecting a substantial number of HIV-infected patients were not subject to epidemiologic surveillance, as they were not included in the AIDS case definition. For reporting purposes, the revision adds to the definition most of those severe non-infectious, non-cancerous HIV-associated conditions that are categorized in the CDC clinical classification systems for HIV infection among adults and children.[4,5]

Another limitation of the old definition was that AIDS-indicative diseases are diagnosed presumptively (i.e., without confirmation by methods required by the old definition) in 10%–15% of patients diagnosed with such diseases; thus, an appreciable proportion of AIDS cases were missed for reporting purposes.[6,7] This proportion may be increasing, which would compromise the old case definition's usefulness as a tool for monitoring trends. The revised case definition permits the reporting of these clinically diagnosed cases as long as there is laboratory evidence of HIV infection.

The effectiveness of the revision will depend on how extensively HIV-antibody tests are used. Approximately one third of AIDS patients in the United States have been from New York City and San Francisco, where, since 1985, <7% have been reported with HIV-antibody test results, compared with >60% in other areas. The impact of the revision on the reported numbers of AIDS cases will also depend on the proportion of AIDS patients in whom indicator diseases are diagnosed presumptively rather than definitively. The use of presumptive diagnostic criteria varies geographically, being more common in certain rural areas and in urban areas with many indigent AIDS patients.

To avoid confusion about what should be reported to health departments, the term "AIDS" should refer only to conditions meeting the surveillance definition. This definition is intended only to provide consistent statistical data for public health purposes. Clinicians will not rely on this definition alone to diagnose serious disease caused by HIV infection in individual patients because there may be additional information that would lead to a more accurate diagnosis. For example, patients who are not reportable under the definition because they have either a negative HIV-antibody test or, in the presence of HIV antibody, an opportunistic disease not listed in the definition as an indicator of AIDS nonetheless may be diagnosed as having serious HIV disease on consideration of other clinical or laboratory characteristics of HIV infection or a history of exposure to HIV.

Conversely, the AIDS surveillance definition may rarely misclassify other patients as having serious HIV disease if they have no HIV-antibody test but have an AIDS-indicative disease with a background incidence unrelated to HIV infection, such as cryptococcal meningitis.

The diagnostic criteria accepted by the AIDS surveillance case definition should not be interpreted as the standard of good medical practice. Presumptive diagnoses are accepted in the definition because not to count them would be to ignore substantial morbidity resulting from HIV infection. Likewise, the definition accepts a reactive screening test for HIV antibody without confirmation by a supplemental test because a repeatedly reactive screening test result, in combination with an indicator disease, is highly indicative of true HIV disease. For national surveillance purposes, the tiny proportion of possibly false-positive screening tests in persons with AIDS-indicative diseases is of little consequence. For the individual patient, however, a correct diagnosis is critically important.

The use of supplemental tests is, therefore, strongly endorsed. An increase in the diagnostic use of HIV-antibody tests could improve both the quality of medical care and the function of the new case definition, as well as assist in providing counselling to prevent transmission of HIV.

REFERENCES

1. World Health Organization. Acquired immunodeficiency syndrome (AIDS): WHO/CDC case definition for AIDS. WHO Wkly Epidemiol Rec 1986;61:69–72.
2. Haverkos HW, Gottlieb MS, Killen JY, Edelman R. Classification of HTLV-III/LAV-related diseases [Letter]. J Infect Dis 1985;152:1095.
3. Redfield RR, Wright DC, Tramont EC. The Walter Reed staging classification of HTLV-III infection. N Engl J Med 1986;314:131–32.
4. CDC. Classification system for human T-lymphotropic virus type III/lymphadenopathy-associated virus infections. MMWR 1986;35:334–39.
5. CDC. Classification system for human immunodeficiency virus (HIV) infection in children under 13 years of age. MMWR 1987;36:225–30,235.
6. Hardy AM, Starcher ET, Morgan WM, et al. Review of death certificates to assess completeness of AIDS case reporting. Pub Hlth Rep 1987;102(4):386–91.
7. Starcher ET, Biel JK, Rivera-Castano R, et al. The impact of presumptively diagnosed opportunistic infections and cancers on national reporting of AIDS [Abstract]. Washington, DC: III International Conference on AIDS, June 1–5, 1987.

APPENDIX 14–A

Laboratory Evidence For or Against HIV Infection

1. For Infection:

When a patient has disease consistent with AIDS:
a. a serum specimen from a patient ≥15 months of age, or from a child <15 months of age whose mother is not thought to have had HIV infection during the child's perinatal period, that is repeatedly reactive for HIV antibody by a screening test (e.g., enzyme-linked immunosorbent assay [ELISA]), as long as subsequent HIV-antibody tests (e.g., Western blot, immunofluorescence assay), if done, are positive; **OR**
b. a serum specimen from a child <15 months of age, whose mother is thought to have had HIV infection during the child's perinatal period, that is repeatedly reactive for HIV antibody by a screening test (e.g., ELISA), plus increased serum immunoglobulin levels and at least one of the following abnormal immunologic test results: reduced absolute lymphocyte count, depressed CD4 (T-helper) lymphocyte count, or decreased CD4/CD8 (helper/suppressor) ratio, as long as subsequent antibody tests (e.g., Western blot, immunofluorescence assay), if done, are positive; **OR**
c. a positive test for HIV serum antigen; **OR**
d. a positive HIV culture confirmed by both reverse transcriptase detection and a specific HIV-antigen test or in situ hybridization using a nucleic acid probe; **OR**
e. a positive result on any other highly specific test for HIV (e.g., nucleic acid probe of peripheral blood lymphocytes).

2. Against Infection:

A nonreactive screening test for serum antibody to HIV (e.g., ELISA) without a reactive or positive result on any other test for HIV infection (e.g., antibody, antigen, culture), if done.

3. Inconclusive (Neither For nor Against Infection):

a. a repeatedly reactive screening test for serum antibody to HIV (e.g., ELISA) followed by a negative or inconclusive supplemental test (e.g., Western blot, immunofluorescence assay) without a positive HIV culture or serum antigen test, if done; OR

b. a serum specimen from a child <15 months of age, whose mother is thought to have had HIV infection during the child's perinatal period, that is repeatedly reactive for HIV antibody by a screening test, even if positive by a supplemental test, without additional evidence for immunodeficiency as described above (in 1.b) and without a positive HIV culture or serum antigen test, if done.

APPENDIX 14-B

Definitive Diagnostic Methods for Diseases Indicative of AIDS

Diseases	Definitive Diagnostic Methods
cryptosporidiosis cytomegalovirus isosporiasis Kaposi's sarcoma lymphoma lymphoid pneumonia or hyperplasia *Pneumocystis carinii* pneumonia progressive multifocal leukoencephalopathy toxoplasmosis	microscopy (histology or cytology).
candidiasis	gross inspection by endoscopy or autopsy or by microscopy (histology or cytology) on a specimen obtained directly from the tissues affected (including scrapings from the mucosal surface), not from a culture.
coccidioidomycosis cryptococcosis herpes simplex virus histoplasmosis	microscopy (histology or cytology), culture, or detection of antigen in a specimen obtained directly from the tissues affected or a fluid from those tissues.
tuberculosis other mycobacteriosis salmonellosis other bacterial infection	culture.

Diseases	Definitive Diagnostic Methods
HIV encephalopathy* (dementia)	clinical findings of disabling cognitive and/or motor dysfunction interfering with occupation or activities of daily living, or loss of behavioral developmental milestones affecting a child, progressing over weeks to months, in the absence of a concurrent illness or condition other than HIV infection that could explain the findings. Methods to rule out such concurrent illnesses and conditions must include cerebrospinal fluid examination and either brain imaging (computed tomography or magnetic resonance) or autopsy.
HIV wasting syndrome*	findings of profound involuntary weight loss >10% of baseline body weight plus either chronic diarrhea (at least two loose stools per day for ≥30 days) or chronic weakness and documented fever (for ≥30 days, intermittent or constant) in the absence of a concurrent illness or condition other than HIV infection that could explain the findings (e.g., cancer, tuberculosis, cryptosporidiosis, or other specific enteritis).

---

*For HIV encephalopathy and HIV wasting syndrome, the methods of diagnosis described here are not truly definitive, but are sufficiently rigorous for surveillance purposes.

APPENDIX 14–C

Suggested Guidelines for Presumptive Diagnosis of Diseases Indicative of AIDS

Diseases	Presumptive Diagnostic Criteria
candidiasis of esophagus	a. recent onset of retrosternal pain on swallowing; **AND** b. oral candidiasis diagnosed by the gross appearance of white patches or plaques on an erythematous base or by the microscopic appearance of fungal mycelial filaments in an uncultured specimen scraped from the oral mucosa.
cytomegalovirus retinitis	a characteristic appearance on serial ophthalmoscopic examinations (e.g., discrete patches of retinal whitening with distinct borders, spreading in a centrifugal manner, following blood vessels, progressing over several months, frequently associated with retinal vasculitis, hemorrhage, and necrosis). Resolution of active disease leaves retinal scarring and atrophy with retinal pigment epithelial mottling.
mycobacteriosis	microscopy of a specimen from stool or normally sterile body fluids or tissue from a site other than lungs, skin, or cervical or hilar lymph nodes, showing acid-fast bacilli of a species not identified by culture.
Kaposi's sarcoma	a characteristic gross appearance of an erythematous or violaceous plaque-like lesion on skin or mucous membrane. (**Note:** Presumptive diagnosis of Kaposi's sarcoma should not be made by clinicians who have seen few cases of it.)

Diseases	Presumptive Diagnostic Criteria
lymphoid interstitial pneumonia	bilateral reticulonodular interstitial pulmonary infiltrates present on chest x-ray for ≥2 months with no pathogen identified and no response to antibiotic treatment.
Pneumocystis carinii pneumonia	a. a history of dyspnea on exertion or nonproductive cough of recent onset (within the past 3 months); **AND** b. chest x-ray evidence of diffuse bilateral interstitial infiltrates or gallium scan evidence of diffuse bilateral pulmonary disease; **AND** c. arterial blood gas analysis showing an arterial pO_2 of <70 mm Hg or a low respiratory diffusing capacity (<80% of predicted values) or an increase in the alveolar-arterial oxygen tension gradient; **AND** d. no evidence of a bacterial pneumonia.
toxoplasmosis of the brain	a. recent onset of a focal neurologic abnormality consistent with intracranial disease or a reduced level of consciousness; **AND** b. brain imaging evidence of a lesion having a mass effect (on computed tomography or nuclear magnetic resonance) or the radiographic appearance of which is enhanced by injection of contrast medium; **AND** c. serum antibody to toxoplasmosis or successful response to therapy for toxoplasmosis.

Chapter 15

AIDS and HIV Infection: Surveillance and Epidemiology in the United States, 1981–1985

Richard M. Selik
James W. Curran

DEFINITION OF AIDS

The Centers for Disease Control (CDC) first defined acquired immunodeficiency syndrome (AIDS) in 1981, before the discovery of its cause, human immunodeficiency virus (HIV).[1-4] The CDC modified the definition of AIDS slightly in 1985 to take into account the results of tests for HIV infection. To maintain a consistent basis for monitoring trends in the epidemic of HIV infection in the United States, the CDC continued to use its definition of AIDS for national reporting of some of the severe late manifestations of HIV infection. Briefly stated, the CDC defined a case of AIDS as an illness characterized by one or more opportunistic diseases (infections and cancers)[5-7] that are at least moderately predictive of an underlying defect in T-lymphocyte-mediated immunity, occurring in the absence of known causes of reduced resistance to those diseases (other than HIV-induced immunodeficiency). Unlike some of the diseases used as markers for AIDS, which may recur multiple times, AIDS itself is considered to persist for the remainder of the patient's life, so that no more than one case of AIDS can occur in a person. It is clear that this strict case definition does not describe the full spectrum of manifestations of HIV infection, which may include diffuse, generalized lymphadenopathy and other nonspecific symptoms,[8] other opportunistic infections or cancers, or merely laboratory evidence of immunodeficiency of antibody to HIV in persons who have no symptoms.[9]

INCIDENCE AND MORTALITY

Between June 1, 1981, and Jan. 20, 1986, the CDC received reports of 16,574 cases of AIDS. Although cases were first reported to the CDC[10,11] and in the scientific literature[12-15] in 1981, cases were first diagnosed as early as 1978. The reported incidence of AIDS by date of diagnosis continues to increase (Table 15–1). Cases of AIDS have been reported to the CDC among residents of every state in the United States, as well as the District of Columbia, Puerto Rico, and three trust territories. Approximately 57% of case reports originated in New York and California; the crude annual incidence rates in New York City and San Francisco have been more than tenfold greater than in the rest of the United States. The highest incidence rates (82 to 269 per 100,000 annually between 1983 and 1984) have been in single men in San Francisco and Manhattan, intravenous drug users in New York City and New Jersey, hemophilia A patients, and Haitians who entered the United States after 1977.[16] Men accounted for 92% of AIDS cases; of the men, 79% were reported to be homosexual or bisexual (Table 15–2). Of heterosexual men and women with AIDS, 64% were reported to have abused drugs intravenously, especially heroin and cocaine.[14,17,18] Approximately 4% of reported patients with AIDS did not appear to belong to groups having increased prevalence of HIV infection, although histories were inadequate for many of these individuals. The ethnic distribution of reported AIDS patients was 60% white (non-Hispanic), 25% black (non-Hispanic), and 14% Hispanic. Over 90% of AIDS patients were under age 50 at the time of

Table 15–1 Reported cases of AIDS, deaths, and case-fatality rates by half-year of diagnosis, 1979–1985, as of Jan. 20, 1986, United States

		Cases	Known Deaths	Case-Fatality Rate (%)
1979	Jan.–June	3	2	67
	July–Dec.	9	8	89
1980	Jan.–June	18	15	83
	July–Dec.	29	27	93
1981	Jan.–June	83	72	87
	July–Dec.	174	147	84
1982	Jan.–June	361	278	77
	July–Dec.	632	465	74
1983	Jan.–June	1,181	855	72
	July–Dec.	1,534	1,129	74
1984	Jan.–June	2,338	1,556	67
	July–Dec.	3,017	1,662	55
1985	Jan.–June	3,842	1,463	38
	July–Dec.[a]	3,339	737	22
Totals[b]		16,574	8,423	51

[a]Data collection is largely incomplete for the most recent six months.
[b]Totals include eight patients diagnosed before 1979, of whom four are known to have died, and six diagnosed in January 1986, of whom three have died.

Table 15-2 Reported cases of AIDS by patient group as of Jan. 20, 1986, United States

	Males No. (%)	Females No. (%)	Total No. (%)
Adults/adolescents, patient group[a]			
Homosexual or bisexual men[b]	11,998 (79)	— (—)	11,998 (73)
Intravenous drug abusers	2206 (14)	572 (53)	2778 (7)
Persons with a blood clotting-factor disorder	128 (1)	4 (0)	132 (1)
Persons with heterosexual contact[c]	27 (0)	158 (15)	185 (1)
Recipients of blood or blood component transfusions	162 (1)	101 (9)	263 (2)
None of the above/other[d]	747 (5)	240 (22)	987 (6)
Total	15,268 (100)	1,075 (100)	16,343 (100)
Children,[e] patient group[a]			
Children with a blood clotting-factor disorder	11 (9)	0 (0)	11 (5)
Children with a parent with AIDS or at increased risk for AIDS[f]	88 (69)	87 (84)	175 (76)
Recipients of blood or blood component transfusions	22 (17)	10 (10)	32 (14)
Children in none of the above groups	6 (5)	7 (7)	13 (6)
Total	127 (100)	104 (100)	231 (100)

[a]Groups listed are ordered hierarchically; cases with multiple characteristics are tabulated only in the group listed first.
[b]1320 (11%) of homosexual men also reported having abused drugs intravenously.
[c]Persons in this group had heterosexual contact with a person who was at increased risk for AIDS or who actually developed AIDS.
[d]This group includes 399 persons born in countries in which most AIDS cases have not been in the groups listed above but in which heterosexual contact is thought to play a major role in transmission.
[e]Children include patients under 13 years of age at diagnosis.
[f]Epidemiologic data suggest that these cases are due to transmission from infected mother to child before, at, or shortly after birth.

diagnosis; the median age was 35 years. Two hundred thirty-one (1.4%) of the cases were in children under 13 years of age. Of these 231 children, 175 (76%) were born to mothers who had a documented HIV infection or who belonged to a group having an increased prevalence of HIV infection. Of these 175 children, 62% had a mother who abused drugs intravenously, and another 10% had a mother with a male sex partner who abused drugs intravenously.

More than 70% of AIDS patients died within three years after diagnosis. No case reports have been published documenting full clinical and immunologic recovery of patients fitting the case definition of AIDS, so the case-fatality rate may be higher yet. This rate varied with the presenting opportunistic disease. Patients with Kaposi's sarcoma, but with no opportunistic infection, tended to survive longer than patients with opportunistic infections (Table 15–3).[19,20]

EARLY STUDIES SUGGESTING SEXUAL TRANSMISSION

After the first reports of cases in California and New York, the CDC formed an internal task force to establish surveillance and conduct epidemiologic and laboratory studies. The CDC physician-epidemiologists interviewed over 30 AIDS patients in New York and California and conducted a brief survey of nitrite inhalant ("popper") use and sexual activity among homosexual and heterosexual men attending sexually transmitted disease (STD) clinics. These interviews revealed no clear potential risk factors; rather, homosexual AIDS patients were sexually active, gave histories of frequent use of prescription and illicit drugs, and had experienced many previous infections. Over 85% of homosexual and bisexual men, as compared with 15% of heterosexual men, reported using nitrite inhalants within the past 5 years.[21] The close correlation in this survey between

Table 15–3 Reported cases of AIDS, deaths, and case-fatality rates by disease category, June 1, 1981, to Jan. 20, 1986, United States

Disease Category[a]	Cases (%)	Deaths (%)	Case-Fatality Rate
Both KS and PCP	920 (6)	598 (7)	65%
KS without PCP	3056 (18)	1167 (14)	38%
PCP without KS	9539 (58)	4986 (59)	52%
Other diseases without KS or PCP	3059 (18)	1672 (20)	55%
Total	16,574 (100)	8423 (100)	51%

[a]KS, Kaposi's sarcoma; PCP, *Pneumocystis carinii* pneumonia; other diseases, other opportunistic infections and cancers used as markers for AIDS in the case definition. The disease categories are ordered hierarchically; cases with multiple diseases are tabulated only in the category listed first.

the reported frequency of nitrite usage among homosexual men and the reported number of sexual partners suggested that the use of nitrites might be associated with other hypothetical risk factors.

In collaboration with other investigators, the CDC conducted a national case control study of AIDS in homosexual men in New York and California. Using logistic regression techniques to analyze data from this study, the CDC found that the characteristic that best distinguished cases of Kaposi's sarcoma or *Pneumocystis carinii* pneumonia from their matched controls was the number of male sex partners. The median number of partners per year for AIDS patients, 61, was twice as great as for controls.[22]

In another epidemiologic investigation, a cluster of cases of Kaposi's sarcoma and *P. carinii* pneumonia in homosexual men in southern California was discovered.[23] Of the first 19 reported cases, nine were in patients from the Los Angeles area with histories of direct sexual contact with at least one other person who developed AIDS. One of the individuals linked to this cluster was a nonresident of California who had sexual contact with eight other men with AIDS. The findings of these two studies strengthened the hypothesis that a sexually transmissible agent was causing AIDS, which has subsequently been identified as HIV.[1-4]

AIDS AND HIV INFECTION

Since the discovery of HIV, and the development of tests for serum antibody to this virus, it has been possible to study the natural history of HIV infection and to better characterize the spectrum of its manifestations. A cohort of 6875 homosexual men, who enrolled in a hepatitis B study at the San Francisco City Clinic for sexually transmitted diseases between 1978 and 1980, was studied to determine the incidence and prevalence of HIV infection and its manifestations. In a representative sample of cohort members, prevalence of antibody to HIV, measured by an enzyme immunosorbent assay (EIA), increased from 4% in 1978 to 73% by August 1985.[24,25] Of the men in the sample who consented to have their earliest specimens tested, 31 had antibody to HIV at the time they enrolled in the hepatitis B study between 1978 and 1980. By August 1985, two (6%; 95% confidence bounds 1% to 21%) had developed AIDS and eight (26%) had developed AIDS-related conditions (ARC) (e.g., generalized lymphadenopathy, oral candidiasis, persistent fever, diarrhea, or weight loss, hematologic abnormalities). Symptomatic illness due to HIV infection thus had occurred in 10 (32%; 95% confidence bounds 17% to 51%) of the 31 men after a follow-up period averaging 61 months, while 68% remained asymptomatic.

A representative sample of 474 of the cohort members was studied between 1984 and 1985. For each man with AIDS, nine others had AIDS-related illness due to HIV, and 18 had asymptomatic HIV infection. If the experience in this sample were extrapolated to the entire United States, it would be estimated that at least 460,000 persons had become infected with HIV infection by the beginning of 1986. This estimate is based on the Jan. 20, 1986 total of 16,574 reported AIDS cases multiplied by a factor of 28. Since the infection first entered many areas of the country more recently than it did in San Francisco, and since reporting of AIDS cases is not complete, the actual number of infected persons in the country may be two or three times greater, i.e., more than a million.[26,27]

PERSISTENCE OF HIV INFECTION

Studies indicate that HIV infection persists for many years, perhaps for as long as an infected individual lives. In investigations of cases of transfusion-associated AIDS, HIV was isolated from cultures of lymphocytes obtained from 22 of 23 seropositive blood donors an average of 28 months after the implicated donations.[28] All but one of the seropositive blood donors were asymptomatic at the time of donation, and 15 of 22 remained so when the virus was isolated 1 to 4 years later. In another study, HIV was isolated from the blood of eight (67%) of 12 homosexual men who had been asymptomatic and seropositive for two to nearly six years.[29] The presence of antibody, therefore, should be considered persumptive evidence of current infection and infectiousness.

MODES OF TRANSMISSION OF HIV

HIV has been isolated from blood, semen,[30] saliva,[31] tears,[32] breast milk,[33] and urine and is likely to be in some other body fluids, secretions, and excretions, but epidemiologic evidence has implicated only blood and semen in transmission. Increased risk of HIV infection has been documented in populations exposed by one or more of four routes: sexual contact, intravenous drug administration with contaminated needles, administration of blood or clotting-factor blood products, and perinatal transmission from infected mothers to their infants. Several studies have identified specific behavioral risk factors for AIDS and HIV infection in homosexual men.[22,34-36] An increased number of sex partners was the risk factor most consistently associated with acquisition of infection or AIDS in homosexual men. In addition, receptive anal intercourse and other practices associated with rectal trauma often differentiated cases from controls in these studies of homosexual men.

In studies of heterosexual transmission, HIV infection was most closely associated with being a steady sex partner of a person who had evidence of HIV infection such as AIDS or antibody to HIV infection.[37-39] Currently, 1% of patients with AIDS have no identified risk factors except for heterosexual contact with persons with evidence of HIV infection or in groups at increased risk. Of men with AIDS interviewed in New York City who had no other risk factor, 20% had a history of contact with prostitutes, a possible indicator of heterosexual transmission.[40] Studies in central African countries have shown that contact with prostitutes and large numbers of heterosexual partners are risk factors for AIDS in heterosexual men.[42-44]

Among intravenous drug abusers, the sharing of needles and syringes, presumably contaminated with infectious blood, has been implicated as a risk factor for AIDS and HIV infection.[45,46] In some developing countries, HIV infection has been associated with the number of injections received for therapeutic purposes, suggesting that reuse of nonsterile needles and syringes may contribute to transmission.[47–50]

Transfusion-associated AIDS has been caused by receipt of a unit of whole blood or blood component from a donor infected with HIV. Usually the donor has been asymptomatic at the time of donation. Patients who received blood components from large numbers of donors were more likely to be exposed. Blood components implicated in transmission have included red blood cells, platelets, and plasma.[51,52] HIV infection has been transmitted to persons with hemophilia through pooled plasma products, specifically clotting factor concentrates and cryoprecipitate.[53–56] HIV seroprevalence increases with severity of hemophilia and increased use of clotting factor therapy.

Most infants with AIDS were born to mothers with AIDS or at increased risk of AIDS. The occurrence of symptoms shortly after birth and the absence of cases in older children suggest transmission *in utero* or during or shortly after birth.[57–60] HIV antibody has been found in an infant of a mother who had acquired HIV infection postpartum from a blood transfusion.[61] It has been hypothesized that transmission occurred from mother to infant as a result of breast-feeding or other close mother-to-infant contact.

Of the 16,574 cases of AIDS reported by Jan. 20, 1986, 701 (4.2%) were in health care workers (HCWs). All but 28 (4.0%) of these HCWs belonged to groups known to be at increased risk for AIDS (e.g., homosexual men, intravenous drug users). In the completed investigations of cases outside high-risk groups, no specific occupational exposures could be documented. In five separate studies, a total of 1498 HCWs have been tested for antibody to HIV.[62] In these studies, 666 (44.5%) of the HCWs had direct parenteral (needlestick or cut) or mucous membrane exposure to patients with AIDS or HIV infection. Most of these exposures were to blood. None of the HCWs whose initial serologic tests were negative developed evidence of HIV infection. In these five studies, 26 HCWs were seropositive when first tested; all but three of these persons belonged to groups recognized to be at increased risk for AIDS.[63] Since one of the three was tested anonymously, epidemiologic information was available on only two. Although these two HCWs were reported as having HIV infection that was probably occupationally related,[63,64] no serum sample had been obtained before or shortly after exposure for either HCW, so the onset of infection could not be determined. In England, a nurse seroconverted after accidentally injecting herself with blood from an AIDS patient.[65]

Although there is no evidence that HCWs infected with HIV have transmitted infection to patients, the risk of such transmission may exist when there is both a high degree of trauma to the patient that provides a portal of entry for the virus (e.g., during invasive procedures) and exposure of the patient's open tissue to blood or serous fluid from an infected HCW, as could occur if the HCW sustains a needlestick or scalpel injury during an invasive procedure.

RECOMMENDATIONS FOR PREVENTION

Of all the known modes of transmission of HIV infection, the most progress has been made in preventing transmission through blood and blood products. In March 1983, the United States Public Health Service advised that members of groups at increased risk for AIDS voluntarily refrain from donating blood.[66] Serologic tests for antibody to HIV were licensed in March 1985 and are being used to screen blood and plasma donations in virtually every collection center in the United States. These tests are necessary, because some infected persons are not aware that they are at increased risk and thus continue to donate blood.[67,68]

Preliminary results reported by the Food and Drug Administration (FDA) showed repeatable enzyme-linked immunosorbent assay (ELISA) reactivity in 0.25% of the first 1.1 million units of donated blood tested.[69] This prevalence of repeatable ELISA reactivity is consistent with a low level of infectiousness among current blood and plasma donors and indicates that discarding these units will decrease the risk of virus transmission and have minimal effect on blood supplies.

HIV is sensitive to heat in vitro.[70-72] Heat-treated clotting-factor concentrates have been developed and are commercially available. The National Hemophilia Foundation has recommended that all patients with hemophilia be treated with these products. Preliminary follow-up studies of seronegative hemophiliacs suggest that these products do not transmit HIV infection.

The factors that influence sexual transmission of HIV are similar to those related to other sexually transmitted infections. Voluntary testing for serum antibody to HIV may help persons to recognize whether they are infected, particularly when they are asymptomatic. However, persons with frequent exposure to possible sources of infection may have a high probability of being infected regardless of negative test results. The likelihood that a given sexual encounter is with an infected (and infectious) partner encompasses two distinct situations: risk of exposure from steady partners, and risk of exposure from occasional partners. Spouses and other steady sex partners of infected persons must receive accurate information about their own infection status and about their risk of becoming infected. Personal counseling for both partners may be necessary while they address this difficult situation. For steady sex partners of infected persons, reducing exposures means avoiding sexual activity that involves contact with the infected person's body fluids (e.g., semen, blood, saliva, and vaginal or rectal secretions) in any body orifice (e.g., vagina, rectum, mouth) or on injured skin of the uninfected partner. Condoms, diaphragms, and spermicides theoretically offer some protection, but their efficacy is unproved. For individuals who have been occasional partners of persons known to be infected or at high risk of being infected, discontinuing sexual relations with such persons may be easier than it is for steady partners. In groups in which the prevalence of HIV infection is high, the only certain way to avoid risk of infection is to restrict sexual intercourse to a partner known to be uninfected or to avoid sexual intercourse completely.

Preventing transmission among intravenous drug users will be as challenging as preventing transmission among homosexual men. Effective drug treatment programs and enforcement of drug laws will both play important roles in preventing AIDS by decreasing illicit drug use and discouraging sharing of needles and syringes. Widespread education of school children, combining information on AIDS and drug abuse, should be undertaken, especially where intravenous drug abuse is common.

The risk of HIV infection and AIDS in infants born to infected mothers has not yet been quantified precisely, but it is substantial enough to warrant recommending that women with clinical or serologic evidence of infection should be counseled about this risk to allow them to make an informed choice concerning reproduction. If they wish to avoid this risk, they should be assisted in choosing the most effective means acceptable to them to avoid bearing children. Women in groups with an increased prevalence of HIV infection, such as intravenous drug users, who are able to have children should be counseled and offered a serologic test for HIV. Clinical settings most appropriate for this include those that provide services specifically directed toward high-risk groups (e.g., drug detoxification, methadone maintenance), and those related to reproduction (e.g., family planning, gynecologic, and obstetric services). The Public Health Service has issued recommendations to assist in prevention of perinatal transmission of HIV infection.[73]

Despite the low occupational risk of transmission of HIV to HCWs even when needlestick injuries occur, more emphasis must be given to precautions to prevent needlestick injuries in HCWs caring for any patient, since such injuries continue to occur even during the care of patients known to be infected with HIV. Summaries of these and related precautions for HCWs have been published.[62,74]

UPDATE ADDENDUM

As of December 5, 1988, CDC had received reports of 79,823 AIDS cases in the United States and U.S. territories. Of the 26,332 of these diagnosed since the 1987 revision of the case definition, 7,252 (28%) met only the new criteria of the revised definition.[75] Sixty-one percent of all cases were homosexual or bisexual men, and an additional 7% were homosexual/bisexual men with a history of intravenous-drug abuse. Heterosexual intravenous-drug abusers accounted for 19% of cases.

REFERENCES

1. Barre-Sinoussi F, Chermann JC, Rey F, et al. Isolation of a T-lymphotropic retrovirus from a patient at risk for acquired immune deficiency syndrome. Science 1983;220:868.
2. Gallo RC, Salahuddin SZ, Popovic M, et al. Frequent detection and isolation of cytopathic retroviruses (HTLV-III) from patients with AIDS and at risk for AIDS. Science 1984;224:500.

3. Levy J, Hoffman AD, Kramer SM, et al. Isolation of lymphocytopathic retroviruses from San Francisco patients with AIDS. Science 1984;225:840.
4. Ratner L, Gallo RC, Wong-Staal F. HTLV-III, LAV, and ARV are variants of the same AIDS virus. Nature 1985;313:636.
5. Selik RM, Haverkos HW, Curran JW. Acquired immune deficiency syndrome (AIDS) trends in the United States, 1978–1982. Am J Med 1984;76:493.
6. Centers for Disease Control. Revision of the case definition of acquired immunodeficiency syndrome for national reporting—United States. MMWR 1985;34:373.
7. Centers for Disease Control. Update on acquired immune deficiency syndrome (AIDS)—United States. MMWR 1982;31:507.
8. Centers for Disease Control. Persistent, generalized lymphadenopathy among homosexual males. MMWR 1982;31:249.
9. Kornfield H, Vande Stowe RA, Lange M, et al. T-lymphocyte subpopulations in homosexual men. N Engl J Med 1982;307:729.
10. Centers for Disease Control. *Pneumocystis* pneumonia—Los Angeles. MMWR 1981;30:250.
11. Centers for Disease Control. Kaposi's sarcoma and *Pneumocystis* pneumonia among homosexual men—New York City and California. MMWR 1981;30:305.
12. Hymes KB, Greene JB, Marcus A, et al. Kaposi's sarcoma in homosexual men—a report of eight cases. Lancet 1981;II:598.
13. Gottlieb MS, Schroff R, Schanker HM, et al. *Pneumocystis carinii* pneumonia and mucosal candidiasis in previously healthy homosexual men. N Engl J Med 1981;305:1425.
14. Masur H, Michelis MA, Greene JB, et al. An outbreak of community-acquired *Pneumocystis carinii* pneumonia. N Engl J Med 1981;305:1431.
15. Siegal FP, Lopez C, Hammer GS. Severe acquired immunodeficiency in male homosexuals, manifested by chronic perianal ulcerative herpes simplex lesions. N Engl J Med 1981;305:1439.
16. Hardy AM, Allen JR, Morgan WM, Curran JW. The incidence rate of acquired immunodeficiency syndrome in selected populations. JAMA 1985;253:215.
17. Centers for Disease Control. Update on Kaposi's sarcoma and opportunistic infections in previously healthy persons—United States. MMWR 1982;31:294.
18. Masur H, Michelis MA, Wormser GP, et al. Opportunistic infection in previously healthy women. Initial manifestations of a community-acquired cellular immunodeficiency. Ann Intern Med 1982;97:533.
19. Riven BE, Monroe JM, Hubschman BP, Thomas PA. AIDS outcome: a first follow-up (letter). N Engl J Med 1984;311:857.
20. Moss AR, McCallum G, Volberding PA, Bacchetti P. Mortality associated with mode of presentation in the acquired immune deficiency syndrome. JNCI 1984;73:1281.
21. Centers for Disease Control, Task Force on Kaposi's Sarcoma and Opportunistic Infections. Epidemiologic aspects of the current outbreak of Kaposi's sarcoma and opportunistic infections. N Engl J Med 1982;306:248.
22. Jaffe H, Keewhan C, Thomas PA, et al. National case-control study of Kaposi's sarcoma and *Pneumocystis carinii* pneumonia in homosexual men: I. Epidemiologic results. Ann Intern Med 1983;99:145.
23. Centers for Disease Control. A cluster of Kaposi's sarcoma and *Pneumocystis carinii* pneumonia among homosexual male residents of Los Angeles and Orange Counties, California. MMWR 1982;31:305.

24. Jaffe HW, Darrow WW, Echenberg DF, et al. The acquired immunodeficiency syndrome in a cohort of homosexual men: A six-year follow-up study. Ann Intern Med 1985;103:210.
25. Centers for Disease Control. Update: acquired immunodeficiency syndrome in the San Francisco cohort study, 1978–1985. MMWR 1985;34:573.
26. Curran JW, Morgan WM, Hardy AM, et al. The epidemiology of AIDS: Current status and future prospects. Science 1985;229:1352.
27. Curran JW. The epidemiology and prevention of the acquired immunodeficiency syndrome. Ann Intern Med 1985;103:657.
28. Feorino PM, Jaffe HW, Palmer E, et al. Transfusion-associated acquired immunodeficiency syndrome: Evidence for persistent infection in blood donors. N Engl J Med 1985;312:1293.
29. Jaffe HW, Feorino PM, Darrow WW, et al. Persistent infection with human T-lymphotropic virus type III/lymphadenopathy-associated virus in apparently healthy homosexual men. Ann Intern Med 1985;102:627.
30. Zagury D, Bernard J, Leibowitch J, et al. HTLV-III in cells cultured from semen of two patients with AIDS. Science 1984;226:449.
31. Groopman JE, Salahuddin SZ, Sarngadharan MG, et al. HTLV-III in saliva of people with AIDS-related complex and healthy homosexual men at risk for AIDS. Science 1984;224:447.
32. Fujikawa LS, Salahuddin SZ, Palestine AG, et al. Isolation of human T-cell leukemia/lymphotropic virus type III (HTLV-III) from the tears of a patient with acquired immunodeficiency syndrome (AIDS). Lancet (in press).
33. Thiry L, Sprecher-Goldberger S, Jonckheer T, et al. Isolation of AIDS virus from cell-free breast milk of three healthy virus carriers. Lancet 1985;II:891.
34. Goedert JJ, Sarngadharan MG, Biggar RJ, et al. Determinants of retrovirus (HTLV-III) antibody and immunodeficiency conditions in homosexual men. Lancet 1984;II:711.
35. Mayer KH, Ayotte D, Stoddard AM, Groopman JE. Sexual practices and other lifestyle variables associated with HTLV-III seropositivity in homosexual men with and without generalized lymphadenopathy (abstr). In: The International Conference on Acquired Immunodeficiency Syndrome: Abstracts. Philadelphia: The American College of Physicians, 1985.
36. Melbye M, Biggar RJ, Ebbesen P, et al. Seroepidemiology of HTLV-III antibody in Danish homosexual men: Prevalence, transmission, and disease outcome. Br Med J 1984;289:573.
37. Kreiss JK, Kitchen LW, Prince HE, et al. Antibody to human T-lymphotropic virus type III in wives of hemophiliacs: Evidence for heterosexual transmission. Ann Intern Med 1985;102:623.
38. Redfield RR, Markham PD, Salahuddin SZ, et al. Frequent transmission of HTLV-III among spouses of patients with AIDS-related complex and AIDS. JAMA 1985;253:1571.
39. Redfield RR, Markham PD, Salahuddin SZ, et al. Heterosexually acquired HTLV-III/LAV disease (AIDS-related complex and AIDS): Epidemiologic evidence for female-to-male transmission. JAMA 1985;254:2094.
40. Rabkin C, Lekatsas A, Walker JA, et al. Acquired immunodeficiency syndrome in heterosexual males associated with sexual contacts. Presented at the International Conference on Acquired Immunodeficiency Syndrome, Atlanta, April 17, 1985.
41. Clumeck N, Robert-Guroff M, Van De Perre P, et al. Seroepidemiological studies

of HTLV-III antibody prevalence among selected groups of heterosexual Africans. JAMA 1985;254:2599.
42. Clumeck N, Sonnet J, Taelman H, et al. Acquired immunodeficiency syndrome in African patients. N Engl J Med 1984;310:492.
43. Van de Perre P, Rouvroy D, Lepage P, et al. Acquired immunodeficiency syndrome in Rwanda. Lancet 1984;II:62.
44. Piot P, Quinn TC, Taelman H, et al. Acquired immunodeficiency syndrome in an heterosexual population in Zaire. Lancet 1984;II:65.
45. Weiss SH, Ginzburg HM, Goedert JJ, et al. Risk for HTLV-III exposure, and AIDS among parenteral drug abusers in New Jersey. Presented at the International Conference on Acquired Immunodeficiency Syndrome, Atlanta, April 16, 1985.
46. Cohen H, Marmor M, Des Jarlais D, et al. Behavioral risk factors for HTLV-III/LAV seropositivity among intravenous drug abusers. Presented at the International Conference on Acquired Immunodeficiency Syndrome, April 16, 1985, Atlanta, Georgia.
47. Mann JM, Francis H, Kapita BM, et al. Household transmission of HTLV-III in Zaire. Presented at the International Conference on Acquired Immunodeficiency Syndrome, Atlanta, April 15, 1985.
48. Kapita BM, Mann JM, Francis H, et al. HTLV-III seroprevalence among hospital workers in Kinshasa, Zaire. Presented at the International Conference on Acquired Immunodeficiency Syndrome, Atlanta, April 17, 1985.
49. Pape JW, Liautaud B, Thomas F, et al. AIDS in Haiti. Presented at the International Conference on Acquired Immunodeficiency Syndrome, Atlanta, April 17, 1985.
50. Pape JW, Liautaud B, Thomas F, et al. Characteristics of the acquired immunodeficiency syndrome (AIDS) in Haiti. N Engl J Med 1983;309:945.
51. Curran JW, Lawrence DN, Jaffe H, et al. Acquired immunodeficiency syndrome (AIDS) associated with transfusion. N Engl J Med 1984;310:69.
52. Peterman TA, Jaffe HW, Feorino PM, et al. Transfusion-associated AIDS in the United States. Presented at the International Conference on Acquired Immunodeficiency Syndrome, Atlanta, April 16, 1985.
53. Centers for Disease Control. *Pneumocystis carinii* pneumonia among persons with hemophilia A. MMWR 1982;31:365.
54. Centers for Disease Control. Changing patterns of acquired immunodeficiency syndrome in hemophilia patients—United States. MMWR 1985;34:241.
55. Jason J, McDougal JS, Holman RC, et al. Human T-lymphotropic retrovirus type III/lymphadenopathy-associated virus antibody: Association with hemophiliacs' immune status and blood component usage. JAMA 1985;253:3409.
56. Gjerset GF, McGrady G, Counts RB, et al. Lymphadenopathy-associated virus antibodies and T-cells in hemophiliacs treated with cryoprecipitate or concentrate. Blood 1985;66:718.
57. Thomas PA, Jaffe HW, Spira TJ, et al. Unexplained immunodeficiency in children: A surveillance report. JAMA 1984;252:639.
58. Oleske J, Minnefor A, Cooper R, et al. Immune deficiency syndrome in children. JAMA 1983;249:2345.
59. Rubinstein A, Sicklick M, Gupta A, et al. Acquired immunodeficiency with reversed T4/T8 ratios in infants born to promiscuous and drug-addicted mothers. JAMA 1983;249:2350.
60. LaPointe N, Michaud J, Pekovic D, et al. Transplacental transmission of HTLV-III virus. N Engl J Med 1985;312:1325.

61. Ziegler JB, Cooper DA, Johnson RO, Gold J. Postnatal transmission of AIDS-associated retrovirus from mother to infant. Lancet 1985;I:896.
62. Centers for Disease Control. Recommendations for preventing transmission of infection with HTLV-III/LAV in the workplace. MMWR 1985;34:682.
63. Centers for Disease Control. Update: evaluation of human T-lymphotropic virus type III/lymphadenopathy-associated virus infection in health care personnel—United States. MMWR 1985;34:575.
64. Weiss SH, Saxinger WC, Rechtman D, et al. HTLV-III infection among health care workers: association with needlestick injuries. JAMA 1985;254:2089.
65. Anonymous. Needlestick transmission of HTLV-III from a patient infected in Africa. Lancet 1984;II:1376.
66. Centers for Disease Control. Prevention of acquired immunodeficiency syndrome (AIDS): Report of inter-agency recommendations. MMWR 1983;32:101.
67. Curran JW. The epidemiology and prevention of the acquired immunodeficiency syndrome. Ann Intern Med 1985;103:657.
68. Ward JW, Grindon AJ, Feorino PM, et al. Laboratory and epidemiologic evaluation of an enzyme immunoassay for antibodies to human T-lymphotropic virus, type III. JAMA 1986;(in press).
69. Centers for Disease Control. Update: Public Health Service Workshop on human T-lymphotropic virus type III antibody testing—United States. MMWR 1985;34:477.
70. Centers for Disease Control. Update: Acquired immunodeficiency syndrome (AIDS) in persons with hemophilia. MMWR 1984;33:589.
71. Spire B, Dormont D, Barre-Sinoussi, et al. Inactivation of lymphadenopathy-associated virus by heat, gamma rays, and ultraviolet light. Lancet 1985;I:188.
72. Martin LS, McDougal JS, Loskoski SL. Disinfection and inactivation of the human T-lymphotropic virus type III/lymphadenopathy-associated virus. J Infect Dis 1985;152:400.
73. Centers for Disease Control. Recommendations for assisting in the prevention of perinatal transmission of HTLV-III/LAV and AIDS. MMWR 1985;34:722.
74. Garner JS, Simmons BP. Guideline for isolation precautions in hospitals. Infect Control 1983;4:245.
75. Centers for Disease Control. Revision of the CDC surveillance case definition for acquired immunodeficiency syndrome. MMWR 1987;36:1S.

Chapter 16
Clinical Manifestations of Kaposi's Sarcoma

Bijan Safai

Kaposi's sarcoma represents a potential model for a virally associated human tumor. Before the epidemic of acquired immunodeficiency syndrome (AIDS), Kaposi's sarcoma was considered a rare tumor occurring in cluster distribution of immune dysfunction, genetic predisposition, and possibly repeated and persistent infections in a given host. In the spring of 1981, a sudden increase in the incidence of Kaposi's sarcoma was observed among homosexual men in New York and California. Later it became clear that this increase is part of an AIDS epidemic manifesting with opportunistic infections and Kaposi's sarcoma.

In the AIDS epidemic, Kaposi's sarcoma appears to be a more aggressive type—involving skin, lymph nodes, and the gastrointestinal (GI) tract—and has a course similar to that seen in African children. Much interest has been generated in the study of this disease since the epidemic of Kaposi's sarcoma–AIDS, and it is hoped that investigative work will provide better insight into this interesting tumor.

HISTORY

Kaposi's sarcoma was first described in 1872 as "idiopathic, multiple pigmented sarcomas of the skin" by Moriz Kaposi.[1] Within the next 15 years the entity was recognized in many countries, and its characteristics were well appreciated. Kaposi described the disseminated form of the disease in 1887, and de Amicis described involvement of the tumor in a five-year-old child in 1882.

In 1914 Hallenberger described a case involving an African.[2] However, the prevalence of the disease in Africa was not appreciated until 20 years later, when Smith and Elmes reviewed a series of 500 tumors in which 10 cases (2%) were

---

Supported in part by National Institutes of Health Grants CA 22507, CA 17404, CA 16599, and CA 31643 and funds from Ancell, Mirsky and Simm.

diagnosed as Kaposi's sarcoma.[3] Over the next three decades several other reviews of Kaposi's sarcoma in Africa appeared, culminating in 1961 in a conference on the disease held in Kampala, Uganda. The presentations were later published in a monograph edited by Ackerman and Murray in 1963.[4]

In June 1981, an increased occurrence of Kaposi's sarcoma and *Pneumocystis carinii* pneumonia was noted in homosexual men. Subsequently, other opportunistic infections were found in this population of patients, and the disease complex was renamed AIDS. This syndrome is widely expanding both in numbers of patients and in heterogeneity of the patient population. Cases of AIDS have been reported in heterosexuals, Haitians, intravenous (IV) drug abusers and hemophiliacs, transfusion recipients, spouses of AIDS patients, and children.[5] These patients are centered mostly in New York City, San Francisco, and Los Angeles, but many other reports continue to accrue from other U.S. cities and Europe as well.[6]

EPIDEMIOLOGY

Incidence

Kaposi's sarcoma is generally considered to be a rare tumor except in certain geographic regions. In the United States the incidence is well below 1%. Reviewing a 38-year experience at the Mayo Clinic, Reynolds et al. reported only 70 cases, or 0.067% of tumors diagnosed at that institution.[7] Dorn and Cutler[8] and Oettle[9] estimate an even lower incidence (0.02%) in the United States.

The above is in sharp contrast to the experience in Africa, where it has been estimated that Kaposi's sarcoma accounts for about 9% of all neoplasms in Uganda.[9,10]

Geographic Location and Race

It has long been argued whether or not the American Kaposi's sarcoma is characterized by a geographic localization along racial lines. The majority of patients in America have ancestry going back to Eastern Europe or Italy or are Jewish. Rothman has used this finding to argue in favor of a racial predisposition to developing the disease.[11] Bluefarb presented data showing that the geographic origin of the patient is most important, since he states that the vast majority of patients are directly of Eastern European or Italian extraction.[12] It would seem that the greatest concentration of cases in Europe is from Eastern Europe and Italy, and there are many North American cases occurring in native descendents of immigrants from these European regions.

The African form of Kaposi's sarcoma has shown very sharp geographic localization. The areas affected include Zaire, Kenya, and Tanzania—predominantly the hill and open savannah bush country at an altitude of 1200 to 1500

m. However, even within this endemic belt, native blacks are far more frequently affected than nonblacks. Scattered cases from around the world have been reported (from Western Europe, Armenia, India, China, and Japan), but the disease is distinctly not as frequent in those areas as it is in North America. The cases of Kaposi's sarcoma in homosexuals have been reported initially from New York City and San Francisco—cities with large homosexual populations.

Age

Until 1979 the non-African Kaposi's sarcoma cases showed the highest incidence in the fifth, sixth, seventh, and eighth decades, accounting for about 80% of cases. The recent cases among the homosexual population are showing a higher incidence in younger adults, with most patients in their 30s.[5]

The African Kaposi's sarcoma, as analyzed by Davies and Lothe, shows peak incidence in the first decade, rare cases in the second decade, and then a progressive incidence throughout adult life.[13]

Sex

Most investigators report a strong male predominance of 10 to 15 males to 1 female even in the African variety.[7,9,11,14] A lower male-to-female ratio of 3:1 was noted in a review of cases of Kaposi's sarcoma in Memorial Sloan-Kettering Cancer Center.[15] Of interest is reversal of the sex ratio among the white population of South Africa and Algeria.[10,16,17]

Clinical Manifestations and Course of Disease

Most patients with Kaposi's sarcoma present with asymptomatic macules or nodules. As lesions become more numerous they may interfere with daily activities due to marked edema. Involvement of internal organs may reveal itself by a patient complaining of GI hemorrhage or diarrhea and leading to weight loss and emaciation.

Several authors have reported patients complaining of pruritus of the affected areas,[18,19] and there is even a report of pruritus preceding the appearance of the lesions.[20] However, Bluefarb[12] considered both these presentations to be distinctly unusual, and in the patients we examined, pruritus has not been a notable feature.

Patients with lesions on their feet may frequently complain of pain on walking, and even spontaneous pain has been reported.[21]

In terms of initial manifestation of the disease, patients present with a single or, more frequently, multiple red to violaceous macules, papules, or nodules (Figure 16–1). With time the macular and patch stage progresses to the plaques and nodule stage.

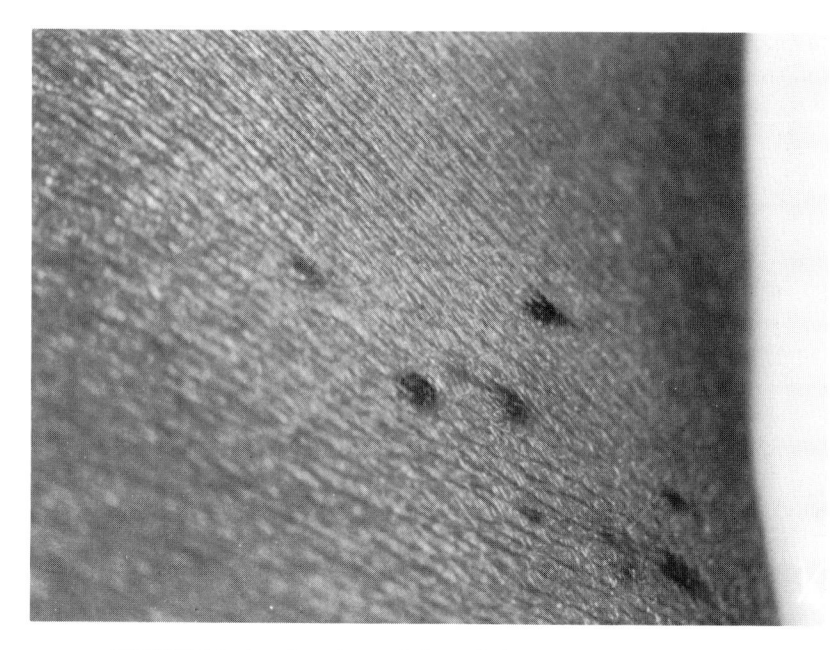

FIGURE 16–1 *Purple nodules of classic Kaposi's sarcoma.*

Initially the lesions may appear unilateral, but with progression bilateral involvement is generally seen. In the older literature the lower limb, usually the foot or ankle, was the site of initial involvement (75% of cases) (Figure 16–2).[14] The hand or forearm was reported as the initial site in about 15% of cases, and the remainder of cases reported the first lesion on the head or trunk. Solitary nodules on the penis,[14] ear,[19] mouth,[22] eye-lid,[22] conjuctiva,[23] and nose[24] have been reported as initial manifestations.

In Kaposi's original description the course of the disease was stated to be rapidly fatal within two or three years.[1] However, in a later publication on the subject he modified this view with the realization that most European cases were quite protracted.[25] It is now well appreciated that in the older heterosexual patients the course of the disease is usually indolent, with the slow development of an increasing number of lesions. The average survival time in the American series is reported to be 8 to 13 years; however, there are also a number of cases of spontaneous regression and survival up to 50 years.[7,9,14,17,26–28]

New lesions develop most frequently on the lower extremities, followed by involvement of the upper extremities and occasionally by lesions on the head, trunk, and internal organs.[7] It is thought that the development of new lesions is not the result of metastases from a primary lesion but rather of multifocal origin, a point recognized by Kaposi himself.[1] Metastases, while seen in aggressive forms of disease, are considered quite rare.

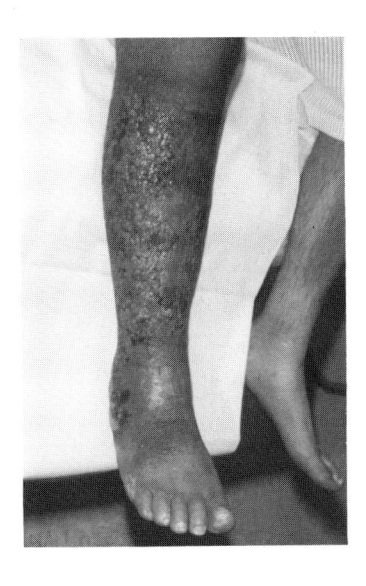

FIGURE 16-2 *Violaceous confluent plaques of classic Kaposi's sarcoma, with lymphedema.*

Involvement of internal organs is probably more frequent than clinically appreciated, with estimates ranging from 10% to 70% of patients showing internal involvement.[29,30] The most common site is the bowel, which is most reliably diagnosed by endoscopy, since the lesions may not be sufficiently protuberant to cause radiologic defects. Other sites frequently involved are the adrenal, pericardium, lymph nodes, and liver.

Some patients will relate the spontaneous regression of one or more nodules of Kaposi's sarcoma, and cases of spontaneous regression of all lesions have been noted.[21] There are three hypothesized mechanisms by which tumor regression is thought to occur: (1) autoamputation of pedunculated lesions by ingrowth of normal epithelium, (2) autoinfarction and fibrosis, and (3) hemorrhagic regression in which bleeding into the tumor is followed by fibrosis.

As mentioned above, the course in the North American and European patients is chronic and progressive, but most patients do not die as a result of Kaposi's sarcoma, succumbing instead to a second malignancy or one of the other diseases that befall the elderly.[31]

From the extensive experience of cases of Kaposi's sarcoma in Africa, the description of four clinical patterns has evolved[26]: (1) nodular, (2) infiltrative, (3) florid, and (4) lymphadenopathic.

The nodular form is similar to that form described above in the older North American or European patient. Involvement begins with a solitary lesion with progression of the disease to other parts of the body, but the overall distribution is on distal extremities. These patients, like their American counterparts, have a chronic, indolent course with prolonged survival.

A worse prognosis is seen among patients with the infiltrative type of disease. These cases show either a fungating mass whose surface is composed of a com-

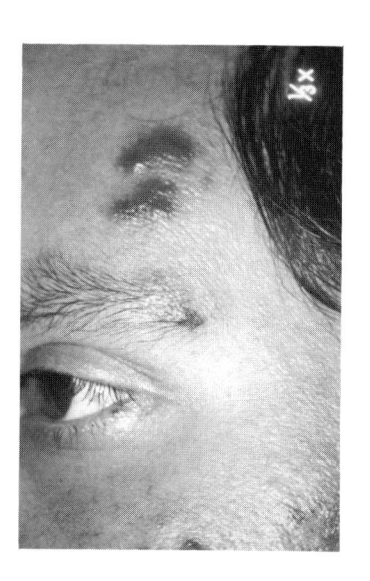

FIGURE 16–3 Reddish purple nodules on the face in AIDS-associated Kaposi's sarcoma.

bination of tumor mass, granulation tissue, hemorrhage, and necrosis or a nonulcerated tumor with involvement in the deep tissue planes and bones. Both these forms are more frequent on the foot, with extension to involve the draining lymph nodes and the development of woody edema due to infiltration of the deep dermis with tumor.

The florid type usually occurs in patients over age 50 years, with the disease accelerating after years of apparent quiescence. Lymph node involvement can be marked, as can presence of lesions in the mouth and significant edema.

Lymphadenopathic Kaposi's sarcoma is almost unique to African children and young adults. Here females account for one quarter of the cases. Cutaneous findings are not at all outstanding.[32,33] Lymphadenopathy is prominent, and on presentation lymphoma and tuberculosis are considered. The prognosis of this form is very poor, and on autopsy remarkably little visceral involvement is found.[34]

In contrast to the cutaneous lesions of the classic Kaposi's sarcoma patients, those in the homosexual men tend to be smaller, pink, and located on the upper trunk and head and neck (Figure 16–3).[31] Some observers have noted that a distinctive feature of the lesions in homosexuals is the arrangement of elongated lesions following the lines of cleavage, as seen in pityriasis rosea (Figure 16–4).[32,35] In addition to the skin findings, striking lymph node involvement is seen. Violaceous nodules on the oral mucosa are frequent, and visceral involvement is found frequently (Figure 16–5). The GI tract is the most common extracutaneous site, but lesions in the lungs, liver, pancreas, adrenal gland, spleen, testis, and larynx have been reported.[31] These patients also present with systemic complaints of fever, weight loss, malaise, and anorexia.

The clinical course in these latter patients has been by and large that of progressive disease and debilitation due to cellular immune deficiency and op-

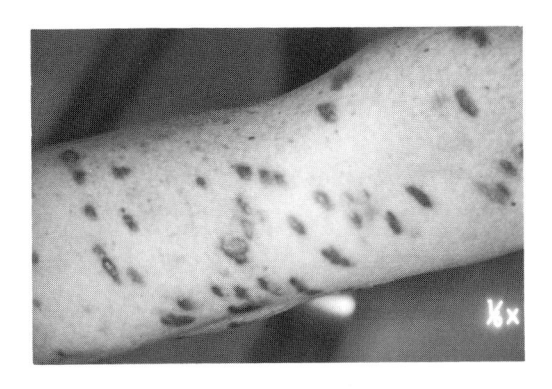

FIGURE 16–4 *Reddish purple nodules of AIDS-associated Kaposi's sarcoma, distributed along skin lines.*

portunistic infections. The mortality rate among the AIDS–Kaposi's sarcoma patients is in the range of 20%.[5]

Histopathology

The histologic features of Kaposi's sarcoma vary according to the age of the lesion. The two constant elements that are the common denominator of all the varieties are the spindle cell and the vascular component.[36]

The spindle cell resembles a fibroblast with elongated tapering ends and a basophilic, central nucleus. Usually the spindle cells are arranged in broad bands with the vascular areas in between bands. Mitoses are infrequent, and there is little pleomorphism.

The vascular component is composed of vascular slits as well as mature endothelial-lined vessels at the periphery. Vascular slits are very characteristic and are scattered throughout the tumor and appear like vacuolated macrophages on light microscopy.

A helpful microscopic feature is the presence of extravasated red blood cells and hemosiderin between the spindle cells. Phagocytosis of red blood cells by interspersed macrophages may be prominent (Figure 16–6).

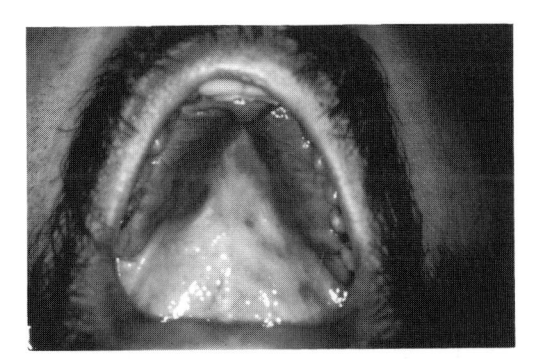

FIGURE 16–5 *Purple confluent tumors involving gingivae in Kaposi's sarcoma in AIDS.*

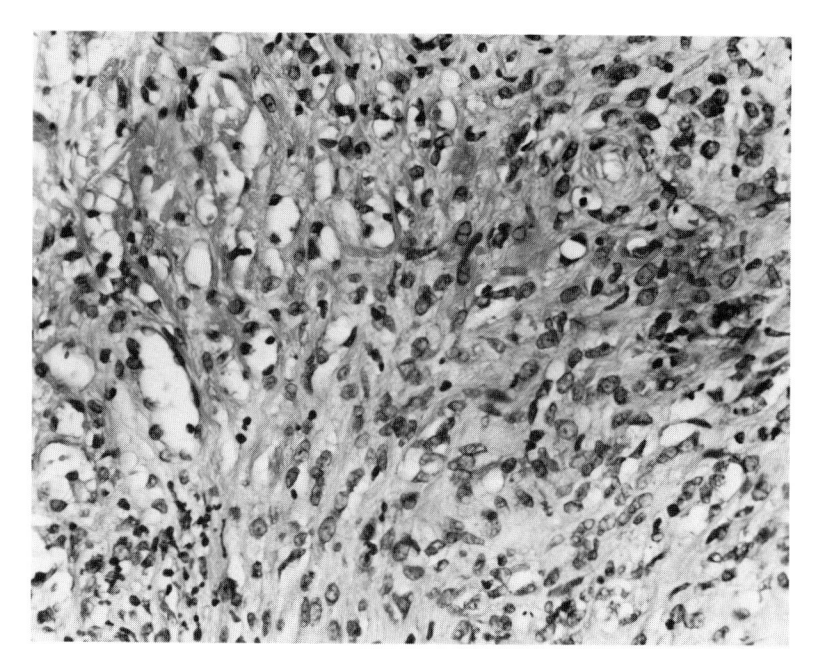

FIGURE 16–6 *Kaposi's sarcoma. Extravasated erythrocytes between spindle cells.*

An inflammatory infiltrate composed of lymphocytes, histiocytes, and plasma cells is present in varying degrees. It is important to keep in mind the chronological changes that occur in the development of Kaposi's sarcoma.[20] Early macular lesions are subtle, with the presence of abnormal and dilated vessels surrounding the normal, superficial vasculature. The inflammatory infiltrate may be sparse and is usually mixed with the presence of plasma cells around the new vessels. Neutrophils are absent, and nuclear atypia and mitoses are rare (Figure 16–7).

The plaque lesions show more extensive involvement, with neoplastic proliferation from the superficial to the deep dermis and, at times, into the adipose tissue. The infiltrate is more prominent than that described above for the macular lesion, with the addition of more spindle cells coursing between the collagen bundles and more extravasated red blood cells. Phagocytized hemosiderin is more conspicuous, but nuclear atypia and mitoses can still be subtle.

The nodules show a marked increase in the spindle cell population, with more extravasation of red blood cells, nuclear atypia, pleomorphism, and mitoses. Staining for iron to demonstrate hemosiderin is of diagnostic importance, and this may be seen within the spindle cells.[37] The spindle cells produce little collagen but do produce significant reticulum fibers, and a Foot stain for reticulum will aid in their recognition.

Attempts have been made to distinguish histologically between Kaposi's sarcoma in the older heterosexual and the younger homosexual, but no appreciable difference has been found between the two types.

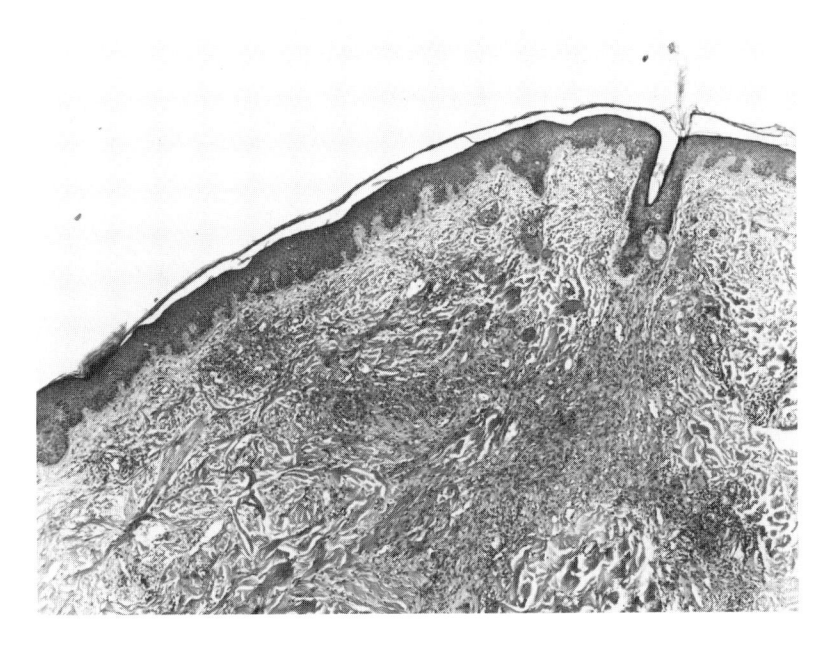

FIGURE 16–7 *Kaposi's sarcoma. Aggregates of spindle-shaped cells and erythrocytes in dermis.*

Involvement of the lymph nodes shows replacement of the normal architecture with irregular vascular spaces, fascicles of spindle cells, extravasated red blood cells and plasma cells in varying degrees. Again, no differences could be detected between the two forms of Kaposi's sarcoma.[31,38]

Classification

The diversity of clinical and histopathological features and the small number of cases, especially in nonendemic areas, has made the clinical classification of Kaposi's sarcoma very difficult. The classifications proposed by Reynolds et al.[7] and by Slavin et al.[39] both suffer from lack of uniformity and have clear limitations. A classification proposed by Taylor et al. summarized in their Table 1, however, seems to be more comprehensive, covering all aspects of the disease.[26] It accounts for clinical preservation, cause of the disease, frequency of extracutaneous tumors, response to therapy, and, in most cases, the histopathology as well.

In the same report these authors describe three basic histological patterns for Kaposi's sarcoma, characterized by variations in the quantity of vascular component, spindle cells, fibrosis, and nuclear pleomorphism in the tumor: (1) the "mixed cell pattern" is characterized by a mixture in equal proportions of spindle cells, vascular slits, and well-formed vascular channels; (2) the "monocellular pattern" features proliferation of 1 cell type, usually the spindle cells; and (3) the "anaplastic pattern" features tumors marked by cellular pleomorphism and frequent mitoses.

Correlation between the clinical types and the histologic patterns revealed that although the mixed cell pattern is seen in all four clinical types, it appears most frequently in the nodular, florid, and lymphadenopathic types. The monocellular pattern may be seen in patients with the nodular, florid, and infiltrative types of clinical disease, while the anaplastic variant has been noted only in the florid type.

The four clinical types identified by Taylor have not been as clearly defined in the European and North American populations as in the African population.

Associated Conditions

Several studies have been published analyzing the association between Kaposi's sarcoma and second primary malignancies. Moertel reviewed the literature relating the development of second neoplasms among patients with lymphoreticular tumors. Among 565 such cases, 51 of these patients developed Kaposi's sarcoma—an incidence of 9%, which is markedly in excess of the proportion of Kaposi's sarcoma generally seen in American patients.[40] In a review from the Mayo Clinic, only two cases of Kaposi's sarcoma were noted of 4475 cases of lymphoreticular neoplasms.[41]

The reverse occurrence, that of a lymphoreticular neoplasm developing in patients with Kaposi's sarcoma, showed 5 cases of 70 patients with Kaposi's sarcoma in one study[7] and 9 of 63 patients in another.[42]

In a recent study, reviewing a period from 1949 to 1975 at Memorial Sloan-Kettering Cancer Center, 92 patients with Kaposi's sarcoma were followed, among whom 34, or 37%, developed a second primary malignancy.[15,43] Of these patients, 58% had a second malignancy involving the lymphoreticular system. This latter figure is in contrast to an incidence of 8% of all patients with one primary malignancy developing a second cancer involving the lymphoreticular system. Other malignancies reported in association with Kaposi's sarcoma from the latter study included neoplasms of the GI tract (two cases), skin (four cases), breast (two cases), and urinary tract (one case).

Several reports have suggested that reduced immunity may play a role in the development and course of Kaposi's sarcoma. The occurrence of Kaposi's sarcoma in a patient with systemic lupus erythematosus during immunosuppressive therapy was reported.[44] An increased incidence of Kaposi's sarcoma has also been reported in patients with disorders of the immune system, such as immunodeficiencies, plasma cell dyscrasias, thymoma, or polymyositis.[45-50] Also reported are cases of renal transplant recipients who developed Kaposi's sarcoma during the course of immunosuppressive therapy. The Kaposi's sarcoma nodules regressed when therapy was tapered down or discontinued.[51]

In contrast to the above, homosexual men with Kaposi's sarcoma have not shown the development of second primary malignancies to the same extent as classic Kaposi's sarcoma patients. These patients, however, have contracted many opportunistic infections with organisms such as cytomegalovirus (CMV), herpes simplex, *Mycobacterium avium–intracellularis, Candida albicans, Cryptococcus neoformans, P. carinii, Toxoplasma gondii, Cryptosporidium* and *Isospora belli*.[35,52-54] These patients also have histories of infections including syphilis, gonorrhea, amebiasis, giardiasis, and hepatitis A and B.

Laboratory Findings

Routine laboratory tests are usually unremarkable in patients with classic Kaposi's sarcoma, and their immunologic profile also appears very close to normal. Minor abnormalities have been seen in the more aggressive infiltrative type of classic Kaposi's sarcoma in Africa. In contrast, the younger homosexual patients with Kaposi's sarcoma tend to be anemic, leukopenic, or thrombocytopenic. These patients have also demonstrated profound cellular immune deficiency manifested by reversal of helper/suppressor T cell ratios with decreased or lack of functional T cell activity in a variety of immunologic assays, elevated levels of immunoglobulins, and abnormally high titers of antibodies to Epstein-Barr virus (EBV) and CMV.

Cell of Origin and Etiology

The cell of origin of Kaposi's sarcoma has been the subject of interest for several decades, and many cell types have been suspected. Recent data, however, support the hypothesis that endothelial cells are the cell of origin of this disease. It has been shown that the antibodies to blood factor VIII stain tumor tissues in Kaposi's sarcoma of both classic and epidemic form,[55] thus indicating the possible endothelial cell origin of Kaposi's sarcoma.

As for the etiology of Kaposi's sarcoma, a multifactorial cause is the most popular hypothesis at present; this has been described in a recent article by Safai et al.[15] A close sociologic association has been observed between Kaposi's sarcoma and CMV.[56] In addition, CMV-DNA sequences and antigens have been found in Kaposi's sarcoma tumor tissues.[57] These observations and many others suggest the possible involvement of CMV in development of Kaposi's sarcoma.

The cluster distribution of Kaposi's sarcoma in endemic areas suggests a possible role for genetic factors in the development of the disease. Although infrequency of familial Kaposi's sarcoma cases negates involvement of such factors, recent data[58,59] demonstrate increased frequency of HLA-DR5 in both classic and epidemic forms of Kaposi's sarcoma. Because of the preliminary nature of these data, further investigation is needed to define the role of genetic factors in this disease.

Conclusion

Available data strongly suggest the involvement of CMV in Kaposi's sarcoma. Much work is necessary to clarify the role of CMV or other viruses in the etiology of this tumor. The increased incidence of HLA-DR5 in Kaposi's sarcoma patients is intriguing, but the actual HLA association with the development of this disease needs further investigation. To identify the cell of origin and the etiopathogenetic mechanisms involved, it is important to try to grow Kaposi's sarcoma tumors in tissue cultures and laboratory animals. Availability of new conditioned media and methodology available to further immunosuppress the laboratory animals may in fact allow such approaches. The intriguing association of second primary malignancies with Kaposi's sarcoma also deserves further investigations and may provide important information concerning the host-tumor interaction.

REFERENCES

1. Kaposi M. Idiopathisches multiples Pigmensarkom der Haut. Arch Dermatol Syph (Berlin). 1872;4:265.
2. Hallenberger O. Multiple angiosarkome der Haut bei einem Kammerunneger. Arch Schiffs Trop Hyg 1914;18:647.
3. Smith EC, Elmes BGT. Malignant disease in the natives of Nigeria. An analysis of 500 tumors. Ann Trop Med Parasitol 1934;28:461.
4. Ackerman LV, Murray JF. Symposium on Kaposi's sarcoma. Basel: S. Karger, 1963.
5. Haverkos HW, Curran JW. The current outbreak of Kaposi's sarcoma and opportunistic infections. CA 1982;32:330.
6. Thomsen HK, Jacobsen M, Malchow-Moller A. Lancet 1981;2:688.
7. Reynolds WA, Winkelmann RK, Soule EH. Kaposi's sarcoma. Medicine 1965;44:419.
8. Dorn HF, Cutler SJ. Morbidity from cancer in the United States. I. Variation in incidence by age, sex, marital status and geographic region (monogr. no. 29). Washington, D.C.: U.S. Public Health Service, 1955; 121.
9. Oettle AG. Geographical and racial differences in the frequency of KS as evidence of environmental or genetic causes. Acta Un Int Cancer 1962;18:330.
10. Rothman S. Medical research in Africa. Arch Dermatol 1962;85:311.
11. Rothman S. Remarks on sex, age and racial distribution of Kaposi's sarcoma and on possible pathogenetic factors. Acta Un Int Cancer 1962;18:322.
12. Bluefarb SM. Kaposi's sarcoma. Springfield, Ill.: Charles C. Thomas, 1957.
13. Davies JNP, Lothe F. Kaposi's sarcoma in African children. In: Ackerman LV, Murray JF, eds. Symposium on Kaposi's sarcoma. Basel: S. Karger, 1963; 81.
14. Lothe F. Kaposi's sarcoma in Ugandan Africans. Acta Pathol Microbiol Scand (suppl) 1963;161:1.
15. Safai B, Mike V, Giraldo G, et al. Association of Kaposi's sarcoma with second primary malignancies: Possible etiopathogenic implications. Cancer 1980;45:1472.
16. Oettle AG. Geographic and racial differences in frequency of Kaposi's sarcoma as evidence of environmental or genetic causes. In: Ackerman LV, Murray JF, eds. Symposium on Kaposi's sarcoma. Basel: S. Karger, 1963; 330.

17. Palmer PES. Haemangiosarcoma of Kaposi. Acta Radiol Rev (suppl 316:6) 1972;12:640.
18. Meyers DS, Jacobson VC. Multiple hemorrhagic sarcoma of Kaposi. Am J Pathol 1927;3:321.
19. Symmers D. Kaposi's sarcoma. Arch Pathol 1941;32:764.
20. Dorffel J. Histiogenesis of multiple idiopathic hemorrhagic sarcoma of Kaposi. Arch Dermatol Syph (Berlin) 1932;26:608.
21. Templeton AC. Kaposi's sarcoma in cancer of the skin, vol 2. Philadelphia: WB Saunders, 1976;1183.
22. McLaren DS. Kaposi's sarcoma of the eyelids of an African child. Arch Ophthalmol 1960;63:859.
23. Mortada A. Conjunctival regressing Kaposi's sarcoma. Br J Ophthalmol 1967;51:275.
24. Hansson CJ. Kaposi's sarcoma. Clinical and radiotherapeutic studies on 23 patients. Acta Radiol (Stockh) 1940;21:457.
25. Kaposi M. Zur nomenclatur des idiopathischen Pigmentsarkom Kaposi. Arch Dermatol Syph (Berlin) 1894;29:164.
26. Taylor JF, Templeton AC, Vogel CL, et al. Kaposi's sarcoma in Uganda: A clinicopathological study. Int J Cancer 1971;8:122.
27. Rothman S. Some clinical aspects of Kaposi's sarcoma in the European and North American populations. Acta Un Int Cancer 1962;18:364.
28. Keen P. The clinical features of Kaposi's sarcoma in the South African Bantu. Acta Un Int Cancer 1962;18:380.
29. Ecklund RE, Valaitis J. Kaposi's sarcoma of lymph nodes. Arch Pathol 1962;74:224.
30. Cox FX, Helwig EB. Kaposi's sarcoma. Cancer 1959;12:289.
31. Urmacher C, Myskowski P, Ochoa M Jr, et al. Outbreak of Kaposi's sarcoma with cytomegalovirus infection in young homosexual men. Am J Med 1982;72:569.
32. Gottlieb GJ, Ackerman AB. Kaposi's sarcoma: An extensively disseminated form in young homosexual men. Hum Pathol 1982;13:882.
33. Dutz W, Stout AP. Kaposi's sarcoma in infants and children. Cancer 1960;13:684.
34. Lothe F, Murray JF. Kaposi's sarcoma. Autopsy findings in the African. In: Ackerman LV, Murray JF, eds. Symposium on Kaposi's sarcoma. Basel: S. Karger, 1963.
35. Myskowski PL, Romano JF, Safai B. Kaposi's sarcoma in young homosexual men. Cutis 1982;29:31.
36. Lever WF, Schaumberg-Lever G. Histopathology of the skin, 5th ed. Philadelphia: JB Lippincott, 1975.
37. Hashimoto K, Lever WF. Kaposi's sarcoma. Histologic and electron microscopic studies. J Invest Derm 1964;43:539.
38. Amazon K, Rywlin AM. Subtle clues to diagnosis by conventional microscopy: Lymph node involvement in Kaposi's sarcoma. Am J Dermatopathol 1979;1:173.
39. Slavin G, Cameron HM, Forbes C, Morton-Mitchell R. Kaposi's sarcoma in East African children: A report of 51 cases. J Pathol 1970;100:187.
40. Moertel CG. Multiple primary malignant neoplasms, vol 7. Recent results in cancer research. Berlin: Springer-Verlag, 1966.
41. Moertel CG, Hagedorn AB. Leukaemia or lymphoma and coexistent primary malignant lesion. A review of the literature and a study of 120 cases. Blood 1957;12:788.
42. O'Brien PH, Brasfield R. Kaposi's sarcoma. Cancer 1966;19:1497.
43. Safai B, Good RA. Kaposi's sarcoma. A review and recent developments. Clin Bull 1980;10:62.
44. Klein MB, Pereira FA, Kantor I. Kaposi's sarcoma complicating systemic lupus erythematosus treated with immunosuppression. Arch Dermatol 1974;110:602.

45. Kapadia SB, Krause JR. Kaposi's sarcoma after long-term alkylating agent therapy for multiple myeloma. South Med J 1977;70:1011.
46. Mazzaferri EL, Penn GM. Kaposi's sarcoma associated with multiple myeloma. Report of a patient and review of the literature. Arch Intern Med 1968;122:521.
47. Dantzig PI. Kaposi's sarcoma and polymyositis. Arch Dermatol 1974;110:605.
48. Law IP. Kaposi's sarcoma and plasma cell dyscrasia. JAMA 1974;229:1329.
49. Ettinger DS, Humphrey RL, Skinner MD. Kaposi's sarcoma associated with multiple myeloma. Johns Hopkins Med J 1975;137:88.
50. Mandel EM, Lask D, Gafter U, et al. Multiple myeloma associated with Kaposi's sarcoma. Acta Haematol 1977;58:120.
51. Myers BD, Kessler E, Levi J, et al. Kaposi's sarcoma in kidney transplant recipients. Arch Intern Med 1974;133:307.
52. Gottlieb MS, Schroff R, Schanker HM, et al. Pneumocystis carinii pneumonia and mucosal candidiasis in previously healthy homosexual men. N Engl J Med 1981;305:1425.
53. Masur H, Michelis MA, Greene JB, et al. An outbreak of community-acquired *Pneumocystis carinii* pneumonia. Initial manifestation of cellular immune dysfunction. N Engl J Med 1981; 305:1431.
54. Siegal FP, Lopez C, Hammer GS, et al. Severe acquired immunodeficiency in male homosexuals, manifested by chronic perianal ulcerative herpes simplex lesions. N Engl J Med 1981;305:1439.
55. Guarda LG, Silva EG, Ordonez NG, Smith L Jr. Factor VIII in Kaposi's sarcoma. Brief Sci Rep 1981;76:197.
56. Giraldo G, Beth E, Henle W, et al. Antibody patterns to herpes viruses in Kaposi's sarcoma: II. Serological associations of American Kaposi's sarcoma with cytomegalovirus. Int J Cancer 1978;22:126.
57. Giraldo G, Beth E, Huang E. Kaposi's sarcoma and its relationship to cytomegalovirus. III. CMV, DNA and CMV early antigens in Kaposi's sarcoma. Int J Cancer 1980;26:23.
58. Friedman-Kien AE, Laubenstein LJ, Rubinstein P, et al. Disseminated Kaposi's sarcoma in homosexual men. Ann Intern Med 1982;96:693.
59. Pollack MS, Safai B, Myskowski PL, et al. Frequency of HLA and Gm immunogenetic markers in Kaposi's sarcoma. Tissue Antigens 1983;21:1.
60. Koziner B, Denny T, Myskowski PL, et al. Letter. N Engl J Med 1982;306:933.

Chapter 17

Neurology in AIDS

Michael Grundman
Mitchell S. Felder
Hyman Donnenfeld
Joseph C. Masdeu

Neurologic symptoms occur in up to two-thirds of all acquired immunodeficiency syndrome (AIDS) patients during their lifetime,[1,2] and 75% to 90% of AIDS patients will have neuropathologic changes at autopsy.[3–5] About 10% of patients with AIDS will present with a neurologic complaint as their initial manifestation of the disease.[1] The neurologic complications of AIDS can be divided into those secondary to human immunodeficiency virus (HIV) itself and those related to superinfections, neoplasms, associated cerebrovascular disease, and metabolic or toxic causes (Table 17–1).

NEUROPATHOGENESIS

The often early and consistent involvement of the nervous system in AIDS is not only of great clinical importance but of scientific interest as well. The neuropathogenicity of HIV has been reviewed.[6,7] The exact mechanism whereby HIV enters the central nervous system (CNS) has not yet been delineated. In the CNS, HIV has been noted in macrophages and multinucleated giant cells (of macrophage origin), less frequently in glial cells, and rarely in neurons.[8,9] One theory suggests that HIV proliferates and infects monocytes and macrophages in the periphery, which then transport the virus across the blood-brain barrier (analogous to a kind of Trojan horse). Once within the CNS, the infected monocytes and macrophages release proteolytic enzymes and chemotactic factors, inducing further inflammatory cell infiltration. The surrounding neurons and glia are then injured by the intense inflammation and toxic inflammatory cell by-products. Another theory proposes that HIV enters the brain directly through endothelial gaps in brain capillaries. HIV then binds to brain cells containing T4 receptors,

Table 17-1 Neurologic complications in AIDS, by etiology

HIV induced
    Aseptic meningitis
    HIV encephalopathy
    Vacuolar myelopathy
    Distal symmetric peripheral neuropathy
    Acute demyelinating polyradiculopathy (Guillain-Barré syndrome)
    Chronic inflammatory demyelinating polyradiculopathy
    Cranial neuropathies
    Mononeuritis multiplex
    Autonomic neuropathy
    Polymyositis

Other viral related
    CMV (encephalitis, retinitis, cranial neuropathy, progressive polyradiculopathy)
    Herpes zoster virus (encephalitis, cranial neuropathy, myelitis, radiculitis)
    Herpes simplex type I (encephalitis, cranial neuropathy)
    Herpes simplex type II (encephalitis, cranial neuropathy, myelitis, radiculitis)
    Papovavirus: JC virus (progressive multifocal leukoencephalopathy)

Nonviral related
    Protozoa
        Toxoplasma gondii (cerebral abscess, encephalitis)
        Acanthamoeba (very rarely)
    Fungi
        Cryptococcus neoformans (meningitis, cryptococcoma)
        Others *(Candida, Aspergillus, Coccidioides, Histoplasma)* rarely
    Bacteria (rarely)
        Listeria (meningitis, abscess)
        Nocardia (abscess)
        Escherichia coli (meningitis)
    Mycobacteria
        M. tuberculosis (abscess, meningitis)
        M. avium-intracellulare (encephalitis, meningitis)
    Spirochetes
        Treponema pallidum (neurosyphilis)

Neoplasms of the CNS
    Primary CNS lymphoma
    Metastatic systemic lymphoma to the CNS
    Metastatic Kaposi's sarcoma (rare) to the CNS

Cerebrovascular complications
    Infarction
        Possible causes:
            Cardiac embolism
            Cerebral granulomatous angiitis
            Circulating hypercoagulants (lupus anticoagulant)
    Hemorrhage
        Possible causes:
            Thrombocytopenia
            Intracerebral neoplasm

Metabolic/Toxic
    Hypoxic encephalopathy (e.g., pneumocystis carinii pneumonia [PCP])
    Drug-induced delirium (psychoactive medications, AZT, DHPG)
    Vincristine-induced neuropathy
    Vitamin deficiency–induced peripheral neuropathies (B_{12}, folate, thiamin)
    Electrolyte abnormalities

enters the cells (astrocytes and oligodendroglia), and replicates. The degeneration of oligodendroglia (the myelin-forming cells of the CNS) results in the diffuse demyelination characteristic of HIV encephalopathy. Budding forms of HIV virions have been noted in neuroglia, indicating infection and replication of the virus within these cell types.[10]

There may be still another way in which HIV causes neuronal dysfunction. Neuroleukin is a neurotrophic growth factor that shares a partial sequence homology with a highly conserved region of the HIV envelope protein (gp120). Viral lysates of HIV or a recombinant fragment of gp120 can inhibit the neurotrophic activity of neuroleukin. It is postulated that the HIV envelope protein may interact with the neuroleukin receptor on certain populations of brain neurons and interfere with the normal trophic functions of neuroleukin.[11]

Aside from its direct effects on the nervous system, HIV also weakens the immune system, such that other viruses and microorganisms are able to proliferate within the nervous system with little restraint. These infectious agents are normally eradicated by the immune system in a similar way, namely, through cell-mediated immunity. Several immune mechanisms crucial to disposing of these organisms are abnormal as a result of HIV infection and decimation of the T4 lymphocyte population. One way CNS infection may normally be controlled is through T4 lymphocyte activation of antigen-specific cytotoxic T cells and macrophages. These latter cells then attack targets bearing specific antigens to which they have been activated. Without T4 cells, the antigen-specific cytotoxic T cells and macrophages are not recruited. T4 lymphocytes also induce class II major histocompatibility complex (MHC) antigens on glia, which can then serve as antigen-presenting cells to other lymphocytes. This mechanism may serve to amplify the immune response within the CNS. Again, since T4 lymphocytes are deficient or lacking, the immune response to infectious agents within the CNS is muted. T4 lymphocytes also induce class I MHC antigen expression in neurons. This expression, which normally assists T effector lymphocytes in recognizing neurons bearing foreign antigens, may fail to occur in AIDS patients. Finally, since T cell help is required for B cell activation and differentiation in the development of effective antigen-specific antibody responses, there is frequently an ineffective polyclonal B cell activation. Abnormal polyclonal B cell activation may result in cross-reacting antibodies against self-antigens. Such a mechanism may underly the postinfectious polyneuropathies seen in patients with AIDS-related complex (ARC) and AIDS.[7]

CLINICAL SYNDROMES

HIV-Induced Neurologic Disease in AIDS

Aseptic Meningitis

Acute aseptic meningitis may be associated with primary HIV infection. It occurs in 5% to 10% of AIDS patients, often at the time of HIV seroconversion.[12,13]

Clinical features may include headache, fever, meningismus, photophobia, and occasionally cranial neuropathies or other transient neurologic deficits. The cerebrospinal fluid (CSF) reveals a mononuclear pleocytosis (mean 41 white blood cells [WBC]/mm³) and elevated protein (mean 65 mg/dl). CSF pleocytosis may persist for 6 to 12 months in some cases. HIV was isolated from the CSF in half the patients tested in one report.[13]

HIV Encephalopathy (AIDS Dementia)

Sixty-five percent or more of AIDS patients may undergo clinically evident progressive dementia over weeks to months.[2] Neuropathologic changes consistent with HIV encephalopathy are present in 90% of autopsied patients.[4] HIV encephalopathy may be present at diagnosis or may be the only manifestation of AIDS. The majority of patients with HIV encephalopathy develop severe global intellectual impairment within two months of the onset of mental symptoms. A significant number, however, will have a protracted course of mild to moderate impairment in intellectual function for four to seven months before the onset of severe intellectual impairment. Early cognitive symptoms of HIV encephalopathy include forgetfulness, loss of concentration, confusion, and slowness of thought. Motor abnormalities may also be seen early and include difficulty with balance, weakness of the lower extremities, and deterioration in handwriting. Apathy or social withdrawal is by far the most common early behavioral change, although dysphoria and psychotic behavior may also be present early. In the late stages the clinical picture is dominated by global dementia with associated motor findings, including hypertonia, ataxia, quadriparesis or paraparesis, myoclonus, and incontinence. In the later stages of HIV encephalopathy, up to 20% of patients may have seizures.[2]

The dementia of AIDS is thought to be a direct result of infection of the brain with HIV (hence the name HIV encephalopathy). On gross examination the brains of these patients show mild to marked atrophy. Histopathologic changes are most prominent in the subcortical white and gray matter, with sparing of the cortex. The most frequent findings include diffuse white matter pallor, vacuolation or multifocal rarefaction, gliosis of the white matter and subcortical gray, focal necrosis, microglial nodules, multinucleated giant cells (Figure 17–1 C), and perivascular inflammation (infiltrates of lymphocytes and macrophages).

Computer tomography (CT) scanning of patients with HIV encephalopathy may reveal atrophy, ventricular dilatation, and diffuse hypodensity of the white matter (Figure 17–1 A and B). T2-weighted magnetic resonance imaging (MRI) scanning often shows diffuse or multifocal white matter hyperintensities in the absence of mass effect in addition to atrophy. Positron emission tomography (PET) studies in these patients are characterized by relative subcortical hypermetabolism early, followed by subcortical and cortical hypometabolism as the disease progresses.[16] Electroencephalograms (EEG), when abnormal, most frequently show diffuse slowing. Improvement of cognitive function in AIDS-related dementia has been reported in a few patients receiving treatment with azidothymidine (AZT) at a dose of 250 mg every 4 hours.[30]

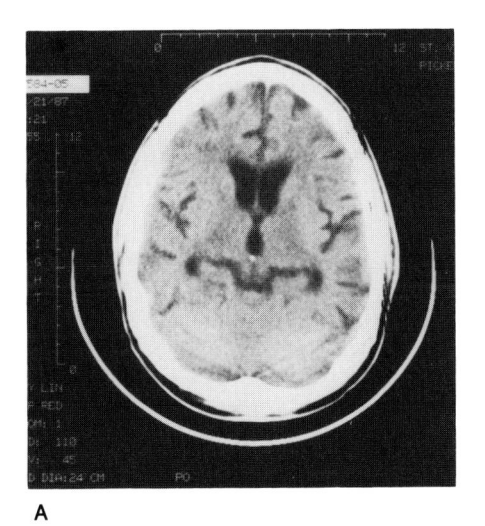

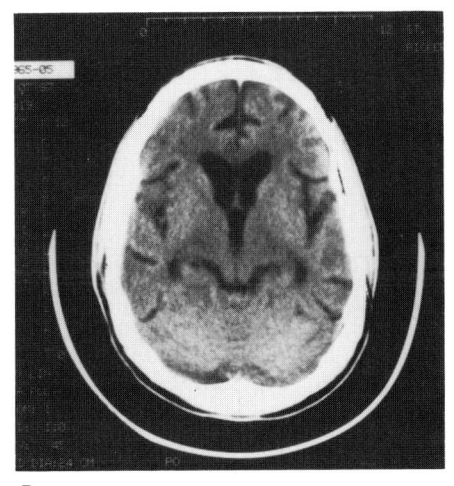

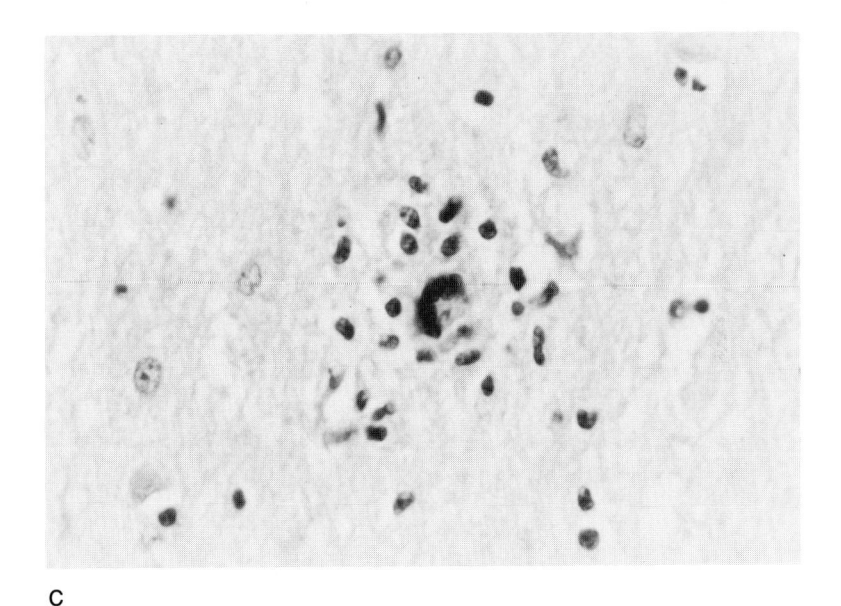

FIGURE 17–1 (A and B) HIV encephalopathy. These two CT scans were taken five months apart. Note the progressive enlargement of the sulci and ventricular system from A to B. The white matter on the later scan (B) is diffusely hypodense compared with the earlier scan (A). (C) HIV encephalopathy. This microscopic section of cerebral white matter contains a small microglial nodule, in the center of which is a multinucleated giant cell. This is a common finding in HIV encephalopathy. (Courtesy Carol K. Petito, M.D., Department of Pathology, The New York Hospital–Cornell University Medical College.)

Vacuolar Myelopathy

Frequently seen with the cognitive changes of HIV encephalopathy are the motor findings alluded to above (hypertonia, progressive paraparesis, pyramidal tract findings). Sometimes, however, patients may have prominent motor findings (paraparesis and ataxia) with minimal intellectual decline. Neuropathologic examination in both instances may reveal vacuolar degeneration of the spinal cord, most prominent in the lateral and posterior columns. Greatest involvement usually occurs at the thoracic level. This pathologic picture is called *vacuolar myelopathy*. The etiology of this myelopathy is unclear, but its frequent occurrence in association with HIV encephalopathy suggests a primary role for HIV.

Peripheral Neuropathies Associated with HIV

Peripheral nerve disease is common in AIDS patients. The most common neuropathy in patients with AIDS is a distal symmetric peripheral neuropathy.[14] This type of neuropathy usually begins with distal sensory loss, which spreads proximally. Pain on the soles of the feet and paresthesias are frequent complaints. Weakness, when present, usually affects only the intrinsic foot muscles, although more extensive distal weakness in the lower extremities may be present in advanced cases. Ankle jerks are typically absent or hyporeflexic, with normal reflexes elsewhere. Trophic changes may occur including hair loss, thinning of the skin, pedal edema, and reddish discoloration of the skin. Neurophysiologic studies and sural nerve biopsies are suggestive of a dying-back axonopathy. Treatment is currently limited to pain-relieving medications including amitriptyline (Elavil) and carbamazepine (Tegretol). The usefulness of AZT in treating this disorder has not yet been determined.

Demyelinating polyradiculopathies (Guillain-Barré syndrome and chronic inflammatory demyelinating polyradiculopathy [CIDP]) occur more frequently in seropositive asymptomatic patients and patients with ARC rather than patients with established AIDS. CIDP patients usually present with subacute or chronic progressive weakness in the proximal and distal muscles of the extremities. Tendon reflexes are hyporeflexic or absent. Sensory loss is mild, with vibratory sense being preferentially affected. Nerve conduction studies show prolonged F responses and slowed nerve conduction velocities in a patchy distribution. Sural nerve biopsies reveal internodal demyelination and mononuclear cell infiltration. CSF abnormalities usually occur in 90% of patients in the form of a mild CSF pleocytosis and elevated CSF protein. Plasmapheresis appears beneficial and is recommended.[15]

Mononeuropathy multiplex, like CIDP, is more common in ARC than AIDS. These patients usually present with an abrupt onset of mononeuropathy and then periodically develop mononeuropathies in other locations. Common mononeuropathies include facial palsy, other cranial neuropathies, foot drop, and patchy sensory abnormalities. Plasmapheresis has been suggested for the treatment of mononeuropathy multiplex as well.[17] Autonomic neuropathy has also been described in AIDS patients. Patients with AIDS may be at increased risk for syncopal reactions and cardiopulmonary arrest in response to invasive procedures.[18] Polymyositis is a rare complication of HIV infection. AIDS patients with this complication present with myalgias, proximal weakness, and elevated creatine phosphokinase (CPK). Muscle biopsies show fiber necrosis and inflammatory infiltrates. The role of immunosuppressive agents in this situation must be considered with caution.

Other Viral Diseases Affecting the Nervous System in AIDS

Cytomegalovirus Infections

Cytomegalovirus (CMV) can cause encephalitis (or myelitis) in AIDS patients and may occur in conjunction with HIV encephalopathy. Up to one-third of AIDS patients will have evidence of CMV involvement in the CNS at autopsy.[5] The clinical features do not allow clear differentiation of CMV encephalitis from HIV encephalopathy. CT scanning may reveal white matter hypodensities or enhancement in the subependymal regions. Virus isolation from the CSF is rare, and the radiologic features are not specific. Histopathologic features include small areas of necrosis in the subependymal region, microglial nodules, and cytomegalic inclusions (Figure 17–2). Most commonly affected are the basal gan-

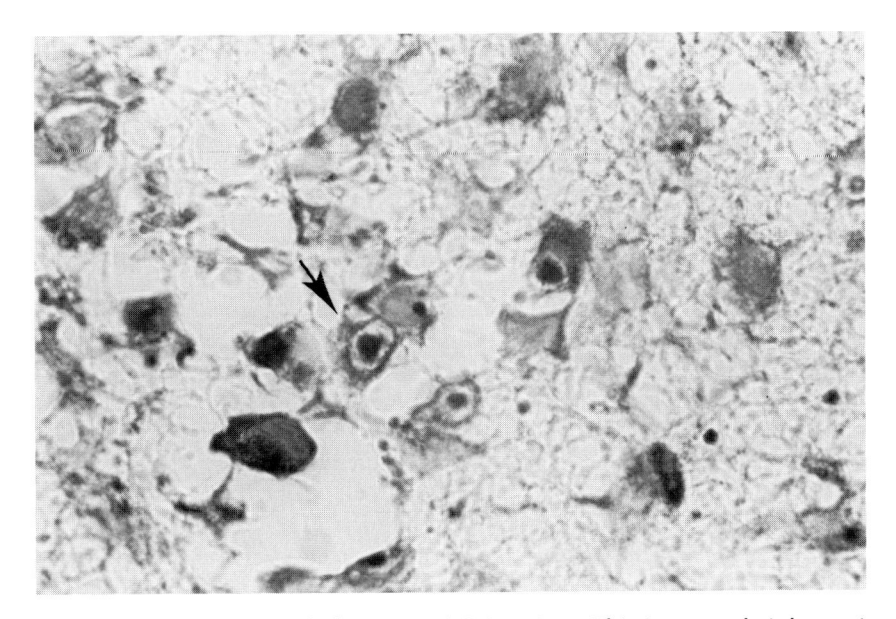

FIGURE 17–2 *CMV encephalitis in an AIDS patient. This is a cresyl violet–stained section of the subependymal tissue adjacent to the temporal horn. Note the abnormally large cells (cytomegaly). The nuclei contain a prominent inclusion producing a halo effect.*

glia, diencephalon, and brain stem. Spinal cord involvement is less common. Compared with HIV encephalopathy, CMV encephalitis usually shows less gliosis and multinucleated cells and greater predilection for gray matter. The efficacy of treatment of CMV encephalitis with the acyclovir analog 9- (1,3-dihydroxy-2-propoxymethyl) guanine (DHPG), which has been used effectively in the treatment of CMV retinitis, is not known. DHPG appeared helpful in the treatment of CMV encephalitis in one recently reported case.[32] CMV can also cause a hemorrhagic retinitis in AIDS patients and, when left untreated, can lead to blindness. DHPG appears to be effective for this condition. Leukopenia often occurs to a mild degree with DHPG, and the drug must be stopped if severe leukopenia develops.

A progressive polyradiculopathy has been described in which CMV appears to be implicated.[14,19] It is characterized by early impairment of bladder and rectal sphincter control and sacral sensory loss. Commonly, there is progression to areflexic paraplegia and more rostral spread of weakness, sensory loss, and areflexia. The role of DHPG in this condition is also undetermined.

Herpes Virus Infections

Encephalitis has been described in AIDS with both herpes simplex (types 1 and 2) and herpes zoster viruses. Herpes simplex encephalitis (predominantly type 1) occurs infrequently in AIDS patients, with an incidence of perhaps 2% to 3%; herpes zoster encephalitis probably occurs even less frequently.[5] Herpes encephalitis presents differently in AIDS patients than in immunocompetent patients. In AIDS patients, the temporal course is often more prolonged with slow progressive worsening over weeks; the inflammatory response is only mild or moderate. The infection is not confined to the temporal lobes, and CT scans do not show temporal lobe abnormalities.[21] Patients may present with headache, fever, confusion, and focal neurologic findings. Concurrent infections with other viruses (e.g., CMV) may occur. Encephalitis, cerebral angiitis, radiculomyelitis, and cranial neuropathies have been temporally related to cutaneous herpes zoster. Diagnosis of CNS herpes infection is difficult. CSF may be helpful if viral cultures are positive but is otherwise nonspecific. Recent cutaneous lesions consistent with herpes zoster may be suggestive. Acyclovir is the treatment of choice for suspected herpes virus infections.

Progressive Multifocal Leukoencephalopathy

Progressive multifocal leukoencephalopathy (PML) occurs in 2% to 6% of AIDS patients.[5,20] It may occur as the initial manifestation of HIV infection. PML is an infectious, demyelinating disease caused by a papovavirus (JC virus). Patients most frequently present with focal findings including hemiparesis or monoparesis, limb incoordination, ataxia, visual loss, and cognitive impairment. CT scans show hypodense, nonenhancing white matter lesions. MRI is more sensitive than CT at detecting lesions that appear as white matter hyperintensities on T2-weighted images. The gross pathologic examination may reveal large areas of abnormal white matter that appears granular and mottled; alternatively, lesions may have a smaller peppered appearance. Microscopically, demyelination is found in the presence of enlarged oligodendrocytes with eosinophilic intranuclear inclusions and bizarre astrocytes (Figure 17–3). The typical oligodendroglial inclusions in the absence of multinucleated cells helps distinguish demyelinating lesions in PML from those seen with HIV encephalopathy. Prognosis is poor, and there is no effective treatment.

Nonviral Infectious Diseases Affecting the Nervous System in AIDS

Toxoplasmosis

Cerebral toxoplasmosis occurs commonly in AIDS, affecting approximately 14% of homosexuals with the disease. It accounts for 50% to 70% of focal lesions seen on CT in these patients.[5,22] The infectious agent is *Toxoplasma gondii*, an intracellular parasite common in humans. In immunocompetent humans, ac-

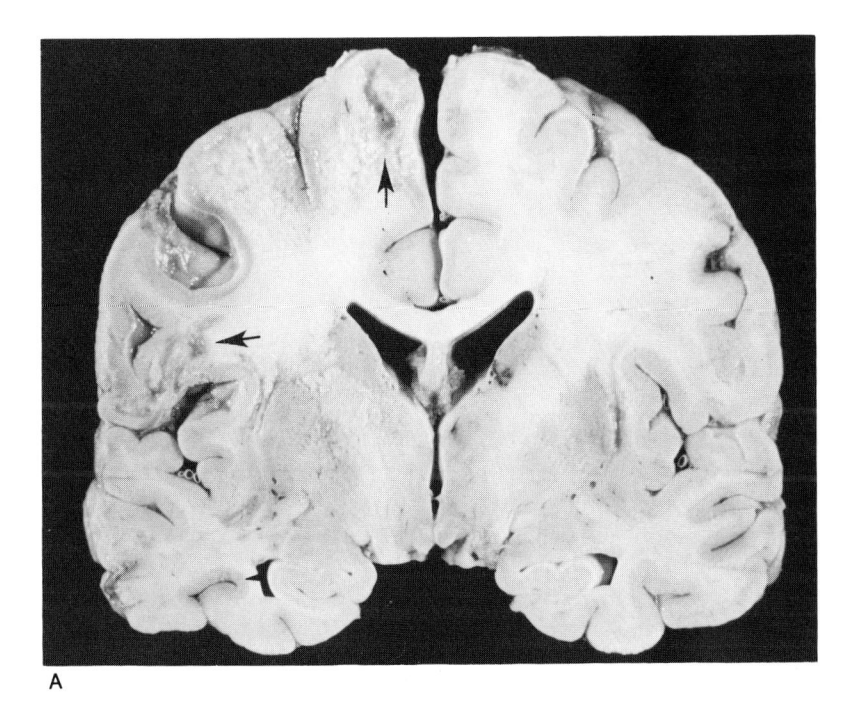

FIGURE 17–3 *Three examples of PML in an AIDS patient. (A) This coronal section of the cerebral hemisphere reveals large zones of degeneration confined primarily to the white matter of the frontal gyri and the internal capsule. (B) This hematoxylin-eosin-stained section of the white matter demonstrates markedly enlarged oligodendroglial nuclei, each with a large central eosinophilic inclusion and a small rim of compressed chromatin. (C) Myelin-stained section of white matter. Note the small- to moderate-sized areas of demyelination.*

B

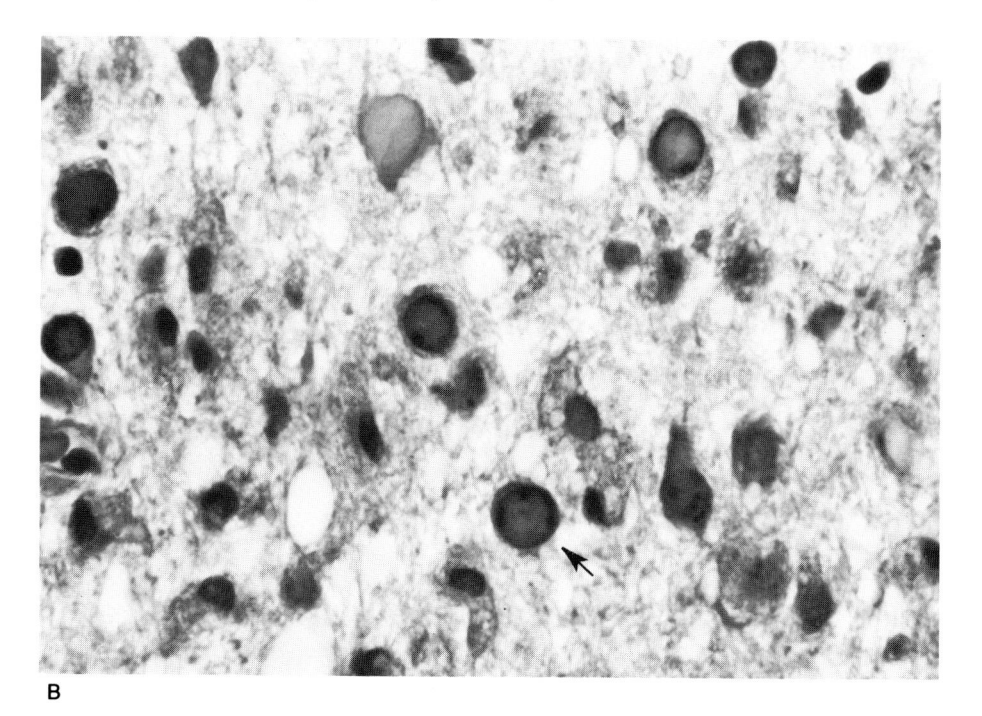

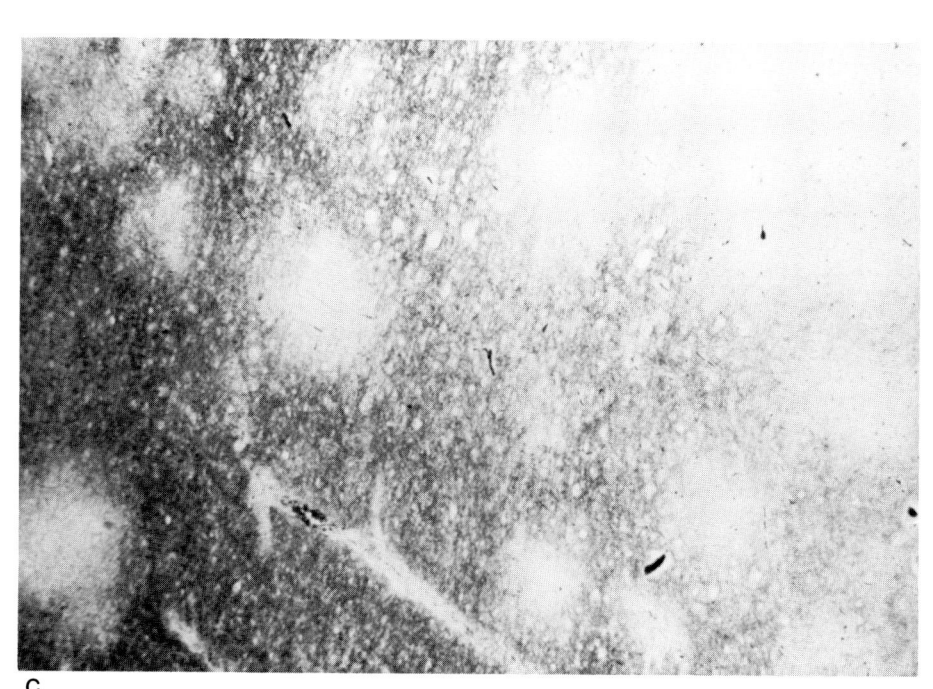

C

quired toxoplasmosis infection is usually subclinical. When symptomatic, toxoplasmosis may cause a mononucleosis-like syndrome, lymphadenopathy, or uveitis with chorioretinitis. Neurologic sequelae are rare. In contrast, neurologic manifestations of toxoplasmosis consisting of focal deficits (70%), seizures (38%), mental status changes (40%), and headaches (45%) occur frequently in AIDS patients.[23] Pathologically, multiple abscesses are found. Untreated, the lesions usually appear necrotic with a variable amount of inflammation (Figure 17–4 C). At this stage, routine microscopic sections often reveal *T. gondii* tachyzoites. Encysted organisms may be found within the viable adjacent tissue.

Toxoplasma lesions are usually multiple, bilateral, and hypodense on noncontrast CT. After contrast, the lesions often show ring enhancement with surrounding edema and a hypodense center (Figure 17–4 A and B). MRI is more sensitive than CT at detecting *Toxoplasma* lesions. The lesions are hyperintense on T2-weighted images and invariably multiple.[22] The main differential diagnosis in patients who present with focal deficits is primary CNS lymphoma. Progressive multifocal leukoencephalopathy, tuberculosis (TB), herpes encephalitis, CMV, cryptococcomas, unusual bacterial abscesses, and strokes occur less frequently.

When the lesions have the characteristic appearance of toxoplasmosis on CT or MRI, a therapeutic trial may be attempted. Treatment is with pyrimethamine (100 mg oral loading dose followed by a single 25 mg oral dose daily) and sulfadiazine (1 g by mouth every six hours). Folinic acid (10 mg orally daily) is also given to reduce the incidence of bone marrow suppression and leukopenia. Improvement both clinically and by CT criteria often starts within days of initiating treatment. Allergy to sulfa drugs or bone marrow suppression may occur, requiring discontinuance of the sulfadiazine. Substitution for sulfadiazine with clindamycin (600 mg four times daily) may be an effective alternative in these instances, but this remains to be proved.[24,25] Most investigators agree that *Toxoplasma* therapy, when effective, should be continued indefinitely. After clinical improvement and radiographic resolution of the lesions, some recommend gradually tapering doses to 25 mg of pyrimethamine and 1 g of sulfadiazine every other day, while others advocate lifelong treatment at maximal doses.[23] If any lesions grow or there is lack of clear improvement with anti-*Toxoplasma* therapy, brain biopsy should be undertaken and specific therapy directed toward the underlying etiology. Steroids are not recommended unless they appear absolutely necessary (e.g., there is such mass effect as to place the patient at risk of herniation). Steroids complicate the interpretation of therapeutic trials against *Toxoplasma* by their capacity to diminish the mass effect of many different types of intracerebral lesions without specificity. In addition, they may exacerbate infection in AIDS patients by further impairing cell-mediated immunity.[24] Despite a generally good response against *Toxoplasma* with therapy, the 12-month death rate for these patients approaches 100%, usually as a result of other opportunistic infections.[23]

Cryptococcosis

Cryptococcal infection occurs in up to 11% of patients with AIDS, usually in the form of cryptococcal meningitis.[5] Most commonly these patients present with

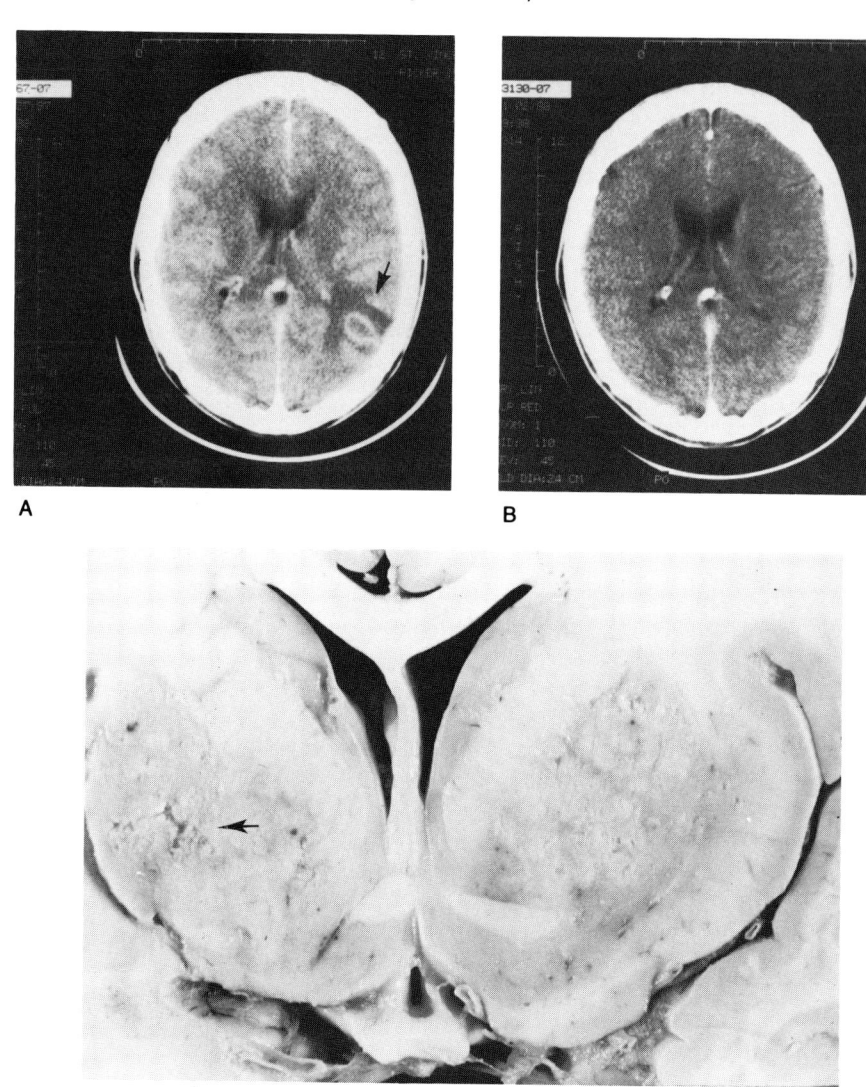

FIGURE 17–4 (**A** and **B**) CT scans of toxoplasmosis in an AIDS patient. Note the ring-enhancing lesion seen with contrast in **A**. CT scan with contrast was done two months after the patient started therapy with pyrimethamine and sulfadiazine shows resolution of the lesion on CT (**B**). (**C**) Toxoplasmosis in an AIDS patient. Note the extensive necrotizing lesions in the putamen on each side.

headache and fever. Meningismus, photophobia, mental status changes, and seizures may occur but are not consistent findings. Patients frequently have symptoms for weeks before presentation.[26] CSF often has an elevated pressure, low glucose, and elevated protein. Pleocytosis may be minimal in AIDS patients with cryptococcal meningitis; 69% of patients may have less than 20 WBCs/mm^3.[26]

CSF should be sent for cryptococcal antigen, India ink stain, and fungal culture. Cryptococcal antigen in the CSF is found in over 95% of patients with culture-proved cryptococcal meningitis. In AIDS patients, fungal cultures are almost always positive in cryptococcal meningitis because the infection is usually well established and many organisms are present. Fungal cultures of the CSF may be negative with intracerebral cryptococcomas in the absence of meningitis. Cryptococcal antigen in the serum is very common in cryptococcal infection as well and should also be obtained. CT scan is not helpful in the diagnosis of cryptococcal meningitis, since scans are usually normal or show only atrophy.

On gross pathological examination the brain may appear normal. Alternatively, there may be a gelatinous exudate within the subarachnoid space, often at the base of the brain. Cysts of gelatinous material may be seen in brain sections, particularly in the deep gray structures. Within the gelatinous material are the cryptococcal organisms (Figure 17–5 A and B).

Treatment of cryptococcal meningitis may consist of a six-week course of either amphotericin B alone (0.4 to 0.6 mg/kg/day) or amphotericin B (0.3 to 0.6 mg/kg/day) in combination with flucytosine (75 to 150 mg/kg/day). Patients who have end-of-treatment CSF cryptococcal antigen titers of 1:8 or greater are more likely to experience a relapse. Following a six-week course, amphotericin B (100mg) should be administered once weekly to prevent relapse. In patients who are not responsive to intravenous (IV) amphotericin, intrathecal therapy may be an option. Common side effects of amphotericin include renal impairment, fever, chills, hypokalemia, and hypomagnesemia. Side effects attributed to flucytosine include leukopenia, thrombocytopenia, and elevated liver transaminases.[23] Flucytosine should be administered with caution to patients with impaired renal or liver function or bone marrow suppression.

Mycobacterial Infections

Mycobacterium tuberculosis involvement of the CNS has been described in AIDS and ARC patients who are IV drug abusers or Haitians.[23,29] Patients may present with either focal cerebral lesions or meningitis. The tuberculous lesions respond to anti-TB therapy. Treatment of CNS TB consists of isoniazid (300 mg daily), ethambutol (800 mg daily) and rifampin (600 mg daily). Steroids are controversial but may be useful in tuberculous meningitis when there is hydrocephalus.

Mycobactrium avium intracellulare (MAI) is a frequent pathogen in AIDS patients, but CNS infections are rare. CNS involvement tends to occur in those with disseminated MAI. Patients may present with encephalitis, meningitis, or cerebral abscesses. There is no effective treatment.

Bacterial Infections

Listeria infections of the CNS occur rarely in AIDS. Pons et al.[23] described three patients with CNS *Listeria* infections and AIDS. Two patients had meningitis, and one had a brain abscess. Treatment with IV ampicillin resulted in clinical improvement.

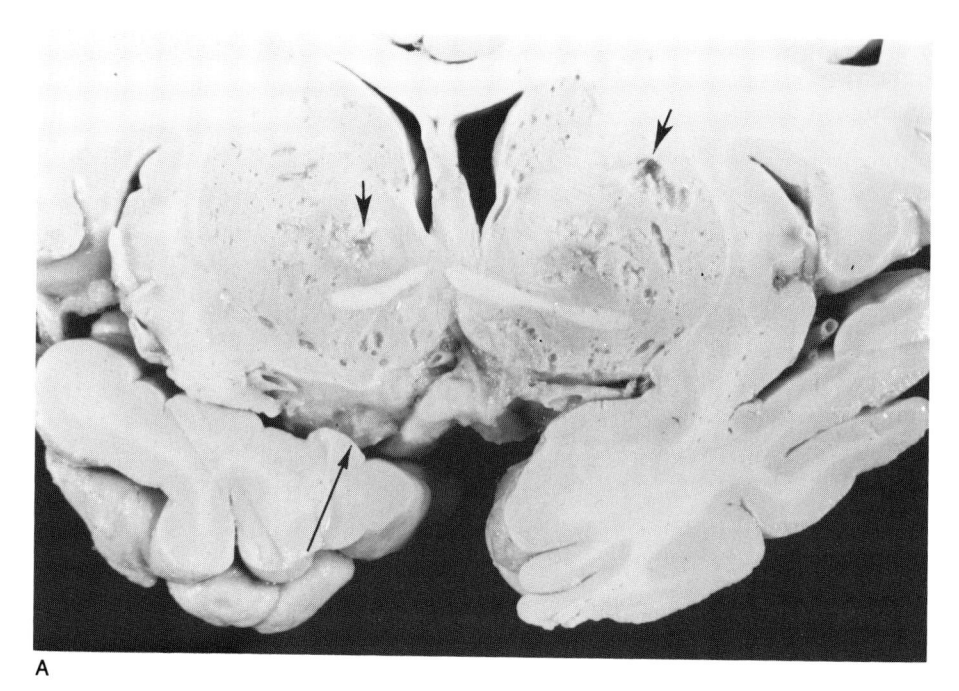

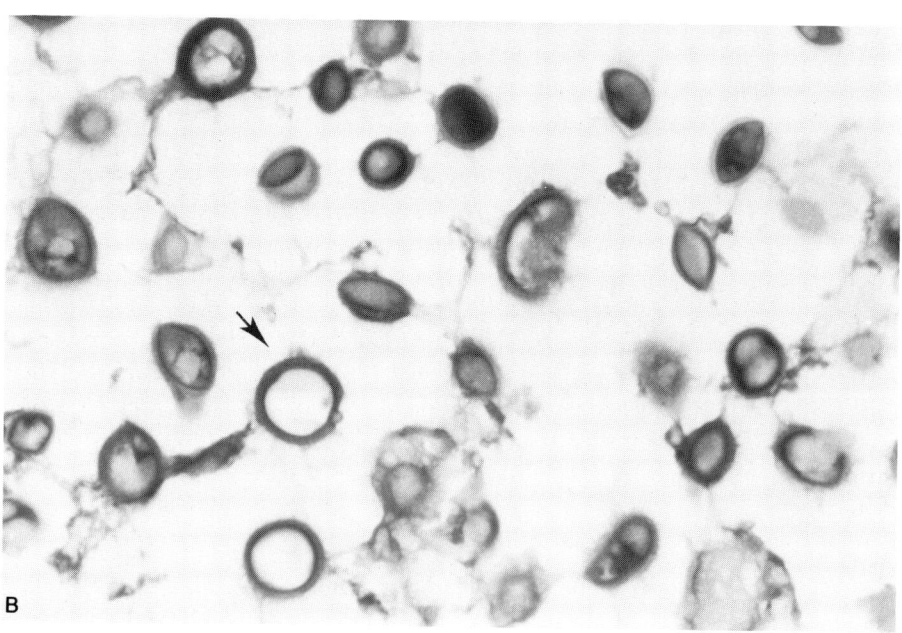

FIGURE 17–5 *Cryptococcal infection of the CNS in an AIDS patient. (A) A coronal section of the cerebral hemisphere with macrocystic changes, resulting in the "swiss cheese appearance" of the striatum, internal capsule, and basal forebrain* (**short arrows**). *Also note the leptomeningeal clouding secondary to cryptococcal meningitis at the base of the brain in the region of the optic chiasm* (**long arrow**). *(B) A hematoxylin-eosin-stained section of a cryptococcal cyst showing numerous round and oval shaped forms with thick capsules.*

Neurosyphilis

Neurosyphilis is another potential infectious complication in AIDS patients. In the Johns Hopkins series,[13] one patient of 186 with HIV infection had active neurosyphilis; he had previously been treated for neurosyphilis. In another series, three patients with meningovascular syphilis were seen who were at high risk for HIV infection, but they refused serologic testing.[1] Johns et al. have reported on several patients with neurosyphilis and AIDS who were previously treated with parenteral penicillin for either gonorrhea or syphilis. They suggest that the course of syphilis may be altered in AIDS patients and that neurosyphilis may be an early complication in AIDS.[31] They recommend lumbar puncture in the evaluation of HIV-seropositive patients with syphilis and question the adequacy of the currently recommended treatment regimens for syphilis in this population.

Neoplastic Disease Affecting the Nervous System in AIDS

Primary CNS Lymphoma

Primary CNS lymphoma occurs in up to 5% of patients with AIDS[5] and accounts for between 10% and 25% of focal lesions seen on CT scan.[22] Patients with CNS lymphoma frequently present with focal neurologic deficits and impaired mentation (Figure 17–6).[27] This impairment may in part be explained by location of the tumor, cerebral edema, or coexisting diseases (e.g., HIV encephalopathy, viral encephalitis, toxoplasmosis, cryptococcal meningitis). Seizures may eventually develop in up to one-third of patients. CT scans may show a hyperdense mass that enhances homogeneously with contrast. Alternatively, these lesions may also appear hypodense, enhance irregularly, show periventricular enhancement, or have ringlike enhancement. Lesions may be single or multiple. Their appearance is generally indistinguishable from toxoplasmosis. A solitary lesion on MRI favors lymphoma over toxoplasmosis, since toxoplasmosis lesions are invariably multiple on MRI.[22] Although CSF cytology may be useful in diagnosis if lumbar puncture can be performed safely, it is relatively insensitive for CNS lymphoma. Stereotactic biopsy is more reliable. Given the similar appearance of CNS lymphoma to toxoplasmosis on CT and its lower prevalence, many patients with CNS lymphoma will receive a trial with anti-*Toxoplasma* medications before biopsy. Patients with CNS lymphoma have a poor prognosis, with most dying within one month. Delay in diagnosis and inadequate therapy may contribute to this rapid decline. Treatment consists of radiation therapy. So et al.[27] have reported survival up to five months and definite CT improvement using radiation therapy to the brain at 4000 cGy over three weeks. Systemic chemotherapy may induce further immunosuppression in these patients, and its effectiveness is questionable.

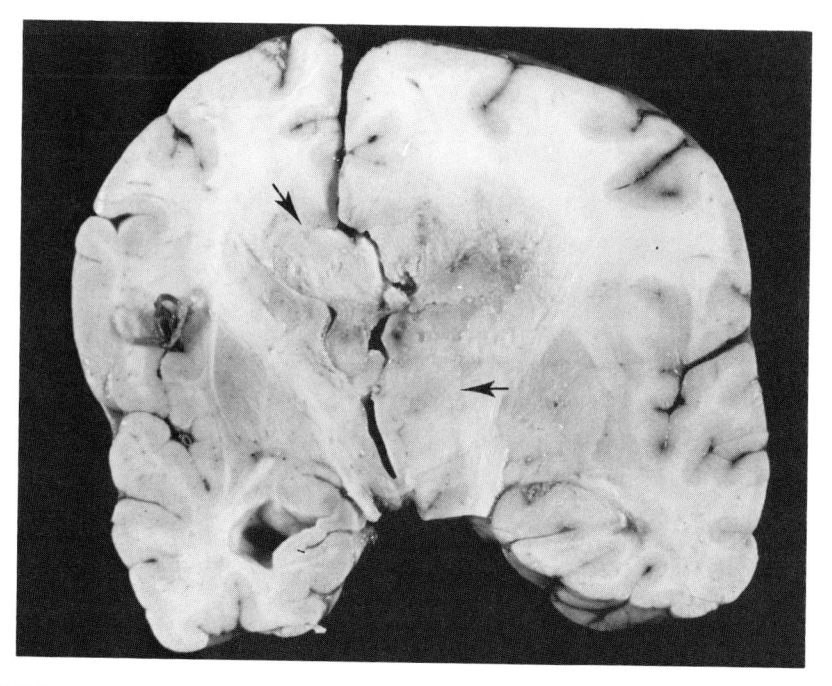

FIGURE 17–6 CNS lymphoma in an AIDS patient. This coronal section reveals lymphoma in the corpus callosum, fornix, and right dorsal thalamus.

Systemic Non-Hodgkin's Lymphoma

Lymphomatous metastasis of systemic non-Hodgkin's lymphoma to the CNS occurs in AIDS patients, and the clinical manifestations usually reflect leptomeningeal or dural involvement.[27] These patients most frequently present with cranial neuropathy, radiculopathy, or myelopathy. CSF cytology often shows the characteristic lymphoma cells. Intrathecal chemotherapy using methotrexate or arabinosyl cytosine (Ara-C) is the primary therapy for leptomeningeal lymphoma. Epidural compression of the spinal cord or cauda equina usually causes back pain, paraparesis, and sphincter disturbances. In patients with acute compressive myelopathy secondary to lymphoma, myelography or MRI of the spine should be obtained and radiation therapy to the appropriate region started.

Kaposi's Sarcoma

Involvement of the nervous system in Kaposi's sarcoma appears to be remarkably rare despite its frequent occurrence in AIDS patients. In three patients reported with metastatic Kaposi's sarcoma to the nervous system, two patients had brain metastases and one had metastatic Kaposi's sarcoma to the brachial plexus.[28]

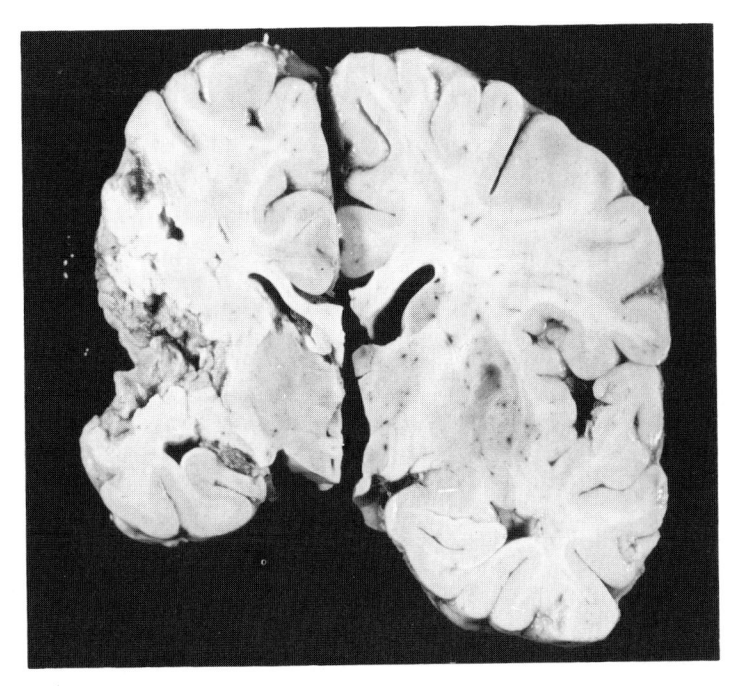

FIGURE 17-7 *Cerebral infarction in an AIDS patient. Four months before death the patient had sudden onset of right hemiplegia. The left cerebral hemisphere, shown in this section, revealed a massive infarction. An organized thrombus was found in the left internal carotid artery. Myocarditis and endocardial disruption, also found at autopsy, was the presumed source of the embolus.*

Cerebrovascular Disease in AIDS

Cerebrovascular complications in AIDS patients are common (Figure 17-7). Levy et al.[1] found that 18 of 94 unselected patients with AIDS had cerebral infarctions at autopsy. The explanation for the high frequency of infarctions is unknown. Some infarctions appear to be embolic from the heart (nonbacterial thrombotic endocarditis), but other possible etiologies include cerebral vasculitis, circulating immune complexes, or lupus-type anticoagulants. Intracranial hemorrhage may occur in the setting of lymphoma, rarely with Kaposi's sarcoma (often within the tumor itself), and with thrombocytopenia.

REFERENCES

1. Rosenblum ML, Levy RM, Bredesen DE. Central nervous system dysfunction in acquired immunodeficiency syndrome. In: Rosenblum ML, Levy RM, Bredesen DE, eds. AIDS and the nervous system. New York: Raven Press, 1988;29-63.

2. Navia BA, Jordan BD, Price RW. The AIDS dementia complex: I. Clinical features. Ann Neurol 1986;19:517–24.
3. Navia BA, Cho E-S, Petito CK, Price RW. The AIDS dementia complex: II. Neuropathology. Ann Neurol 1986;19:525–35.
4. de la Monte SM, Ho DD, Schooley RT, et al. Subacute encephalomyelitis of AIDS and its relation to HTLV III infection. Neurology 1987;37:562–9.
5. Neilson SL, Davis RL. Neuropathology of acquired immunodeficiency syndrome. In: Rosenblum ML, Levy RM, Bredesen DE, eds. AIDS and the nervous system. New York: Raven Press, 1988;155–79.
6. Ho DD, Pomerantz RJ, Kaplan JC. Pathogenesis of infection with human immunodeficiency virus. N Eng J Med 1987;317:278–86.
7. Houff SA. Neuroimmunology of human immunodeficiency virus infection. In: Rosenblum ML, Levy RM, Bredesen DE, eds. AIDS and the nervous system. New York: Raven Press, 1988;347–75.
8. Koenig S, Gendelman HE, Orenstein JM, et al. Detection of AIDS virus in macrophages in brain tissue from AIDS patients with encephalopathy. Science 1986;233:1089–93.
9. Pumarola-Sune T, Navia BA, Cordon-Cardo C, et al. HIV antigen in the brains of patients with the AIDS dementia complex. Ann Neurol 1987;21:490–6.
10. Gyorky F, Melnick JL, Gyorkey P. Human immunodeficiency virus in brain biopsies of patients with AIDS and progressive encephalopathy. J Infect Dis 1987;155:870–6.
11. Apatoff BR, Lee MR, Gurney ME. Trophic effects of neuroleukin on central neurons and functional interactions with HIV envelope protein. Ann Neurol 1987;22:156.
12. Gabuzda DH, Hirsch MS. Neurologic manifestations of infection with human immunodeficiency virus. Ann Intern Med 1987;107:383–91.
13. McArthur JC. Neurologic manifestations of AIDS. Medicine 1987;66:407–37.
14. Miller RG, Kiprov DD, Parry G, Bredesden DE. Peripheral nervous system dysfunction in acquired immunodeficiency syndrome. In: Rosenblum ML, Levy RM, Bredesen DE, eds. AIDS and the nervous system. New York: Raven Press, 1988;65–78.
15. Cornblath DR, McArthur JC, Kennedy PGE, et al. Inflammatory demyelinating peripheral neuropathies associated with human T-cell lymphotropic virus type III infection. Ann Neurol 1987;21:32–40.
16. Rottenberg DA, Moeller JR, Strother SC, et al. The metabolic pathology of the AIDS dementia complex. Ann Neurol 1987;22:700–6.
17. Rosenblum ML, Bredesen DE, Levy RM. Algorithms for the treatment of AIDS patients with neurological diseases. In: Rosenblum ML, Levy RM, Bredesen DE, eds. AIDS and the nervous system. New York: Raven Press, 1988;389–95.
18. Craddock C, Bull R, Pasvol G, et al. Cardiopulmonary arrest and autonomic neuropathy in AIDS. Lancet 1987;2:16.
19. Eidelberg D, Sotrel A, Hannes V. Progressive polyradiculopathy in acquired immune deficiency syndrome. Neurology 1986;36:912–6.
20. Berger JR, Kaszovitz B, Post JD, et al. Progressive multifocal leukoencephalopathy associated with human immunodeficiency virus infection. Ann Intern Med 1987;107:78–87.
21. Dix RD, Bredesen DE. Opportunistic viral infections in acquired immunodeficiency syndrome. In: Rosenblum ML, Levy RM, Bredesen DE, eds. AIDS and the nervous system. New York: Raven Press, 1988;221–61.

22. De La Paz R, Enzmann D. Neuroradiology of acquired immunodeficiency syndrome. In: Rosenblum ML, Levy RM, Bredesen DE, eds. AIDS and the nervous system. New York: Raven Press, 1988;121–53.
23. Pons VG, Jacobs RA, Hollander H. Nonviral infections of the central nervous system in patients with acquired immunodeficiency syndrome. In: Rosenblum ML, Levy RM, Bredesen DE, eds. AIDS and the nervous system. New York: Raven Press, 1988;263–83.
24. Navia BA, Petito CK, Gold JWM, et al. Cerebral toxoplasmosis complicating acquired immune deficiency syndrome: Clinical and neuropathological findings in 27 patients. Ann Neurol 1986;19:224–38.
25. Navia BA, Price RW. Infections in AIDS and in other immunosuppressed patients. In: Kennedy PGE, Johnson RT, eds. Infections of the nervous system. Stoneham, Mass.: Butterworths, 1987.
26. Zuger A, Louie E, Holzman RS, et al. Cryptococcal disease in patients with the acquired immunodeficiency syndrome. Diagnostic features and outcome of treatment. Ann Intern Med 1986;104:234–40.
27. So YT, Choucair A, Davis RL, et al. Neoplasms of the central nervous system in acquired immunodeficiency syndrome. In: Rosenblum ML, Levy RM, Bredesen DE, eds. AIDS and the nervous system. New York: Raven Press. 1988;285–300.
28. Levy RM, Bredesden DE, Rosenblum ML. Neurological manifestations of the acquired immunodeficiency syndrome (AIDS): Experience at UCSF and review of the literature. J Neurosurg 1985;62:475–95.
29. Bishburg E, Sunderdam G, Reichman LB, Kapila R. Central nervous system tuberculosis with the acquired immunodeficiency syndrome and its related complex. Ann Intern Med 1986;105:210–13.
30. Schmitt FA, Bigley JW, McKinnis R, et al. Neuropsychological outcome of zidovudine (AZT) treatment of patients with AIDS and AIDS-related complex. N Engl J Med 1988;319:1573–78.
31. Johns DR, Tierney M, Felsenstein D. Alteration in the natural history of neurosyphilis by concurrent infection with the human immunodeficiency virus. N Eng J Med 1987;316:1569–72.
32. Masdeu JC, Small CB, Weiss L, et al. Multifocal cytomegalovirus encephalitis in AIDS. Ann Neurol 1988;23:97–99.

Chapter 18

Case Presentations of AIDS in the United States

AIDS in Prostitutes

Joyce Wallace

Early in the acquired immunodeficiency syndrome (AIDS) epidemic it was appreciated that AIDS was linked with promiscuity.[1-3] In infectious disease, in this case a sexually transmitted disease, those who have the most exposure will be more likely to have the disease. In 1982 we undertook two studies to determine if women who were very sexually active with diverse partners were as likely to contract AIDS as sexually active homosexual men.

STUDY 1

The first study grew out of treating a 27-year-old prostitute, who, three months before the study, had *Pneumocystis carinii* pneumonia. Six other prostitutes were alerted to the problem by the patient, and a seventh prostitute was referred to us by another physician. Their age, intravenous drug history, and T4:T8 cell ratios are listed in Table 18–1.

Patient 1 had AIDS as defined by the Centers for Disease Control (CDC). She had the following opportunistic infections: *P. carinii* pneumonia, molluscum contagiosum, herpes simplex, and thrush. Her lifetime sexual contacts numbered about 15,000. During the year before her illness appeared, in addition to sexual intercourse she performed anal fellatio on approximately 20% of her 1000 clients that year. She very rarely had rectal intercourse. She never used intravenous (IV) drugs, but she had a two-year relationship with a sexual partner who used IV drugs. This relationship ended approximately five years before her illness. Her latest consort was studied and found to have normal immunologic parameters. The patient died two months after this study. Her T cell ratio was 0.3 (Table 18–1, patient 1).

Table 18–1 Study of eight self-referred female prostitutes (in 1982)[a]

Patient No.	Age (yr)	Length of IV Drug Use	T3 (%)	T4 (%)	T8 (%)	T4:T8[a]
1	27		56	14	40	0.3
2	21		66	31	48	0.64
3	31	Occasionally	73	51	22	2.32
4	21	1 year	75	52	36	1.44
5	24		72	51	30	1.7
6	36	4 years	60	54	17	3.18
7	35		88	48	40	1.2
8	25		38	18	28	0.64

[a]Mean = 1.43; median = 1.31.

Another prostitute who reported some malaise and weight loss had an abnormally low T cell ratio of 0.64 (Table 18–1, patient 2). She also had a penicillinase-producing gonococcus infection in the throat and mild lymphadenopathy. She was the only patient studied who had a high asialo GM1 antibody level.* She also had an abnormally high IgM antispermatoza level. (See Table 18–2, patient 5).

Patient 8, Table 18–1, reported malaise and weight loss and had a low T4:T8 ratio (0.64). Five of the other women had normal ratios and were normal on physical examination, even though three had been IV drug users. Patients 3, 4, and 6 worked as call girls (few partners), and one had only begun this work in the past year (patient 6). The mean T4:T8 ratio in this group was 1.43. It is significant that in this group of eight women, three had abnormally depressed T4:T8 ratios. Control group data were supplied by Ortho Pharmaceutical Company. Forty "normal females" between 25 and 30 years of age were tested. The mean for this group was 1.71 ± 0.43, with a range between 0.9 and 2.7.

There was a significant difference between the group of eight prostitutes studied and the control groups. The prostitute group, however, comprised self-selected concerned individuals (patients 2 through 8) and one dying patient (1) and was therefore felt not to be representative of prostitutes as a group.

It was important to survey a group of non-self-selected, non-drug-using prostitutes. We were able to do this through the New York City Department of Health, which in 1982 was involved in a program to determine the incidence of penicillinase-producing *Neisseria gonorrhoeae* (PPNG) in the prostitute population.

Small teams of health workers were sent to brothels. As part of the testing, gonorrhea cultures and serologic blood tests for syphilis were obtained. On repeat visits the workers informed the patients of our experiment and obtained permission to obtain extra blood for T cell analysis. These specimens, although obtained from volunteers, reflected sampling among active New York City pros-

---

*Asialo GM1 is a neutral glycolipid found on the walls of lymphocytes.

Table 18-2 Prostitute study: Female prostitutes examined for sperm and asialo GM1 antibody[a] (in 1985)

Patient	T4/T8		Immune Complexes	Sperm Antibody ELISA			Sperm Agglutinin	Asialo GM1 Antibody
				IgG	IgM	IgA		
B.R.	2.32		125	0.426	*0.945*	0.206	*1:40*	0.281
B.J.	2.1	Low NK	0	0.459	0.443	0.255	0	*0.308*
F.M.	NA			0.375	0.326	0.224	0	0.261
J.S.	NA		*350*	0.404	0.306	0.196	0	*0.293*
S.V.	0.64		0	0.457	0.647	0.214	0	*0.372*
N.C.	1.21		*300*	0.350	*0.900*	0.227	*1:40*	0.262
1	1.75		0	0.280	0.164	0.236	0	0.235
3	1.19		0	0.402	0.238	0.257	0	0.234
4	1.43		0	*0.644*	0.463	0.196	0	0.255
5	3.5		0	0.420	0.236	0.178	0	0.260
6	2.11		*8000*	*0.675*	0.490	*0.493*	*1:40*	*0.327*
7	2.17		*270*	0.463	0.397	*0.293*	0	0.258
8	1.88		0	0.450	0.336	*0.274*	0	0.237
10	1.54		0	0.412	*0.542*	*0.376*	*1:80*	0.244
26	1.8		*8000*	*0.641*	*0.513*	*0.474*	*1:20*	*0.266*
27	2.13		0	0.452	*0.498*	*0.292*	0	0.210

[a]Positive values are italicized
NK, natural killer.
NA, not available.

titutes. The women were asked their age and whether they were using or had ever used IV drugs. All 25 women denied IV drug use and had no physical signs of IV drug use (track marks or venipunctures). All the women were presumed to be healthy because they were actively working.

There was no statistical difference in the mean ratios between the control group and the randomly selected prostitute group. Note, however, that one of 25 subjects had a depressed T4:T8 ratio (Table 18–3, patient 21a and b). This woman (#21) was evaluated during the two months after the initial T4:T8 determination. She had malaise, a 30 lb. weight loss in one year, and posterior cervical lymphadenopathy. This constellation was first incriminated as AIDS related in May 1982. Her T4:T8 was 0.26 initially and repeated 0.08 two months later. It is noteworthy to find such an aberrant ratio even in one person of 25 patients. The chance of finding this type of abnormality in apparently healthy individuals in the general population is nil.[4,5]

This patient had an abnormally high antibody titer to cytomegalovirus (CMV (1:128) and a high titer to Epstein-Barr virus (EBV) (viral capsid antigen [VCA] 1:160). Although this patient's steady sexual partner was an IV drug user, his T cell ratio was normal. This patient was examined again one year after the initial visit; she then had more energy and had gained 15 lbs. Her results then were as follows: CMV, 1:256; T3 lymphocytes, 42 (N 65% to 82%); T4, 23% (N 30% to 55%); T8, 17% (N 10% to 25%); T4:T8, 1.35; and natural killer (NK) cell

Table 18-3 Random sampling of 25 New York City prostitutes seen in brothels in 1982

Patient No.	Age (yr)	T3 (%)	T4 (%)	T8 (%)	T4/T8
1	33	53	35	20	1.75
2	36	54	40	25	1.6
3	31	64	37	31	1.19
4	29	59	40	28	1.43
5	42	59	49	14	3.5
6	22	55	40	19	2.11
7	26	35	26	12	2.17
8	23	51	30	16	1.88
9	27	64	46	25	1.84
10	21	53	37	24	1.54
11	35	69	36	31	1.16
12	27	83	56	34	1.65
13	29	48	33	19	1.74
14	37	67	36	36	1.0
15	31	72	55	27	2.04
16	45	66	45	26	1.73
17	32	61	46	17	2.71
18	29	83	51	42	1.21
19	26	79	47	29	1.62
20	25	53	38	17	2.24
21a	30	64	8	31	0.26
21b[a]	30	36	2	24	0.08
22	23	75	49	32	1.53
23	29	41	27	15	1.8
24	28	50	34	16	2.13
25	28	54	33	26	1.27

[a] 21b is a repeat of 21a two months later.

number 4 (N 10% to 25%). Pokeweed and phytohemagglutinin response was normal.

Taking both these groups together, the overall rate of immunodeficiency as measured by having inverted T cell ratios in the 33 women studied in 1982 is 5/33 (15%). This is similar to the rate of human immunodeficiency virus (HIV) antibody positivity in New York City prostitutes as measured in 1985 (see Table 18-4).

The other abnormalities that have been demonstrated in sexually active homosexual men are the presence of antispermatazoa antibodies, high circulating immune complexes, and asialo GM1 antibodies.[6] Vasectomized heterosexual men demonstrate antisperm antibodies as well but do not have the same high levels as the homosexual men. Furthermore, they do not have the same high levels of asialo GM1 antibodies.[7]

Figure 18-1 shows the levels of sperm antibody previously described in homosexual and heterosexual men alongside the values of the female prostitutes in our study. The levels of sperm antibody were not as high as those found in

Table 18–4 Clinical presentation in 62 infants and children with symptomatic HIV infection

Symptom	Number	%
Anemia (microcytic hypochromic)	60	97
Thrombocytopenia	24	34
Chronic pneumonia (interstitial)	42	68
Failure to thrive	55	89
Opportunistic infection		
P. carinii	18	29
Mycobacterium avium intracellulare (MAI)	3	5
CMV	8	13
Aspergillosis	3	5
Adenovirus	3	5
Herpes simplex virus	6	10
Candida		
Mucocutaneous	50	81
Disseminated (including esophagitis)	8	13
Toxoplasmosis	2	3
LIP	22	36
Recurrent bacterial sepsis	28	45
Hepatosplenomegaly	46	74
Lymphadenopathy	44	71
Recurrent febrile episodes	60	97
Diarrhea	54	87
Encephalopathy	40	65
Skin rash (eczemalike)	13	20
Chronic parotid swelling	8	13
Cardiomyopathy	3	5
Nephropathy/nephritis	3	5

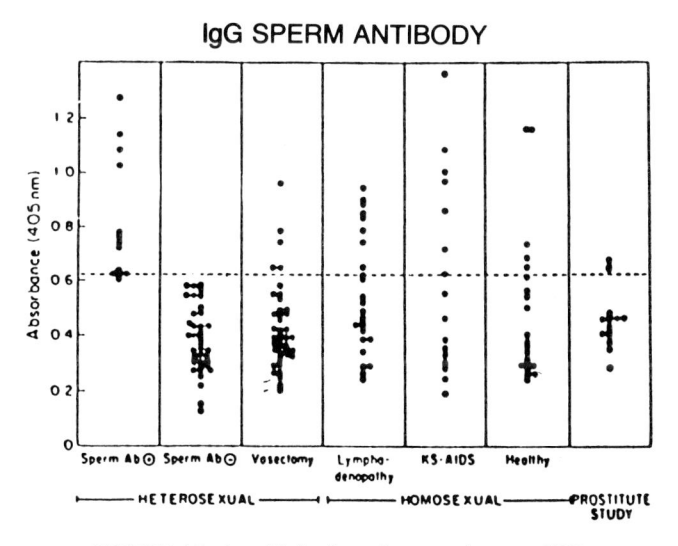

FIGURE 18–1   *Eight female prostitutes, 1982.*

healthy homosexual men and were well below those found in homosexual men with lymphadenopathy or AIDS.

Because sperm might stimulate the production of an antilymphocyte factor, studies were undertaken to measure asialo GM1 antibodies. These antibodies were not elevated in the women studied. Note that the one woman who had an anti-asialo GM1 level approaching the abnormal was the one with the lowest T cell ratio (Table 18–3). We now believe that anti-asialo GM1 may be a nonspecific marker for HIV infection as one of many immune globulins that have become elevated in HIV infection.

The methods used in laboratory evaluations for the study are described below.

Lymphocyte Subsets

Production growth and characterization of the hybridoma-secreting monoclonal antibodies OKT 3, OKT 4, and OKT 8 have been discussed.[8,9] In brief, the monoclonal antibody OKT 3 recognizes a surface antigen present on the majority of normal peripheral T cells. The OKT 4 and OKT 8 sets constitute 55% to 65% and 30% to 40%, respectively, of the peripheral T cell pool.

Mononuclear cells were isolated from heparinized peripheral blood on Ficoll-Hypaque gradients. Lymphocytes positive for OKT 3, OKT 4, and OKT 8* were identified by a direct immunofluorescence assay using a 30 H cytofluorograph (Ortho Instruments, Westwood, Mass.). The means of the percentages of OKT 4/OKT 8 ratios were compared in the different groups using Student's t-test.

Sperm Antibody Assay

IgG antibody to spermatozoa was determined by an enzyme-linked immunosorbent assay (ELISA). Briefly, 0.05 ml of serum diluted 1:5 in phosphate-buffered saline (PBS) was admixed with an equal volume of motile spermatozoa (5×10^7 ml), purified as described previously,[10] and incubated at 37°C for 60 minutes. The spermatozoa were then washed three times with PBS and fixed to wells of a microtiter plate with 0.25% glutaraldehyde. Bound IgG was quantitated using alkaline phosphatase conjugated swing IgG antibody to human IgG (heavy chain specific, Medical Technology Corp., Hackensack, N.J.) as previously described.[11]

Antibody to Asialo GM1

IgG antibody to asialo GM1 was determined by ELISA using asialo GM1 (1.2 µg/well) fixed to wells of polyvinyl microtiter plates.[12]

---

*Supplied by Gideon Goldstein, M.D., Ph.D., Ortho Pharmaceutical Corporation.

Circulating Immune Complex Assay

Circulating immune complexes (CICs) were quantitated by an ELISA using Raji cells fixed to polystyrene microtiter plate wells.[13]

STUDY 2

After our first study and the survey performed in 1982, we were not able to study prostitutes again until the spring of 1985. This was not intentional. In 1983 it was clear that this type of study would be difficult to perform within an institution or other formal setting. Proposals to major institutions to use their equipment, such as a van for on-site phlebotomy, were rejected.

During 1984 and 1985 several developments made a new survey possible. One was the elucidation of HIV as the cause of the disease. A test for the antibody became available in research laboratories. Another was a grant from the Cancer Research Institute, which had financed a project that included a study of ten women who practiced anal coitus as contrasted to age-and experience-matched controls who practiced only vaginal coitus. The search for controls who were neither prostitutes nor IV drug users for the five most promiscuous anal-receptive women was fruitless, since this subgroup of women had had thousands of partners. We asked that the funds remaining from that project be used to look for HIV antibodies in prostitutes. An additional factor that facilitated this survey was the increasing public awareness of AIDS. Many prostitutes were now anxious to have the test. Also, it had become clear that the two groups most affected by this disease, homosexual men and IV drug users, had a high incidence of antibodies to HIV. DesJarlais found an 85% incidence of antibodies in men in a drug detoxification program. We found a 40% incidence of antibody in a study of women who had become drug addicts.[14]

Prostitution can be the means of financing a drug habit, and therefore it seemed even more important to look at prostitutes as a group.

In April and May of 1985, I and my assistant canvassed areas of Manhattan frequented by streetwalkers. During five separate excursions in a station wagon with M.D. plates, outfitted with my medical license and phlebotomy equipment, we approached approximately 75 streetwalkers. The women were invited to become patients for the purpose of learning whether they had any antibody to the virus associated with AIDS. Those who participated signed consent forms. Twenty-two female prostitutes, one male transvestite prostitute, and two male pimps agreed to become patients. They were each given a letter describing the project, which included an office phone number and address. The patients were questioned about their age, the length of time they worked as prostitutes, their use of IV drugs, and the IV drug use of their sexual partners. Our sample includes only four IV drug users. Perhaps this sample is skewed because drug users are suspicious and less willing to cooperate with a project of this type. Two subjects could not be studied because their antecubital veins were excessively scarred. Only three patients eventually requested their test results.

Sera samples were sent to the National Cancer Institute in Washington, the National Bacteriological Laboratory in Stockholm, and the Harvard School of Public Health. The first two laboratories did ELISA testing with Western blot for confirmation. The Harvard School of Public Health, looking for breakdown of antibody into ways that might offer insight into the difference among antibodies, performed membrane immunofluorescence (MIF), and radio immunoprecipitation and sodium dodecyl sulfate-electrophoresis (RIP/SOS-PAGE, or RIPA). The concordance of results between the three laboratories is perfect. Of the 22 women studied, four were positive for the presence of antibody (19%). Two of the four admitted to IV drug use, and one had a boyfriend who was an IV drug user. The three men (the transvestite prostitute and the two pimps) were negative for the antibody.

In 1986, more streetwalkers were willing to participate in this study, attributable to the increased awareness of AIDS. This made it possible to recruit at least one of three streetwalking prostitutes. Forty-three volunteers were evaluated, including two who had been seen in the previous year. This time there were six current or former IV drug users. Of these six, two were infected (33%). In addition, another two women who denied IV drug use showed antibodies to HIV. The rate of seropositivity to HIV in the women studied in 1986 was 9% (4/43).[15]

In 1987, two of three women approached agreed to be studied. We recruited 67 volunteers. Eight of these women had used IV drugs. Of these eight, four were positive for antibodies to HIV. Four of the 67 studied in 1987 were infected (6%).[15]

Of the 131 streetwalkers evaluated from 1985 through July 1987, 12 demonstrated seropositivity (9%). Eliminating IV drug-abusing prostitutes from this group resulted in a seropositivity rate of 4.6%.[15] In 1988 we examined another 33 prostitutes and found 2 who are seropositive (4.5%). Thus, we have noted a high seropositivity rate among prostitutes, though it has not increased between 1982 and 1988.

Former Drug-Abusing Women (Including Prostitutes)

The rate of 6% seropositivity in nondrug-using prostitutes can be compared with the rate of 42% for former drug-abusing women noted in another study.[15] A group of 110 former drug abusers were studied during 1983, 1984, and 1985 for signs of AIDS.[5] (Thirty-five women [31%] admitted to having worked as prostitutes.) Although none of these women had AIDS, 87% of the seropositive group had lymphadenopathy, low white blood cell counts, anemia, excretion of abnormal RNA nucleosides, past history of other sexually transmitted diseases, hepatitis B infection, sperm antibodies, T4 lymphocyte suppression, and low T4:T8 ratios. The above findings are all associated with HIV infection. A disquieting finding of this study is that the people who were seropositive had an average of three times as many sexual partners as those who were seronegative.

ANTI-ASIALO GMI ANTIBODY

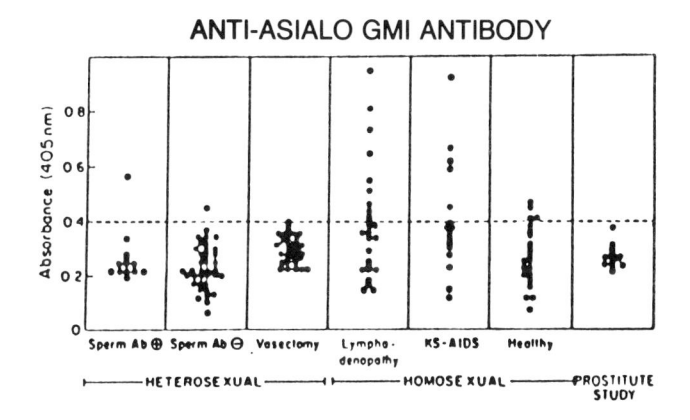

[Scatter plot: Absorbance (405 nm) vs. groups: Sperm Ab⊕, Sperm Ab⊖, Vasectomy (HETEROSEXUAL); Lymphadenopathy, KS-AIDS (HOMOSEXUAL); Healthy (PROSTITUTE STUDY)]

FIGURE 18-2 *Sample of women in brothels.*

The mean number of partners for infected women was 3062, with a median of 30. The mean number of partners for members of the seronegative group was 1047, with a median of 25. This raises the question of whether drug abuse and sexual activity are additive risks for AIDS.

Studies of anti-HIV antibody prevalence in prostitutes working in other cities have shown widely varying differences. In Kigali, Rwanda, the heart of the African endemic area, 29 of 33 (87%) prostitutes were seropositive.[17] Researchers in cities in eastern Africa are now reporting seropositivity.[18] In London and Paris, recent reports show no seropositivity,[19,20] yet prostitutes in Pardenone, Italy, were seropositive in 10 of 24 (42%) cases studied.[21] In Athens there is a 6% (12/200) rate of seropositivity.[22] In the United States, reports from Miami, when women sought attention at a medical facility known for its AIDS work, 10 of 40 (25%) were seropositive.[23] They may, however, represent a self-selected group. In Seattle, where all prostitutes were examined as they entered a detention center, all were negative for anti-HIV antibodies.[24] Note that the Seattle figure was originally reported as 5%[24] but was corrected after Western Blot testing.

The positivity rate of 19% in 1985 is not very different from the positivity rate (of immunodeficiency) of 15% in 1982 (see Table 19-4). Yet there still are men who ascribe their AIDS solely to the use of prostitutes and deny other high-risk behavior. Perhaps the long incubation period of this disease obscures female-to-male transmission in this country. Female-to-male transmission is obvious in Africa, and female-to-male transmission may become more evident in the United States. AIDS in America is currently a male disease (90%) because the earliest carriers of the virus were primarily male drug addicts and gay men. At present 17% of new cases in New York City are women. The next group to contract this disease should be heterosexual men who catch it from women who caught it by heterosexual transmission or in IV drug use.

Women, especially prostitutes, act as depositories of seminal fluid, which has been shown to be exquisitely capable of holding large numbers of viral particles. Saliva is probably a much less effective fluid for virus transmission. Indeed, the difficulty in culturing the virus from saliva has been noted. Researchers have found the virus in vaginal secretions.[25,26] Men must be advised that if they engage in casual sexual encounters, they should put a barrier between mucous membranes. Likewise, women should make sure that their male sexual partners use condoms. Additionally, spermicidal jelly may offer some protection against the AIDS virus, but the widespread use of condoms is necessary. Since condoms have been known to tear, perhaps the safest prophylactic measure is to place a small amount of 9% Nonoxynl 9 spermicide (Virucide) inside the condom. Condoms are less likely to break when worn with "head space" or with a reservoir tip. Women may use in addition the "female condom" or the Today Sponge, which is impregnated with Nonoxynl 9.

Studying prostitutes is limited in that it tells us the group's rate of infection but not if the prostitutes are infecting their clients. To investigate whether or to what extent they are transmitting the disease to their male clients, it is necessary to study their customers as well. Our preliminary studies in self-selected customers of New York City prostitutes show a seropositivity rate of 1%. Three of 340 men who have not admitted having had sex with men or using IV drugs are infected.[27] One question arising from these results is whether this rate will be different when larger numbers are studied.

REFERENCES

1. Wallace JI, Coral FS, Rim IR, et al. T-cell ratios in homosexuals (letter). Lancet 1982;1:908.
2. Kornfeld H, VanDe Stowe RA, Lange M, et al. T-lymphocyte subpopulations in homosexual men. N Eng J Med 1982;307:729–31.
3. Curran J. CDC control study. Reported at the American Society of Microbiology meeting, New York City, Sept. 10, 1982.
4. Reinherz E, Schlossman SF. The differentiation and function of human T lymphocytes. Cell 1982;19:821–27.
5. Reinherz E, O'Brian C, Rosenthal P, Schlossman SF. The cellular basis for viral-induced immunodeficiency: Analysis by monoclonal antibodies. J Immunol 1980; 125:1269–74.
6. Witkin SS, Sonnabend J. Immune responses to spermatazoa in homosexual men. Fertil Steril 1983;39:337.
7. Witkin SS, Bongiovanni AM, Yu IR, et al. Humoral immune responses in healthy heterosexual, homosexual and vasectomized men and in homosexual men with the acquired immune deficiency syndrome. AIDS Res 1983/4;1:31–44.
8. Kung PC, Goldstein G, Reinherz EL, Schlossman SF. Monoclonal antibodies defining distinctive human T-cell surface antigens. Science 1979;206:347–49.
9. Thomas Y, Sosman J, Irigoyeu OH, et al. Interactions among human T cell subsets. Int J Immunopharmacol 1981;3:193–201.
10. Witkin SS, Zelikovsky G, Bongiovanni AM, et al. IgA antibody to spermatazoa in seminal and prostate fluids of subfertile men. J Am Med Assoc 1982;247:1014.
11. Witkin SS, Zelikovsky G, Good RA, Day NK. Demonstration of 11S IgA antibodies to spermatozoa in human seminal fluid. Exp Immunol 1981;44:368–74.

12. Witkin SS, Sonnabend J, Richards JM, Purtilo D. Inductions of antibody to asialo GM1 by spermatazoa and its occurrence in the sera of homosexual men with acquired immonodeficiency syndrome (AIDS). Exp Immunol 1983;54:346–50.
13. Witkin SD, Zelikovsky G, Bongiovanni AM, et al. Sperm-related antigen, antibodies and circulating immune complexes in sera of recently vasectomized men. J Clin Invest 1982;70:33.
14. Wallace JJ, Mann J, Beatrice S. HIV-1 exposure among clients of prostitutes. IV International Conference on AIDS. Abstract 7833. Stockholm, Sweden: June 15, 1988.
15. Wallace JI, Christonikos N, Mann J. HIV exposure in New York City streetwalkers (prostitutes). Presented at the Third International AIDS Conference, Washington, D.C., June 4, 1987.
16. International Conference on AIDS in Children, Adolescents and Heterosexual Adults. An Interdisciplinary Approach to Prevention, Atlanta, February 19–21, 1987.
17. Van De Perre P, Carael M, Robert-Guroff M, et al. Female prostitutes: A risk group for infection with human T-cell lymphotropic virus type III. Lancet 1985;2:524–27.
18. Kreiss JK, Koech D, Plummer FA, et al. AIDS virus infection in Nairobi prostitutes. N Engl J Med 1986;314:414–18.
19. Barton SE, Underhill GS, Gilchrist C, et al. HTLV-III antibody in prostitutes. Lancet 1985;2:1424.
20. Brenky-Fandeux D, Fibourg-Blanc A. HTLV-III antibody in prostitutes. Lancet 1985;1424.
21. Tirelli U, Vaccer E, Carbone A, et al. HTLV-III antibody in prostitutes. Lancet 1985;2:1421.
22. Papaevangelou G, Roumeliotou-Karayannis A, Kallinikos G, Papoutsakis G. LAV/HTLV-III infection in female prostitutes. Lancet 1985;2:1018.
23. Handsfield H, Kobayashi J, Fischl M, et al. Heterosexual transmission of human T lymphotropic virus type III/LAV-associated virus. MMWR 1985;34:561–63.
24. Handsfield H. Third International AIDS Meeting. Washington, D.C., June 4, 1987.
25. Vogt MW, Craven DE, Crawford DF, et al. Isolation of HTLV-III/LAV from cervical secretions of women at risk for AIDS. Lancet 1986;2:525–7.
26. Wofsy CB, Hauer LB, Michaelis BA, et al. Isolation of AIDS-associated retrovirus from genital secretions of women with antibodies to the virus. Lancet 1986;2:527–9.
27. Wallace JJ, Mann J, Beatrice S. HIV-1 exposure among clients of prostitutes. IV International Conference on AIDS. Abstract 4055. Stockholm, Sweden: June 13, 1988.

AIDS in Children

Anthony B. Minnefor
James M. Oleske

From time to time, a "new" disease appears on the medical scene and captures the medical community's attention and imagination because of its severity, unique features, or public health impact. Some, such as Kawasaki disease and toxic shock syndrome, were first encountered in infants, children, or adolescents. Others, like Lyme disease and legionnaires' disease, initially appeared in older patients. The latter situation pertained in the case of acquired immunodeficiency syndrome (AIDS).[1-4] From the earlier reports and studies, a distinct and unusual syndrome has emerged. The Centers for Disease Control (CDC) surveillance and clinical requirements for the diagnosis of adult AIDS have been presented (in Chapter 14).

The first indication that infants and children could be affected came from investigators in California, who reported the case of a 20-month-old, prematurely born, white male with transfusion-associated AIDS.[5] The infant had received multiple transfusions of irradiated blood products for anemia and hyperbilirubinemia secondary to Rh sensitization. Hepatosplenomegaly was noted at four months of age. The child subsequently developed neutropenia, autoimmune hemolytic anemia, thrombocytopenia, hypergammaglobulinemia, in vitro evidence of T cell dysfunction, and opportunistic infection. Investigation revealed that 1 of the 19 persons who had donated blood to this infant was a 48-year-old man who subsequently developed ultimately fatal AIDS. He was apparently well at the time of his donation but was presumably in the incubation period of his illness, when the putative etiologic agent for AIDS was already present in the blood. Subsequently, CDC received reports on four infants under two years of

---

The authors thank Mrs. Gail Thompson for her invaluable secretarial help in the preparation of this manuscript.

age with unexplained immune deficiency and opportunistic infection.[6] None of these infants was known to have been given blood or blood products or to have been sexually abused before their illness. All four, however, resided in households with recognized risks for AIDS—a Haitian mother (2) and a mother who was a prostitute and an intravenous (IV) drug abuser (2). These reports also commented on six other young children with similar illness who are still under investigation. Twelve additional children aged one to four years with T cell dysfunction, but without documented serious opportunistic infection, were also mentioned. Seven of the nine mothers on whom information was available were IV drug abusers.

In this chapter we will present data on our experience and that of others with AIDS in infants and children. In 1979, when we first began to encounter pediatric patients with otherwise-unexplained immune deficiencies, some of these individuals fit CDC's working definition of AIDS, while others would now be classified as having AIDS-related complex (ARC). None of the children we reported on had cystic fibrosis, sickle cell anemia, or underlying malignancy, nor did any demonstrate recognized laboratory or clinical patterns for known congenital immune defects or infection.

Since our first report on the subject, considerably more data have accumulated.[7] This has permitted a far better understanding of AIDS in the pediatric age group. We have chosen to present some instructive cases from our experience, followed by a discussion of the literature.

It is not surprising that the Newark, N.J., metropolitan area did, and continues to, experience an epidemic of pediatric AIDS. Unlike other major population centers with a high incidence of adult AIDS, over 50% of New Jersey patients are male IV drug abusers.[8] With what is currently known about heterosexual transmission of human immunodeficiency virus (HIV), the concomitant higher rate of infection in women and their offspring was predictable.

CASE 1

Case 1 was a black male born at term by cesarean section. His birth weight was 8 lb. He was well until five months of age (April 1982), when he developed a cough with fever; interstitial pneumonia was diagnosed radiographically. Over the next two weeks respiratory failure ensued, and he required ventilatory support. Lung biopsy showed *Pneumocystis carinii*. The patient was treated with trimethoprim/sulfamethoxazole and pentamidine but did not improve. He died seven weeks after hospitalization. Autopsy revealed thymic hypoplasia with depletion of T cell areas in the reticuloendothelial system. This infant's parents, natives of Haiti, are both in good health. Immunologic studies demonstrated lymphopenia and reversal of helper/suppressor T cell ratios in both parents.

This child's symptoms most closely resembled AIDS as it appears in adults. Immunologic studies and autopsy findings were nondiagnostic for any known congenital immune deficiency syndrome. Both parents were in good health despite laboratory studies consistent with AIDS. Although being a Haitian is no longer "officially" listed as a risk factor, the incidence of AIDS in Haitians seems disproportionately high.

CASE 2

Case 2 was a 27-month-old black male noted at birth (October 1980) to have hepatomegaly, but he was otherwise healthy until one month of age, when he presented with failure to thrive, significant hepatosplenomegaly, anemia, pyoderma, atopic dermatitis, and adenopathy. He was hospitalized four times for recurrent febrile illnesses; one included *Salmonella* gastroenteritis. Extensive evaluation ruled out Wiskott-Aldrich syndrome and Leiner's disease as well as other defined congenital immune defects. Serial immunologic evaluation demonstrated a progressive depression of cellular immune functions with a reversal of helper/suppressor T cell ratios and a polyclonal hypergammaglobulinemia. The patient developed thrush and interstitial pneumonia in December 1982. Lung biopsy demonstrated lymphocytic interstitial pneumonia (LIP), and skin biopsy showed atopic dermatitis. The mother frequently abused IV heroin and cocaine with some weight loss, but she had normal immunologic function.

Follow-up demonstrated a progressive decline in the patient's cellular immune function, increasing hypergammaglobulinemia, and worsening clinical status. This patient, one of our cases with LIP, died.

CASE 3

Case 3 was a 24-month-old Hispanic male who first presented at nine months of age (March 1982) because of recurrent high fever, hepatosplenomegaly, pneumonia, and lymphadenopathy associated with failure to thrive and a mild eczema-like rash. Between nine and 20 months of age he had four admissions for recurrent febrile illness, one of which was associated with *Salmonella* sepsis and enteritis and another with esophageal candidiasis. Extensive laboratory evaluation documented persistently elevated Epstein-Barr virus (EBV) titers associated with progressive depression of cellular immunity and polyclonal hypergammaglobulinemia. Biopsy studies demonstrated a normally reactive bone marrow, follicular hyperplasia of lymph nodes with prominence of immunoblasts and plasma cells, lymphoid cell infiltration of portal tracts of the liver, and LIP. An extensive evaluation at the National Institutes of Health Research Hospital (before the availability of HIV serology) failed to determine a specific diagnosis. At birth, the patient had mild enlargement of his liver and jaundice, but he was discharged from the nursery without apparent problems. His mother had no known risk factors for AIDS and had normal immunologic studies. His father was an IV drug user with recent weight loss and adenopathy. His paternal uncle, a household contact, was a homosexual and a drug abuser who had been diagnosed as having AIDS.

This child was exposed to two adult males in his household who were potential sources for AIDS. Recognized persistent EBV infection syndromes have been ruled out. Persistent infection with EBV, *Candida*, *Salmonella*, and LIP in conjunction with an expanding immune defect made a strong case for AIDS.

CASE 4

Case 4 was a 28-month-old black female identical twin who was first hospitalized at seven weeks of age (October 1980), along with her twin, for *Salmonella* septicemia. Her twin recovered rapidly without sequelae, but patient 4 required a two-month hospitalization because of malabsorption, failure to thrive, anemia, and oral and esophageal moniliasis. She had four subsequent admissions for progressive interstitial pneumonia, continued failure to thrive with malabsorption, pneumococcal sepsis, hepatosplenomegaly, and mild atopic dermatitis. A bone marrow examination showed an increase in lymphocytes and plasmacytic cells. A duodenal biopsy showed severe blunting of villi with elongated cysts and diffuse lymphoplasmacytic infiltration. A lung biopsy revealed LIP. Serial studies demonstrated increasing depression of cell-mediated immunity associated with polyclonal hypergammaglobulinemia. Immunologic evaluation of the patient's twin was normal. Her mother was a prostitute and occasional drug user but refused further evaluation.

Illness occurring in only one of identical twins is a strong argument against congenital immune defect. As did four other patients, this infant had problems with *Salmonella* infections and also had LIP.

CASE 5

Case 5 was a 22-month-old black male who was well until six months of age (June 1981), when he was admitted to hospital for fever, cough, interstitial pneumonia, failure to thrive, mild eczemalike skin rash, and oral and esophageal candidiasis. He was admitted five more times for progression of his interstitial pneumonia, recurrent febrile episodes, chronic oral candidiasis, and failure to thrive. He had cortical brain atrophy on computed tomography (CT) scan of the head and an abnormal electroencephalogram (EEG) but a normal cerebrospinal fluid (CSF) study. Extensive serial evaluations during these hospitalizations revealed elevated cytomegalovirus (CMV) titers with isolation of CMV from the urine and adenovirus from the stool. He had progressive deterioration of cell-mediated immunity functions and polyclonal hypergammaglobulinemia. His mother was a heavy IV drug abuser with weight loss, chronic diarrhea, and depressed cell-mediated immunity with a reversed helper/suppressor T cell ratio. The father was also an IV drug abuser but appeared to be in good health and had normal immune functions.

The progressive immune impairment associated with deep-tissue *Candida* infections and interstitial pneumonia in a child cared for by a mother with laboratory and clinical evidence of AIDS supports the diagnosis of AIDS in the child. Like some of our other patients, this child had neurologic impairment manifested by cortical brain atrophy and seizure activity. Although no specific neurologic diagnosis has been established for these children, the presence of central nervous system (CNS) involvement is comparable to a similar predisposition in adults with AIDS.[9,10]

CASE 6

Case 6 was a 5-year-old black female who died in 1979 from gram-negative sepsis. She first became ill at six months of age with anemia, hepatosplenomegaly, and failure to thrive associated with thrombocytopenia and *Salmonella* and pneumococcal sepsis. At two years of age she had a splenectomy for steroid-unresponsive anemia and thrombocytopenia. At four years of age she continued to have bouts of *Salmonella* and pneumococcal sepsis and was noted to have chronic interstitial infiltrates on chest x-ray study. Immunologic studies at four years of age demonstrated depressed cell-mediated immunity and dysgammaglobulinemia. Autopsy demonstrated diffuse depletion of T-lymphocyte-dependent areas of the reticuloendothelial system and LIP in lung tissue. Her mother, 16 years old at delivery, was promiscuous and an IV drug abuser who also had idiopathic thrombocytopenia when the patient was born. The mother refused follow-up studies.

At first this child was thought to have Nezelof's syndrome. The immunologic findings of depressed cellular immunity with elevated IgM are compatible with both Nezelof's syndrome and AIDS. The presence of family risk factors, multiple blood transfusions, thrombocytopenia, and LIP suggest to us that, in retrospect, this child may represent one of the first examples of AIDS.

CASE 7

Case 7 was a full-term black female infant who was well until three months of age (September 1980), when she was hospitalized for pneumonia. At four months, she was seen in consultation for shortness of breath, cough, and oral moniliasis of one week's duration. A CT scan of the head showed cortical brain atrophy, and an EEG was abnormal. Increasing respiratory distress developed with hypoxia, necessitating lung biopsy, which revealed *P. carinii*. Depression of T cell numbers and function was noted. The infant continued to deteriorate despite appropriate therapy and died at five months of age. At death, CSF cultures were positive for *C. albicans*. The father was an IV drug addict who, when first hospitalized for bacterial lung abscess, had a low helper/suppressor T cell ratio with depressed mitogen response. He was subsequently diagnosed as having AIDS associated with oral candidiasis, weight loss, adenopathy, and interstitial pneumonia.

This child died three months before the onset of symptomatic AIDS in his father. The mother, in good health, denied IV drug abuse. When the child was first seen, a diagnosis of alveolar proteinosis was considered because of massive respiratory tract secretions. However, the clinical course, immunologic defects, and epidemiologic setting indicate that this child had AIDS.

CASE 8

This 5-year-old black female was admitted to hospital in December 1984 with a five-day history of fever, diarrhea, vomiting, and a "wheezy" pneumonia. (Her only previous hospitalization was at one year of age for asthma.) Initial laboratory evaluation showed trace blood and protein in the urine. The pneumonia failed to respond to bronchodilators and antibiotics, and there was progressive abdominal distention with generalized edema. The patient received prednisone for suspected nephrotic syndrome and was transferred for further evaluation.

Fever and respiratory distress persisted; edema and thrush developed. Laboratory data revealed a panhypogammaglobulinemia and a marked reversal in the helper/suppressor T cell ratio. A renal biopsy revealed focal glomerulosclerosis. Shortly thereafter a lung biopsy revealed *P. carinii*. The patient's condition deteriorated further, and she subsequently died of gram-negative peritonitis. An HIV antibody test was later reported as positive.

This patient is one of three children we have identified with clinical manifestations of HIV-associated nephropathy. She also represents our first patient in whom the disease may have been acquired secondary to sexual abuse. Sexual transmission was first considered because of the late age of disease onset. Suspicions were heightened when it was learned that the patient's live-in stepfather (who was an IV drug abuser) had sexually abused the patient's 15-year-old sister.

DISCUSSION

From rather tentative initial acceptance, there is now overwhelming agreement in the scientific and public health community on the existence of pediatric AIDS as a distinct entity. Early reluctance was based in part on concerns about distinguishing between congenital immune defects and congenital infections of the "classic" variety. This was compounded by incomplete data on the epidemiology of the disease, mode of transmission, and, most important, absence of confirmation of the suspected viral etiology for AIDS. All this has changed. Now, coupled with a steadily increasing clinical experience, a much clearer picture of pediatric AIDS has emerged.[11]

The CDC now defines pediatric AIDS as "an illness in a child under 13 years of age, who has had a reliably diagnosed disease at least moderately indicative of underlying cellular immunodeficiency and no known cause of reduced resistance reported to be associated with that disease." In addition to the exclusions mentioned elsewhere for adults, congenital infections such as toxoplasmosis, CMV, herpes simplex, and so on must be excluded as *primary* causative agents in the observed clinical picture. The high incidence of LIP in pediatric AIDS qualifies it as an opportunistic infection equivalent, and if the other criteria are met, it is sufficient to establish the diagnosis.[12] At present HIV seropositivity or viral isolation are not essential requirements. These tests can be useful in those instances where one of the rare congenital combined immune deficiency diseases such as Nezelof's syndrome is under strong consideration. It and other congenital defects would not be expected to be associated with HIV infection.[13]

It seems clear that most pediatric HIV infections and AIDS are acquired perinatally from infected women.[14,15] Transfusion-related infection (e.g., neonates, hemophiliacs) should diminish in parallel with donor screening and treatment of infused products. As noted earlier, sexual abuse can be a risk factor, and IV drug abuse or sexual acquisition must be considered in some older children who are functioning as emancipated minors.

Although the mechanisms are not clearly defined, HIV most likely is transmitted from infected mothers to their fetuses or offspring in utero, labor, and delivery or possibly shortly postpartem. Cesarean section does not seem to be protective (suggesting transplacental infection). There are also clinical and virologic data to implicate breast milk of infected mothers in transmission to a nursing infant.[16] It is too early to quantitate the risk to a fetus born of an HIV-positive mother. In one study, however, 65% of the infants had serologic or clinical evidence of infection. Other data put the risk much lower.[17] It is clear that additional studies are required before the rate of transmission and variables associated with it can be stated more definitively. What is evident, however, is that women need not be symptomatic to transmit potentially lethal infection to their offspring. Data regarding fetal wastage or even teratogenic potential of HIV are not available. Any such surveys must take into account the high rate of IV drug abuse and promiscuity (prostitution) in many women and the associated high rate of exposure to potentially harmful chemical substances and other infectious agents. Horizontal spread of HIV from casual contact in a household setting has not been corroborated but should not be entirely dismissed as a possibility until the molecular epidemiology of AIDS is further studied.[18]

In view of the aforementioned epidemiology, CDC has made the following recommendations. Counseling services and testing for antibody to HIV should be offered to pregnant women and women who may become pregnant in the following groups: (1) those who have evidence of HIV infection, (2) those who have used IV drugs for nonmedical purposes, (3) those who were born in countries where heterosexual transmission is thought to play a major role, (4) those who have engaged in prostitution, (5) those who are or have been sex partners of IV drug abusers, bisexual men, men with hemophilia, men who were born in countries where heterosexual transmission is thought to play a major role, or men who otherwise have evidence of HIV infection. Since detectable antibodies to HIV may take two to four months to develop, this should be taken into account, along with whether the woman is continuously exposed and requires repeat testing.[17]

The incubation period for HIV appears to vary with the route of transmission. In infants born to high-risk parents, the median time to onset of symptoms is four months. For transfusion-associated AIDS in children, the median time is eight months. (This is considerably shorter than the 28-month median in transfused adults.)[11] Evidence suggests that infants of high-risk parents are born with manifestations of the disease, including hepatosplenomegaly and small size for gestational age.[17]

The most constant abnormalities in children are failure to thrive (or low birth weight), chronic interstitial pneumonitis, and hepatosplenomegaly. These and other prominent features in childhood AIDS are listed in Table 18–4. Differences between adult and pediatric AIDS are more quantitative than qualitative; however, some additional observations are worthy of special note. Kaposi's sarcoma is rare, and *hepatitis B* infection is much less frequently encountered. The degree of lymphopenia is not as profound, but hypergammaglobulinemia seems more pronounced than in adults with AIDS. Chronic pneumonitis in which LIP alone is found is regularly seen in children and only rarely in adults. Serious bacterial infections with common pathogens (*Streptococcus pneumoniae, Haemophilus influenzae,* and *Salmonella* sp.) are more of a problem in children. This has been associated with significant abnormalities in humoral responses and supports the concept that both B cells and T cells play a role in poor specific antibody production.[19]

Perhaps the most disturbing recent observation in both the adult and pediatric population has been the detection of HIV in the brains of affected individuals.[9,10] Children manifest a progressive encephalopathy, which may be the first clinical sign of illness. Major features include loss of motor milestones or intellectual abilities, weakness with pyramidal tract signs, ataxia, and seizures. Most patients do not demonstrate opportunistic infection of the CNS at postmortem examination, providing strong evidence that HIV can cause a primary, persistent, and progressive infection of the brain.

Conventional antimicrobial therapy and supportive measures have resulted in morbidity and mortality roughly comparable to that of adult AIDS patients. (Onset earlier than one month of age carries a particularly poor prognosis.) A few infants have reached school age and are able to attend classes. Intravenous gammaglobulin given at least monthly has dramatically reduced the incidence of bacterial sepsis. Attempts to intervene with antiviral agents or immunomodulators are just beginning, and no data are currently available.

CONCLUSION

Pediatric AIDS patients currently only represent a very small number relative to the epidemic at large (less than 300 reported cases.) However, their number is expected to grow steadily in those geographic areas and social circumstances in which females are likely to be exposed to the causative agent. At present, there is even less reason for optimism concerning control and management of AIDS in children than there is for AIDS in adults.

REFERENCES

1. Gottlieb MS, Schroff R, Schanker RM, et al. *Penumocystis carinii* pneumonia and mucosal candidiasis in previously healthy homosexual men. Evidence of a new acquired cellular immunodeficiency. N Engl J Med 1981;305:1425.
2. Mildvan D, Mathur A, Enlow R, et al. Opportunistic infections and immune deficiency in homosexual men. Ann Intern Med 1982;96:700.
3. Vieira J, Frank E, Spira T, Landesman SH. Acquired immune deficiency in Haitians. N Engl J Med 1983;308:125.
4. Lederman MM, Ratnoff OD, Scillian JJ, et al. Impaired cell-mediated immunity in patients with classic hemophilia. N Engl J Med 1983;308:79.
5. Centers for Disease Control. Possible transfusion-associated acquired immune deficiency syndrome (AIDS). California. MMWR 1982;31:652.
6. Centers for Disease Control. Unexplained immunodeficiency and opportunistic infections in infants. New York, New Jersey, California. MMWR 1982;31:665.
7. Oleske J, Minnefor A, Cooper R, et al. Immune deficiency syndrome in children. JAMA 1983;249:2345.
8. Curran J, Morgan W, Hardy A, et al. The epidemiology of AIDS: Current status and future prospects. Science 1985;229:1352.
9. Shaw G, Harper M, Hahn B, et al. HTLV-III infection in brains of children and adults with AIDS encephalopathy. Science 1985;222:177.
10. Epstein L, Sharer L, Joshi V, et al. Progressive encephalopathy in children with acquired immune deficiency syndrome. Ann Neurol 1985;17:488.
11. Rogers M. AIDS in children: A review of the clinical, epidemiologic and public health aspects. Pediatr Infect Dis 1985;4:230.
12. Centers for Disease Control. Pediatric AIDS. MMWR 1985;34:373.
13. Ammann A, Kaminsky L, Cowan M, Levy J. Antibodies to AIDS-associated retrovirus distinguish between pediatric primary and acquired immunodeficiency diseases. JAMA 1985;253:3116.
14. Rubinstein A, Sicklick M, Gupta A, et al. Acquired immunodeficiency with reversed T4/T8 ratios in infants born to promiscuous and drug-addicted mothers. JAMA 1983;249:2350.
15. Scott G, Fischl M, Klimas N, et al. Mothers of infants with acquired immunodeficiency syndrome. JAMA 1985;253:363.
16. Ziegler J, Cooper D, Johnson R, Gold J. Postnatal transmission of AIDS-associated retrovirus from mother to infant. Lancet 1985;1:896.
17. Centers for Disease Control. Recommendations for assisting in the prevention of perinatal transmission of HTLV-III/LAV and AIDS. MMWR 1985;34:721.
18. Kaplan J, Oleske J, Getchell J, et al. Evidence against transmission of human T-lymphotropic virus/lymphadenopathy-associated virus (HTLV-III/LAV) in families of children with the acquired immunodeficiency syndrome. Pediatr Infect Dis 1985;4:468.
19. Bernstein L, Krieger B, Novick B, et al. Bacterial infection in the acquired immunodeficiency syndrome of children. Pediatr Infect Dis 1985;4:472.

AIDS in Prisoners

Gary P. Wormser

Prison inmates are a growing population whose complex medical and social needs present a serious challenge to the health care profession. In 1984 one of approximately every 500 Americans was incarcerated in a state or federal prison. The prison population nationally had reached an all-time high of 454,136 inmates, with 32,276 confined in New York State alone.[1,2]

Prisoners as a group differ from the general population in regard to several important demographic features pertinent to the epidemic of acquired immunodeficiency syndrome (AIDS). First, the vast majority of prisoners are young men. For example, in 1981 when AIDS was first described, the median age of inmates in prisons in the New York State correctional system was 27.8 years, and 96% were male.[2] Second, a background of illicit drug use is very common in these individuals. A survey in 1978 by the Department of Justice found that 61% of inmates had used heroin, methadone, cocaine, marijuana, amphetamines, or barbiturates without medical sanction.[3] In a 1975 study of more than 1400 detainees of New York City prisons, 41% were found to have used illicit drugs, and more than 80% of those inmates abused heroin.[4] Third, homosexual activity during confinement is known to take place and may well occur with greater frequency than it does among civilians. In one study in which inmates from 17 different federal facilities were surveyed, 30% of prisoners admitted to homosexual activity in prison.[5]

The similarity of many of these characteristics of prisoners to those of AIDS patients diagnosed throughout the United States (Table 18–5)[6] is so striking as

---

I gratefully thank the following people for their many contributions to the research efforts described in this chapter: Drs. J. Hanrahan, L. Krupp, E. Gelberg, S. Cunningham-Rundles, E. Allen, G. Gavis, R. E. Stahl, R. Yarrish, F. Duncanson, and R. Broaddus, and Mss. B. Maguire and S. Gamble. In October 1986, the contract between Westchester County Medical Center and the New York State Correctional System was discontinued.

Table 18-5 Comparison of prisoners in the New York State correctional system with AIDS patients diagnosed in the United States

	Prisoners[a]	AIDS Patients
Median age (yr)	28	34
Percent male	96	94
History of IV drug abuse (%)[b]	50	24
Homosexuality (%)	Not known	73

[a]All figures are approximations.
[b]Includes both heterosexual and homosexual IV drug abusers.

to suggest that prisoners are likely to be a high-risk group for AIDS. Evidence to support this conjecture came in late 1981 when the first prisoner with the syndrome was identified. The first report of this event appeared in the medical literature in 1982.[7] In 1983, Wormser et. al.[8] described in detail seven previously healthy male inmates from the New York State correctional system who were diagnosed to have AIDS and *Pneumocystis carinii* pneumonia between September 1981 and June 1982. The seven prisoners had a mean age of 29 years and had been incarcerated for 18 months on average before AIDS was diagnosed. All the inmates were heterosexual before incarceration and vehemently denied homosexual contact while in prison. However, all readily admitted to use of intravenous (IV) narcotics with a mean reported duration of use of 12 years (range, 7 to 25 years). Like other AIDS patients, these prisoners had profound defects in cellular immune function as indicated by cutaneous anergy, lymphopenia, and inversion of the normal ratio of helper to suppressor T cell lymphocyte populations. Since this report, an escalating number of cases of AIDS have been diagnosed among New York State prisoners, mirroring (and possibly surpassing) the epidemic among high-risk civilians, with an annual incidence rate of 329 cases per 100,000 for the year 1985. There is no evidence that this incidence rate has stabilized.

Westchester County Medical Center (WCMC), through a contractual agreement, acts as a referral hospital for three county and 11 state correctional facilities (over 11,000 inmates). Approximately one-third of New York State's total prisoner population is in the catchment area served by this medical center. Almost half of all New York State prisoners with AIDS have been hospitalized at WCMC or use its outpatient services. As of December 1984, 73 prisoners with AIDS had been seen at WCMC. Among these patients, the initial diagnostic manifestations of the syndrome (Table 18–6) were *P. carinii* pneumonia in 50 (69%), cerebral toxoplasmosis in eight (11%), Kaposi's sarcoma in four (5%), cryptococcal meningitis in three (4%), brain lymphoma in two (3%), cryptosporidiosis in two (3%), and other opportunistic infections in four (5%). Over 90% of these patients were men, and, in the large majority of cases, the only identified risk factor for AIDS was IV drug use before incarceration. Indeed, the low frequency of Kaposi's sarcoma found in these patients is consistent with the

Table 18-6 Initial manifestation of AIDS in 73 prisoners seen at Westchester County Medical Center between Nov. 1981 and Dec. 1984

Criterion for AIDS	%
P. carinii pneumonia	69
CNS toxoplasmosis	11
Kaposi's sarcoma	5
Cryptococcal meningitis	4
Brain lymphoma	3
Cryptosporidiosis	3
Miscellaneous	5

observation that homosexuality is a relatively unimportant risk factor for prisoners with AIDS.[6]

Certain features peculiar to the New York State prison system make prisoners with AIDS unique and permit studies not possible in other populations with AIDS (Table 18-7). They are (1) in the prison setting, laboratory studies and medical examinations are routinely performed on entry; (2) the date of discontinuation (or reduction) of IV drug use is known; (3) the size of the population is precisely known; and (4) postmortem examinations are required by law. These characteristics proved useful in helping to address some difficult issues well before the discovery of the etiologic agent of AIDS. The first issue was whether AIDS was acquired in prison, or did inmates have the disease before incarceration? Prisoners with AIDS may well be the only group of AIDS patients for whom systematic retrospective reviews of medical records are possible. The second issue concerned the incubation period of AIDS in IV drug abusers, a group especially hard to evaluate, since most of these individuals regularly and continuously engage in high-risk behavior until AIDS symptoms begin. In contrast, IV drug abusers who are prisoners have an interrupted exposure history, stopping or drastically reducing IV drug use at the time of incarceration.

It was reasoned that if AIDS actually predated entry into the state corrections system, some laboratory abnormality might be discovered through retrospective inspection of the routine blood tests done on all prisoners when they entered the system. To this end, we studied the entrance total leukocyte counts on 19 prisoners who were diagnosed with AIDS between November 1981 and January

Table 18-7 Features associated with incarceration in the New York State correctional system pertinent to AIDS

- Date of discontinuation (or reduction) of IV drug use known
- Postmortem examinations required by law
- Laboratory studies and medical examinations routinely performed on entry
- Size of population precisely known

1983.[9] We chose to study leukocyte counts, since anecdotal experience had suggested that these counts were usually depressed in AIDS patients. Five prisoners were excluded, three because they had symptoms on entry, one because no leukocyte count was done, and one because he lacked an identifiable risk factor for AIDS. The 14 remaining prisoners were all heterosexual IV drug abusers before incarceration.

Each prisoner with AIDS was matched with three controls of the same age (within three years), sex, and race and with a similar date of entry into the New York State correctional system and a history of IV drug abuse. The three control prisoners chosen were those with an identification number closest to that of an index case who met each of the five matching criteria.

The 14 inmates with AIDS first developed symptoms of the disease 12.4 ± 7.6 months (mean $\pm$ SD) after the leukocyte counts were done. Nevertheless, 12 (86%) of these 14 AIDS patients had entrance leukocyte counts of <5000 cells/mm^3, versus only 6 (14%) of the 42 controls (<0.00001 by Fisher exact test). The mean leukocyte count for the AIDS inmates was 4430 cells/mm^3, compared with 6320 cells/mm^3 for the controls ($P < 0.005$ by F exact test for matched samples).

These findings are consistent with the premise that these inmates were infected before the entrance laboratory test. They also suggest that leukopenia is a typical (but nondiagnostic) laboratory abnormality associated with the incubation period of AIDS. Since all but three denied participation in high-risk activities (IV drug use or homosexual acts) following incarceration, it was deduced that most, if not all, were infected before entering prison. Since the mean interval from time of incarceration to onset of AIDS was 22.6 months (4 to 36 months) for these 14 prisoners, it is reasonable to conclude that the incubation period in IV drug abusers with AIDS may be more than two years, a figure consistent with the results of other studies done on recipients of contaminated blood transfusions.[10] Furthermore, most of these prisoners had been incarcerated between 1979 and 1981, around the time of, or shortly after, entry of human immunodeficiency virus (HIV), the etiologic agent of AIDS, into the United States. This information, plus the study findings, suggest that the mean incubation period from onset of HIV infection to development of AIDS for this specific group of IV drug abusers was approximately two to four years.

Inclusion of New York State prisoners in the AIDS epidemic also helped to clarify an early controversy over whether AIDS was a new illness or one that had been merely overlooked by the medical community. This came about because, unlike most other patient groups with AIDS, New York State prisoners who die are required by law to undergo a postmortem examination. At present the most common cause of death among prisoners in New York State is AIDS, and at postmortem examination there is usually clear evidence of an opportunistic infection.[11,12] If undiagnosed cases of AIDS had been occurring in the general population before recognition of the syndrome, it stands to reason that some prisoners would have also been affected and very likely would have died of it. Review of postmortem records on all 168 prisoners who died from nontraumatic causes during approximately five years preceding the first recognized case of

AIDS in a New York State prisoner, however, failed to show anything suggesting AIDS.[8] Additionally, even for the three prisoners who had an unexplained respiratory death, there was no evidence of *P. carinii* pneumonia on subsequent reexamination of lung tissue using special stains for this organism. These observations, along with other data, have helped to establish that AIDS is genuinely a new illness in the United States.[13]

An additional feature of the prison population is that it is a well-defined group for whom population sizes are known and incidence figures can be calculated. This information has helped to strengthen the association of lymphoma and AIDS. Lymphomas, especially non-Hodgkin's lymphomas, had been suspected to be an important clinical manifestation of AIDS based on their occurrence in homosexual men at risk for AIDS.[14,15] The total number of homosexual men is, however, unknown, and thus it is impossible to compute exact incidence or prevalence figures for lymphoma in this group. Therefore, it has never been conclusively established that homosexual men have a greater frequency of this neoplasm than does the general population.

Ahmed et al.[16] determined the incidence rate of non-Hodgkin's lymphomas among New York State prisoners based on patients seen at WCMC. Among the general population aged 20 to 49 years, the annual incidence of non-Hodgkin's lymphoma is approximately 3.8 per 100,000. In contrast, among the prisoners studied of the same age group, the incidence rate was 21.5 to 67.2 per 100,000, representing a relative risk 5.7 to 17.7 times higher than in the general population. Similar to the experience with AIDS in prisoners, non-Hodgkin's lymphoma occurred almost exclusively in the prisoner subpopulation that included former IV drug abusers. Indeed, in this group the relative risk of non-Hodgkin's lymphoma may be as high as 164-fold greater than in the general population. These data support the theory that non-Hodgkin's lymphoma is another manifestation of AIDS.

In summary, New York State prisoners are a group well established to be at risk for AIDS. So far, the principal explanation for the elevated incidence of AIDS in this population appears to be IV drug use before incarceration. Because New York State prisoners with AIDS differ from other risk groups in regard to several important epidemiologic features associated with incarceration, certain studies of this patient population may be done that are difficult, if not impossible, to do in other risk groups. Results of these investigations have given insight into the date of onset of AIDS in the United States, the incubation period of AIDS, the association of leukopenia with prodromal AIDS, and the occurrence of non-Hodgkin's lymphoma as another manifestation of the expanding clinical spectrum of HIV infection.

REFERENCES

1. U.S. Department of Justice. Memo and census report of state and federal correctional facilities. Washington, D.C.: U.S. Government Printing Office, Aug. 6, 1984.

2. Krupp LB, Gelberg EA, Wormser GP. Prisoners as medical patients. Am J Public Health 1987;77:859–60.
3. Barton WI. Drug histories and criminality of inmates of local jails in the United States: Implication for treatment and rehabilitation of the drug abuser in a jail setting. Int J Addic 1982;17:417–44.
4. Novick LF, Dello Penna R, Schwartz MS, et al. Health status of the New York City prison population. Med Care 1977;15:205–16.
5. Nacci PL, Kane TR. Sex and sexual aggression in federal prisons: Progress reports. Washington, D.C.: U.S. Department of Justice, 1982.
6. Jaffe HW, Bregman DJ, Selik RM. Acquired immunodeficiency syndrome in the United States: The first 1000 cases. J Infect Dis 1983;148:339–45.
7. Hanrahan JP, Wormser GP, Maguire GP, et al. Opportunistic infections in prisoners. N Engl J Med 1982;307:498.
8. Wormser GP, Krupp LB, Hanrahan JP, et al. Acquired immunodeficiency syndrome in male prisoners. New insights into an emerging syndrome. Ann Intern Med 1983;98:297–303.
9. Hanrahan JP, Wormser GP, Reilly AA, et al. Prolonged incubation period of AIDS in intravenous drug abusers: Epidemiologic evidence in prison inmates. J Infect Dis 1984;150:263–6.
10. Curran JW, Lawrence DN, Jaffe H, et al. Acquired immunodeficiency syndrome (AIDS) associated with transfusions. N Engl J Med 1984;310:69–75.
11. De Lorenzo LJ, Maguire GP, Wormser GP, et al. Persistence of *Pneumocystis carinii* pneumonia in the acquired immunodeficiency syndrome. Evaluation of therapy by follow-up transbronchial lung biopsy. Chest 1985;88:79–83.
12. Stahl RE. General pathology of AIDS. In: Wormser GP, Stahl RE, Bottone EJ, eds. AIDS, acquired immune deficiency syndrome and other manifestations of HIV infection. Park Ridge, N.J.: Noyes Publications, 1987;838–66.
13. Auerbach DM, Bennett JV, Brachman PS, et al. Report of the Centers for Disease Control task force on Kaposi's sarcoma and opportunistic infections: Epidemiological aspects of the current outbreak of Kaposi's sarcoma and opportunistic infections. N Engl J Med 1982;306:248–52.
14. Levine AM, Meyer PR, Begandy MK, et al. Development of B-cell lymphoma in homosexual men: Clinical and immunologic findings. Ann Intern Med 1984;100:7–13.
15. Ziegler JL, Beckstead JA, Volberding PA, et al. Non-Hodgkin's lymphoma in 90 homosexual men. Relation to generalized lymphadenopathy and the acquired immunodeficiency syndrome. N Engl J Med 1984;311:565–70.
16. Ahmed T, Wormser GP, Stahl RE, et al. Malignant lymphomas in a population at risk for acquired immune deficiency syndrome. Cancer 1987;60:719–23.

Chapter 19

AIDS in Europe, and the Immunodeficiency of AIDS

Bo Hofmann
Jan Gerstoft
Bjarne Ørskov Lindhardt

By December 1987, cases of acquired immunodeficiency syndrome (AIDS) had been reported from all Western European countries.[1] The total number of reported cases was above 10,000 (Table 19–1). In Europe, homosexual men comprised the major risk group, representing 59% of all AIDS cases. Five percent were without known risk factors (18% of these had a geographic origin from outside Europe), 20% were intravenous (IV) drug abusers, 3% were hemophiliacs, and 8% were recipients of transfusion or other blood products.

Three hundred and eighty-two of the patients came from Africa, and they were predominantly located in Belgium, France, and Switzerland. However, at least half of these African patients presumably contracted the disease outside Europe, since they reported symptoms before entrance. The IV drug abusers were predominantly located in Southern Europe. In Northern Europe, including the United Kingdom and The Netherlands, homosexual men accounted for more than 80% of the cases.

In retrospect, the number of diagnosed AIDS cases per capita in France, Switzerland,[2] and Denmark[3] by 1980 to 1981 matched or even exceeded those in the United States. Also suggesting a relatively early appearance of human immunodeficiency virus (HIV) in Europe are a number of case reports documenting the occurrence of AIDS-like syndromes as far back as 1976. However, the virus might not by then have reached subgroups allowing rapid propagation, and the import of HIV to Europe from the United States during the first part of the 1980s[4] remains the only epidemiologically well-documented intercontinental travel of the virus.

The authors appreciate the helpful critical review and suggestions of Arne Svejgaard, M.D., D.Sc., Tissue Typing Laboratory, University Hospital, Copenhagen, during the preparation of this chapter.

Table 19-1 Total number of AIDS cases reported in 18 European countries and estimated rates per million population

Country	July 1984	July 1985	July 1987	December 1987	1987 Rates per Million
Austria		18	93	139	18.3
Belgium		99	255	277	28.0
Bulgaria			1	1	.1
Czechoslovakia			7	8	.5
Denmark	28	48	176	228	44.7
Finland		6	19	24	4.9
France	180	392	1980	3073	55.3
German Democratic Republic			4	6	.4
German Federal Republic	79	220	1133	1669	27.4
Greece	2	9	49	88	8.8
Hungary			5	8	.8
Iceland			4	4	20.0
Ireland			19	33	9.4
Israel			39	47	10.7
Italy	8	52	870	1411	24.6
Luxembourg		1	7	9	22.5
Malta			6	7	17.5
The Netherlands	21	66	308	420	28.8
Norway		11	49	70	16.7
Poland			2	3	.1
Portugal			67	90	8.7
Romania			2	3	.1
Spain	14	38	508	789	20.2
Sweden	7	27	129	163	19.4
Switzerland	28	63	266	355	53.8
United Kingdom	54	176	870	1227	21.6
USSR			3	3	0
Yugoslavia			11	26	1.1
Total	421	1226	6882	10181	

The epidemic in Europe has not progressed as rapidly as in the United States. The number of cases has doubled approximately every ten months, not every six months as observed during the beginning of the epidemic in the United States. This might be related to differences in lifestyle among high-risk groups.

The epidemiology of AIDS in Europe led, by 1983, to the important identification of the African connection. Apart from this, findings and routes of transmission have been similar to those in the United States. As of 1988, a generalized heterosexual spread among Europeans had not been identified.

PREVALENCE OF HIV ANTIBODIES

The recognition of HIV as the probable cause of AIDS, and the subsequent development of a widely applicable serologic test, has provided researchers with a powerful tool for investigating the epidemiology of AIDS. Despite some differences in the techniques used to detect antibodies to HIV, it is generally agreed that the presence of antibodies as measured by a screening procedure (radioimmunoassay [RIP], enzyme-linked immunosorbent assay [ELISA], and a confirmatory Western blot) is a sign of ongoing retroviral infection.

The incidence of AIDS in Denmark is one of the highest in Europe, and the first cases of AIDS in Europe were reported in Denmark. Likewise, seropositivity existed as early as 1978,[5] with patients still being seropositive and clinically healthy eight years later. In a study performed in December 1981, 250 homosexuals enrolled through a gay organization were serologically investigated.[4] Twenty-two individuals (9%) had antibodies to HIV, and the seroconversion rate from December 1981 through February 1983 was 1% per month. Three years after the initial investigation, 9% of the initial seropositive individuals had developed AIDS, and 9% had developed AIDS-related complex (ARC).

Another study investigated homosexuals in two Danish sauna clubs between June 1982 and March 1983.[6] Forty of 171 persons (23%) had antibodies to HIV. During follow-up, a conversion rate of 3% per month was observed. In a four year follow-up period, three of these anti-HIV-positive individuals had developed AIDS.[7]

Gerstoft et al.[8] investigated 64 promiscuous healthy homosexuals at venereal disease clinics in Copenhagen between October 1982 and May 1983. Twenty-one (33%) had antibodies to HIV. In this study, a significant association was found between HIV antibodies and lymphadenopathy, cytomegalovirus (CMV) isolation, low skin test score, and verified fever within a two-month period before investigation. On the other hand, no significant differences occurred in the total number of T cells, CD8 positive cells, CD4 positive cells, or CD4/CD8 ratio between seropositive and seronegative individuals. Forty-eight members of this cohort were reinvestigated in 1985, and the seropositivity rate had increased to 60%. Of the seronegative group, 35% had converted during a median observation period of 30 months. Of the 21 individuals originally seropositive, three individuals (14%) had developed AIDS, and three (14%) had developed ARC. In addition, low CD4 cell counts and inverted CD4/CD8 ratios were significantly associated with seropositivity. This emphasizes the long course of HIV infection.

In 1984 free screening clinics were established by the Danish Health Authorities. On average, one-third of the homosexual males who attended the clinics had antibodies to HIV. A pronounced fluctuation in the rate of seropositivity was observed. During periods of pronounced media attention to AIDS, the rate of seropositivity decreased, probably because people of lower risk also attended the clinics.

After Denmark, France, and Belgium, Switzerland has the highest incidence of AIDS in Europe. In France, rates of seropositivity among asymptomatic homosexuals were 18% to 20% in two studies[9,10] at VD clinics. In Switzerland, 10% of healthy homosexual males had antibodies[11] in 1985. In the United Kingdom, 53 of 308 (17%) homosexuals at risk visiting a VD clinic between 1982 and 1984 were seropositive.[12] At another VD clinic, 4 of 107 (4%) homosexual males were positive in March 1982. This figure rose to 26 of 124 (21%) in July 1985.[13] A large German multicenter survey revealed a rate of seropositivity of 204/814 (25%) among homosexuals investigated during 1984. In contrast to the high incidence of AIDS in Denmark, the incidence in the other parts of Scandinavia at that time was still low.

The high prevalence of AIDS in IV drug abusers in Central and Southern Europe is reflected in the high prevalence of HIV antibodies in these populations. At that time, HIV was not introduced to Danish drug abusers before 1983. The study of antibodies to HIV in hemophiliacs reflects the source of factor VIII preparation. Hemophiliacs treated with commercial preparations, usually containing American products, have a far higher incidence of antibodies to HIV than those treated with local, noncommercial factor VIII preparations.[14]

In summary, HIV infection is generally spreading in Europe, although at different rates in different countries. Positive measures are needed to restrict the spread of HIV from high-incidence areas to low-incidence ones.

IMMUNODEFICIENCY OF AIDS

AIDS is characterized by deficient cellular immunity, which leads to infections with opportunistic microorganisms usually combatted by the T lymphocytes. It is important to determine the exact nature of this immunodeficiency, since an understanding of the immunologic mechanisms involved can provide a basis for rational treatment of the disease.

HIV is lymphotropic for CD4 positive cells,[15] that is, mostly T helper lymphocytes. After becoming infected with HIV, some individuals develop HIV-related clinical symptoms, and some of those individuals later develop AIDS. If the infection proceeds to AIDS, the general course is a gradual, eventually almost complete disappearance of the CD4 positive cells, both in peripheral blood and lymphatic tissues. At the same time, the lymphocyte proliferative response to mitogens and antigens disappears. These events are most probably due to a slow and continuous spread of the HIV infection, which is probably accelerated by activation of CD4 positive cells occurring during recurrent infections with other microorganisms.

Function of T Cell Subsets from Patients with AIDS

Experiments have shown that the decreased responsiveness of the AIDS virus to mitogens and antigens cannot solely be explained by a decreased number of CD4 positive cells. Peripheral blood mononuclear cells (PBMC) from AIDS patients with a decreased number of helper cells and severely decreased responses to mitogens and antigens were depleted by monoclonal antibodies and complement for either CD4 positive or CD8 positive T lymphocytes (Figure 19–1) and then studied in a proliferative assay. Previous studies had shown that CD8 positive lymphocytes from normal controls respond with about 50% of the response of unseparated lymphocytes.[16] In contrast, the mitogen response of the CD8 cells from AIDS patients was very low compared with that of CD8 positive cells from controls.[15] These cells' lack of response cannot be explained by infection of HIV, since HIV infects only the the CD4 positive cells,[15] but it shows that other mechanisms in addition to low numbers of CD4 cells are involved in the decreased responsiveness of AIDS lymphocytes.

The ability of CD4 positive AIDS cells to respond to mitogens was investigated by increasing the number of CD4 positive cells to the same concentration as in controls after depletion for CD8 positive cells. The responses were increased in five of six experiments but remained significantly lower than the response of CD4 positive cells from normal controls.[16] Some of these CD4 positive AIDS cells might be infected with HIV, but the number of infected cells in peripheral blood has been reported to be very low, so additional abnormalities are probably also involved in the decreased proliferative responses of the CD4 positive AIDS cells.

Other investigators[17] have reported normal lymphocyte transformation of CD4 positive and CD8 positive cells from patients with AIDS. The differences in results are probably due to differences in the two groups of patients investi-

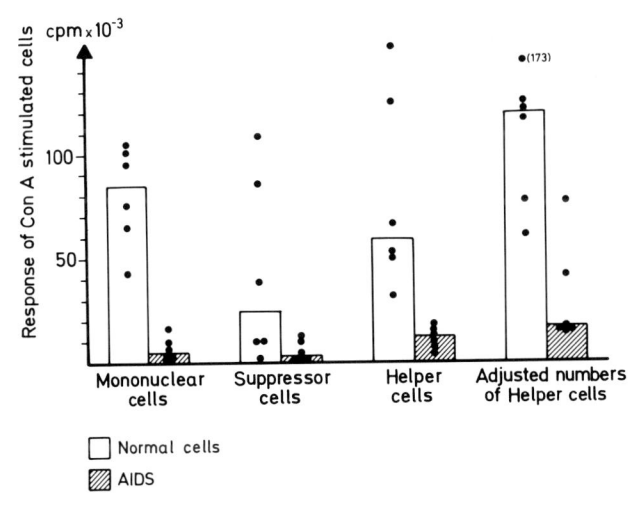

FIGURE 19–1 *Both mononuclear cells, CD8 enriched suppressor cells, and CD4 enriched helper cells from patients with AIDS showed decreased proliferative responses to Con A. The last columns show that even if the CD4 numbers from controls and patients were adjusted to 20,000 the responses are still decreased.*

gated, because our patients were selected to have low numbers of CD4 positive cells and decreased responses to mitogens and antigens, while the other group of patients included patients with Kaposi's sarcoma, who are usually less immunosuppressed.

Function of AIDS Accessory Cells

To study the function of accessory antigen-presenting cells, a group of AIDS patients were typed for their class II major histocompatibility antigens (HLA-DR) and matched with controls with known HLA-DR types. Six pairs of patients and controls with identical HLA-DR types and without mutual stimulation in mixed lymphocyte culture (MLC) were found. It was then possible to mix cells from the AIDS patients with cells from the HLA-DR identical controls without the interference of an allogeneic response since patients and controls shared the "same" tissue type. Highly irradiated cells from the controls or from the HLA-DR-matched patients were added to cultures of mitogen-stimulated purified T cells from the controls. Figure 19–2 suggests that AIDS cells could support the mitogen response of control T cells to the same extent as autologous cells.[18] One of the controls had a high transformation response to tuberculin (PPD), and the response to this antigen could also be restored by AIDS cells. Therefore the

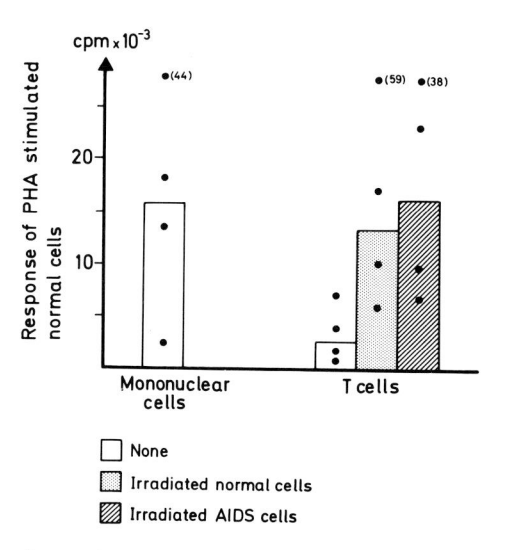

FIGURE 19–2 *The first column shows the responses of normal lymphocytes before monocyte depletion, the next three columns show the same cells after depletion. In the second of the three columns, irradiated cells from the same person were added and in the third column irradiated HLA-DR compatible lymphocytes from an AIDS patient were added. It appears that AIDS lymphocytes were able to "present" PHA to normal lymphocytes.*

function of the antigen-presenting cells from AIDS patients seems to be normal. In agreement with this observation, C. Enk et al.[19] have found a normal production of interleukin-1 (IL-1) in AIDS cells. Prince et al. have shown that AIDS monocytes have a decreased ability to "present" CD3 antibodies indicating that other parts of the antigen presentation may be impaired.[20]

Finally, the ability of AIDS cells to stimulate normal responder cells in MLC was investigated. AIDS cells appeared to have a very low stimulatory capacity in MLC.[18] Because AIDS cells presented antigen normally, the decreased stimulatory capacity in MLC was unexpected but might be due to low numbers of dendritic cells. This would be consistent with the decreased number of Langerhans cells found in the skin of AIDS patients.[21] However, the concentration of dendritic cells in the blood is largely unknown.

Active Suppression of the Proliferative Responses by AIDS Cells or Soluble Factors

Cellular suppression of the proliferative response seems to occur in other infectious diseases; e.g., mononucleosis, and thus it seemed possible that the high proportion of CD8 positive "suppressor" cells in patients with AIDS could lead to suppression of the proliferative response of AIDS cells. To investigate this possibility, AIDS lymphocytes were depleted for CD8 positive cells. As shown in Figure 19–1, this led to an increase of the proliferative response to mitogen in only one of six experiments.[15] Accordingly, the CD8 positive AIDS "suppressor" cells do not seem to be responsible for the severely decreased mitogen responses of AIDS cells. PBMC subsets other than the CD8 positive may have suppressor properties, and in some rheumatic diseases certain soluble factors are also known to have suppressive properties. To investigate this, irradiated and nonirradiated AIDS cells were added to cultures of cells from HLA-DR identical controls as described above. Figure 19–3 shows that AIDS cells could not suppress the responses of the normal cells to mitogen and allogeneic cells but could perhaps suppress the responses to antigens.[18] Other investigators have reported that AIDS cells have suppressive properties when added to B lymphocytes in a PWM-driven plaque-forming assay.[17]

To investigate the possible role of suppressive factors produced by AIDS cells, supernatants from mitogen-stimulated cultures of AIDS cells were added to cultures of normal cells. The responses of these cultures were not suppressed by supernatants from AIDS cultures.[18] This contradicts the observation that serum from AIDS patients can suppress normal lymphocytes' proliferative response.[22] A possible explanation for this discrepancy might be that the suppressive factor found in serum came from HIV.

We investigated whether addition of a lysate of HIV virus to normal lymphocytes could decrease the proliferative response of these cells and found that low concentrations of HIV lysate severely decreased the proliferative response of lymphocytes stimulated with mitogens or antigens.[24] Similar results have been

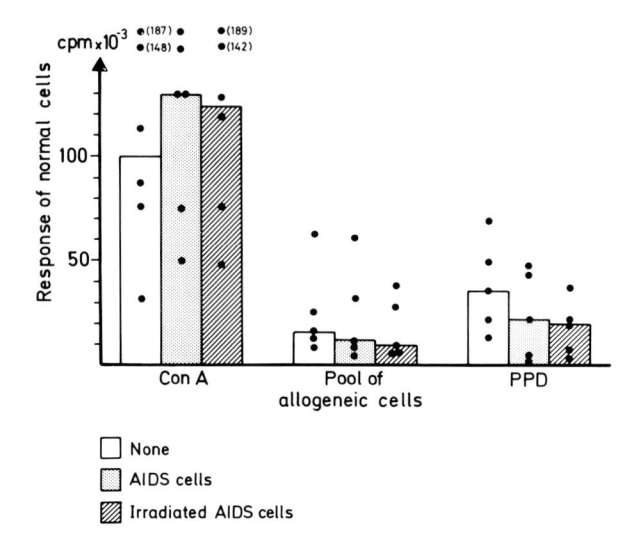

FIGURE 19–3 *The first three columns show the responses of Con A stimulated normal lymphocytes without or with addition of either nonirradiated or radiated AIDS lymphocytes. The next three columns show the lymphocytes stimulated with allogeneic cells instead of Con A, and the last three columns show the cells stimulated with PPD. It appears that the AIDS cells did not suppress the responses to Con A and to allogeneic cells.*

found by other groups.[25] Mann et al.[26] have suggested that the suppression is due to the glycoprotein pg120. Thus, active suppression by any AIDS cell subset does not seem to be responsible for the decreased proliferative response but may be involved in the decreased response in the B lymphocyte plaque-forming assay. However, it seems possible that HIV proteins are partly responsible for the suppression of lymphocyte proliferation in AIDS.

Role of Cytokines for Decreased Transformation Responses of AIDS Cells

In addition to IL-1, other cytokines (e.g., interleukin-2 [IL-2]) are required for a normal lymphocyte transformation to take place. To investigate the role of cytokines in AIDS, highly irradiated cells from controls were added to HLA-DR-identical AIDS cells. The responses of the AIDS cells were significantly increased but still subnormal compared with the responses of cells from controls.[18] The responses were increased to the same extent when supernatants from mitogen-stimulated cultures of normal cells or commercially available IL-2 were added. IL-2 is produced both by the CD4 positive and CD8 positive cells. When IL-2 was added to AIDS lymphocytes depleted for either CD4 positive or CD8 positive cells, the responses were increased, but neither of the responses of CD8 positive cells nor the response of CD4 positive cells were normalized.[23] Using a murine assay for IL-2, a decreased content of IL-2 has been found in supernatants from cultures of mitogen-stimulated AIDS cells.[17] Moreover, a decreased expression of the IL-2 receptor on mitogen-stimulated AIDS cells has also been reported.[17]

To investigate whether the decreased proliferative responses were due to blockage or to failure of the membrane receptors to transmit signals to the metabolic stimulatory inositol-trisphosphate and diacylglycerol pathways, the membrane receptors were bypassed by stimulating AIDS lymphocytes with a calcium ionophore A23187 and a phorbol ester PMA. We found a normal increase in intracellular calcium and a normal expression of IL-2 receptors, indicating that the function of the inositol-trisphosphate pathway was normal. In contrast, we found a decreased production of IL-2 and a decreased proliferative response, indicating that the diacylglycerol/protein kinase C pathway or a later step of activation was defective.

It appears from these experiments that the nature of the functional CD4 and CD8 cell deficiency in patients with AIDS seems at least partly related to a deficient IL-2 release, but lack of IL-2 cannot be the only explanation for these cells' low responses because exogenously added IL-2 does not normalize the responses completely. In addition, lack of IL-2 cannot explain the responsiveness of the CD8 positive AIDS cells even when IL-2 was added. Further studies must concentrate on the regulatory mechanisms for IL-2 production and on metabolic disturbances in this regulation.

CYTOTOXIC T LYMPHOCYTES IN AIDS

The T lymphocyte–mediated major histocompatibility complex (MHC)-restricted cytotoxicity in AIDS is of considerable interest. It represents a defensive mechanism that, in the normal host, is important for the eradication of a number of the infections observed in the AIDS patient. Further, cytotoxic T cells operating against HTLV-1 (the other major human retrovirus) have been demonstrated. A decreased cytotoxicity against CMV-infected fibroblasts has been reported in AIDS patients.[27] The response was, however, unrestricted in the majority of the investigated patients.

We addressed the capabilities of the MHC-restricted cytotoxic T lymphocyte in the cell-mediated lympholysis system.[28] In this assay, allogeneic lymphocytes were used as targets (and inducers). The inducer mechanisms and the effector cells are, however, similar to those involved in generating MHC-restricted cytotoxicity against viral infected cells.

In brief, responder PBMC from AIDS patients and controls were incubated with irradiated (2200 rad) PBMC from the allogeneic stimulator for six days.

On the sixth day the cytotoxicity of the responder cells toward PHA-blasted target cells from the allogeneic stimulator was measured using ^{51}Cr release assay. The ability to produce alloreactive cytotoxic cells was reduced ($P<0.01$) among AIDS patients. Adding IL-2 to the responder cultures gave rise to a significant increase in the cytotoxicity among patients and controls ($P<0.01$). After IL-2 was added, the AIDS patients still showed decreased cytotoxic capability compared with controls who did not receive IL-2 (Figure 19–4).

The host defense toward HIV infection has not been delineated. A possible role for cytotoxic T lymphocytes must be anticipated. These cells could also be involved in the destruction of the immune system by eliminating infected cells such as CD4 positive cells and the dendritic cells in the follicular clusters of the lymph nodes. Because the majority of the cytotoxic cells are CD8 positive, the infiltration of the follicular centers with CD8 positive lymphoblasts could represent a morphologic correlate to the hypothesis.

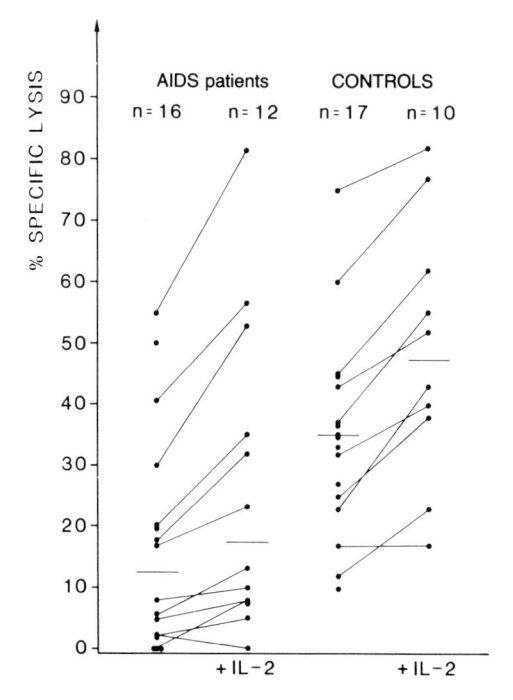

FIGURE 19–4 *The graph shows that the specific lysis of $_{51}$Cr labelled allogeneic PHA blasts by lymphocytes from either AIDS patients or controls was significantly ($p<0.01$) reduced in patients. Addition of IL-2 increased the responses of patients and controls, but the cytotoxic capability of patient lymphocytes was still decreased compared with controls.*

PROGNOSTIC FACTORS FOR DEVELOPMENT OF AIDS

A large number of individuals both in the United States and Europe are HIV-antibody positive, but fortunately only a proportion of these have developed AIDS. An incubation time of several years makes the search for prognostic factors for the development of AIDS crucial.

Our studies of a cohort of 60 individuals have shown that a stabilized proliferative response to PWM can subdivide the anti-HIV-positive individuals into two groups. In the group with low responses to PWM, a high occurrence of AIDS cases seems to indicate a correlation between a low response to PWM and a poor prognosis.[29] Others have found evidence that a low PWM response together with low numbers of CD4 positive cells indicate a poor prognosis.[30]

OPPORTUNISTIC INFECTION

The well-known consequence of T4 cell deficiency is opportunistic infection. Note that this clinical picture differs partially from that of congenital T cell deficiencies, which are characterized by lethal virus infections. A likely explanation for the difference is that patients with AIDS have acquired the immunodeficiency at a time when they already were immune to viral infections such as measles, and the humoral antibody responses to these infections seem to remain intact. In general, there is polyclonal activation of many B cell clones in AIDS patients, giving a broad spectrum of autoantibodies, including lymphocytotoxic antibodies, but the primary antibody response to new antigens is impaired.[31]

Many of the opportunistic infections occurring in AIDS patients can be successfully treated with antibiotics. Unfortunately, severe allergic reactions among some of the patients, especially to sulfomethoxazole, have restricted the use of antibiotics prophylactically. It would be valuable to find markers that could help to ascertain the group of patients especially at risk of infections, so prophylactic treatment could be given to this group only. *Pneumocystis carinii* infection is one of the most life threatening of the opportunistic infections occurring in AIDS patients. We examined a group of nine AIDS patients and six ARC patients for antibodies to *P. carinii* and found that the AIDS patients had only low levels of IgM antibodies to *P. carinii* and that the ARC patients had higher levels of IgM as well as IgA antibodies. None of four patients with *P. carinii* infection had IgM antibody to *P. carinii*, while nine of 11 patients with Koposi's sarcoma, other opportunistic infections, or ARC had such antibodies.[32] This preliminary finding has been confirmed in a group of 36 AIDS patients and indicates that AIDS patients without IgM antibody to *P. carinii* may be at high risk of becoming infected with *P. carinii*. However, further investigations are needed to clarify the mechanism.

REFERENCES

1. WHO surveillance center for AIDS. Paris. AIDS surveillance in Europe. Report No. 16. Situation by 31st December 1987.
2. Update: Acquired immunodeficiency syndrome (AIDS)—United States. MMWR 1983;32:465–7.
3. Gerstoft J, Nielsen JO, Dickmeiss E, et al. The acquired immunodeficiency syndrome (AIDS) in Denmark. A report from the Copenhagen Study Group of AIDS on the First 20 Danish Patients. Acta Med Scand 1985;217:213–24.
4. Melbye M, Bigger RJ, Ebbesen P, et al. Seroepidemiology of HTLV-III antibodies in Danish homosexual men: Prevalence, transmission, and disease outcome. Br Med J 1984;289:573–5.
5. Arendrup M, Lindhardt BO, Krogsgaard K, et al. Antibodies to HIV in patients with acute hepatitis B in the period 1975–1984. Scand J Infect Dis 1987;19:167–72.
6. Hofmann B, Platz P, Odum N, et al. Occurrence of anti-HTLV-III antibodies in Danish high risk homosexuals in 1982–83—seroconversion rate and risk of AIDS. AIDS Res 1986;2:1–3.
7. Hofmann B, Kryger P, Strandberg NS, et al. Sexually transmitted diseases, HIV antibodies, and subsequent development of AIDS in visitors of homosexual sauna clubs in Copenhagen in 1982–83. J Sex Trans Dis 1988;15:1–4.
8. Gerstoft J, Lindhardt BØ, Petersen CS, et al. Antibodies to human T-cell lymphotropic virus type III in promiscuous healthy homosexual men. Relation to immunological and clinical findings. Eur J Clin Invest 1985;15:290–95.
9. Mathez D, Leibowitch J, Matherson S, et al. Antibodies to HTLV-III associated antigens in populations exposed to AIDS virus in France. Lancet 1984;2:460.
10. Brun-Vezinet F, Barre-Sinoussi F, Sainot AG, et al. Detection of IgG antibodies to lymphadenopathy virus in patients with AIDS or lymphadenopathy syndrome. Lancet 1984;1:1253–6.
11. Schupbach J, Hallet O, Vogt M, et al. Antibodies to HTLV-III in Swiss patients with AIDS and pre-AIDS and in groups at risk for AIDS. N Engl J Med 1985;312:265–70.
12. Cheingson-Popov R, Weiss RA, Dalgleish A, et al. Prevalence of antibodies to human T-lymphotropic virus type III in AIDS and AIDS-risk patients in Britain. Lancet 1984;2:477–80.
13. Carne CA, Sutherland J, Feras RB, et al. Rising prevalence of human T-lymphotropic virus type III (HTLV-III) infection in homosexual men in London. Lancet 1985;1:1261–2.
14. Lindhardt BØ, Gerstoft J, Ulrich K, et al. Antibodies againt HTLV-III in Danish haemophiliacs; relation to source of factor VIII used in treatment on immunological parameters. Scand J Haematol 1985;35:379–85.
15. Safa B, Sarnagadharan M, Groopmann J, et al. Seroepidemiological studies of human T-lymphotropic retrovirus type III in acquired immunodeficiency syndrome. Lancet 1984;1:1438–40.
16. Hofmann B, Ødum N, Platz P, et al. Immunological studies in acquired immunodeficiency syndrome. Functional studies of lymphocyte subpopulations. Scand J Immunol 1985;21:235–43.
17. Lane HC, Depper JM, Greene WC, et al. Qualitative analysis of immune function in patients with acquired immunodeficiency syndrome. N Engl J Med 1985;313:79–84.

18. Hofmann B, Ødum N, Jakobsen BK, et al. Immunological studies in AIDS II, active suppression or intrinsic defect—investigated by mixing AIDS cells with HLA-DR identical normal cells. Scand J Immunol 1986;23:669–78.
19. Enk C, Gerstoft J, Moller S, et al. Interleukin-1 activity in AIDS. Scand J Immunol 1986;23:491–97.
20. Prince HE, Moody DJ, Shubin BI, et al. Defective monocyte function in AIDS: evidence from a monocyte-dependent T-cell proliferative system. J Clin Immunol 1985;5:21–25.
21. Belsito D, Sanchez M, Bauer R, et al. Reduced Langerhans cell Ia antigen and ATPase activity in patients with acquired immunodeficiency syndrome. N Engl J Med 1984;310:1279.
22. Cunningham-Rundles S, Michelis MA, Massur H. Serum suppression of lymphocyte activation in vitro in acquired immunodeficiency disease. J Clin Immunol 1983;3:156.
23. Hofmann B, Odum N, Fugger L, et al. Immunological studies in AIDS: the effect of TCGF and indomethacine on the in vitro lymphocyte response. Cancer Detect Prevent 1987;suppl 1:619–26; and in: Nieburgs HE, Bekesi JG. Immunobiology of cancer and AIDS. New York: Alan R Liss, 1987.
24. Hofmann B, Langhoff E, Lindhardt BØ, et al. Patient antibodies against a potent suppressive factor associated with HTLV-III and possible therapeutic consequences. AIFO 1986;11:619–21.
25. Pahwa S, Pahwa R, Saxinger C, et al. Influence of the human T-lymphotropic virus/lymphadenopathy-associated virus on function of human lymphocytes: evidence for immunosuppressive effects and polyclonal B-cell activation by banded viral preparations. Proc Natl Acad Sci USA 1985;82:8198–02.
26. Mann DL, Lasane F, Popovic M, et al. HTLV-III large envelope protein (gp120) suppresses PHA-induced lymphocyte blastogenesis. J Immunol 1987;138:2640–44.
27. Rook AH, Masur H, Lane HC, et al. Interleukin-2 enhances the depressed natural killer and cytomegalovirus-specific cytotoxic antivity of lymphocytes from patients with the acquired immunodeficiency syndrome. J Clin Invest 1983;72:398–403.
28. Gerstoft J, Dickmeiss E, Mathisen L. Cytotoxic capabilities of lymphocytes from patients with the acquired immunodeficiency syndrome. Scand J Immunol 1985;22:463–70.
29. Hofmann B, Lindhardt BØ, Gerstoft J, et al. The lymphocyte transformation response to PWM as a highly predictive parameter for the development of AIDS and AIDS-related symptoms in homosexual men with antibodies to HIV. Br Med J 1987;295:293–96.
30. Fishbein DB, Kaplan JE, Spira TJ, et al. Unexplained lymphadenopathy in homosexual men. JAMA 1985;254:930–5.
31. Ammann AJ, Schiffman G, Abrams D, et al. B-cell immunodeficiency in acquired immune deficiency syndrome. JAMA 1984;251:1447–9.
32. Hofmann B, Ødum N, Platz P, et al. Humoral responses to *Pneumocystis carinii* in patients with acquired immunodeficiency syndrome and immunocompromised homosexuals. J Infect Dis 1985;152:15.

Chapter 20

Opportunistic Infections in AIDS Patients

Jonathan W. M. Gold
Donald Armstrong

Acquired immunodeficiency syndrome (AIDS) is the result of progressive, irreversible destruction of immune function.[1-3] It is caused by infection with the human immunodeficiency virus (HIV-1), one of five known human retroviruses.[4,5] Retroviruses are transmitted by sexual contact, by transfusion of blood and blood products from infected donors, and by accidental or purposeful injections with contaminated needles and syringes. They can also be transmitted in the perinatal period and by breast milk.

Infection with HIV-1 is occurring worldwide. Different transmission patterns predominate in different parts of the world: heterosexual spread predominates in Central Africa[6] and other developing areas while homosexual and contaminated-needle transmission (among intravenous drug users) predominates in the developed countries of the west. Transmission by transfusion of contaminated blood products has occurred in all regions. Individuals at risk for HIV infection and, therefore, AIDS include homosexual men, intravenous drug users, recipients of infected blood products (including transfused patients and those with hemophilia who received concentrated, pooled clotting factors), sexual partners of infected people, and infants of infected mothers.

As HIV infection becomes more common and spreads into different populations, it is having important effects on the epidemiology and clinical features of a number of other infectious diseases, such as tuberculosis, syphilis, malaria, measles, and infections due to human T-lymphotropic virus I and II (HTLV-I and HTLV-II), *Streptococcus pneumoniae*, *Haemophilus influenzae*, and *Campylobacter jejuni*.[7-9]

Massive efforts are underway to prevent the spread of HIV. Such efforts include education in techniques of risk reduction as well as development of vaccines, although a practical vaccine does not seem likely soon. In addition, treatments that ameliorate, delay, or prevent progression of immunodeficiency in infected individuals are being developed. At present, however, the infections that complicate AIDS are by far the most important causes of morbidity and mortality in AIDS patients. Much of the medical management of AIDS patients focusses on the diagnosis, prevention, and treatment of these infections.

IMMUNE DEFECTS IN HIV INFECTED PATIENTS AND THE ASSOCIATED INFECTIOUS AND NEOPLASTIC COMPLICATIONS

The primary immunologic defect in AIDS patients is loss of the T-helper lymphocyte, as a result of direct infection of this cell by HIV. This leads to profound disregulation of immune function and an increased susceptibility to infections with certain microorganisms and to neoplastic diseases (especially Kaposi's sarcoma [KS] and B-cell lymphoma). Most of these microorganisms are familiar to physicians caring for patients with neoplastic diseases and other immunosuppressed patients.[10] The occurrence of these microorganisms in an HIV infected person heralds the development of clinically significant immunologic dysfunction.[11] These organisms are generally obligate or facultative intracellular parasites that often cause latent infections. In fact, many of the infectious complications of AIDS are due to reactivation of latent infections acquired in the distant past. These organisms often persist and their treatment must be prolonged, often for months or even for life. The presence of latent infection in AIDS patients can be detected by serologic testing (e.g., toxoplasma, cytomegalovirus [CMV]), by skin

Table 20–1 Infectious complication of AIDS: Organisms that take advantage of T-cell defects

Parasites	Bacteria	Fungi	Viruses
Pneumocystis carinii	Mycobacterium avium-complex	Candida albicans	Cytomegalovirus
Toxoplasma gondii	M. tuberculosis	Cryptococcus neoformans	Herpes simplex virus
Cryptosporidium	Salmonella	Histoplasma capsulatum	Varicella zoster virus
Isospora belli		Coccidioides immitis	Papovavirus (JC)
	Reported but uncommon:		
	Legionella		
	Nocardia asteriodes		
	Listeria monocytogenes		

testing for delayed hypersensitivity (although many patients are anergic), or by history (e.g., a history of exposure to tuberculosis or a history of recurrent herpes). Thus it is possible to identify patients at high risk for certain infectious complications and observe them for early signs so treatment can be administered early, when it is most effective. High risk patients can also be offered prophylaxis, and efforts are underway to develop effective prevention for these infections.

B-cell dysfunction is a secondary consequence of T-helper lymphocyte depletion.[12] AIDS patients have normal or increased levels of circulating immunoglobulins but fail to develop antibodies in response to challenge with new or recall antigens. Consequently, attempts at serodiagnosis of infectious diseases often fail because rising antibody titers may not occur. Since preexisting antibodies are usually maintained, serologic tests are often useful for recognizing a history of prior infections (such as toxoplasmosis or CMV).

Response to vaccines is impaired, and, strikingly, there is a greatly increased risk of infections that take advantage of defective antibody responses, including *S. pneumoniae* and *H. influenzae*.[9,13] This increase in frequency of infection is seen in AIDS patients and HIV infected patients without AIDS.

SPECIFIC INFECTIOUS COMPLICATIONS OF AIDS

Table 20.2 lists opportunistic infections seen in 780 patients at Memorial Sloan-Kettering Cancer Center (MSKCC) and gives an indication of the relative frequency of such infections.

Table 20–2 Opportunistic infections in 780 patients with AIDS at Memorial Sloan-Kettering Cancer Center, 1981 through June 1988

Infection	Number of Patients[a]
Pneumocystis carinii	362
Disseminated	3
Cytomegalovirus (CMV)[b]	224
Retinitis	35
Adrenalitis	17
Mycobacterium avium-complex (disseminated)	151
Cryptococcosis	36
CNS toxoplasmosis	32
Cryptosporidiosis	29
Mycobacterium tuberculosis	25
Salmonellosis	22
Histoplasmosis	6

Candidiasis[c] (oral and esophageal): 336 recorded cases.

[a]Many patients have more than one infection and recurrent or relapsing infections, especially with *Pneumocystis carinii*, are common.
[b]Most cases of CMV are recognized at autopsy.
[c]Information on candidiasis is not uniformly recorded. Invasive candidiasis is rare.

Pneumocystis carinii pneumonia

Pneumocystis carinii pneumonia (PCP) is the most commonly diagnosed serious infection in AIDS patients. Characteristically, it presents as pneumonia with gradually progressive shortness of breath, cough, and fever. The chest x-ray shows bilateral interstitial-alveolar infiltrates, and the diagnosis is made by demonstration of characteristic cysts in respiratory secretions, most often obtained by bronchoalveolar lavage.[14] Presentation is often atypical in AIDS patients and a very high index of suspicion is required. Chest x-rays are often normal or nearly normal. Atypical presentations including nodular disease, cavitary disease, and pneumothoraces are being increasingly encountered. Patients receiving aerosol pentamidine prophylaxis may have a modified illness with upper lobe involvement. Often respiratory symptoms are minimal or absent, and fever may be the only sign. The most sensitive sign in PCP is a decreased diffusion capacity determined by pulmonary function testing or by a decrease in arterial pO_2 following exercise (the normal response is an increase). In febrile patients with known or suspected HIV infection, an abnormal diffusion capacity or a decreased post-exercise arterial blood pO_2 should lead to evaluation for PCP. This will usually be examination of expectorated sputum which if negative should be followed by bronchoscopy with bronchoalveolar lavage. Various stains such as methenamine silver, gram weigert, and Toludine blue have been used. Monoclonal antibody direct fluorescent antibody studies have also been successful. Diagnosis may be difficult in patients receiving aerosol pentamidine prophylaxis. Falsely negative bronchoalveolar lavage may occur and transbronchial biopsy may be necessary to make the diagnosis.

PCP is treated with trimethoprim-sulfamethoxazole or pentamidine. Trimetrexate is under investigation as an alternative therapy in people unable to tolerate or failing to respond to the other drugs.[15] Aerosolized pentamidine also appears to be an effective treatment in mild cases, but cannot be recommended since the distribution may be inadequate due to lung disease and dissemination is increasingly reported.[16,17]

Because of the frequency with which PCP occurs in AIDS patients and the very high frequency of relapses (20 to 30% of patients with one episode will have a second episode; three and even four episodes may occur), several strategies for prophylaxis are being investigated. Trimethoprim-sulfamethoxazole is effective prophylaxis but is limited because of the high frequency of adverse reactions (including rash and neutropenia).[18] Aerosol pentamidine is widely used by physicians, although studies to determine its efficacy are not yet completed.[19]

Cytomegalovirus

CMV is commonly isolated from AIDS patients, and evidence of tissue involvement is more common in patients at autopsy than is recognized during life. It causes disseminated infection; the most common recognized forms are chorioretinitis, enterocolitis, and pneumonia. Adrenalitis is often present at autopsy and sometimes causes clinically detectable adrenal insufficiency.[20]

Chorioretinitis is recognized from its typical fundoscopic appearance with hemorrhage, exudate, and endovascular cuffing. Untreated, it can rapidly lead to decreased vision and ultimately blindness.

Enterocolitis usually is associated with fever, diarrhea, and cramping abdominal pain. It is diagnosed by detecting typical inclusion bodies on endoscopically obtained biopsy specimens.

CMV pneumonitis is similarly diagnosed by demonstration in pulmonary tissue of typical inclusion bodies, identified by culture or immunologic staining as CMV, and surrounded by signs of inflammatory reaction.

Although not currently licensed, ganciclovir (DHPG) is effective treatment for retinitis, enterocolitis, and, probably, pneumonia due to CMV.[21] Marrow suppression is a side effect, and treatment often must be maintained indefinitely as relapse is common. Foscarnet (phosphonoformate) is currently under investigation for treatment of CMV infection. It has appeared to be effective in treating CMV retinitis, although controlled studies are not available.

Mycobacterium avium-complex

Infection with M. avium-complex (MAC; also *M. avium-intracellulare* or MAI) has developed in half of AIDS patients at MSKCC. The infection is a late complication in many AIDS patients with median survivals from the time of diagnosis of around three months. Symptoms are often surprisingly mild despite bacteremia and may include fevers, rigors, cramping abdominal pain, and diarrhea. Massively enlarged mesenteric nodes which may be palpable are often present. Blood cultures are the most sensitive way to make the diagnosis and are positive in nearly all cases. Bone marrow, liver, lymph nodes, and gastrointestinal biopsy also may be positive. Stool smears for acid fast bacilli (AFB) are positive in half of disseminated cases. These should be followed by blood culture. Gastrointestinal biopsy may resemble Whipple's disease because of infiltration of the lamina propria with histiocytes, which have phagocytosed huge numbers of organisms and may be seen in the endoscopic biopsy.

Despite in vitro susceptibility to a variety of drugs including ansamycin, clofazimine, ethionamide, and sometimes ethambutol and cycloserine, the response of MAC to drug therapy is very disappointing. Few patients show clinical improvement and many are unable to tolerate combined drug treatment.[22]

Tuberculosis

In countries where tuberculosis is endemic, it is a major complication of AIDS. The recent increase in reported cases of tuberculosis in the United States marks the first rise in the incidence of tuberculosis since the beginning of the twentieth century.[8] This increase is due mainly, although not entirely, to reactivation of tuberculosis in HIV infected people.

Tuberculosis should be considered in HIV infected people with positive tuberculin tests, radiographic evidence of healed tuberculosis, or prior exposure. Isoniazid prophylaxis should be considered for such individuals.

The disease has some features suggestive of primary tuberculosis, although most cases arise from reactivation of a prior infection. Lymphatic disease, especially of the cervical and hilar nodes, is common. The disease may progress rapidly. Diagnosis is by identification of *M. tuberculosis* in respiratory secretions or tissue. *Mycobacterium tuberculosis* has been isolated from the blood of AIDS patients.[23] However, this is uncommon. The usefulness of blood cultures for the diagnosis of tuberculosis appears limited.

Initial treatment regimens should take into consideration the possibility of isoniazid (INH) resistance. The final selection of drugs is guided by antimicrobial sensitivity results.

Herpes Simplex

Individuals at risk for ulcerative herpes simplex infection usually have histories of genital or oral herpes. Severe, persistent, ulcerative perianal herpes simplex infection was one of the first infections recognized among AIDS patients. Other forms of herpes infections include herpetic esophagitis. Herpes simplex is sometimes isolated from the brain and lungs of AIDS patients and may cause encephalitis. The appearance of the persistent, raw, painful ulcers is highly suggestive, and the diagnosis is easily confirmed by virus isolation.[3] Treatment with topical acyclovir may be adequate treatment for the mildest cases of herpes simplex, but oral or even intravenous treatment is often needed.

Salmonella

Salmonella gastroenteritis, which must be looked for in AIDS patients, is often complicated by bacteremia. Relapses of bacteremia and disseminated infection may occur when treatment is discontinued. Prolonged suppressive antimicrobial therapy, generally with amoxicillin or ampicillin, is usually given. Ceftriaxone, cefoperazone, and ciprofloxacin appear to be acceptable alternatives. If a decision to stop treatment is made, patients must be carefully monitored for relapse.[24,25]

Candida sp.

Thrush is very common in AIDS patients. It may cause dryness or discomfort in the mouth or may be asymptomatic. Progression to candida esophagitis is common and presents with characteristic retrosternal pain on swallowing. This may occur in the absence of thrush. Disseminated candidiasis is rare, even at autopsy, probably reflecting the relatively normal functioning of polymorphonuclear leukocytes in AIDS patients. Treatment of thrush is with topical antifungal agents such as clotrimazole or nystatin. Candida esophagitis usually responds to ketoconazole. Ketoconazole absorption requires an acid pH in the stomach. Treatment failure may be due to administration of antacids, H_2 antagonists, or to achlorhydria, which is seen in some AIDS patients. Herpes simplex and CMV esophagitis may resemble candida esophagitis and require esophagoscopy and biopsy. Initially empiric treatment with nystatin or ketoconazole is generally indicated in patients with symptoms of candida esophagitis, with further diagnostic procedures reserved for patients who do not respond.

Cryptosporidium sp.

Cryptosporidium sp., a cause of diarrhea in a variety of domestic animals, has been a cause of acute, self-limited diarrhea in veterinarians. Prior to the AIDS epidemic, cryptosporidiosis was a rarely recognized cause of severe diarrhea in severely immunocompromised patients. In AIDS patients, cryptosporidia may cause self-limited diarrhea; chronic diarrheal illness that waxes and wanes; or prolonged, profound, unrelenting watery diarrhea. Diagnosis is usually made by detecting the organisms in wet mounts or acid fast stains. It should also be looked for in intestinal biopsies from patients with severe diarrhea. There is no effective treatment for this infection.[26,27] *Isospora belli* is another parasite that causes diarrhea in AIDS patients. Recent studies suggest that treatment with trimethoprim-sulfamethoxazole is effective.[28]

Cryptococcus neoformans

Cryptococcal meningitis presents either as an acute or subacute illness. A high index of suspicion is necessary as symptoms may be minimal. The disease usually involves the central nervous system (CNS) and blood, and bone marrow cultures may also be positive for *Cryptococcus neoformans*. Titers of cryptococcal antigen can be extraordinarily high. Over 1:100,000 is not uncommon, and serum titers frequently exceed those in the CSF. Treatment is with amphotericin B with or without 5 flucytosine. Relapses occur when treatment is stopped, so that most patients require maintenance therapy with amphotericin B indefinitely. Fluconazole, an imidazole derivative, is being studied for both initial treatment and maintenance therapy of cryptococcal meningitis.[29]

Toxoplasma gondii

Toxoplasmosis in AIDS patients is usually a CNS disease due to reactivation of a latent, earlier infection. Acute infection in adults is asymptomatic or produces lymphadenopathy. The diagnosis should be suspected in seropositive patients with evidence on CT scan of multiple or solitary nodules. Lack of antibody makes the diagnosis of CNS toxoplasmosis unlikely. Brain biopsy to diagnose lymphoma, bacterial brain abscess, or tuberculoma may be considered in patients with CNS mass lesions who do not appear to have toxoplasmosis.

Treatment is with sulfadiazine and pyrimethamine, generally for the life of the patient because relapse in patients off treatment is common. Clindamycin and pyrimethamine may be effective alternative therapy in the sulfa-intolerant patient, but controlled studies are lacking. Many clinicians give folinic acid to patients receiving pyrimethamine, although the usefulness of this drug in preventing marrow suppression is not entirely clear.

Rising antibody titers are seldom documented in AIDS patients with toxoplasmosis, although most patients have antibodies prior to the onset of disease. About 20% of AIDS patients in New York City are infected with toxoplasma. In many continental European cities, such as Paris and Brussels, 90% of people are infected. The risk of developing CNS toxoplasmosis in seropositive AIDS patients is about 30% over two years. Unfortunately, although it is easy to identify patients at risk, there is no known safe and effective prophylaxis at this time.[30,31]

OTHER CNS INFECTIONS

AIDS Dementia Complex

The AIDS dementia complex is a direct consequence of HIV infection of the brain, not a complicating infection. Many AIDS patients have subtle neurologic abnormalities and the frequency of AIDS dementia complex is believed to be very high. Severe cases are associated with profound CNS dysfunction. Anecdotal reports suggest that some patients improve with zidovudine, and a recent study of infected children showed reversal of atrophy and improved performance with zidovudine treatment.[32]

Brain abscesses are common in intravenous drug users who also have a high frequency of AIDS. Diagnosis depends on biopsy; however, many patients are treated empirically unless drainage is indicated for treatment.

Progressive multifocal leukoencephalopathy (PML) is caused by a papovavirus (JC virus). The CT scan shows multifocal hypodense areas in the white matter, and definitive diagnosis is by brain biopsy. However, there is no effective treatment for this disease.[33]

A variety of painful and debilitating peripheral neuropathies and myelopathies are also common in AIDS patients.

Infections Taking Advantage of B-Cell Defect

Impaired B-cell function in AIDS patients limits the usefulness of serologic diagnosis, impairs the response to polysaccharide vaccines, such as the pneumococcal vaccine, and is associated with a small but significant increase in the number of infections with encapsulated organisms, especially *H. influenzae* and *S. pneumoniae*. Other infections have been reported, including B beta-hemolytic streptococci and *Branhamella catarrhalis,* but they are rare and their relationship to immune deficiency is, therefore, not certain at this time.[13,34,35]

Pneumonia due to these encapsulated organisms may be typical lobar pneumonia, but diffuse interstitial alveolar infiltrates mimicking PCP may occur. Simultaneous infections with *Pneumocystis carinii* and bacteria also may occur. Diagnosis is readily established by gram stain and culture of respiratory secretions. The frequency of bacteremia due to these organisms is high in AIDS and other HIV-infected patients with pneumonia. Because of the likelihood of these bacterial pneumonias, initial treatment of AIDS patients with pneumonia, especially with acute onset, should usually cover *H. influenzae* and *S. pneumoniae* until a definitive diagnosis is made. Trimethoprim-sulfamethoxazole, generally the drug of choice for treatment of PCP, is adequate coverage for both these organisms. When pentamidine is the initial therapy, it is often advisable, at first, to provide coverage for these two organisms with, for example, ampicillin or cefuroxime. In patients with extensive KS, *S. aureus* should be covered, as it may be isolated from respiratory secretions and blood of patients with pulmonary KS and pneumonia.[34]

As the epidemiology of HIV infection evolves and as treatments modify its natural history, physicians will need to be on the lookout for different patterns of infection and neoplastic complications. For the foreseeable future, the diagnosis, treatment, and prevention of these complications will be the principal form of management of AIDS patients.

REFERENCES

1. Gottlieb MS, Schroff R, Schanker HM, et al. *Pneumocystis carinii* pneumonia and mucosal candidiasis in previously healthy homosexual men: evidence of a new acquired cellular immunodeficiency. N Engl J Med 1981;305:1425–1431.
2. Masur H, Michelis MA, Greene JB, et al. An outbreak of community-acquired *Pneumocystis carinii* pneumonia: initial manifestation of cellular immune dysfunction. N Engl J Med 1981;305:1431–1438.
3. Siegal FP, Lopez C, Hammer GS, et al. Severe acquired immunodeficiency in homosexual males, manifested by chronic perianal ulcerative herpes simplex lesions. N Engl J Med 1981;305:1439–1444.
4. Barre-Sinoussi F, Chermann JC, Rey F, et al. Isolation of a T lymphotropic retrovirus from a patient at risk for acquired immune deficiency syndrome (AIDS). Science 1983;224:868–871.
5. Gallo RC, Salahuddin SZ, Popovic M, et al. Frequent detection and isolation of cytopathic retroviruses (HTLV-II-I) from patients with AIDS and at risk for AIDS. Science 1984;224:500–502.
6. Quinn TC, Mann JM, Curran JW, Piot P. AIDS in Africa: an Epidemiologic Paradigm. Science 1986;234:955–963.
7. Lupton GP, Tramont E. Seronegative secondary syphilis in a patient infected with

the human immunodeficiency virus (HIV) with Kaposi sarcoma: a diagnostic dilemma. Ann Intern Med 1987;107:492–495.
8. Tuberculosis, final data—United States, 1986. MMWR 1988;36:817–820.
9. Simberkoff MS, El-Sadr W, Schiffman G, Rahal JJ Jr. *Streptococcus pneumoniae* infections and bacteremia in patients with acquired immune deficiency syndrome, with report of a pneumococcal vaccine failure. Am Rev Respir Dis 1984;130:1174–1176.
10. Gold JWM. Clinical spectrum of infections in patients with HTLV-III-associated diseases. Cancer Research 1985; (supplement) 45:4652s–4654s.
11. Revision of the CDC surveillance case definition for acquired immunodeficiency syndrome. MMWR 1987;36:3s–15s.
12. Lane HC, Masur H, Edgar LC, Whalen G, Rook AH, Fauci AS. Abnormalities of B-cell activation and immunoregulation in patients with acquired immunodeficiency syndrome. N Engl J Med 1983;309:453–458.
13. Polsky B, Gold JWM, Whimbey E et al. Bacterial pneumonia in patients with the acquired immunodeficiency syndrome. Ann Intern Med 1986;104:511–514.
14. Stover DE, Zaman MB, Hajdu SI, et al. Bronchoalveolar lavage in the diagnosis of diffuse pulmonary infiltrates in the immunosuppressed host. Ann Intern Med 1984;101:1–7.
15. Allegra CJ, Chabner BA, Tuazon CU, et al. Trimetrexate for the treatment of *Pneumocystis carinii* pneumonia in patients with the acquired immunodeficiency syndrome. N Engl J Med 1987;317:978–985.
16. Montgomery AB, Debs RJ, Luce JM, et al. Preliminary communications: Aerosolized pentamidine as sole therapy for *Pneumocystis carinii* pneumonia in patients with acquired immunodeficiency syndrome. Lancet 1987;2:480–483.
17. Armstrong D, Bernard E. Aerosol pentamidine. (Editorial) Ann Intern Med 1988; 109(11):852–854.
18. Gordin FM, Simon GL, Wofsy CB, et al. Adverse reactions to trimethoprim-sulfamethoxazole in patients with the acquired immunodeficiency syndrome. Ann Intern Med 1984;100:495–499.
19. Bernard EM, Donnelly HJ, Tsang SF, et al. Aerosolized pentamidine is effective in the prevention and treatment of *Pneumocystis carinii* pneumonia in the rat model. 86th Annual Meeting, American Society for Microbiology, Washington, D.C., March 23–28, 1986.
20. Tapper ML, Rotterdam HZ, Lerner CW, et al. Adrenal necrosis in the acquired immunodeficiency syndrome. Ann Intern Med 1984;100:239–241.
21. Masur H, Lane HC, Palestine A, et al. Effect of 90(1,3-Dihydroxy-2-Propoxymethyl) Guanine on serious cytomegalovirus disease in eight immunosuppressed homosexual men. Ann Intern Med 1986;104:41–44.
22. Hawkins CC, Gold JWM, Whimbey E, et al. Treatment of disseminated *Mycobacterium avium-intracellulare* infections in patients with the acquired immune deficiency syndrome. Ann Intern Med 1986;105:184–188.
23. Kiehn TE, Gold JWM, Brannon P, et al. *Mycobacterium tuberculosis* bacteremia detected by isolator lysis-centrifugation blood culture system. J Clin Microbiol 1985;21:647–648.
24. Jacobs JL, Gold JWM, Murray HW, et al. Salmonella infections in patients with the acquired immune deficiency syndrome. Ann Intern Med 1985;102:186–188.
25. Glaser JB, Morton-Kute L, Berger SR, et al. Recurrent *Salmonella typhimurium* bacteremia associated with the acquired immune deficiency syndrome. Ann Intern Med 1985;102:189–193.

26. Current WL, Reese NC, Ernst JV, et al. Human cryptosporidiosis in immunocompetent and immunodeficient persons. N Engl J Med 1983;308:1252-1257.
27. Soave R, Johnson WD Jr. *Cryptosporidium* and *Isopora belli* infections. J Infect Dis 1988;157:225–229.
28. DeHovitz JA, Pape JW, Boncy M, et al. Clinical manifestations and therapy of Isopora belli infection in patients with acquired immunodeficiency syndrome. N Engl J Med 1986;315:87–90.
29. Kovacs JA, Kovacs AA, Polis M, et al. Cryptococcosis in the acquired immunodeficiency syndrome. Ann Intern Med 1985;103:533–538.
30. Wong B, Gold JWM, Brown AE, et al. Central-nervous-system toxoplasmosis in homosexual men and parenteral drug abusers. Ann Intern Med 1984;100:36–42.
31. Luft BJ, Remington JS. Toxoplasmic encephalitis. J Infect Dis 1988;157:1–6.
32. Snider WD, Simpson DM, Nielson S, et al. Neurologic complications of acquired immune deficiency syndrome: analysis of 50 patients. Ann Neurol 1983;14:403–418.
33. Miller JR, Barrett RE, Britton CB, et al. Progressive multifocal leukoencephalopathy in a male homosexual with T cell immune deficiency. N Engl J Med 1982;307:1436–1438.
34. Whimbey E, Gold JWM, Polsky B, et al. Bacteremia and fungemia in patients with the acquired immunodeficiency syndrome. Ann Intern Med 1986;104:511–514.
35. Witt DJ, Craven DE, McCabe W. Bacterial infections in adult patients with the acquired immune deficiency syndrome (AIDS) and AIDS related complex. Am J Med 1987;82:900–906.

Chapter 21

Treatment of Opportunistic Infections in Patients with AIDS

Jeffrey Kocher
Richard B. Roberts

Eight years after recognition of acquired immunodeficiency syndrome (AIDS), the greatest source of morbidity and mortality for patients continues to be infectious complications. Recent progress in defining and isolating the etiologic retrovirus, human immunodeficiency virus (HIV), has surpassed gains in our ability to provide curative therapy for many of the opportunistic infections. The spectrum of microbial agents infecting the AIDS patient has been well defined, and although reports of novel organisms previously unrecognized in this population can be expected to arise from time to time, our familiarity with the majority of clinical syndromes has allowed earlier diagnosis and treatment.

Most relevant pathogens in AIDS patients require an effective cell-mediated (T lymphocyte/mononuclear phagocyte) immune response for successful eradication. Examples include the following: (1) bacteria—*Mycobacterium tuberculosis*, *M. avium-intracellulare* (MAI), *Salmonella* sp., (2) viruses—*Herpes zoster*, *Herpes simplex*, cytomegalovirus (CMV), polyomavirus, (3) fungi—*Cryptococcus neoformans*, *Candida albicans*, *Aspergillus*, (4) protozoa—*Pneumocystis carinii*, *Toxoplasma gondii*, *Cryptosporidium*. Other organisms that take advantage of depressed cellular immunity, such as *Listeria monocytogenes*,[1] *Legionella* sp,[2] and *Actinomycetales*,[3] have been observed less commonly than might have been predicted.

Recent evidence has confirmed the clinical importance of immunoglobulin defects, which appear to place AIDS patients at increased risk for infection with *Streptococcus pneumoniae* and *Hemophilus influenzae*. Finally, iatrogenic factors such as in-dwelling catheters, drug-induced leukopenia, invasive diagnostic procedures, and broad-spectrum antibiotic therapy expose these patients to infection with *Staphylococcus aureus*, *S. epidermidis*, aerobic gram-negative bacilli, and disseminated fungi.[4]

Table 21-1 Therapy of opportunistic infections in patients with AIDS

Organism	Therapeutic Agents	Response/Comments	Experimental Therapy
Protozoa			
P. carinii	SMZ-TMP plus folinic acid or pentamidine	Good but 30% relapse rate	Trimetrexate DFMO Aerosol pentamidine
Cryptosporidium sp.	No single reliable agent	Unpredictable	Furazolidone DFMO Spiramycin Transfer factor Bovine colostrum
Toxoplasma gondii			
Brain abscess	Sulfadiazine plus pyrimethamine plus folinic acid	Good but chronic therapy indicated to prevent relapse	
Chorioretinitis	Sulfadiazine-pyrimethamine plus clindamycin		
Fungi			
Cryptococcus neoformans	Amphotericin B plus 5-FC	Good but long-term amphotericin B indicated to prevent relapse	Fluconazole
Candida sp.			
Mucocutaneous	Nystatin or clotrimazole or ketoconazole	Good but frequent relapses	
Disseminated	Amphotericin B	Highly dependent on associated factors such as neutropenia	
Aspergillus sp.	Amphotericin B	Poor	
Histoplasma capsulatum	Amphotericin B	Consider maintenance ketoconazole	

Bacteria			
MAI	Multidrug regimens including ansamycin plus clofazimine Isoniazid, ethambutol, ethionamide, amikacin, cycloserine, ciprofloxacin	Poor but may have symptomatic improvement	Gamma-interferon Tumor necrosis factor Transfer factor Granulocyte-monocyte colony stimulating factor
M. tuberculosis	Isoniazid plus rifampin or, if resistance likely, isoniazid, rifampin, streptomycin, and pyrazinamide	Good in pulmonary tuberculosis and lymphadenitis	
Salmonella	Standard antibiotic therapy	Good but long-term therapy indicated to prevent relapses	
Streptococcus pneumoniae Hemophilus influenzae Listeria monocytogenes	Standard antibiotic therapy Standard antibiotic therapy Standard antibiotic therapy	Response generally good if bacterial etiology is recognized and treated promptly	
Viruses			
Herpes simplex	Topical, oral, or parenteral acyclovir	Good but frequent relapses	
Herpes zoster	Acyclovir or vidarabine	Shortens healing and lessens chance of dissemination	
CMV		Transient improvement	Gangcyclovir Foscarnet
Papovavirus JC	ARA-C	Transient response in some patients	

Difficulties in the therapy of these infections are due to a number of factors: (1) persistence of the HIV-related immune suppression, (2) limitations of available diagnostic techniques, (3) inadequate chemotherapeutic agents and attendant toxicity, (4) multiple and repeated opportunistic infections, and (5) progressive debility due to HIV neurologic disease.

Our experience with a large number of AIDS patients over the last eight years has been marked by the growing awareness that in many instances opportunistic infections can be suppressed but not eradicated with current therapeutic modalities and that prolonged suppressive therapy to curtail recurrences is desirable. Despite our expanded knowledge of the spectrum of disease, improvements in diagnosis, such as the use of blood isolation techniques for mycobacteria, and some advances in therapeutic options, the clinical course of AIDS patients continues to be marked by severe recurrent and multiple infections.

BACTERIAL INFECTIONS

M. tuberculosis in AIDS patients is presumed to be reactivated disease in many instances, since it occurs with much greater frequency among patients born in areas of endemic tuberculosis, such as Haiti or Africa. *M. tuberculosis* may present as localized adenitis or pulmonary disease but appears to disseminate more readily in AIDS patients. In Haitians, *M. tuberculosis* has frequently preceded other manifestations of AIDS by as much as 17 months.[5] Response to therapy with conventional antituberculous drugs has generally been good, but in view of the high incidence of drug resistance in Haiti (up to 33%), a regimen of isoniazid, rifampin, streptomycin, and pyrazinamide may be appropriate pending susceptibility testing.[6] Initial evaluation of all HIV infected patients should include mantoux skin testing.

MAI, one of the most commonly encountered pathogens in AIDS, has been found at autopsy in up to 50% of patients. Diagnosis of disseminated disease has been facilitated by use of blood culture systems such as the *Dupont Isolator,* and continuous high level bacillemia is common.[7,8]

Sensitivity patterns of MAI isolates have varied somewhat among institutions, but in general MAI is resistant to conventional antituberculous drugs.[9] Agents that may have in vitro activity against clinical isolates include cycloserine, ethionamide, ethambutol, amikacin, and ciprofloxacin. In vitro synergy of multidrug combinations has been demonstrated but is of uncertain clinical significance.[10] Clofazimine (Lamprene) and ansamycin are investigational agents active against MAI in vitro that have been used widely. Isolates from The New York Hospital have been 92% sensitive to 1 µg/ml of clofazimine and 100% sensitive to 2 µg/ml of ansamycin.[11]

Clofazimine is available from Ciba-Geigy and has been useful in the treatment of lepromatous leprosy. It is well absorbed (70%), metabolized by the liver, and has a prolonged tissue half-life of approximately 70 days. Tissue deposition with crystal formation causing infarction has been reported. Recommended oral dosage ranges from 100 mg three times per week to 300 mg daily. Ansamycin (LM427) is a rifamycin derivative that may be obtained from the Food and Drug Administration (FDA) (301-443-6797). It is more active in vitro against both rifampin-sensitive and rifampin-resistant strains of mycobacteria. Despite low serum levels, ansamycin is concentrated fivefold in lung and twofold in kidney, liver, and spleen.

Our recent observations suggest that bacillemia may be eradicated in a significant number of patients (33%) employing a four-drug regimen of isoniazid, ethambutol, ansamycin, and clofazimine.[12] Symptomatic improvement may occur during therapy, with resolution of fever, sweats, and malaise. In addition, patients may gain weight and have improvement in hepatic enzyme abnormalities. In our experience, however, patients whose blood is sterilized on therapy do not have a markedly improved prognosis, and the mean survival from diagnosis remains short (6.5 months).[12] Despite eradication of bacillemia, persistent intracellular infection is probably the rule and has been demonstrated by bone marrow biopsy and at autopsy. The role of immunomodulatory therapy using gamma-IFN or tumor necrosis factor in an attempt to enhance intracellular killing of MAI is under investigation.

Given the potential for at least transient clinical response, it is reasonable to treat symptomatic patients. Asymptomatic patients may benefit from therapy, but evidence that treatment prolongs their survival is lacking, and any decision to treat should be reviewed if drug toxicity occurs.

Pneumococcal pneumonia and sepsis has been reported to occur with increased frequency in AIDS patients. *H. influenzae* has also been noted as a cause of pneumonia, presumably due to impaired opsonizing antibody production.[13] Bacterial pneumonias may be patchy or diffuse on chest x-ray film and indistinguishable from *P. carinii*. If patients with alveolar infiltrates are given pentamidine as empiric therapy for presumed *P. carinii* pneumonia, they should also receive an antibiotic active against *S. pneumoniae* and *H. influenzae* pending culture results of blood and respiratory secretions.

Salmonella typhimurium has caused severe gastroenteritis and persistent bacteremia in AIDS patients. Patients may be prostrate or relatively asymptomatic despite ongoing bacteremia. These infections have been difficult to eradicate, and prolonged courses of antibiotics (four to six weeks) are frequently necessary to prevent prompt relapse. Those patients who relapse despite an adequate course of intravenous (IV) therapy are candidates for long-term oral suppression.[14]

VIRAL INFECTIONS

Members of the herpes virus group regularly cause severe, protracted, and recurrent infection in AIDS patients. CMV causes a wide variety of clinical syndromes, including fever of undetermined origin (FUO), adrenalitis, colitis, hepatitis, pneumonia, necrotizing retinitis, and possibly encephalitis. The virus is often recovered from the blood and urine of AIDS patients without apparent disease, and, in general, histopathologic confirmation of tissue invasion should be sought to corroborate culture results. DHPG (gancyclovir) is a guanosine analog with impressive in vitro activity against CMV. Recent reports have demonstrated significant improvement in patients with CMV retinitis, but relapse within a month of terminating therapy has been the rule.[15] Limited evidence also suggests transient improvement in patients with other disseminated CMV syndromes.[16] The major toxicity encountered at the dosages used (2.5 to 5 mg/kg every eight hours) has been leukopenia. Efforts are underway to define the role and toxicity of long-term maintenance regimens. Other currently available antiviral compounds have not demonstrated efficacy in AIDS patients with CMV infection.[17,18]

Herpes simplex viral infections are most commonly seen as chronic perianal and genital ulcerations in persons with AIDS. The ulcers may be very extensive and are easily diagnosed by viral culture. Patients not responding to topical 5% acyclovir frequently respond to IV therapy. Relapses are quite common, and long-term suppression with oral acyclovir (600–800 mg per day) is helpful. Subsequent episodes may respond to repeated courses of IV acyclovir. Other syndromes due to herpes simplex include encephalitis, pneumonia, and esophagitis. The clinical picture of herpetic esophagitis is indistinguishable from candida infection, and patients with oral thrush may have herpetic lesions of the esophagus.

Dermatomal and ophthalmic *Herpes zoster* may precede the onset of opportunistic infections of Kaposi's sarcoma. A greatly increased number of cases of ophthalmic *Herpes zoster* has been noted among young homosexuals at risk for AIDS.[19] *Zoster* infections in AIDS patients tend to be more severe, with delayed healing and a higher incidence of local complications. Recent evidence demonstrating the superiority of acyclovir (10 mg/kg every eight hours) over vidarabine for treatment of *Herpes zoster* in immunologically compromised non-AIDS patients suggests that IV acyclovir may be the drug of choice for persons with AIDS as well.[20,21]

Progressive multifocal leukoencephalopathy (PML) is a subacute demyelinating disease in which patients present with focal motor and sensory deficits, cerebellar dysfunction, or personality changes. Infection with the papovavirus JC has been documented in several AIDS patients by brain biopsy demonstrating oligodendrocyte intranuclear inclusions and viral particles.[22] No clinical benefit has been obtained with Idoxuridine or vidarabine; however, a transient improvement was seen in 50% of patients treated with cytosine arabinoside (ARA-C).[23]

HIV appears to be directly responsible for clinically important neurologic disease. Virus has been recovered from brain, cerebrospinal fluid (CSF), and peripheral nerve of patients with syndromes including aseptic meningitis, subacute encephalopathy, myelitis, and peripheral neuropathy.[24] An etiologic role for the virus is further substantiated by the finding of local HIV antibody production in CSF.[25] Thus, central nervous system (CNS) penetration will be an important consideration in designing therapeutic trials of new antiviral compounds.

Case History

This 26-year-old homosexual male developed clumsiness of his right hand for several weeks. Past history revealed intermittent fever and headaches for eight months. Head computed tomography (CT) showed a nonenhancement hypodense lesion of the left motor strip. Two lumbar punctures were normal except for elevated gammaglobulin. Bone marrow and lymph node biopsies showed reactive patterns. His three-week hospital course was complicated by *P. carinii* pneumonia. Intravenous (IV) sulfamethoxazole-trimethoprim (SMX-TMP) was discontinued after 13 days of therapy because of fever and rash. Laboratory studies revealed a white blood cell count of 5.1/mm^3, hematocrit of 33%, an erythrocyte sedimentation rate of 68/mm/h, elevated liver function tests, CMV 1:128, Epstein-Barr virus (EBV) 1:320, hepatitis B surface antibody positive, and negative Sabin-Feldman to toxoplasmosis. Oral thrush was controlled with mycostatin.

The patient was readmitted one week after discharge for persistent fever, headache, increasing right arm weakness, speech and word finding difficulties, and a gait disturbance to the right. Physical examination revealed generalized adenopathy, oral thrush, dysarthria, right cranial nerve VII and arm weakness, inability to perform rapid alternating movements on the right, and a positive Rhomberg to the right. A cerebral arteriogram was normal. A CT-guided needle aspirate of the lesion yielded scanty material. Rare oligodendrocytes containing acidophilic nuclear inclusion bodies consistent with PML were seen. Electron microscopy of these cells revealed intranuclear viruslike particles.

Therapy with a continuous IV infusion of ARA-C (60/mg/m^2 daily for five days) was given. One week later, objective neurologic improvement was observed with disappearance of the paresthesia, a more fluent speech pattern, and an increase in the right hand, arm, and leg motor function. However, right-sided weakness again progressed, and a second course of ARA-C was administered three weeks later without a clinical response. Over the next month, weakness and dysarthria became progressively worse, and the patient was admitted for alpha-interferon therapy. A CT scan at that time showed no change from the previous examination. After ten days of therapy, fever and leukopenia developed and the interferon was discontinued. Over the next two weeks, the patient's clinical course was marked by fever, leukopenia, progressive neurologic deterioration, and coma. Consent for a postmortem examination was not obtained.

PROTOZOAL INFECTIONS

P. carinii pneumonia (PCP) has been diagnosed in approximately 60% of AIDS patients and is the most common life-threatening infection.[26,27] The presentation in AIDS patients tends to be more subtle and subacute than in persons with other causes of immunosuppression.[28] Diagnosis can be delayed unless it is recognized that patients may have atypical or normal chest x-ray films and normal resting arterial oxygen saturation. Gallium scanning has proved to be a useful adjunct in patients with mild respiratory symptoms and equivocal chest x-ray films. The organism can be readily demonstrated in bronchoalveolar lavage, thus avoiding the need for transbronchial biopsy in many cases. The diagnostic yield of bronchoalveolar lavage can be improved by the use of giemsa and toluidine blue stains in addition to methenamine silver stain. Several studies have recently demonstrated that examination of sputum specimens induced with hypertonic saline can lead to diagnosis in 55% of patients.[28a,28b] Furthermore, diagnostic yields are improved when induced sputums were stained by indirect immunofluorescence using a specific monoclonal antibody.[28c] Broader application of these techniques will reduce the need for bronchoscopy.

Survival of AIDS patients with initial episodes of PCP is similar to other immunosuppressed patients; however, resolution of clinical signs and symptoms is slower in the person with AIDS. Delayed clearing of cysts from lung tissue has been demonstrated by serial transbronchial biopsy. In one study, cysts were present in 9 of 10 patients following 9 to 21 days of therapy, and in 4 of 6 patients evaluated between 22 and 29 days.[29] These observations, coupled with a relapse rate of approximately 25%, have prompted us to treat all patients for 21 days. Longer courses of therapy have been successful when resolution is delayed. SMX-TMP and pentamidine have demonstrated similar efficacy.[30,31]

We treat patients initially with SMX-TMP, but up to 60% of AIDS patients will develop drug-related toxicity.[32] The most common adverse reactions are fever, hypersensitivity rash, bone marrow suppression, elevated hepatic enzymes, and gastrointestinal intolerance. Pentamidine, an aromatic diamidine, may be given safely intravenously in a dose of 4 mg/kg daily if infused slowly over one to two hours with monitoring of vital signs. Serious adverse effects occur with pentamidine, including hypotension, hypoglycemia, marrow suppression, azotemia, hypocalcemia, elevated hepatic enzymes, and hallucinations. Hypoglycemia is often severe, and its onset can be delayed until after a course of therapy is complete. This complication may be more common in patients who develop azotemia during treatment.[33] Late diabetes mellitus has been noted occasionally.

Retrospective analysis has shown that patients who fail to respond to initial therapy and are subsequently switched to the alternate drug have a poor prognosis for survival. Combined SMX-TMP and pentamidine for treatment failures does not appear to improve outcome and undoubtedly compounds toxicity. Anecdotal reports and personal experience suggest there is a role for the use of corticosteroids in patients presenting with severe hypoxemia.

Progress toward defining less toxic alternative therapy has been hampered by the difficulties of drug evaluation in the lung cell tissue culture system required for laboratory support of *P. carinii*. An improved pentamidine bioassay technique using a strain of *Candida tropicalis* has enhanced understanding of the drug's pharmacokinetics and tissue distribution. Following a 4 mg/kg dose IV over one hour, peak plasma levels are in the range of 0.5 to 3.2 µg/ml and decline rapidly, with a mean elimination half-life of 17 ± 4 minutes. After repeated dosing, there is a second, more prolonged elimination phase, and the half-life of urinary excretion is in the range of five days. The highest tissue levels of pentamidine after IV or intramuscular (IM) administration are found in the liver and spleen, followed by the kidney and adrenal; lung levels are much lower.[34] Aerosol administration of pentamidine is being evaluated as a means of limiting toxicity and increasing efficacy.[35] Studies in rats have demonstrated that aerosol administration leads to higher lung drug levels and diminished drug concentration in kidney and liver.[36] Another observation of interest is that liposome-encapsulated pentamidine, given by either the IV or aerosol route, leads to an increased lung to kidney concentration ratio.[37] Finally, comparative trials of SMX-TMP and trimetrexate with leukovorin in patients with moderately severe PCP are in progress.

The 25% recurrence rate of PCP in the AIDS population has prompted the search for effective prophylactic regimens. Initial use of SMX-TMP was disappointing because of frequent hypersensitivity reactions. Fansidar (sulfadoxine-pyrimethamine) has a prolonged half-life that allows dosing once a week. A group of 33 homosexual AIDS patients with a history of PCP were given Fansidar weekly and observed. Although 22 patients had a history of SMX-TMP allergy, only 5 had to discontinue taking Fansidar because of rash or leukopenia. None of the patients who continued taking the drug developed PCP, and after a mean follow-up of 48 weeks, 20 patients remained alive.[38] Fansidar has been associated with the development of Stevens-Johnson Syndrome and concern over this, as well as possible marrow toxicity of both Fansidar and SMX-TMP, has prompted trials of prophylactic aerosol pentamidine. Aerosolized pentamidine given in doses of 300 mg every four weeks appears to be effective, but long-term toxicities need to be defined. Dissemination of pneumocystis to other organs may be a hazard of this approach.

TOXOPLASMOSIS

Cerebral toxoplasmosis has been noted frequently in AIDS patients. The clinical presentation is not specific, but focal neurologic signs or seizures are present in most patients. Multiple or single contrast-enhancing mass lesions are found on CT scan. CSF usually demonstrates a mild mononuclear cell pleocytosis with elevated protein but may be entirely normal.[39,40]

Serologic data have been compatible with reactivated rather than primary disease. IgM antibodies are absent in most patients and IgG (Sabin-Feldman dye test or IFA [immunofluorescent antibody]) is present at variable levels. Few AIDS patients will have fourfold rises in IgG IFA or titers greater than 1000.[41] Complement-fixing antibodies are frequently negative. We routinely obtain baseline IFA titers on patients with HIV infection to identify those at risk for subsequent CNS toxoplasmosis.

The diagnosis is confirmed by brain biopsy. Routine histopathology may be negative, and the yield is enhanced by use of an immunoperoxidase stain and mouse inoculation. Brain biopsy in this patient group seems to have a high morbidity rate, and we frequently treat patients with characteristic CT scans and positive serologies empirically. Follow-up CT scans in 12 to 14 days generally show significant improvement in toxoplasmosis lesions. Patients not responding may then require biopsy. Patients respond well to sulfadiazine (6 to 8 daily) plus pyrimethamine (25 to 50 mg daily), but relapses follow discontinuation of even prolonged therapy. Drug-induced bone marrow suppression can be ameliorated in some cases by folinic acid, 6 mg daily. *Toxoplasma* chorioretinitis is also seen in AIDS patients. Clindamycin may be useful with sulfadiazine in the treatment of chorioretinitis.[42]

Case History

A 33-year-old white homosexual male was admitted for progressive neurologic symptoms over one week. Six months before this second admission, he was admitted because of progressive shortness of breath and intermittent low-grade fever for one month. Physical examination revealed a temperature of 37.5°C, generalized adenopathy, and a normal chest examination. Laboratory studies revealed a hematocrit of 35%, a white blood cell count of 12.3/mm³, a platelet count of 175,000/mm³, pO$_2$ of 76 mm Hg on room air, and bilateral diffuse interstitial infiltrates. Bronchoscopy was normal, but lavage and biopsy were positive for *P. carinii*.

He received IV SMX-TMP, three ampules four times daily, with a clinical response and improvement in chest x-ray films and blood gases. Fever (40°C), leukopenia (white blood cell count 2.6 mm³), and a diffuse maculopapular rash were noted on day 8 of SMX-TMP, and pentamidine (4 mg/kg daily) was substituted. Fever, nausea, and vomiting occurred eight days later, and pentamidine was discontinued. During this hospitalization, the patient developed oral thrush and esophagitis, which responded to mycostatin and ketoconazole. Serologic studies revealed CMV, 1:64; EBV, 1:640; and Sabin-Feldman dye test, 1:1024 (complement fixation, 1:8). Identical results were obtained two weeks later. Circulating immune complexes were 75 μg/ml.

Over the ensuing five months, fatigue, anemia, and leukopenia persisted. One week before admission, the patient developed poor motor control of his left hand and would walk to the left. Four days before admission, he sideswiped five parked cars on the left and backed into a parked police car on the left. He also noted difficulty in remembering events, understanding what was read, and dressing apraxia. In retrospect, he recalled early morning and late afternoon headaches. Physical examination revealed normal temperature, whitish exudates by funduscopic examination, and right parietal lobe signs. Laboratory data included a hematocrit of 28.3%, a white blood cell count of 2.8 mm³, an erythrocyte sedimentation rate of 94 mm/h, normal chest film, and a ring-enhancing lesion in the right parietal area on head CT. A brain biopsy revealed *Toxoplasma gondii* with abscess formation. Sabin-Feldman dye test was 1:1024, and complement fixation was 1:4.

Because of the patient's previous hypersensitivity reaction to SMX-TMP, he was given pyrimethamine (loading dose 100 mg followed by 25 mg twice daily), folinic acid (6 mg every day), and IV clindamycin (900 mg every eight hours). Decadron was slowly tapered postoperatively. On the seventh hospital day, fever and a diffuse maculopapular rash were noted. Prophylactic dilantin was discontinued, with prompt disappearance of both findings. Repeat head CT two weeks postoperatively revealed marked reduction in brain edema but no change in the size of the abscess. Clinically the patient continued to improve, with a decrease in headaches and partial return of parietal lobe function.

Case History

This 32-year-old white male homosexual was well until February 1982, when he developed fever, cough, and shortness of breath. He was admitted to another hospital, where the diagnosis of PCP was made on transbronchial biopsy. He was treated with SMX-TMP and discharged in good condition after three weeks. The Sabin-Feldman dye test at discharge was positive at 1:128, but the complement-fixation test and IgM titer by enzyme-linked immunosorbent assay (ELISA) were negative. He did well, except for a brief episode of poorly characterized pleuritis, until late June, when he developed fever, generalized weakness, and scotomata in both eyes. On July 2, 1982, he was evaluated at the National Institutes of Health (NIH), where he was noted to have intermittent fever and bilateral chorioretinitis. His immunologic evaluation revealed markedly decreased natural killer cell activity, decreased interferon levels, elevated levels of circulating immune complexes, absent T cell response to mitogen stimulation, anergy to multiple delayed hypersensitivity skin tests, reversal of the normal helper/suppressor T cell ratio, and mild neutropenia with a lymphocytopenia. In addition, CMV was cultured from throat, urine, and blood samples. The Sabin-Feldman dye test was positive at 1:256, and IgM titer by ELISA was 2 (on a scale of 0 to 10). Because of the significant CMV excretion, it was felt that the retinitis represented CMV chorioretinitis, and no specific therapy was given.

Between Aug. 8 and Aug. 20, 1982, the patient received five plasmaphareses, with improvement in his sense of well-being. On Aug. 5, the Sabin-Feldman dye test was positive and the IgM titer by ELISA was four. He had progressive visual loss and was treated with a brief course of intraocular steroid injections without benefit. He was admitted to The New York Hospital on Sept. 3, 1982, for rapid progression of bilateral blindness over the previous two weeks. On admission, he was cachetic and febrile to 39.2°C and had diffuse cervical and axillary adenopathy and an extensive, multifocal, bilateral chorioretinitis and vitriitis. His visual acuity was reduced to only finger counting bilaterally. Laboratory studies revealed a hemoglobin 9.4g/dL, a white blood cell count of 4.1 mm³, a platelet count of 157,000 mm³, hepatitis A and B antibody positive and hepatitis B surface antigen negative, antinuclear antibody (ANA) 2+, total complement (CH_{50})-180, CMV 1:1024, EBV 1:5120, polyclonal elevation of IgG and IgA, normal chest x-ray film, and negative cultures of throat, blood, and urine for CMV. The Sabin-Feldman dye test was 1:8000, the complement-fixation test was 1:512, and the IgM titer by ELISA was 2 positive. The patient was started empirically on systemic amphotericin B, pyrimethamine, sulfadiazine, and clindamycin and underwent a left diagnostic vitrectomy.

Cultures of the vitreous fluid were negative for bacteria, mycobacteria, fungi and viruses. Gram's stain, potassium hydroxide (KOH) preparation, and AFB smear were unrevealing. About 0.5 ml of the vitreous fluid was inoculated intraperitoneally into laboratory mice. On sacrifice of the mouse six weeks later, *Toxoplasma* cysts were found in the brain and spleen. The Sabin-Feldman dye test performed on the mouse was positive at 1:1024. After three days, amphotericin B was discontinued and the patient continued taking pyrimethamine, 50 mg daily, and sulfadiazine, 1.5

g four times daily. Clindamycin was also discontinued because of gastrointestinal side effects. After three months of chemotherapy, visual acuity markedly improved, as did the chorioretinitis. The patient's ophthalmologist discontinued treatment with pyrimethamine and sulfadiazine because of apparent complete resolution of chorioretinitis. Three months later the patient was admitted to the hospital in coma with multiple contrast-enhancing lesions on CT scan. Postmortem examination confirmed *Toxoplasma* brain abscess with intraventricular rupture.

CRYPTOSPORIDIUM

Cryptosporidium sp. is a coccidian protozoan that causes enteritis in animals and humans. Recognized initially in immunocompromised patients and animal handlers, it is now known to be a cause of transient diarrheal illness in healthy persons worldwide.[43] Cryptosporidial infection in AIDS patients is generally severe and persistent. Patients develop profuse watery diarrhea, malabsorption, and weight loss. Cryptosporidia have been found throughout the epithelial surfaces of the gastrointestinal tract, including the biliary system.[44,45] Organisms can be demonstrated by acid-fast- or auramine-stained smears of stool, by sucrose flotation concentration, and by histopathology.[46] Small bowel biopsies reveal cryptosporidia adherent to the microvillus border, epithelial cell flattening, and villous atrophy.

Therapy of cryptosporidial infection in AIDS patients has been frustrating. Various antibiotics active against other protozoans have been ineffective. Occasional patients have shown some benefit from furazolidone, 400 to 600 mg daily. DFMO (alpha-diflouromethylornithine) has also been used with limited success. Spiramycin, a macrolide antibiotic, appears to have a beneficial clinical and parasitologic effect, but owing to the variable natural course of untreated infection, blinded, controlled trials are necessary to establish efficacy.[47] The observation that a small number of patients with *Cryptosporidium* infection improved after therapy with oral bovine transfer factor, derived from *Cryptosporidium*-immune calves, is intriguing.[48]

Case History

A 30-year-old black homosexual male was admitted three times over a nine-month period to The New York Hospital. His first admission was due to renal failure secondary to immune complex deposition requiring hemodialysis until his death. Renal biopsy demonstrated focal proliferative glomerulonephritis with intense immune-complex-mediated vascular injury by immunofluorescence. Circulating immune complexes were 8000 µg/ml. Persistent oral and esophageal candidiasis and herpes perianal ulceration were noted, requiring ketoconazole and acyclovir therapy, respectively.

The second admission, which spanned five months, was noted for nausea, vomiting, abdominal pain, and voluminous watery diarrhea, with a 60 lb weight loss requiring total parenteral nutrition (TPN). Because of a right lower lobe infiltrate on admission, a transbronchial biopsy was performed, which revealed nonspecific inflammation and few *P. carinii*. The clinical course was not consistent with PCP, and therefore only oral prophylactic SMX-TMP was given for two weeks. An extensive gastrointestinal investigation including small bowel biopsy revealed 2 to 3 μm protozoa embedded on the brush border of the small intestine and replacing intestinal microvilli at the epithelial cell junction. The morphologic forms included trophozoites and schizonts consistent with *Cryptosporidium*. Oocysts were also demonstrated by acid-fast stain in repeated stool examinations employing sucrose flotation. The patient was placed on furazolidone, 150 mg four times daily. The clinical response over a period of eight weeks of therapy included abatement of the diarrhea and a 30 lb weight gain. TPN was discontinued, and the patient was able to subsist on oral feedings. Two stool examinations were negative for cryptosporidium oocysts.

The third and final admission was precipitated by recurrent diarrhea, cachexia, and severe rectal pain due to herpes perianal ulceration. The patient was given IV acyclovir and oral furazolidone with some clinical improvement. However, fever and bilateral pulmonary infiltrates were noted three weeks after admission, and *P. carinii* was demonstrated by Gram-Weigert stained smear in bronchial lavage. IV SMX-TMP was instituted, but the patient developed leukopenia (white blood cell count 1.1 mm^3) and acute respiratory distress syndrome and died 72 hours later. Consent for autopsy was denied.

FUNGAL INFECTIONS

Cryptococcus neoformans causes meningitis, fungemia, and pneumonia in AIDS patients. Meningitis has been the most common syndrome, although blood cultures are often simultaneously positive. There may be a remarkable lack of inflammatory response, and it is not unusual to find numerous organisms with few leukocytes in the CSF. India ink stained preparation is diagnostic in more than 80% of cases, and CSF cultures are virtually always positive. Extremely high titers (1:10,000) of both serum and CSF cryptococcal antigen have been noted.[49]

Most patients respond initially to systemic amphotericin B and 5 flourocytosine (5-FC), but relapse is common after treatment is discontinued. We have treated patients with daily amphotericin B and 5-FC for six to eight weeks while monitoring sequential cultures as well as CSF and serum cryptococcal antigen. If response is adequate, we follow patients at home while they take amphotericin B three times a week until evidence of active disease has resolved. Long-term maintenance with once- or twice-weekly amphotericin B is then indicated. 5-FC is excreted by the kidneys, and toxic levels will occur in patients with nephrotoxicity unless appropriate dose reductions are made. Management is more difficult if 5-FC levels are not rapidly available.

Fluconazole is a triazole antibiotic that has demonstrated good CSF penetration in animal models. Early clinical studies with fluconazole have shown encouraging results in cryptococcal meningitis. It has demonstrated efficacy both in treatment and in long-term prophylaxis of recurrences following initial acute therapy with amphotericin B.

Oral *C. albicans* has been the most common mycotic infection in patients with AIDS or AIDS-related complex (ARC). Thrush occurring in the HIV-positive lymphadenopathy patient has a particularly ominous prognosis for rapid progression to full-blown AIDS and has been shown to correlate with severely impaired lymphocyte gamma-interferon production in vitro.[50,51] *Candida* esophagitis should be suspected in any patient with symptoms of odynophagia or dysphagia, even in the absence of thrush.

Patients not responding promptly to empiric therapy for presumed *Candida* esophagitis should have diagnostic endoscopy performed to exclude other pathology, such as *Herpes simplex* infection or Kaposi's sarcoma. Oral nystatin, clotrimazole trouches, and ketoconazole are generally effective, but long-term therapy is frequently needed to prevent relapse. Severe cases respond well to amphotericin B in doses of 0.3–0.4 mg/kg/day.

Disseminated *Candida* infections do not commonly arise de novo in AIDS patients but may result from catheter-initiated sepsis, broad-spectrum antibiotic regimens, or severe neutropenia. Other fungi that have been noted, although less commonly, are *Aspergillus, Coccidioides immitis, Blastomyces dermatitidis,* and *Histoplasma capsulatum*. *Histoplasma* should be considered in the FUO patient with a history of residence in an endemic region. Organisms can be demonstrated by stained preparation and culture of bone marrow or liver and may also be found within monocytes on peripheral blood smears. Circulating antigen detection techniques should also be helpful. Ketoconazole has proved effective for both progressive cavitary and disseminated histoplasmosis; however, in these severely immunocompromised patients, amphotericin B is the preferred treatment.

CONCLUSION

Impressive gains have been made since the discovery of HIV, the etiologic agent of AIDS. Nonetheless, the epidemic has continued to grow and mounting evidence now suggests that the vast majority of the more than one million infected persons in the United States will become symptomatic. It is clear that physicians will be confronted with greater numbers of opportunistic infections in the coming months and years.

Experience gained to date has facilitated the earlier diagnosis of many infections. Pitfalls in diagnosis have been recognized, such as an atypical inflammatory response, i.e., lack of granuloma formation in disseminated MAI and cryptococcosis. Serologic confirmation is also hampered by the absence of typical IgG and IgM responses to acute exacerbation of latent infections, as in CNS toxoplasmosis.

Extended courses of antibiotics and maintenance regimens have been useful in preventing relapse of some opportunistic infections, but have not apparently changed the overall prognosis of AIDS. Improved therapeutic modalities are needed for this population with severe and persistent immune deficiency.

REFERENCES

1. Real FX, Gold JWM, Krown SE, Armstrong D. *Listeria monocytogenes* bacteremia in the acquired immunodeficiency syndrome (letter). Ann Intern Med 1984;101:883.
2. Schlanger G, Lutwick LI, Kurzman M, et al. Sinusitis caused by *Legionella pneumophilia* in a patient with the acquired immune deficiency syndrome. Am J Med 1984;77:957–60.
3. Holtz HA, Lavery DP, Kapila R. Actinomycetales infection in the AIDS syndrome. Ann Intern Med 1985;102:203–5.
4. Armstrong D, Gold JWM, Dryjanski J, et al. Treatment of infections in patients with the acquired immunodeficiency. Ann Intern Med 1985;103:738–43.
5. Pitchenik AE, Cole C, Russell BW, et al. Tuberculosis, atypical mycobacteriosis and the acquired immunodeficiency syndrome among Haitian and non-Haitian patients in south Florida. Ann Intern Med 1984;101:641–5.
6. Pitchenik AE, Russell BW, Cleary T, et al. The prevalence of tuberculosis and drug resistance among Haitians. N Engl J Med 1982;307:162–5.
7. Kiehn TE, Edwards FF, Brannon P, et al. Infection caused by *Mycobacterium avium* complex in immunocompromised patients: Diagnosis by blood culture and fecal examination. J Clin Microbiol 1985;21:148–73.
8. Wong B, Edwards FF, Kiehn TE, et al. Continuous high-grade *Mycobacterium avium-intracellulare* bacteremia in patients with AIDS. Am J Med 1985;78:35–40.
9. Dutt AK, Stead WW. Long-term results of medical treatment in *Mycobacteria intracellulare* infection. Am J Med 1979;67:449–53.
10. Zimmer BL, DeYoung DR, Roberts GD. In vitro synergistic activity of ethambutol, isoniazid, kanamycin, rifampin and streptomycin against *Mycobacterium avium-intracellulare* complex. Antimicrob Agents Chemother 1982;22:148–50.
11. Horsburgh CR, Cohen DL, Roberts RB, et al. *Mycobacterium avium-intracellulare* isolates from AIDS patients differ from patients without AIDS. Antimicrob Agent Chemother 1986;30:955–57.
12. Kocher J, Scavuzzo D, Horsburgh CR, et al. Therapeutic response in AIDS patients with disseminated *Mycobacterium avium-intracellulare* (Abstr.). Clin Res 1986;34:522A.
13. Polsky B, Gold JWM, Whimbey B, et al. Bacterial pneumonia in patients with the AIDS syndrome. Ann Intern Med 1986;104:38–40.
14. Jacobs JL, Gold JWM, Murray HW, et al. *Salmonella* infections in patients with the acquired immune deficiency syndrome. Ann Intern Med 1985;102:186–8.
15. Felstein D, D'Amico DJ, Hirsch M, et al. Treatment of cytomegalovirus retinitis with 9-(2-hydroxy-1-(hydroxy-methyl ethoxymethyl) guanine. Ann Intern Med 1985;103:377–80.
16. Masur H, Lane CH, Palestine A, et al. Effect of 9-(1,3dihydroxy-2-propoxymethyl) guanine on serious cytomegalovirus disease in eight immunosuppressed homosexual men. Ann Intern Med 1986:104:41–4.
17. Lopez C, Watanabe KA, Fox JJ. 2'-fluoro-6-iodo-aracytosine, a potent and selective anti-herpesvirus agent. Antimicrob Agent Chemother 1980;17:803–6.
18. Gold JWM, Leyland-Jones B, Urmacher C, Armstrong D. Pulmonary and neurologic complications of treatment with FIAC in patients with acquired immune deficiency syndrome. AIDS Res 1984;1:243–52.
19. Sandor EV, Millman A, Groxson, Mildvan D. *Herpes Zoster* ophthalmicus in patients at risk for AIDS. Am J Ophthamol 1986;101:153–55.

20. Shepp DH, Dandliker PS, Meyers JD. Treatment of varicella-zoster virus infection in severely immunocompromised patients. N Engl J Med 1986;314:208–11.
21. King DH, Galasso G, eds. Proceedings of a symposium on acyclovir. Am J Med 1982;73:1–392.
22. Miller JR, Barrett RE, Britton CB, et al. Progressive multifocal leukoencephalopathy in a male homosexual with T-cell immune deficiency. N Engl J Med 1982;307:1436–8.
23. Smith CR, Sima AAF, Salit IE, Gentili F. Progressive multifocal leukoencephalopathy: Failure of cytarabine therapy. Neurology 1982;32:200–3.
24. Ho DD, Rota TR, Schooley RT, et al. Isolation of HTLV III from cerebrospinal fluid and neural tissues of patients with neurologic syndromes related to AIDS. N Engl J Med 1985;303:1493–7.
25. Resnick L, DiMarzo-Veronese F, Schupbach J, et al. Intra blood-brain barrier synthesis of HTLV III specific IgG in patients with neurologic symptoms associated with AIDS or AIDS related complex. N Engl J Med 1985;303:1498–1504.
26. Murray JF, Felton CP, Garay SM, et al. Pulmonary complications of the acquired immunodeficiency syndrome: Report of a National Heart, Lung Blood Institute workshop. N Engl J Med 1984;310:1682–8.
27. Stover DE, White DA, Romano PA, et al. Spectrum of pulmonary diseases associated with the acquired immune deficiency syndrome. Ann Intern Med 1985;78:429–37.
28. Kovacs JA, Hiemenz JW, Macher AM, et al. *Pneumocystis carinii* pneumonia: A comparison between patients with AIDS and patients with other immunodeficiencies. Ann Intern Med 1984;100:663–71.
28a. Pitchenik AE, Ganjei P, Torres A, et al. Sputum examination for the diagnosis of pneumocystis carinii pneumonia in the acquired immune deficiency syndrome. Am Rev Respir Dis 1986;133:226–29.
28b. Bigby TD, Margolskee D, Curtis TL. The usefulness of induced sputum in the diagnosis of the acquired immunodeficiency syndrome. Am Rev Respir Dis 1986;133:515–18.
28c. Kovacs JA, Ng VL, Masur H, et al. Diagnosis of pneumocystis carinii pneumonia: improved detection in sputum with the use of monoclonal antibodies. N Engl J Med 1988;318:589–93.
29. Shelhamer JH, Ognibene FP, Macher AM, et al. Persistance of PCP in lung tissue of acquired immunodeficiency syndrome patients: Treatment for pneumocystis pneumonia. Am Rev Respir Dis 1984;130:1161–5.
30. Winston DJ, Lau WK, Gale RP, Young LS. Trimethoprim-sulfamethoxazole for the treatment of *Pneumocystis carinii* pneumonia. Ann Intern Med 1980;92:762–9.
31. Haverkos HW. Assessment of *Pneumocystis carinii* pneumonia therapy. Am J Med 1984;76:510–18.
32. Gordin FM, Simon GL, Wofsy CB, Mills J. Adverse reactions to trimethoprim-sulfamethoxazole in patients with AIDS. Ann Intern Med 1984;100:495–9.
33. Stahl-Bayliss C, Kalman C, Laskin O. Pentamidine induced hypoglycemia in patients with the acquired immune deficiency syndrome (Abstr.). Clin Res 1985;33:288A.
34. Bernard EM, Donnelly HJ, Maher MP, Armstrong D. Use of a new bioassay to study pentamidine pharmacokinetics. J Infect Dis 1985;152:750–4.
35. Bernard EM, Donnelly HJ, Koo HP, Armstrong D. Aerosol administration improves delivery of pentamidine to the lungs (Abstr.). 25th ICAAC pp. 193.
36. Waldman RH, Pearce DE, Martin RA. Pentamidine isothionate in lungs, liver and kidney of rats after aerosol or intramuscular administration. Am Rev Respir Dis 1973;108:1004–6.

37. Debs R, Straubinger R, Ryan J, et al. Selective lung delivery of pentamidine by liposomes (Abstr.). 25th ICAAC pp. 192.
38. Roberts RB, Madoff L, Scavuzzo D, Kocher J. Fansidar prophylaxis for recurrent *Pneumocystis carinii* pneumonia in AIDS patients (Abstr.). Clin Res 1986;34:524A.
39. Luft BJ, Brooks RG, Cowley FK, et al. Toxoplasmic encephalitis in patients with AIDS. JAMA 1984;252:913–17.
40. Hauser WE, Luft BJ, Conley FK, Remington JS. Central nervous system toxoplasmosis in homosexual and heterosexual adults (letter). N Engl J Med 1982;307:498–9.
41. Wong B, Gold JWM, Brown AE, et al. Central nervous system toxoplasmosis in homosexual men and parenteral drug abusers. Ann Intern Med 1984;100:36–42.
42. Tabbara KF, O'Connor GR. Treatment of ocular toxoplasmosis with clindamycin and sulfadiazine. Ophthalmology 1980;87:129–34.
43. Clinicopathological Conference. Immunodeficiency and cryptosporidiosis. Br Med J 1980;281:1123–7.
44. Soave R, Armstrong D. Cryptosporidium and cryptosporidiosis. Rev Infect Dis 1986;8:1012–23.
45. Guarda LA, Stein SA, Cleary KA, Ordonez NG. Human cryptosporidiosis in the acquired immune deficiency syndrome. Arch Pathol Lab Med 1983;107:562–6.
46. Ma P, Soave R. Three step stool examination for cryptosporidiosis in 10 homosexual men with protracted watery diarrhea. J Infect Dis 1983;147:824–8.
47. Portnoy D, Whiteside ME, Buckley E, MacLeod CL. Treatment of intestinal cryptosporidiosis with spiramycin. Ann Intern Med 1984;101:202–4.
48. Louie E, Borkowsky W, Klesius PH, et al. Treatment of cryptosporidiosis with oral bovine transfer factor (Abstr.). 25th ICAAC 1985;244.
49. Kovacs JA, Kovacs AA, Polis M, et al. Cryptococcosis in the acquired immune deficiency syndrome. Ann Intern Med 1985;103:533–8.
50. Murray HW, Hillman JK, Rubin B, et al. Patients at risk for AIDS-related opportunistic infections: Clinical manifestations and impaired gamma-interferon production. N Engl J Med 1984;313:1504.
51. Roberts RB, Scavuzzo D, Hart C, et al. Prospective monitoring of high risk patients for AIDS (Abstr.). 1986 International Conference on AIDS, p.110.

Chapter 22

Treatment of Kaposi's Sarcoma

Patricia L. Myskowski
Bijan Safai

The therapeutic approaches to Kaposi's sarcoma (KS) are as diverse as the clinical variants of the disease. Before 1981, KS was classified into three different clinical types[1]: classic KS, seen primarily in elderly men of Eastern European extraction[2–4]; African KS, occurring in epidemic areas of Central Africa; and KS of immunocompromised individuals, the result of preexisting malignancy[5] or immunosuppressive drug therapy.[6–8] In 1981, a fourth clinical variant of KS was discovered in young, previously healthy homosexual men as part of acquired immunodeficiency syndrome (AIDS).[9–11] Although these four types of KS share a common histology,[12] the important differences in clinical course and complicating factors (e.g., opportunistic infections) have mandated varied treatment approaches to the disease.[12]

BACKGROUND

KS is a multifocal neoplasm that usually begins as reddish purple patches on the skin. Histopathologic examination of a skin biopsy reveals that the neoplastic process begins in the upper dermis. The characteristic findings of KS include the presence of spindle-shaped cells, often arranged in vascularlike patterns, with extravasated erythrocytes present in slitlike clefts between these bundles of spindle cells.[2] Although the cell of origin of KS is not clear, most authors favor a reticuloendothelial or endothelial origin.[2,12] No differences in histopathologic patterns can be discerned among the different clinical variants of the disease.[12]

Classic KS, as first described by Moritz Kaposi in 1872, is a rare, multicentric neoplasm affecting the lower extremities of elderly men.[13] It is primarily seen in North America and Europe and occurs in individuals of eastern European descent.[14] There is a significant male predominance, with classical KS being three to ten times more frequent in men than women.[15] The disease mainly affects older individuals (mean age 63 years)[16] and runs an indolent course. Skin lesions are usually slow growing, beginning as violaceous patches in the lower legs or feet. Early in the disease, skin lesions may be unilateral patches on the feet but later tend to evolve into reddish purple plaques and nodules on both lower extremities (Plate VII). Lymphedema often occurs with progression of disease. Lymph node and visceral involvement is rare. The mean survival of classic KS patients in the United States is prolonged, with a range of 8 to 13 years being typical; many classic KS patients succumb to second malignancies or one of the (unrelated) illnesses that befall the elderly.[2,12] Thus, for many classic KS patients, their disease is chronic and rarely life threatening. Palliation and local tumor control are foremost concerns, often with radiotherapy or single-agent chemotherapy. Aggressive antitumor regimens, with their potentially dangerous side effects and complications, are often best avoided in this elderly population.[2]

African KS presents a different problem in management.[17,18] This endemic form of KS has been recognized in Africa for many years and is a relatively common tumor in Central Africa. In Uganda, KS constituted nearly 9% of all the malignancies in 1962[15] and continues to be a common problem even today. African KS has been classified into four different types by Taylor.[17] There are three locally aggressive, primarily cutaneous forms that occur in adults; these have been classified as nodular, florid, or infiltrative. Soft tissue and bony involvement may accompany these forms of African KS, and these variants are often managed with chemotherapy or locally destructive means such as surgery. The fourth type of African KS is the lymphadenopathic type, which primarily affects children and young adults (under 25 years of age). This very aggressive and widely disseminated type of KS involves the skin to a lesser degree than do the other forms; it has lymph node and visceral involvement and is usually fatal within a short time. For this reason, the most common therapeutic approach has been aggressive chemotherapy.

A third type of KS affects patients who are immunosuppressed through the use of different medications. The recognition of this variant has provided important information for the development of treatment regimens in AIDS. This group of patients consists primarily of renal transplant recipients but also includes individuals receiving immunosuppressive drugs for the treatment of collagen vascular diseases such as systemic lupus erythematosus and dermatomyositis.[6-8]

Several different immunosuppressive drugs, including prednisone, azathioprine, and cyclophosphamide, have been implicated in the development of this type of KS. Discontinuation of these medications has been reported to result in the spontaneous regression of lesions in several instances.[6-8] Therefore, it appears that as the patients entered a less immunosuppressed state, the KS lesions began to disappear without specific antitumor therapy.

The occurrence of KS as part of AIDS has presented a new dilemma in the choice of treatment.[19-21] This form of epidemic KS initially involved individuals who were quite different from the previously described groups of patients. As first described, epidemic KS involved homosexual and bisexual men, and it continues to occur in that group. Other groups at risk for AIDS, such as intravenous (IV) drug users, hemophiliacs, and blood transfusion recipients, appear to be much less likely to contract epidemic KS.[20] In contrast to the other forms of KS, AIDS-associated KS is a disease of younger men, with a median age of approximately 39 years.[14] The clinical presentations are very different from the classic form of KS and involve the development of multiple reddish purple, often oval-shaped, macules and papules. The lesions are distributed primarily on the upper part of the body, especially the trunk and arms. These lesions tend to follow the skin lines, in a distribution similar to that of pityriasis rosea (Plate VIII).[14] Mucous membrane, lymph node, and gastrointestinal tract involvement may also be evident early in the disease and occasionally may be the first sites of involvement (Plate IX). These skin lesions tend to grow rapidly and may develop into large tumors over a few months, in contrast to the slower growth of classic KS lesions. Epidemic KS may rapidly progress to very large, almost confluent tumor masses, often with accompanying lymphedema. This is especially frequent on the lower extremities, where ulcerated tumors may interfere with ambulation or become the source of secondary bacterial infection. For these reasons, tumor control is crucial in the management of epidemic KS. However, the use of effective cytotoxic therapy is complicated by the patient's profoundly immunosuppressed state as a result of the infection by the AIDS-associated retrovirus, human immunodeficiency virus (HIV). Thus, opportunistic infections may be more likely with aggressive chemotherapy. Another therapeutic avenue has led to efforts toward immune restoration through various immune modulators (e.g., interferon). This potential source of tumor control may be effective by reversing the retrovirus-associated immunosuppression, resulting in regression of KS lesions. For the physician treating epidemic KS, there is a special dilemma: maintaining a balance between the patient's own AIDS-associated immunosuppression and iatrogenic immunosuppression by chemotherapeutic agents.

RADIOTHERAPY

When KS is primarily localized to the skin, physical modalities may offer a logical approach to the disease. Cryosurgery with liquid nitrogen, laser therapy, and surgical excision have all had some success with limited disease, but radiotherapy has emerged as the most effective means of local therapy.[22-28] Radiation therapy has been widely advocated as the treatment of choice for classic KS[25] and is also effective in managing large tumors in AIDS-associated KS.[26,28] KS is a very radiosensitive tumor, and several different regimens of radiation treatment have proved useful. Spot therapy of individual lesions, as well as limited and extended field radiation therapy, have all been shown to be effective means of controlling this disease.

Borok et al. have successfully used whole-leg irradiation, with a megavoltage apparatus, to treat mild to moderate classic KS. Patients were treated with a total dose of 3000 rad given in 20 fractions during a four-week period.[22] Lo et al. have also reported on their experience with 50 patients with classic KS.[23] Patients received different regimens as follows: 21 patients received megavoltage electron for their initial radiotherapy, 12 patients were given supervoltage photons, and 27 patients received a combination of both electron and photons. The authors reported an overall response rate of 93% after a single fractioned radiotherapy course. A single dose of 800 to 1200 rad was necessary to control localized KS lesions.[23] Harwood has also reported his experience with 38 classic KS patients, giving them extended field radiotherapy with cobalt 60 irradiation of at least half a limb.[24] He noted that this was also a safe and effective treatment for cutaneous tumors. Nisce et al. noted a 100% overall response to total skin electron beam therapy in classic KS patients.[25] They treated 20 patients with 400 rad to the entire skin surface with a 3.5 MeV electron beam, once weekly, for six to eight weeks (total dose 2400 rad). Seventeen of these patients (85%) had complete remissions of their skin lesions, with the median duration being 48 months (range 10 to 92 months).[25] Thus radiotherapy has proved to be an effective means of tumor control in classic KS and may provide prolonged remissions of the disease.

The lesions of AIDS-associated KS have also been shown to be sensitive to traditional radiotherapy.[26-28] This approach cannot be used for (most) visceral disease, but it has some value for palliation and cosmetic improvement for the patient with extensive cutaneous KS. Cooper et al. noted that the lesions of AIDS-associated KS were very radiosensitive, similar to classical KS lesions.[26] They used different types of radiation (megavoltage, kilovoltage, or a combination) in 15 patients with AIDS-associated KS. Dosages ranged from 1800 to 3000 rad of total radiation. All patients reported some improvement in symptoms of their skin lesions, with flattening in size and decreased pain being the most commonly reported results. This group of 15 radiation-treated patients was selected from a total group of 182 AIDS-associated KS patients. The authors concluded that there is a small subgroup of individuals who are best managed by radiation therapy. Nisce and Safai have also reported on their experience with 38 patients with AIDS-associated KS treated by radiation therapy.[26] Twenty-seven patients were treated with local radiation therapy, and 11 patients received either subtotal skin electron beam (SSEB) or total skin electron beam (TSEB) therapy. Seven patients received radiation therapy to the cutaneous lesions only, while 20 patients received additional radiation to sites other than the skin. In addition, 12 patients received radiation for oropharyngeal lesions. Even though AIDS-related KS lesions were noted to be very radiosensitive, survival times were not significantly prolonged, and patients frequently died of opportunistic infections unrelated to therapy. There was significant toxicity associated with radiation of oropharyngeal lesions, largely because the lesions were generally extensive, infiltrated, and usually associated with oral candidiasis. The authors concluded that radiotherapy was a potentially effective therapy but was often complicated by opportunistic infections and was limited by toxicity in oral mucosal lesions.[27]

CHEMOTHERAPY

Single-agent and combination chemotherapy regimens have been useful, to varying extents, in all the clinical variants of KS. Chemotherapy has emerged as the main form of therapy in patients with African KS, as well as in classic KS patients with visceral involvement or disseminated skin lesions not controlled by radiation therapy. Several chemotherapeutic agents have also been shown to be helpful in controlling tumors in AIDS-associated KS, and these are:

- *Vinca* alkaloids
  Vinblastine
  Vincristine
  Etoposide
- Actinomycin-D
- Bleomycin
- 1,3-bis (B-chloroethyl)-1-nitrosourea (BCNU)
- Dimethyl-inidazole-triazeno-carboxamide (DTIC)
- Razoxane

Some of the drugs used in the treatment of African and classic KS are now largely of historic interest. The older literature records the use of inorganic arsenic, also known as Fowler's solution, as well as subcutaneous injections of calcium codylate in KS with equivocal results. Hormone therapy, using testosterone proprionate, was also used, without success, in the early search for antitumor effects.[29]

The first chemotherapeutic agent that was used successfully in KS was nitrogen mustard. Early anecdotal reports of the use of intra-arterial infusion with nitrogen mustard preceded Cook's trial of the drug in a large number of patients.[30] He employed intra-arterial infusions with mustine hydrochloride in 75 Ugandan patients with KS and obtained a follow-up of two years in 60 of these patients. Cook noted that 60% of these individuals showed improvement, although most remissions were short. The major side effects found in this regimen included nausea, vomiting, transient decrease in the white blood cell count, and pain and edema in the infused extremity, which lasted approximately ten days.[30]

Kyalwazi administered 2,3,5-tris 1-azire-dinye-p-benzoquinone (triaziquone) to 21 patients orally,[31] with complete regressions seen in 11 patients and partial responses in nine patients. The primary side effects were nausea, vomiting, and bone marrow depression, which were felt to be quite severe. Complete remission was obtained in only two patients, and most remissions were short-lived. The authors also emphasized that lymph node and visceral lesions did not respond to this regimen.[31]

VINCA ALKALOIDS

The *Vinca* alkaloids have been shown to be the most effective single chemotherapeutic agents in disseminated classic and African KS. In addition, these drugs have shown promise in the treatment of AIDS-associated KS tumors. Vinblastine and vincristine are alkaloids that have been obtained from *Vinca rosea*, the common periwinkle plant. These agents disrupt spindle formation in metaphase as their mode of antitumor action. Although their mechanisms of tumor inhibition are similar, the toxic effects of vincristine and vinblastine are somewhat different. The primary side effect of vincristine is neurotoxicity, manifested by muscular weakness, peripheral neuritis, and areflexia; myelosuppression is relatively uncommon. Vinblastine, however, frequently results in myelosuppression, primarily leukopenia, and this is often the dose-limiting toxicity. Neurotoxicity is much less frequent with vinblastine. In addition, alopecia may result from the use of either of these agents.

The first successful use of *Vinca* alkaloids was reported by Scott and Voight in 1966.[32] They treated three American males with classic KS, who had significant involvement of their lower extremities, with vincoleukoblastine, with some response.[32] Goldman et al. also treated five classic KS patients and reported prolonged remission with systemic vinblastine therapy, including one patient who had visceral involvement.[33] Tucker and Winkelmann reviewed the literature of 18 cases treated with vinblastine and included reports of five of their own patients with classic KS. They concluded that vinblastine was an effective antitumor agent, with tumor regression being obtained in most patients. The drug also appeared to be relatively nontoxic and was not myelosuppressive when used in the standard IV dose of 0.1 mg/kg per week.[34] Klein et al. reported their experience with 14 patients with classic KS. Patients were treated with vinblastine administered through a number of routes—intra-arterial, IV, and intralesional. Nine patients had limited cutaneous nodular disease, three had locally invasive disease, and two had systemic involvement by KS. Patients were maintained on low-dose therapy; the longest duration of treatment in any single patient was 900 mg of vinblastine given intravenously over eight years. Side effects were mild and consisted mainly of leukopenia. These authors noted that the majority of patients had good to excellent results from therapy.[35] In addition, Solan et al. reported their experience with four patients with cutaneous classic KS who had long-term remissions of two to seven years after receiving IV vinblastine treatment. They did not note any toxic effects from this chemotherapeutic regimen and emphasized the safety of this drug in the setting of classic KS.[36]

The experience with vinblastine as single-agent chemotherapy has been more limited in AIDS-associated KS; however, it does appear to be an effective approach in some settings.[37] Volberding et al. have reported their experience with vinblastine in the treatment of 38 patients with AIDS-associated KS. They treated patients with 4 to 8 mg of vinblastine weekly and titrated the dose to the total leukocyte count. Ten of their patients had an objective response to therapy, and 19 had stable disease. They found a lower response rate in patients who had anemia, elevated erythrocyte sedimentation rates, or any lymphoma B–like symptoms. They also noted that opportunistic infections were more common in patients who did not respond to therapy. The authors did not feel that opportunistic infections were more common in the vinblastine-treated patients, but they noted that a larger group of individuals would need to be studied before this impression could be confirmed. They concluded that vinblastine was a weak but effective chemotherapeutic agent in AIDS-associated KS.[37]

Vincristine has also been used to a limited extent, but with some encouraging results, in classic, AIDS-associated, and African KS patients. Odom and Goette used intralesional vincristine to treat lesions of classic KS in a 68 year-old man.[38] They injected 0.4 to 0.5 mg of vincristine per lesion, with excellent results.[38] Vogel et al. reported their experience with vincristine in combination with actinomycin D (dactinomycin), compared with actinoymcin D alone, in 24 African KS patients in a randomized clinical trial.[39] They noted that adding vincristine to dactinomycin increased the number of complete responses (10/14) compared with dactinomycin alone (4/10 complete responses). However, the authors could not comment on the use of vincristine alone in this setting.[39]

Vincristine has also shown promise as single-agent chemotherapy for AIDS-associated KS.[40,41] Rieber et al. treated five homosexual/bisexual men with AIDS-associated KS with vincristine, 1.4 mg/m^2 IV weekly, for four weeks and then every other week. They noted four partial responses in this group, with a median response duration of ten weeks.[40] Mintzer et al. treated 23 men with AIDS-associated KS, three of whom had a coexisting immune thrombocytopenia.[41] Patients were treated with vincristine IV, 2 mg per week for two to five weeks and then every two weeks as tolerated. The primary side effect was neurotoxicity, requiring dose reduction to 1 mg weekly in several patients. Five patients died after one or two doses, leaving eighteen evaluable patients. There were 11 partial responses (tumor regression incomplete but greater than 50%) and 7 minor responses (definite tumor regression but less than 50% improvement). The median duration of partial responses was over four months; in addition, all three patients with thrombocytopenia had a significantly increased platelet count. The group concluded that vincristine alone had significant antitumor activity, with little myelosuppression, in AIDS-associated KS.[41]

Vinca alkaloids have also been used in combination with other chemotherapeutic regimens in AIDS-associated KS.[42–47] Laubenstein et al. used etoposide (VP-16), an experimental podophylotoxin, in the treatment of KS in AIDS. They noted a 79% response rate in 32 patients, with almost half experiencing complete remissions. However, most patients appeared to have relatively early disease, since individuals were excluded if they had visceral disease, fever, or weight loss. The median response was approximately ten months.[42] Combination chemotherapy with doxorubicin, blemomycin, and vinblastine (ABV) was also used by these authors in KS patients with more advanced disease. Although response rates were high (80%), most responses were only partial (75%). However, their results were complicated by a very high risk of opportunistic infection (50%) in this group of patients. De Wys et al. have reported similar results in a smaller group of patients using ABV.[43] However, Levine et al. noted a difference in response rates between AIDS-associated and African KS. Only 15% of epidemic KS patients responded to chemotherapy (such as ABV), in contrast to 90% of African KS patients achieving complete response.[44] Volberding has also issued a note of caution in treating AIDS-associated KS patients with combination chemotherapy, since four of seven patients treated by him in this manner developed opportunistic infections.[45] He has suggested that further trials of combination chemotherapy be postponed, pending more results on the efficacy of less immunosuppressive, single-agent regimens.[45,46]

DACTINOMYCIN

Dactinomycin is an antibiotic that exerts its antitumor effect through the inhibition of DNA-directed RNA synthesis. Its major side effects include bone marrow suppression, gastrointestinal disturbances, stomatitis, and alopecia. Kyalwazi et al. first reported the use of the drug to treat African KS patients in 1970.[48] They treated 26 patients with KS (24 with nodular-florid, one with visceral, and one with lymphadenopathic disease) with IV dactinomycin. There were eighteen evaluable patients, of whom 61% were alive and free of disease after chemotherapy. Follow-up time was short (two years), and the drug appeared to be effective for cutaneous disease only.[48] Vogel et al. achieved tumor regression in 9 of 12 patients using dactinomycin (compared with 1 of 10 patients who achieved tumor regression using cyclophosphamide).[49]

BLEOMYCIN

Bleomycin is another antitumor antibiotic; its antitumor effects are the result of scission of DNA. Its common side effects include mucocutaneous ulcerations, nausea, vomiting, and alopecia. The most serious toxicity, however, is pulmonary fibrosis, occurring in 5% to 10% of patients. Yagoda et al. first noted regression of KS lesions in a patient treated with bleomycin.[50] Vogel et al. treated 10 African KS patients with nodular, florid, or infiltrative disease with bleomycin.[51] Six of the patients responded to 300 mg administered over a one-month period. Unfortunately, responses were short-lived, with three of six patients showing tumor progression within two months after stopping the drug. The authors felt that the short duration of response was related to either drug dosage or administration schedule; however, higher doses were not feasible because of the high risk of pulmonary fibrosis.[51] Two additional patients with nodular KS have been reported to have responded to bleomcyin alone.[52]

1-3-BIS(B-CHLOROETHYL)-1-NITROSOUREA

1,3-bis(B-chloroethyl)-1-nitrosourea (BCNU) is another chemotherapeutic agent that has shown some promise in African KS patients. Its antitumor effect is the result of cross-linkage with DNA, and its primary toxic effect is bone marrow suppression. Vogel et al. found BCNU to be somewhat effective in phase II trials.[51] Twenty-one African KS patients were treated with BCNU, 200 mg/m^2 every six to eight weeks, with nine patients (43%) responding. There was, however, one drug-related death in this trial. The authors felt that BCNU might have limited use because of toxicity.[51]

DIMETHYL-IMIDAZOLE-TRIAZENO-CARBOXAMIDE

Dimethyl-imidazole-triazeno-carboxamide (DTIC) is a cell-cycle nonspecific agent; its antitumor actions may occur through cross-linkage with DNA. Its major toxic effect is bone marrow suppression with impairment of immune responses. As a chemotherapeutic agent, DTIC has shown its primary usefulness in the treatment of metastatic melanoma, but there are also a few reports of its efficacy in African KS.[53–55] Vogel et al. treated ten patients with African KS with DTIC, 250 mg/m^2 daily for five days, every six weeks. All patients had been previously treated with at least two other chemotherapeutic agents. They noted a 50% overall response rate without infectious or hemorrhagic complications.[53] DTIC has also proved useful in combination chemotherapy regimens.[54,55] Olweny et al. treated a group of children with lymphadenopathic KS with different treatment regimens.[54] DTIC alone was given to six patients; two complete remissions (lasting 50+ and 66+ months) and two partial responses were observed. DTIC plus vincristine was given to two patients, with one patient having a complete response (lasting 24 months) and one patient having no response. Three other children received dactinomycin, vincristine, and DTIC, resulting in complete remissions in all three patients (3, 6, and 12 months, respectively).[54] DITC, then, has been shown to have some effect in African KS in limited trials.[53–55]

MISCELLANEOUS ANTICANCER DRUGS

Razoxane (1,2 bis(3,5-dioxopiperazine-1-yl)propane) (ICRF-159) is a relatively new anticancer drug that is a derivative of ethylene diaminetetraacetic acid (EDTA). This drug exerts its antitumor effect by arrest in either the late premitotic (G2) or early mitotic (M) phase of the cell cycle. Olweny et al. have demonstrated a 60% overall response rate with razoxane in African KS patients.[56] The drug was administered in a dose of 1gm/m^2 daily, orally for three days every eight hours, and repeated in two weeks. Eighteen patients were treated, with ten patients (55%) having a partial response and one patient having a complete response that lasted five months. The other patients had no response to this agent.

Cyclophosphamide is an alkylating agent that has been widely used in the treatment of various malignancies. However, it has been quite disappointing in the treatment of KS patients. In a comparison trial of this drug with dactinomycin, Vogel et al. noted that only one of ten patients had any response to the treatment.[49] This lack of therapeutic response has been documented in another case.[55]

IMMUNE STIMULATION: TREATMENT WITH BIOLOGIC-RESPONSE MODIFIERS

The potential use of biologic-response modifiers has appeared especially attractive in the treatment of AIDS-associated KS. An interaction between tumor progression and the immune system has been documented in KS, since spontaneous remissions in renal transplant recipients have been reported following discontinuation of immunosuppressive drug therapy.[57] In addition, spontaneous regression of KS lesions has also been seen in the setting of AIDS.[58] These observations provide support for therapeutic trials with immunomodulatory agents in AIDS-related KS. Of the various agents available as immune stimulators, interferon has been especially promising because of its combination of antiviral, antiproliferative, and immunostimulatory actions. Krown et al. were the first to use interferon in AIDS-related KS.[59] The authors treated 12 patients with high-dose recombinant alpha-interferon, at doses of 36 or 54×10^6 units intramuscularly (IM) per day for 28 days. After this 28-day period, patients received injections three times a week for more prolonged periods. Forty percent of patients had major objective responses, with complete responses observed in three of 12 patients. The side effects seen were primarily those of a flulike syndrome, including fever, malaise, and headache. Opportunistic infections were infrequent, especially in patients who responded to the interferon.[59] Groopman et al. conducted a phase II study of 20 patients with AIDS-associated KS, using recombinant alpha-2 interferon. They randomly assigned patients to two groups: a low dose of 1×10^6 units/m^2 subcutaneously per day, or a high dose of 50×10^6 units/m^2 per day. An overall response rate of 30% was noted when both groups were considered, but of the 14 patients who received the higher dose of interferon, 42% had objective responses.[60] Side effects were similar to those of Krown's group in that 75% of patients experienced a flulike syndrome. Mitsuyasu et al. have reported similar response rates (25%) in 60 patients who were treated with high-dose alpha-2 recombinant interferon, 30 million units/m^2 subcutaneously three times a week.[61] Other trials with alpha interferon at lower doses have not been as promising.[62,63] Real et al. noted only 3% (partial) response rates in patients treated with low-dose recombinant alpha interferon of 3 million units IM per day.[62] Gelmann et al. were not encouraged by their use of lower doses of purified alpha interferon. They treated ten patients with either 7.5 million units/m^2 daily for 28 days or 2 courses of 15 million units/m^2 daily for ten days separated by a rest period of ten days. Only two patients had partial responses, and they concluded that this particular treatment regimen was not effective in the therapy of AIDS-related KS.[63]

Some other forms of interferon have been used with limited success in AIDS-associated KS.[64-66] Rios et al. reported the use of lymphoblastoid interferon alpha in 20 patients with KS. Patients received 20 million units/m² IM once a day for 60 days and then three times a week after they were determined to be either stable or responding to therapy. A 66% objective response rate (four complete responses and four partial remissions) were observed. The authors felt that lymphoblastoid interferon alpha showed promising antitumor activity in this setting.[64] Gamma interferon has largely been disappointing in its effect on AIDS-associated KS.[65,66] Odajnyk et al. failed to find any regression of tumor in seven patients treated with gamma interferon, 0.5 million units IM once daily for ten days, followed by a ten-day rest period and then a second course of therapy. In addition, tumor progression was noted in all patients, with three having rapid escalation of previously stable disease.[65] Thus, other types of interferon need further evaluation to establish their role in the treatment of AIDS-associated KS.

MISCELLANEOUS DRUGS

Anecdotal reports have occurred on the use of a few other agents in AIDS-associated KS.[67,68] Dapsone was reported to cause regression of KS lesions in one patient with AIDS.[67] In contrast, isotretinoin did not appear to have any results.[68] Isoprinosine, an immune potentiator, is also currently being studied for possible activity in AIDS-associated KS.

FUTURE DIRECTIONS IN THERAPY

The future direction of therapy against KS and AIDS is likely to involve the use of antiviral agents, probably in conjunction with some immune reconstitution. Antiretroviral agents against HIV are currently being tested, although it is too early to know the effect of these drugs on KS.[69,70] Most exciting of the anti-HIV drugs is azidothymidine.[69] Ribavirin has also shown promise in vitro against HIV. Some studies have suggested that ribavirin therapy can reduce HIV activity in peripheral blood lymphocyte cultures.[70] Interferon has also been shown to inhibit the replication of HIV in vitro, which may account for some of its effectiveness in the treatment of AIDS-associated KS. In addition, a number of other antiviral agents, such as phosphonoformate, are entering clinical trials and may prove to have some activity against HIV.

However, the use of antiviral drugs alone cannot be expected to result in an antitumor response in AIDS-associated KS patients, unless immune recovery accompanies the treatment of HIV. The combination of antiviral drugs and immune modulators needs further investigation. Most promising of these is the combination of alpha-interferon and azidothymidine in KS[71] perhaps because of the synergistic inhibition of HIV by azidothymidine and recombinant interferon-alpha in vitro.[72] Another, theoretically interesting possibility is the use of bone marrow transplantation in KS patients with AIDS. Several trials have been carried on with bone marrow transplantation, but it is too early to tell whether this will be an effective means of therapy.[21]

CONCLUSION

KS, with its varied clinical patterns, provides a true spectrum of disease. At one end of the spectrum is classic KS, an indolent disorder that remains primarily limited to the skin. Therapy of classic KS consists primarily of local control of disease, often through the use of radiation therapy but occasionally through chemotherapy. In contrast, AIDS-associated KS is an aggressive neoplasm that poses a special problem for the physician. Effective tumor control may be crucial, since disseminated disease may sometimes be life threatening. However, the primary limiting factor is the severe immunosuppression by HIV. Some chemotherapeutic regimens have been useful in controlling this disease. In addition, the use of biologic-response modifiers, especially alpha interferon, has proved useful in treating these patients. Radiation therapy may also provide important palliation of cutaneous tumors. Antiviral therapies, as well as new forms of immune restoration, may hold the answer for truly effective treatment of AIDS-associated KS.

Several crucial questions, however, must be answered before effective therapies can be developed. First is the unanswered question of the cell of origin of KS. Next is the possible role of environmental factors, such as cytomegalovirus, in initiating the disease. And last is the poorly understood relationship between the immune system and the behavior of KS. Further investigation is necessary to better understand and develop treatments for this complex disease.

REFERENCES

1. Safai B, Good RA. Kaposi's sarcoma. A review and recent developments. Clin Bull 1980;10:62.
2. Oettle AG. Geographical and racial differences in the frequency of Kaposi's sarcoma as evidence of environmental or genetic causes. Acta Un Int Cancer 1962;18:330.
3. Reynolds WA, Winkelmann RK, Soule EH. Kaposi's sarcoma. Medicine 1965;44:419.
4. Dorn HF, Cutler SJ. Morbidity from cancer in the United States: I. Variation in incidence by age, sex, marital status and geographic region. Public Health Monogr 1955;29:121.
5. Safai B, Mike V, Giraldo G, et al. Association of Kaposi's sarcoma with second primary malignancies. Cancer 1980;4:1472–9.
6. Harwood AR, Osoba D, Hofstader SL, et al. Kaposi's sarcoma in recipients of renal transplants. Am J Med 1979;67:759–65.

7. Stribling J, Weitzner S, Smith GV. Kaposi's sarcoma in renal allograft recipients. Cancer 1978;42:442–6.
8. Klein M, Pereira F, Kantor I. Kaposi's sarcoma complicating systemic lupus erythematous treated with immunosuppression. Arch Dermatol 1974;110:602–5.
9. Centers for Disease Control. Kaposi's sarcoma and pneumocystis pneumonia among homosexual men—New York City and California. MMWR 1981;30:305.
10. Centers for Disease Control. Follow-up on Kaposi's sarcoma and pneumocystis pneumonia. MMWR 1981;30–409.
11. Hymes KS, Cheung TL, Greene JB, et al. Kaposi's sarcoma in homosexual men: A report of eight cases. Lancet 1981;2:598.
12. Gottlieb GJ, Ackerman AB. Kaposi's sarcoma: An extensively disseminated form in young homosexual men. Hum Pathol 1982;13:882.
13. Kaposi M. Idiopathisches multiples Pigmensarkam der Haut. Arch Derm Syph 1972;4:265–73.
14. Myskowski PL, Safai B. Classical and AIDS-associated Kaposi's sarcoma In: J Raaf, ed. Management of soft tissue sarcoma. Chicago: Year Book Medical Publishers, 1986.
15. Rothman S. Remarks on sex, age and racial distribution of Kaposi's sarcoma and on possible pathogenetic factors. Acta Un Int Cancer 1962;18:332.
16. Di Giovanna JJ, Safai B. Kaposi's sarcoma. Review of ninety cases with particular emphasis on the familial occurrences, ethnic background, and prevalence of other diseases. Am J Med 1981;71:779–83.
17. Taylor JF, Templeton AC, Vogel CL, et al. Kaposi's sarcoma in Uganda: a clinicopathological study. Int J Cancer 1971;8:122.
18. Katiku KK, Durosinmi, Etti FA. The treatment of Kaposi's sarcoma by combination chemotherapy in Nigeria. Clin Radiol 1984;35:155–8.
19. Volberding PA. The problem of Kaposi's sarcoma in AIDS. Front Radiat Ther Oncol 1985;19:91–8.
20. Odajnyk C, Muggia FM. Treatment of Kaposi's sarcoma: Overview and analysis by clinical setting. J Clin Oncol 1985;3:1277–85.
21. Mitsuyasu RT, Groopman JE. Biology and therapy of Kaposi's sarcoma. Semin Oncol 1984;11:53–9.
22. Borok T, Farina AT, Leider M. Radiotherapy for Kaposi's sarcoma. J Dermatol Surg Oncol 1979;5:39.
23. Lo TCM, Salzman FA, Smedal MI, Wright KA. Radiotherapy for Kaposi's sarcoma. Cancer 1980;45:684.
24. Harwood AR. Kaposi's sarcoma: An update on the results of extended field radiotherapy. Arch Dermatol 1981;117:775.
25. Nisce LZ, Safai B, Poussin-Rosillo H. Once weekly total and subtotal skin electron beam therapy for Kaposi's sarcoma. Cancer 1981;47:640.
26. Cooper JS, Fried PR, Laubenstein J. Initial observations on the effect of radiotherapy on epidemic Kaposi's sarcoma. JAMA 1984;252:934–5.
27. Nisce LZ, Safai B. Radiation therapy of Kaposi's sarcoma in AIDS. Memorial Sloan-Kettering experience. Front Radiat Ther Oncol 1985;19:133–7.
28. Harris JW, Ree TA. Kaposi's sarcoma in AIDS: The role of radiation therapy. Front Radiat Ther Oncl 1985;19:126–32.
29. Kyalwazi SK. Treatment of Kaposi's sarcoma. East Afr Med J 1969;46:450.
30. Cook J. The treatment of Kaposi's sarcoma with nitrogen mustard. Acta Un Int Cancer 1962;18:494.

31. Kyalwazi SK. Chemotherapy of Kaposi's sarcoma. Experience with Trenimon. East Afr Med J 1968;45:17.
32. Scott WP, Voight JA. Kaposi's sarcoma. Management with vincaleucoblastine. Cancer 1966;19:557.
33. Goldman J, Greenwald ES, Schulman PL. Vinblastine therapy of Kaposi's sarcoma. NYS J Med 1974;74:1828.
34. Tucker SB, Winkelmann RK. Treatment of Kaposi's sarcoma with vinblastine. Arch Dermatol 1976;112:958.
35. Klein E, Schwartz RA, Laor Y, et al. Treatment of Kaposi's sarcoma with vinblastine. Cancer 1980;45:427.
36. Solan AJ, Greenwald ES, Silvay O. Long-term complete remissions of Kaposi's sarcoma with vinblastine therapy. Cancer 1981;47:637.
37. Rieber E, Mittelwan A, Wormser GP, et al. Vinblastine therapy for Kaposi's sarcoma in the acquired immunodeficiency syndrome. Ann Intern Med 1985;103:335–8.
38. Odom RB, Goette DK. Treatment of cutaneous Kaposi's sarcoma with intralesional vincristine. Arch Dermatol 1978;114:1693.
39. Vogel CL, Primack A, Dhru D, et al. Treatment of Kaposi's sarcoma with a combination of actinomycin-D and vincristine: Results of a randomized clinical trial. Cancer 1973;31:1382.
40. Rieber E, Mittelwan A, Wormser GP, et al. Vincristine and Kaposi's sarcoma in the acquired immunodeficiency syndrome (letter). Ann Intern Med 1984;101:876.
41. Mintzer DM, Real FX, Jovino L, Krown SE. Treatment of Kaposi's sarcoma and thrombocytopenia with vincristine in patients with the acquired immunodeficiency syndrome. Ann Intern Med 1985;102:200–2.
42. Laubenstein LJ, Krigel RL, Odajnyk CM, et al. Treatment of epidemic Kaposi's sarcoma with etoposide or a combination of doxorubicin, bleomycin, and vinblastine. J Clin Oncol 1984;2:115–20.
43. De Wys WD, Curran J, Henie W, Johnson G. Workshop on Kaposi's sarcoma: Meeting report. Cancer Treat Rep 1982;66:1387–9.
44. Levine AS. The epidemic of acquired immune dysfunction in homosexual men and its sequelae opportunistic infections; Kaposi's sarcoma and other malignancies: An update and interpretation. Cancer Treat Rep 1982;66:1391–6.
45. Volberding P. Therapy of Kaposi's sarcoma in AIDS. Semin Oncol 1984;11:60–7.
46. Volberding P, Conant MA, Stricker RB, et al. Chemotherapy in advanced Kaposi's sarcoma. Am J Med 1983;74:652–6.
47. Armentrout SA. Cytotoxic chemotherapy in Kaposi's sarcoma. Adv Exp Med Biol 1985;187:159–62.
48. Kyalwazi SK, Bhana D, Master SP. Actinomycin-D in malignant Kaposi's sarcoma. East Afr Med J 1971;48:16.
49. Vogel CL, Templeton CJ, Templeton AC, et al. Treatment of Kaposi's sarcoma with actinomycin-D and cyclophosphamide: Results of a randomized clinical trial. Int J Cancer 1971;8:136.
50. Yagoda A, Krakoff I, LaMonte C, Tan C. Clinical trial of bleomycin. Proc Assoc Cancer Res 1971;12:37.
51. Vogel CL, Clements D, Wanume AK, et al. Phase II-clinical trials of BCNU (NSC-409962) and bleomycin (NSC-125066) in the treatment of Kaposi's sarcoma. Cancer Chemother Rep 1973;57:325.
52. Kim R, Guerrero RC, Ho R. Treatment of Kaposi's sarcoma with bleomycin. Cutis 1979;23:73.
53. Vogel CL, Primack A, Owor R, Kyalwazi SK. Effective treatment of Kaposi's sar-

coma with 5-(3, 3-dimethyl-1-triazeno) imidazole-4-carboxamide (NSC-45388). Cancer Chemother Rep 1973;57:65.
54. Olweny CLM, Toya T, Katongole-Moidde E, et al. Treatment of Kaposi's sarcoma by combination of actinomycin-D, vincristine and imidazole carbozamide (NSC-45388): Results of a randomized clinical trial. Int J Cancer 1974;14:649.
55. Olweny CLM, Kaddumukasa A, Atine I, et al. Childhood Kaposi's sarcoma: Clinical features and therapy. Br J Cancer 1976;33:555.
56. Olweny CLM, Masaba JP, Sikyewunda W, Toya T. Treatment of Kaposi's sarcoma with ICRF-159 (NSC-129943). Cancer Treat Rep 1976;60:111.
57. Grange RW, Jones EW. Kaposi's sarcoma and immune suppressive drug therapy: An appraisal. Clin Exp Dermatol 1978;3:135.
58. Real FX, Krown SE. Spontaneous regression in Kaposi's sarcoma. N Engl J Med 1985;313:1659.
59. Krown SE, Real FX, Cunningham-Rundles S, et al. Preliminary observations on the effect of recombinant leukocyte-A interferon in homosexual men with Kaposi's sarcoma. N Engl J Med 1983;308:1071.
60. Groopman JE, Gottlieb MS, Goodman J, et al. Recombinant alpha-2 interferon therapy for Kaposi's sarcoma associated with the acquired immune deficiency syndrome. Ann Intern Med 1984;100:671–6.
61. Mitsuyasu R, Volberding P, Jacobs A, et al. High dose alpha-2 recombinant interferon (IFN) in the therapy of epidemic Kaposi's sarcoma (KS) in acquired immune deficiency (AIDS) (Abstr. C-196). Proc Am Soc Clin Oncol 1984;3:51.
62. Real FX, Krown SE, Krim M, et al. Treatment of Kaposi's sarcoma (KS) with recombinant leukocyte A interferon (rIFN-alpha A) (Abstr. C-211). Proc Am Soc Clin Oncol 1984;3:55.
63. Gelmann EP, Preble O, Steis R, et al. Human lymphoblastoid treatment of Kaposi's sarcoma in the acquired immune deficiency syndrome: Clinical response and prognostic parameters. Am J Med 1985;78:737.
64. Rios A, Mansell P, Newell G, et al. The use of lymphoblastoid interferon HU IFN alpha-(Ly) in the treatment of acquired immune deficiency syndrome (AIDS)-related Kaposi's sarcoma (Abstr. C-245). Proc Am Soc Clin Oncol 1984;3:63.
65. Odajnyk C, Laubenstein L, Friedman-Kien A, et al. Therapeutic trail of human gamma-interferon (IFN) in patients with epidemic Kaposi's sarcoma (EKS) (Abstr. C-237). Proc Am Soc Clin Oncol 1984;3:61.
66. Krigel RL, Odajnyk CM, Laubenstein LJ, et al. Therapeutic trial of interferon-gamma in patients with epidemic Kaposi's sarcoma. J Biol Response Mod 1985;4:358–64.
67. Poulsen A, Hultberg B, Thomasen K, Wantzin GL. Regression of Kaposi's sarcoma in AIDS after treatment with dapsone (letter). Lancet 1984;1:560.
68. Ziegler JL, Volberding PA, Itri LM. Failure of isotretinoin in Kaposi's sarcoma (letter). Lancet 1984;2:641.
69. Fischl MA, Richman DD, Grieco MH, et al. The efficacy of azidothymidine (AZT) in the treatment of patients with AIDS and AIDS-related complex: a double-blind, placebo-controlled trial. N Engl J Med 1987;17:185–91.
70. McCormick JB, Getchell JP, Mitchell SW, et al. Ribavirin suppresses replication of lymphadenopathy-associated virus in cultures of human adult T lymphocytes. Lancet 1984;2:1367–69.
71. Krown SE, Bundow D, Tong WP, et al. Interferon-alpha plus azidothymidine (AZT) in AIDS-associated Kaposi's sarcoma: a phase 1 trial of the Memorial Sloan-Kettering AIDS treatment and evaluation unit. J Interferon Res 1987;7:674–88.

72. Hartshorn KL, Vogt MW, Chou TC, et al. Synergistic inhibition of human immunodeficiency virus in vitro by azidothymidine and recombinant interferon alpha-A. Antimicrob Agents Chemother 1987;3:168–72.

PART V
Immunologic Evaluation Methods and Controls

Chapter 23

Analysis of Mechanisms of Immune Suppression in AIDS

Susanna Cunningham-Rundles

Since the first published reports on the epidemic of opportunistic infections and rare tumors, now known as the acquired immunodeficiency syndrome (AIDS), much attention has been focused on the altered immunoregulation that is central to the syndrome.[1-6] Evidence linking a T lymphocyte retrovirus, human immunodeficiency virus (HIV), to AIDS transmission has provided an accepted common cause for the etiology and lethality of AIDS while raising many questions concerning the basis of differences in (1) the time required for development of frank AIDS in persons infected with the virus, (2) variation in disease course, (3) potential response to therapy and, most critically, (4) whether a balanced carrier state can occur or be achieved by therapeutic intervention. Immunologic assessment of patients with AIDS or HTLV-HIV/LAV disease has produced significant evidence for marked depression of functional response in patients with the retrovirus and no acute clinical manifestations, as well as evidence for strongly variable immune response among patients with defined AIDS.[7-10]

New approaches to immunologic assessment are needed to determine the functional dynamics of the immune system in patients with AIDS and patients with retroviral disease who do not yet have AIDS. Combined and multivariate analysis may provide one avenue of approach, since the etiology of the AIDS syndrome is complex but depends on recognition of critical variables that are largely unknown. The search for functional markers has provided evidence for immune deregulation at several levels. Both intrinsic defects at the cellular level, and quantitative defects have been described,[11,12] indicating potential variability in evolution and expression.

Efforts to achieve modulation in vitro may also provide valuable information, since such systems can be used to reveal the presence (or apparent absence) of residual or retained functional capacities that could potentially be drawn on to offset the effects of the infecting process. Some approaches to the immunologic substaging of patients with HIV disease or AIDS are presented below.

APPROACHES TO THE STUDY OF IMMUNE MODULATION IN AIDS

Initial studies in patients with AIDS by ourselves and others were chiefly focused on patients with opportunistic infections (AIDS-OI), including *Pneumocystis carinii, Toxoplasma gondii, Entamoeba histolytica, Cryptococcus neoformans, Mycobacterium avium intracellulare (MAI), Mycobacterium tuberculosis, Candida albicans, Cytomegalovirus (CMV), herpes simplex virus (HSV),* and *Epstein-Barr virus (EBV).* Since these infecting processes are known to cause perturbation of the immune system in other settings, it is reasonable to suppose that the extreme depression of functional response observed in vitro in patients with AIDS-OI might be directly caused by the secondary opportunistic infection or at least strongly influenced by its presence. However, when comparison is made between persons infected with the same organism or virus with and without concurrent HIV infection, one observes a marked difference in functional capacity and duration of immune response depressions.

Data are shown in Table 23–1 for the effect of cryptosporidiosis in patients with AIDS-OI, AIDS-associated Kaposi's sarcoma (AIDS-KS), and HIV-associated lymphadenopathy syndrome (LAS). As shown in three patients with AIDS and *P. carinii* pneumonia (AIDS-PCP), cryptosporidiosis did not further depress immune response. The T cell proliferative activity of cases 1 and 2 was actually less than that of case 3. Furthermore, response to *Escherichia coli,* a B cell mitogen that has prognostic significance in AIDS, was clearly strongest in case 3, whereas response in cases 1 and 2 was negative. In AIDS-KS, however, presence of cryptosporidiosis (case 6) was associated with significantly poorer immune response in vitro compared with cases 4 and 5. In LAS, presence of cryptosporidiosis was associated with significant loss of natural killer (NK) function and general loss of proliferative response. Case 10 illustrates opportunistic cryptosporidiosis in immunodeficiency acquired during cancer chemotherapy. Travelers' cryptosporidiosis, shown in case 11, is associated with strongly increased systemic immune response in infection and is in sharp contrast to all other cases. The responses shown here were significantly stronger than that of normal controls.

The data suggest that the meaning and effect of the appearance of cryptosporidiosisis is different in LAS and AIDS-KS than in AIDS-OI because relationship to the state or type of underlying HIV disease may be different. As shown in Table 23–2, resolution of PCP and cryptosporidiosis in AIDS-OI was paradoxically accompanied by a further decline in immune response to levels seen in cases 1 and 2 (see Table 23–1), who had only AIDS-PCP. The data suggest that some infections may actually augment immune response temporarily. In AIDS-OI, this presumably cannot be sustained and leads to peripheral exhaustion, whereas in transient infection of previously healthy persons, immune response returns to baseline normal levels. The presence of opportunistic infection in AIDS-KS has been recognized as a harbinger of poor progress.[8] Data here suggest that this may be for intrinsic reasons.

Table 23-1 Relative effect of multiple infecting agents on immune response in vitro in AIDS and HIV infection

Patient	Diagnosis	Infections	Immune Response[a,b]					
			NK[a]	PHA[b]	ConA	PWM	EC	SA
1	AIDS-OI	HIV, PCP[c]	0.0	2745	315	1700	220	330
2	AIDS-OI	HIV, PCP	3.5	2525	175	455	85	80
3	AIDS-OI	HIV, PCP, Crypto[d]	6.6	6280	685	495	3195	ND
4	AIDS-KS	HIV	0.0	8445	1445	1515	190	245
5	AIDS-KS	HIV	10.2	13,230	2980	6660	220	190
6	AIDS-KS	HIV, Crypto	7.2	7145	560	610	100	300
7	LAS	HIV	20.3	2950	1560	500	815	70
8	LAS	HIV, Crypto	10.1	3110	335	680	180	115
9	LAS	HIV, Crypto	11.8	103	90	50	70	40
10	Cancer	Crypto	7.8	5415	965	1965	680	145
11	Crypto	Crypto	54.2	26,875	23,095	15,858	26,130	26,570
12	Control[e]	None	26.5	20,175	9500	6500	3600	4200

[a] NK activity shown as percentage of ^{51}Cr release against K562 at effector-target ratio 100:1.
[b] Proliferative response given as maximum net cpm to PHA; ConA, concanavalin A; PWM, pokeweed mitogen, EC, E. coli; and SA, S. aureus.
[c] PCP, P. carinii pneumonia.
[d] Crypto, cryptosporidiosis.
[e] Normal responses: PHA >17,000 cpm; ConA >9000; PWM >5600; EC >2000; SA >2000; positive response ≥600 cpm; NK >15%.

Table 23-2 Longitudinal study of immunoresponse in AIDS-OI with cryptosporidiosis

Time (mo)	NK[b]	PHA[c]	ConA	PWM	CA[d]	EC
0[a]	6.6	6280	685	495	505	3,195
1	ND	500	200	130	35	40
2	ND	7685	935	780	65	100
4	8.4	2335	155	85	40	35

[a]Initial identification of cryptosporidiosis patient with PCP.
[b]Percentage of lysis at K562 at effector-target ratio of 100:1.
[c]Proliferative response as described in Table 23-1.
[d]CA, *Candida albicans*.

AIDS patients who present initially with Kaposi's sarcoma have, on average, a longer survival than do patients with AIDS-OI, leading to the hypothesis that AIDS-KS might be subclassified prognostically to reflect these differences. Vadhan-Raj et al.[13] have constructed a model for predicting clinical course in AIDS-KS. End points were response to alpha interferon (IFN-α) therapeutically, development of opportunistic infection, and survival. The logistic regression model for predicting responses to recombinant leukocyte A interferon (rIFNα A) selected the following markers as having significant prognostic value: (1) delayed-type hypersensitivity to recall antigens and (2) better lymphocyte proliferative response to *E. coli*. All patients had very depressed proliferative response compared with healthy controls. The overall P value for the model was 0.01. For prediction of development of OI, the model selected low proliferative response to *E. coli* ($P = 0.000$) and to PHA ($P = 0.039$). Favorable factors predicting survival were absence of serum IFN and better proliferative response to *E. coli*. The survival rate was greater than 60% at 36 months for patients remaining free of infection. The median survival for patients who developed OI was 11 months ($P = 0.01$). Although absolute T cell number, helper/inducer T cell number, and helper/inducer to cytotoxic/suppressor lymphocyte subset ratios were significantly associated with survival, addition of these factors did not add significantly to the predictive power of the model.

The fact that response to *E. coli* alone was associated with survival ($P = 0.019$) suggests either that immune response in vitro is a marker for extent of retroviral infection or that residual immune function directly affects survival potential.

If cellular immune function were a passive reflection of the extent of disease incursion, one would anticipate that absolute number of helper/inducer cells or ratio to cytotoxic/suppressor cells would be equally good or better as a predictor. But this is not the case; neither T cell subset imbalance nor quantitative limitation nor excess are directly linked with lymphocyte activation in vitro. Data shown in Table 23-3 are arranged to show descending strength of response to phytohemagglutinin and associated lymphocyte subpopulations in patients with AIDS. No simple correlation is seen. Absolute T helper numbers do not correlate with activation in a continuous fashion but only with the use of cut-off points.

Table 23–3 Comparison of helper/inducer to cytotoxic/suppressor ratio in AIDS

Patient	Proliferative Response		Lymphocyte Subpopulations		
	PHA	PWM	T4[a]	T8[b]	T4/T8[c]
1	19,976	1342	13.4	48.5	0.28
2	11,680	2049	3.3	40.7	0.08
3	11,419	2389	10.5	73.3	0.14
4	10,412	445	5.5	67.5	0.08
5	8578	586	1.1	24.6	0.04
6	6368	215	18.7	53.4	0.35
7	135	45	6.1	42.3	0.14

[a]Normal range: 21.4% to 64.7%.
[b]Normal range: 12.8% to 49.7%.
[c]Normal range: 1.0 to 3.4.

Among the populations of persons considered at risk for AIDS as a result of life style, homosexual men with LAS constitute a relatively homogenous group. Analysis of immune function in this group has been ongoing since 1981 in this laboratory.[14,15] Of the original group of 90 patients, 17% developed AIDS during the 8- to 19-month follow-up period. The incidence of AIDS in this group is now about 25%. Approximately 15% developed AIDS-KS, a similar incidence rate to that reported by others. Persistent lymphadenopathy is not limited to homosexual men but it is a characteristic of other risk groups and precedes the development of AIDS in about 40% of KS patients and 25% of patients with opportunistic infections. Among patients with LAS, about 70% showed abnormally low response to *E. coli* in vitro, and 19% (17 of 90) could be subgrouped as having the lowest response. Of these, 12 (70%) developed AIDS within 3 to 13 months. These data suggest that patients with LAS or AIDS-KS may be subgrouped according to lymphocyte functional ability and that those criteria define intrinsically different functional immune status.

Assessment of immune function in vitro is usually carried out in this laboratory in culture medium supplemented with pooled normal human serum. However, serum from AIDS patients may contain factors that further modify response. We previously reported that sera from patients with AIDS may completely block lymphocyte activation of normal controls in vitro and that this factor appeared to have anti-T lymphocyte activity.[16] As discussed above, the presence of acid labile IFNα in patients' sera has prognostic significance in patients with AIDS-KS. We have examined stored sera from patients with opportunistic infections, the prodromal syndrome (HIV disease), LAS, and AIDS-KS. Patients in each group had significant levels of IFNα (>10 IU/ml), in contrast to normal controls who did not have serum IFNα. This IFN was unstable at low pH. A close correlation was observed between presence of systemic symptoms, poor functional response in vitro, and level of IFNα in serum. The sudden appearance of IFNα was a harbinger of the development of opportunistic infection.[17]

Table 23–4 Modulation of proliferative response in vitro by alpha interferon[a]

IFN	PHA		
IU/ml	143 µg/ml	12 µg/ml	C. albicans
0	21,358	16,068	8406
32	10,920	15,038	5480
80	11,508	15,028	1532
160	8800	15,655	3522

[a]Response shown as mean cpm ^{14}C thymidine uptake following three- or five-day culture period.

Studies of IFNα in vitro, as shown in Table 23–4, show a concentration-dependent inhibition of proliferation. This inhibition, however, is highly dependent on culture conditions and appears to be virtually insignificant at lower concentrations of lymphocyte activators, as shown for the lower concentration of phytohemagglutinin. In addition, IFNα causes cellular proliferation, which results in enhanced thymidine uptake at higher concentrations (when assessed after at least four days of culture, which allows the signal to develop sufficient amplitude for detection), as indicated by the biphasic response to *C. albicans* plus IFNα in Table 23–4. The proliferating cells have been identified as NK cells. Examination of acid labile IFNα in vitro, as shown in Table 23–5, clearly demonstrates the biologic efficacy of this mediator in recruiting precursor NK cells in a healthy control, leading to augmented NK activity.

Among patients with LAS, mononuclear cells from approximately 60% cannot be induced in vitro to augmented NK activity. This failure to show augmentation is independent of endogenous baseline NK function. This suggests that deregulation of the NK system does occur in vivo and may be related to acid-labile IFN secretion. The role of acid-labile IFN in this process is unknown; however, sustained presence of this mediator may act to down-regulate NK function by feedback inhibition or repression of functional expression. This type of effect can also be observed in patients receiving IFN therapeutically.

Table 23–5 Acid-labile alpha interferon–induced NK activity

	Cytotoxicity (%)[a]		
	100:1	50:1	25:1
Endogenous	25.6	25.4	14.1
IFN-rA[b]	66.3	63.4	ND
Acid-labile IFNα[c]	52.2	64.3	59.3

[a]^{51}Cr release at effector-target ratios as shown.
[b]Recombinant IFNα.
[c]Serum containing equivalent antiviral activity as IFN-rA.
ND: Not done.

When mononuclear cells from AIDS or LAS patients are activated in vitro, the resulting proliferation is much less than seen in controls; however, in some cases, we found that removal of adherent monocytes by Sephadex G-10 filtration markedly improved response.[18] This treatment had no effect on lymphocyte subpopulation balance as detected by flow cytometry with monoclonal antibodies. Interestingly, indomethacin produced a similar effect. This observation led to a systemic evaluation of stored sera for the possible presence of prostaglandin (PGE) and the discovery that PGE was significantly elevated in AIDS and LAS.[19] PGE levels were more elevated in LAS than AIDS, whereas acid-labile IFN was more often detectable in AIDS patients when groups were simultaneously tested for both. The presence of IFNα correlated with PGE in 53% of AIDS cases, whereas PGE correlated with IFNα in only 18% of AIDS cases. Since PGE was more commonly seen in LAS, it may reflect an earlier stage of disease. In vitro analysis of the producer cell indicated that peripheral blood monocytes produced PGE without exogenous stimulation.[19] This activation of the cellular immune system during early phase of infection with HIV may be accompanied by the elaboration of soluble factors, which act as regulatory signals critically affecting cell-cell interactions to down-regulate response.

Positive modulation of immune response in AIDS has been attempted in a number of ways, including cellular replacement, use of biologic response modifiers, and antiretroviral therapy. Agents directed against the retrovirus may also directly modulate the immune system, as in the case of IFNα, which augments NK activity in recipients. Interestingly, despite IFNα's known antiproliferative effects, as shown above, among patients treated with IFNα in vivo, there is a trend toward increased proliferative response, as shown in Table 23–6. For ex-

Table 23–6 Effect of interferon treatment on proliferative response to B cell activators in AIDS-KS[a]

Patient	Pretreatment			Posttreatment		
	CA	EC	SA	CA	EC	SA
1	1629	309	190	3160	1164	540
2	4288	2910	1134	4810	3434	2304
3	168	160	300	3660	746	806
4	240	118	114	2243	1634	825
5	5092	643	550	4965	3190	1395
6	1568	310	444	7876	895	955
7	40	ND	ND	4058	ND	ND
8	602	150	290	402	398	204
9	338	508	370	11,556	323	276
10	105	130	90	9000	2304	300
11	2640	500	678	4390	3940	3965
12	180	158	190	160	203	144
13	108	90	73	78	100	84

[a] Data shown as cpm of maximum response to *C. albicans*, *E. coli*, and *S. aureus*. Responses less than 600 cpm are negative. Normal response is more than 2000 cpm.

ample, before IFN therapy, two of 12 patients had positive lymphocyte response to *E. coli*, and after treatment, eight of the 12 had positive lymphocyte response in vitro. In many patients, these effects were transient; however, the magnitude of the improved response suggests that such changes could reflect a potentially beneficial effect in vivo.

As noted above, response to lymphocyte activators in vitro may be used to characterize patients with AIDS or LAS, and response level may have prognostic significance. A new approach with potential significance might be the capacity to induce in vitro modulation. In this laboratory, studies have been carried out using a purine immunomodulating compound NPT-15392 (erythro-9-(-2-hydroxy-3-nonyl)-c-hydroxy-purine) (Newport Pharmaceuticals), which has been found to have immunomodulating properties. Figure 23–1 shows the effects of adding NPT-15392 at various concentrations to lymphocytes activated with *C. albicans* and *E. coli* in vitro in AIDS-KS. In healthy controls, no significant effect was seen. Not all patients' lymphocyte response could be affected by this compound, suggesting that patients could be subgrouped by this criterion. This kind of approach has the potential possibility of providing an index of modulating capacity.

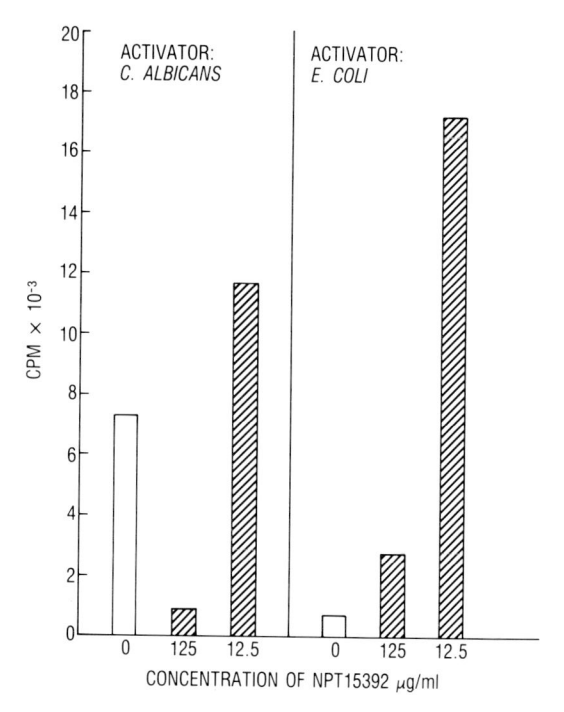

FIGURE 23–1 *Peripheral blood mononuclear cells from a patient with AIDS-KS were cultured in vitro with C. albicans or E. coli alone or with two concentrations of NPT-15392. Results of ^{14}C thymidine uptake after five days of culture are shown.*

In summary, the analysis of immune response in AIDS suggests that immune deregulation evolves differently in different subgroups of patients infected with HIV. Since reception of soluble signals as well as lymphocyte subpopulation balances affect signal transduction, study of these factors and the conditions in which they are produced is essential to meaningful analysis. Furthermore, different patients have varied capacities for modulation in vitro and the study of intrinsic modulatory function may well prove essential to future assessment of immune response in AIDS.

REFERENCES

1. Gottlieb MS, Schroff R, Schanker HM, et al. *Pneumocystis carinii* pneumonia and mucosal candiasis in previously healthy homosexual men: Evidence of a new acquired cellular immunodeficiency. N Engl J Med 1981;305:1425–31.
2. Masur H, Michelis MA, Greene JB, et al. A community acquired outbreak of *Pneumocystis carinii* pneumonia: Initial manifestation of cellular immune dysfunction. N Engl J Med 1981;305:1432–8.
3. Siegal FP, Lopez C, Hammer GS, et al. Severe acquired immunodeficiency in male homosexuals manifested by chronic perianal ulcerative herpes simplex lesions. N Engl J Med 1981;305:1439–44.
4. Masur H, Michelis MA, Wormser GP, et al. Previously healthy women with opportunistic infection vs. the initial manifestation of a community acquired cellular immunodeficiency extension of an emerging syndrome. Ann Intern Med 1983;97:533–9.
5. Vieira J, Frank E, Spira RJ, Landesman SH. Acquired immune deficiency in Haitians: Opportunistic infections in previously healthy Haitians. N Engl J Med 1983;308:125–9.
6. Elliott JH, Hoppes SL, Platt MS, et al. The acquired immunodeficiency syndrome and *Mycobacterium avium intracellular* bacteremia in a patient with hemophilia. Ann Int Med 1983;98:290–3.
7. Wormser GP, Krupp LB, Hanrahan JP, et al. Acquired immunodeficiency syndrome in male prisoners. New insights into an emerging syndrome. Ann Intern Med 1983;98:297–303.
8. Safai B, Johnson KG, Myskowski PL, et al. Natural history of Kaposi's sarcoma in the epidemic of acquired immune deficiency syndrome. Ann Intern Med 1985;103:744–50.
9. Cunningham-Rundles S. Analyses of altered immune function in the acquired immunodeficiency syndrome. In: Ma P, Armstrong D, eds. The acquired immunodeficiency syndrome and infections of homosexual men. New York: Yorke Medical Books, 331–40.
10. Friedman-Kien AE, Laubenstein LJ, Rubinstein P, et al. Disseminated Kaposi's sarcoma in homosexual men. Ann Intern Med 1982;96:693–700.
11. Lane HC, Depper JM, Greene WC, et al. Qualitative analysis of immune function in patients with the acquired immunodeficiency syndrome: Evidence for a selective defect in soluble antigen recognition. N Engl J Med 1985;313:79–83.
12. Cunningham-Rundles A, Safai B, Metroka C, et al. Lymphocyte effector function in vitro in the acquired immune deficiency syndrome. In: Friedman-Kien AE, Lau-

benstein LJ, eds. AIDS: The epidemic of Kaposi's sarcoma and opportunistic infections. New York: Masson, 1984, 153–9.
13. Kafatos FC, Jones CW, Efstratiadis J. Determination of nucleic acid sequence homologies and relative concentrations by a dot hybridization procedure. Nuc Acids Res 1979;7:1541–50.
14. Metroka CE, Cunningham-Rundles S, Pollack MS, et al. Generalized lymphadenopathy in homosexual men. Ann Intern Med 1982;99:585–91.
15. Cunningham-Rundles S, Metroka CE, Safai B, et al. Cytotoxic effector mechanisms in AIDS. In: Gupta S, ed. AIDS-associated syndromes. New York: Plenum Press, 1985;97–110
16. Cunningham-Rundles S, Michelis MA, Masur H. Serum suppression of lymphocyte activation in vitro in acquired immunodeficiency disease. J Clin Immunol 1983;3:156–65.
17. Metroka CE, Sonnabend JA, Cunningham-Rundles S, Krim M. Acid labile interferon alpha in homosexual men: A preclinical marker for opportunistic infection. Clin Res 1984;32:375.
18. Cunningham-Rundles S, Safai B, Metroka CE, Lange M. Modulation of immune response in the acquired immunodeficiency disease syndrome. In: Oppenheim JJ, Jacobs DM, eds. Progress in leukocyte biology, vol. 5. New York: Alan R. Liss, 1986;175–84.
19. Tartar T, Cunningham-Rundles S, Lawrence J. Increased production of PGE by mononuclear leukocytes from patients with lymphadenopathy syndrome and AIDS. In: Recent advances in primary and acquired immunodeficiency disease (submitted for publication).

Chapter 24

Immunologic Responses in AIDS

Patricia Fitzgerald-Bocarsly
Carlos Lopez
Frederick P. Siegal

Acquired immunodeficiency syndrome (AIDS) is characterized by profound deficiencies of the immune system that cause opportunistic infections (OI) or neoplasms in the affected individual. The immunologic aberrations associated with AIDS are now known to follow infection with the causative agent, a retrovirus originally designated lymphadenopathy-associated virus (LAV) or human T lymphotropic virus (HTLV-III) by its discoverers.[1,2] In 1986, the International Committee on the Taxonomy of Viruses recommended that the name human immunodeficiency virus (HIV) be used for this family of viruses, a convention we will adopt in this manuscript.[3] Although one of the targets of HIV is the T4 or Leu-3 positive helper cell, immune functions other than those mediated by T cells are known to be deficient in AIDS patients, and the disease is characterized by a progressive failure of many components of the immune system. In the following discussion, we will summarize and update the immunologic defects that have been described in AIDS.

T CELL–MEDIATED IMMUNITY

Among the earliest immunologic observations of patients with AIDS were that T cell numbers and functions were deficient in patients with either OI or Kaposi's sarcoma (KS).[4–6] These patients were generally found to be lymphopenic, to have inverted ratios of T helper (T4) to T suppressor (T8) cells, and to have low absolute numbers of T4 cells; absolute numbers of T8 cells were typically normal. The inversion of the T4/T8 ratio was accompanied by marked deficiencies in proliferative responses to T cell mitogens phytohemagglutinin (PHA) and concanavalin A (Con A) as well as to the T dependent B cell mitogen, pokeweed mitogen (PWM). Proliferative responses to specific antigens have shown even greater deficiencies than to bulk mitogens.[4-8]

In addition to deficient T helper cell numbers and responses to T cell mitogens, anergy to recall antigens in delayed-type hypersensitivity responses, another function known to be associated with T4 cells,[6,8] was usually but not always observed in patients with OI. Other defects of in vitro T cell responses include defective lymphokine and gamma interferon production,[9] low mixed lymphocyte responses,[10] deficient cytotoxic responses[11] and diminished T cell help for immunoglobulin production.[12]

The deficiencies in T cell numbers and functions can only partially be explained by tropism of HIV for the T4 positive helper cell. Direct involvement of the T4 molecule itself in viral replication has been indicated using monoclonal antibodies against the T4 molecule.[13,14] In 1986, McDougal et al.[15] demonstrated that the T4 molecule serves as a receptor for the virus by complexing of an epitope on T4 to the 100K viral envelope glycoprotein. In vitro studies have confirmed that infected T cells are rapidly killed following HIV infection, although a latent state of virus with concomitant down-regulation of T4 molecules has been described.[16]

Although T4 cells can clearly be infected with and killed by HIV, only a small proportion of peripheral T cells ($<0.01\%$) can be demonstrated to be lytically infected with HIV at a given time, a result which fails to account for the profound T cell deficiencies in AIDS. Recent studies have indicated that mononuclear phagocytes from brain and lung tissues of AIDS patients harbored HIV[17] and that in vitro–infected macrophages from healthy individuals produced large quantities of virus.[17,18] Separate isolates of HIV were found to have differential tropism for macrophages or T cells, with macrophage isolates preferring to infect macrophages and T cell isolates preferring T cells.[17] Like infection of T cells, binding of HIV to monocytes appears to occur through low-density T4 molecules on the cells.[18] Unlike infection of T cells, the infection in monocytes appears to be persistent.[18] Thus, mononuclear phagocytes may serve as primary targets for HIV infection and, through establishment of persistent infection, serve as a stable reservoir for viral infection in vivo. Monocyte abnormalities induced by HIV may contribute to the observed abnormalities in T cell function and number.[17]

In addition to T cells and macrophages,[17-19] other cell types have also been shown to harbor virus. These include Epstein-Barr virus (EBV)—transformed B cell lines,[20] glial cells (leading to so-called AIDS encephalopathy),[21] and antigen-presenting dendritic cells.[22] Thus, a number of different cell types may directly contribute to the pathology associated with AIDS.

B LYMPHOCYTE DEFICIENCIES

Polyclonal activation of B cells leading to elevated serum immunoglobulin (Ig) and circulating immune complexes were among the earliest clinical observations in patients with AIDS. The elevated serum Ig was found to be a consequence of increased levels of spontaneously secreting cells rather than of a few cells overproducing Ig.[12] Despite elevated levels of serum Ig, B cells from patients with AIDS have been found to be deficient in their responses to B cell mitogens, including PWM (even when adequate T cell help is provided), *Staphylococcus aureus* Cowan I, and *Escherichia coli*.[12,23,24]

Pneumococcal immunization of AIDS patients with tetradecavalent polysaccharide or the protein antigen keyhole-limpet hemocyanen led to deficient responses three to four weeks after immunization, as compared with controls.[12] Thus, B cell functional aberrations occur in AIDS; whether these deficiencies are secondary to T helper cell deficiencies or might also in part represent primary immunodeficiencies remains to be determined.

NATURAL KILLER CELLS

Deficient natural killer (NK) cell activity against both K562 tumor target cells and herpes simplex virus type 1(HSV-1) infected target cells were observed by us in the first five AIDS patients studied with advanced AIDS and OI.[6] In subsequent analysis of large numbers of patients at various stages of disease, we have observed that NK activity of most patients was within two standard deviations of the normal mean.[8,25] However, the *mean* NK activity of groups of patients was found to decrease with progressively worse clinical disease. Numbers of large granular lymphocytes or Leu-11 positive cells (a marker for Fc receptors on NK cells) were found to be normal in patients with AIDS,[8] suggesting qualitative rather than quantitative defects. Studies in other laboratories have indicated low NK cell activity in some, but by no means all, patients with AIDS when assessed using cytomegalovirus (CMV)-infected or K562 targets.[11,21] More striking is the observation that NK activity in the majority of AIDS patients with KS or CMV infection was not augmented by in vitro pretreatment of the effector cells with interferon (IFN),[23,26] suggesting that the pool of NK cells available for recruitment or activation was somehow deficient in these patients.

INTERFERON IN AIDS

Interferons (IFNs) are a family of cytokines that have direct antiviral effects, are potent immunoregulators, and can directly inhibit the growth of certain cells. We have been interested in the generation of IFNs by peripheral blood mononuclear cells in response to HSV-1 infected fibroblasts or HSV-1 ultraviolet-inactivated antigen. IFN generated in 14 hour assays by normal individuals was shown to be IFN-alpha in that it was neutralized by antiserum to IFN-alpha but not beta or gamma IFN.[27,28] IFN-alpha release in response to these stimuli is mediated by light-density cells that express HLA-DR antigens but that lack T cell, B cell, macrophage, and NK cell markers.[27,28,29] Because IFN is produced by both HSV-seropositive and seronegative individuals, it reflects a component of the natural, rather than the adaptive, cellular host defense. In contrast, T cell production of IFN-gamma and other lymphokines occurs more slowly and only by cells derived from seropositive individuals and depends on the presence of primed T cells.[30] Thus, IFN-gamma production is an expression of adaptive immunity, detectable only after antigen-specific clonal expansion of T cells.

Several abnormalities in the IFN system have been described in patients with AIDS. In earlier studies, we found that individuals with AIDS, with OI or about to come down with OI, were grossly deficient in their ability to generate IFN-alpha in 14 hour coculture experiments using patients' peripheral blood mononuclear cells and HSV-1 infected fibroblasts.[8] In our initial study, patients with OI made a mean of 21 international units (IU)/ml of IFN as compared with 1400 IU/ml made by normal donors, 457 IU/ml made by AIDS patients with KS but without OI, or 734 by patients with lymphadenopathy. In a subsequent, comprehensive, serial study, we studied IFN generation by five clinically staged groups of individuals, ranging from individuals with probable exposure (71% of whom were later found to be HIV seropositive, category A) to individuals at high risk for OI (categories B through D, of whom >90% were HIV seropositive) to individuals with OI (comprising category E).[25] In this study, mean IFN-alpha generation was found to decrease dramatically with disease category. Deficits of IFN-alpha production such that patients generated $\leq$ 300 IU/ml were closely associated with the presence of OI ($P < 7 \times 10^{-9}$) and were also predictive of subsequent OI in groups of patients not yet meeting the AIDS case definition ($P < 2 \times 10^{-5}$).

An unusual acid-labile IFN-alpha has been described in the serum of many patients with AIDS or prodromal AIDS.[31] Acid-labile IFN-alpha is also seen in patients with systemic lupus erythematosus and other autoimmune diseases and in animal retroviral models. Recent evidence demonstrates that human B cell lines infected with either EBV or human T leukemia virus spontaneously produce both acid-labile and acid-stable IFN-alpha,[32] and EBV-transformed B cells from AIDS patients produce acid-labile IFN alpha. The presence of acid-labile IFN in the serum of many AIDS patients suggested the possibility that this IFN is serving to down-regulate the in vitro IFN production we measured and may lead to the refractoriness of NK cells from many AIDS patients in activation by IFN. We have studied both serum IFN levels and in vitro generation of IFN by patients with AIDS with or without OI and with or without KS as well as individuals with lymphadenopathy (LAD).[33] IFN ($\geq$ 12 IU/ml) was found in the serum of 38% to 57% of patients with LAD, KS, or OI, whereas virtually all the individuals with LAD or KS alone generated normal levels of IFN-alpha in vitro and >90% of the patients with OI failed to generate IFN in vitro. Thus, there does not appear to be a simple correlation between these two phenomena. However, it remains possible that transient levels of IFN in the serum may be involved in the pathogenesis of AIDS or even in the in vitro deficiency we have observed.

Deficiency in IFN-gamma production has also been observed in AIDS patients.[9] In one study, 11 of 16 patients failed to produce normal levels of IFN gamma in response to mitogen, and 13 of 14 failed to generate IFN-gamma in response to specific microbial antigens. These results parallel the deficient proliferative responses to mitogens and antigens and clearly represent a further manifestation of the defective T cell component of immunity consequent to HIV infection.

SUSCEPTIBILITY TO OI IN AIDS

As described above, reduced in vitro production of IFN-alpha by patients' mononuclear cells was closely associated with, and possibly contributed to, the development of the severe OI defining AIDS. In the same study using stratified groups of patients, we confirmed that severe compromise of T cell numbers, particularly absolute numbers of helper (T4) cells, was found to be closely associated with later development of OI ($P < 8 \times 10^{-9}$).[25] Those patients with one but not the other deficit did not have a significantly increased tendency toward OI. In contrast, those with both T cell and IFN-alpha production deficiencies generally went on to develop infections in the follow-up period.

Our results suggest that apparently independent elements of both natural (IFN-alpha) and adaptive (T4 cells) immunity contribute to defense against the pathogens associated with AIDS. So long as either function persists, the host remains selectively resistant to overwhelming attack. Unlike the evidence that HIV infects and kills T helper cells, nothing is known about the mechanism by which the HLA-DR-positive IFN-alpha-producing cells are affected by the virus. Enumeration and purification of IFN-alpha-producing cells has been hampered by the lack of specific cell surface markers for these cells and their apparent paucity in peripheral blood. Only when enriched populations of these cells are obtained will we be able to determine whether they represent direct targets for HIV infection or whether their function is somehow down-regulated before the development of OI.

IMMUNOLOGIC RESPONSES TO HIV

Individuals are clearly able to mount an immune response to HIV in that antibodies to the virus, particularly the p24 or gp41 proteins, can be documented in virtually all patients with AIDS by enzyme immunoassay and Western blot. However, the coexistence of high titers of antibody to HIV and active, progressive disease indicate that antibody is not protective in the presence of established disease.

Recent studies have addressed the in vitro effects of HIV on immune responses and HIV-specific immune responses from seropositive donors. Pahwa et al.[34] reported that disrupted viral preparations were not by themselves mitogenic for normal peripheral mononuclear cells but were able to suppress the proliferative response to both mitogens and antigens. Addition of disrupted virus preparations to mononuclear cell cultures resulted in an impressive number of cells becoming immunoglobulin secreting cells (ISC), suggesting that the virus acts as a polyclonal activation. In contrast, the same viral preparations were able to suppress ISC formation in response to several other polyclonal B cell activators.

In studies of cell-mediated cytotoxicity against HIV-infected cells, sera from healthy seropositive donors mediated significantly higher levels of antibody-dependent cellular cytotoxicity (ADCC) against HIV-infected T cells than did sera from AIDS patients.[35] High ADCC levels correlated with antibody reactivity with the p24 and gp41 proteins of HIV better than did reactivity with gp 120/160. In addition, HLA-restricted cytotoxic T cell activity has been detected by these investigators in peripheral blood of two AIDS patients who had received marrow transplants from their identical twins. A recent study has demonstrated that interleukin-gp41-2 (IL-2)-activated large granular lymphocytes are able to preferentially lyse HIV-infected T cells and could inhibit infection of other T cells, suggesting a potential protective role for NK cells.[36]

CONCLUSION

Infection with HIV often leads to gross abnormalities of the immune system. Although one of the targets of HIV is clearly the T helper cell, the virus leads, either directly or indirectly, to profound deficiencies in humoral and natural immunity as well and can infect a variety of other cell types. Thus, AIDS cannot be considered to be solely a T cell disease.

The question of whether immunodeficiencies in AIDS patients are the result, or cause, of OI has been at least partially answered: Certain immune deficits, such as decreased T4 cells, clearly are a consequence of HIV infection and, together with deficient IFN-alpha production, are necessary prerequisites for the development of OI. In contrast, other immune functions diminish rather late in the course of disease and may not directly predispose the individual to OI.

A thorough understanding of how HIV interacts with the immune system and how (or if) some individuals successfully clear the virus are important areas requiring further investigation. The mechanism of HIV latency and the relative contribution of macrophages, dendritic cells, and T cells both as viral reservoirs and as targets for the lytic infection also is poorly understood and requires further study. The ultimate goals of such research are to design a successful vaccine that will protect individuals from infection and to design immunopotentiating and antiviral therapies that will benefit infected patients.

REFERENCES

1. Barre-Sinoussi F, Chermann J-C, Rey F, et al. Isolation of a T-lymphotropic retrovirus from a patient at risk for acquired immune deficiency syndrome (AIDS). Science 1983;220:868–70.

2. Gallo RC, Salahuddin SZ, Popovic M, et al. Frequent detection and isolation of cytopathic retroviruses (HTLV-III) from patients with AIDS and at risk for AIDS. Science 1984;224:500–3.
3. Coffin J, Haase A, Levy J, et al. Human immunodeficiency viruses (letter). Science 1986;232:697.
4. Gottlieb MS, Schroff R, Schanker HM, et al. *Pneumocystis carinii* pneumonia and mucosal candidiasis in previously healthy homosexual men: Evidence of a new acquired cellular immunodeficiency. N Engl J Med 1981;305:1425–30.
5. Masur H, Michelis MA, Greene JB, et al. An outbreak of community-acquired *Pneumocystis carinii* pneumonia: Initial manifestation of cellular immune dysfunction. N Engl J Med 1981;305:1431–8.
6. Siegel FP, Lopez C, Hammer GS, et al. Severe acquired immunodeficiency in male homosexuals, manifested by chronic perianal ulcerative herpes simplex lesions. N Engl J Med 1981;305:1439–44.
7. Bowen D, Lane H, Fauci A. Immunologic features of AIDS. In: DeVita V, Hellman S, Rosenberg S, eds. AIDS: etiology, diagnosis, treatment and prevention. Philadelphia: J.B. Lippincott Co., 1986;89–109.
8. Lopez C, Fitzgerald PA, Siegal FP. Severe acquired immune deficiency syndrome in male homosexuals: Diminished capacity to make interferon-alpha in vitro associated with severe opportunistic infections. J Infect Dis 1983;148:962–6.
9. Murray HW, Rubin B, Masur H, et al. Impaired production of lymphokines and immune (gamma) interferon in the acquired immunodeficiency syndrome. N Engl J Med 1984;310:883–9.
10. Gupta S, Safai B. Deficient autologous mixed lymphocyte reaction in Kaposi's sarcoma associated with deficiency of Leu-3 positive responder cells. J Clin Invest 1983;71:296.
11. Rook AH, Masur H, Lane HC, et al. 1983. Interleukin-2 enhances the depressed natural killer and CMV-specific cytotoxic activation of lymphocytes from patients with the acquired immunodeficiency syndrome. Clin Invest 1983;72:398.
12. Lane HC, Masur H, Edgar LC, et al. Abnormalities of β lymphocyte activation and immunoregulation in patients with the acquired immunodeficiency syndrome. N Engl J Med 1983;309:453.
13. Klatzmann D, Champagne S, Charmaret S, et al. T-lymphocyte T4 molecules behave as the receptor for human retrovirus LAV. Nature 1984;312:767.
14. Dalgleish A, Beverly P, Clapham D, et al. The CD4 (T4) antigen is an essential component of the receptor for the AIDS retrovirus. Nature 1984;312:763.
15. McDougal J, Kennedy M, Sligh, et al. Binding of HTLV-III/LAV to T4+ T cells by a complex of the 110K viral protein and the T4 molecule. Science 1986;231:382.
16. Folks T, Powell D, Lightfoote M, et al. Induction of HTLV-III/LAV from a nonvirus producing T-cell line: Implications for latency. Science 1986;231:600.
17. Gartner S, Markovits P, Markovitz D, et al. The role of mononuclear phagocytes in HTLV-III/LAV infection. Science 1986;233:215.
18. Nicholson J, Cross G, Callaway C, McDougal J. In vitro infection of human monocytes with human T lymphotropic virus type III/lymphadenopathy-associated virus. J Immunol 1986;137:323.
19. Gyorkey F, Melnick JL, Sinkovics JG, Gyorkey P. Retrovirus resembling HTLV in macrophages of patients with AIDS. Lancet 1985;1:106.
20. Montagnier L, Gruest J, Charmaret S, et al. Adaptation of lymphadenopathy associated virus (LAV) to replication in EBV-transformed B lymphoblastoid cell lines. Science 1984;225:63.

21. Shaw GM, Harper ME, Hahn BH, et al. HTLV-III infection of brains of children and adults with AIDS encephalopathy. Science 1985;227:177.
22. Armstrong JA, Horne R. Follicular dendritic cells and virus-like particles in AIDS-related lymphadenopathy. Lancet 1984;2:370.
23. Vadhan-Raj S, Wong G, Gecco C, et al. Immunological variables as predictors of prognosis in patients with Kaposi's sarcoma and the acquired immunodeficiency syndrome. Cancer Res 1986;46:417.
24. Pahwa S, Quilop M, Lange M, et al. Defective B-lymphocyte function in homosexual men in relation to the acquired immunodeficiency syndrome. Ann Intern Med 1984;101:757.
25. Siegal F, Lopez C, Fitzgerald P, et al. Opportunistic infections in acquired immune deficiency syndrome result from synergistic defects of both the natural and adaptive components of cellular immunity. J Clin Invest 1986;78:115.
26. Frederick W, Epstein J, Gelmann E, et al. Viral infections and cell-mediated immunity in immunodeficient homosexual men with Kaposi's sarcoma treated with human lymphoblastoid interferon. J Infect Dis 1985;152:162.
27. Fitzgerald PA, Schindler TE, Siegal FP, Lopez C. Independence of interferon production and natural killer function and association with opportunistic infections in acquired immune deficiency syndrome. In: Hoshino T, Koren HS, Uchida A, eds. Natural killer activity and its regulation, Amsterdam: Excerpta Medica, 1984;415.
28. Fitzgerald PA, von Wussow P, Lopez C. Role of interferon in natural killers on HSV-1-infected fibroblasts. J Immunol 1982;129:819.
29. Fitzgerald-Bocarsly P, Feldman M, Mendelsohn M, et al. Human mononuclear cells which produce interferon-alpha during NK(HSV-FS) assays are HLA-DR positive cells distinct from cytolytic NK effectors. J Leuk Biol 1988;43:323.
30. Green J, Yeh T, Overall J. Sequential production of IFN-alpha and immunospecific IFN-gamma by human mononuclear leukocytes exposed to herpes simplex virus. J Immunol 1981;127:1192.
31. DeStefano E, Friedman R, Friedman-Kien A, et al. Acid-labile human leukocyte interferon in homosexual men with Kaposi's sarcoma and lymphadenopathy. J Infect Dis 1982;146:451.
32. Boumpas D, Hooks J, Popovis M, et al. Human T-cell leukemia/lymphoma virus I and/or EBV-infected B-cell lines spontaneously produce acid-labile alpha-IFN. J Clin Immunol 1985;5:340.
33. Lopez C, Fitzgerald P, Siegal F. Letter to the editor. J Infect Dis 1984;150:158.
34. Pahwa S, Pahwa R, Saxinger C, et al. Influence of the human T-lymphotropic virus/lymphadenopathy associated virus on functions of human lymphocytes. Proc Natl Acad Sci 1985;82:8189.
35. Rook A, Koenig S, Lane H, et al. Cell-mediated cytotoxicity against HTLV-III/LAV-infected cells. Fed Proc 1986;45:377.
36. Ruscetti F, Mikovits J, Kalyanaraman V, et al. Analysis of effector mechanisms against HTLV-I and HTLV-III infected lymphoid cells. J Immunol 1986;136:3619.

Chapter 25

Epidemiologic Observations of Immunologic Abnormalities in Homosexual Men

Michael Lange
Hardy Kornfeld
Elena Klein
Robert A. Vande Stouwe
Michael H. Grieco

An unprecedented outbreak of opportunistic infections and Kaposi's sarcoma has occurred since 1979, predominantly among homosexuals, parenteral drug abusers, hemophiliacs, and Haitians.[1-5] The cases reported at the time of this writing (January 1983) number approximately 900 and continue to be reported at the rate of approximately two to three cases per day. Approximately half the cases have been reported from the New York metropolitan area, with other foci having been reported in California, Texas, and Florida.

Of the original 19 cases of opportunistic infections described, all patients were found to have suppressed cell-mediated immunity as measured by decreased skin anergy, decreased lymphocyte proliferation to mitogens and antigens, reduced numbers of T lymphocytes, and reduction of helper T lymphocytes with a concomitant increase in suppressor T cells, resulting in a reversal of the helper/suppressor T cell ratio.[1-3]

These abnormal immunologic parameters suggested a profound suppression of cell-mediated immunity that appeared to be acquired. The etiology of this abnormality, which has been called acquired immunodeficiency syndrome (AIDS), was unknown until 1983. Drug abuse, sexual promiscuity, sequential infections

---

We are indebted to the Columbia Health Service, the Gay Men's Health Project, and the volunteers of Columbia University for their help; to Mary Moriarty, Armel Francesco, and Stephen Wechter for technical assistance; and to Marion Pinks for preparation of the manuscript.

leading to immune exhaustion, or indeed an epidemic with a new, as-yet-unrecognized virus were all implicated as potential etiologic factors. The previously known viruses suggested as potential causes of AIDS included cytomegalovirus (CMV), herpes simplex virus (HSV), Epstein-Barr virus (EBV), and hepatitis B virus (HBV).[6,7] It is now known that a retrovirus, termed human immunodeficiency virus (HIV), is responsible for AIDS.

The opportunistic infections as well as Kaposi's sarcoma seen in AIDS occur in a setting analogous to that in renal transplant patients, except that in this latter setting the cause of AIDS is artificially created by the use of corticosteroids, azathioprine, and antilymphocyte globulin.[8] In the transplant patient it is believed that the infections, as well as Kaposi's sarcoma, result from the immune deficiency; further evidence of this effect is that a decrease in immunosuppression, achieved by discontinuing or reducing the dose of medication, has in many cases resulted in improvement of the infections and in some cases has led to reduction or disappearance of Kaposi's sarcoma.[9]

On the hypothesis that cell-mediated immune deficiency precedes clinical disease in AIDS patients, a larger number of the high-risk groups identified may be at risk to develop the severe complications of AIDS. Early recognition of such immune deficiency could lead to earlier identification of the opportunistic infections and Kaposi's sarcoma and result in institution of therapeutic modalities at an earlier date, which, in turn, may lead to increased survival.

To evaluate the presence and extent of possible immune abnormalities, we studied a group of 100 male homosexual volunteers—who did not have evidence of serious underlying illness—in a sequential longitudinal study. Our preliminary results are reported below.

MATERIALS AND METHODS

Eighty-one homosexual volunteers were recruited through a university health service, a homosexual health organization, and newspaper advertising. Twenty heterosexual controls, matched by age and sex and living in the same geographic area, were also recruited.

Informed consent was obtained, after which a questionnaire was administered regarding previous medical history, drug use (recreational drugs—both oral and parenteral), sexual practices, and recurrent symptoms observed during the preceding year. For purposes of definition, symptoms were defined as follows:

1. History of fever: temperature greater than 100°F (37.8°C) for more than one week.
2. Weight loss: unintentional weight loss of more than ten lb.
3. Diarrhea: three or more unformed stools per day for more than one week.
4. Recurrent amebiasis: five or more successfully treated discrete bouts of amebiasis diagnosed by a physician during the previous year. Persistent ame-

biasis: persistently positive stool examinations despite two successive standard treatment regimens.
5. Lymphadenopathy: persistently enlarged nodes outside the inguinal chains.

Lymphocyte Subpopulations

Mononuclear cells were isolated from heparinized peripheral blood on Ficoll-Hypaque gradient. Monocytes were identified by latex-particle ingestion. After washing and suspension in Roswell Park Memorial Institute 1640 medium containing 10% heat-inactivated calf serum, lymphocytes positive for OKT4 and OKT8 were identified by methods previously described.[10]

Delayed Hypersensitivity

Anergy testing was performed on 26 individuals using *Candida* 100 PNU (Greer Laboratories, Lenoir, N.C.); mumps (Eli Lilly, Indianapolis) 0.1 ml; purified protein derivative (PPD) (Connaught Laboratories, Willorodale, Ontario, Canada) 5 toxic units (TU); staphage lysate (Delmont Laboratories, Swarthmore, Pa.); tetanus toxoid at a 1:5 dilution 0.2 LFU (Wyeth, Marietta, Pa.); and trichophytin 1:1000 (Hollister-Stier, Spokane, Wash.).

CMV Serology

Titers of CMV antibody were determined by complement fixation.[11]

Statistical Analysis

The means of the percentages and calculated absolute numbers of OKT4 positive and OKT8 positive lymphocytes and the OKT4:OKT8 ratios were compared in different groups using Student's t test. The applicability of the t test to the data was verified by F tests and graphic inspection of cumulative frequency distributions. Linear regression analysis was used to compare the OKT4:OKT8 ratios with the height of the CMV antibody.

RESULTS

Symptoms

Of 81 homosexual volunteers studied, 50 were asymptomatic and 31 gave a history of 1 or more symptoms by questionnaire. Of these, 2 reported weight loss, 5 had diarrhea, 7 had fever, 11 had lymphadenopathy, 18 had amebiasis, 2 had thrush, and 11 reported more than 1 symptom.

Distribution of T Cell Subsets

Both the asymptomatic and symptomatic homosexuals had an abnormal distribution of T cell subsets as compared with controls. The percentages and absolute counts of OKT4 positive lymphocytes and the ratios of OKT4:OKT8 cells were lower in the homosexuals and were significantly different in all three groups as compared with one another (Figure 25–1 and Table 25–1). Only 14 (17.3%) of the 81 homosexuals tested had ratios within the control range (defined as 1.4 to 2.8 in our laboratory); of these 14, 2 were in the symptomatic and 12 in the asymptomatic group. A total of 15 (6 asymptomatic and 9 symptomatic) subjects had ratios below 0.5. Both percentages as well as the absolute counts of OKT8 positive lymphocytes were significantly higher in homosexuals than in controls, but there was no difference between the 2 groups of homosexuals. Sexual promiscuity was associated with reduced OKT4:OKT8 ratios but became statistically significant (P 0.05) only when volunteers who reported 50 or more sexual partners were compared with those individuals reporting 9 or fewer different partners.

Drug use, including chronic use of amyl and butyl nitrites, was unrelated to OKT4:OKT8 ratios (Figure 25–2). Of 40 volunteers using nitrites at least once a week, 6 (15%) had normal ratios. Eighteen of 23 (78.3%) volunteers who had never used nitrites had low ratios.

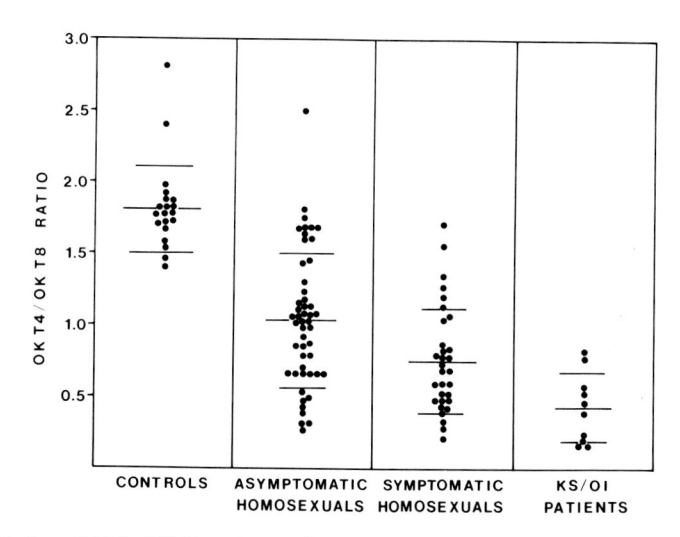

FIGURE 25–1 *OKT4:OKT8 ratios in homosexual men and heterosexual controls.*

Table 25–1 Lymphocyte subpopulations in symptomatic and asymptomatic male homosexuals and heterosexual controls[a]

Group	OKT4 (%)	Absolute OKT4 (cells/mm³)	OKT8 (%)	Absolute OKT8 (cells/mm³)	OKT4:OKT8 Ratio
Controls ($N = 20$)	36.6 ±1.0	813.3 ±60.6	20.5 ±0.8	454.0 ±37.3	1.8 ± 0.1
Asymptomatic homosexuals ($N = 50$)	27.4 ±1.4	643.9 ±41.5	28.8 ±1.1	675.1 ±33.3	1.1 ± 0.1
Symptomatic homosexuals ($N = 31$)	22.4 ±1.6	483.5 ±43.0	31.1 ±1.6	651.2 ±42.5	0.8 ± 0.1

[a]Means ± SEM. The percentage and absolute OKT4 counts and the OKT4:OKT8 ratios were significantly different among all three groups ($P < 0.05$ or less). The percentage and absolute OKT8 counts of symptomatic and asymptomatic homosexuals were higher than controls ($P < 0.01$ or less) but did not differ from each other.

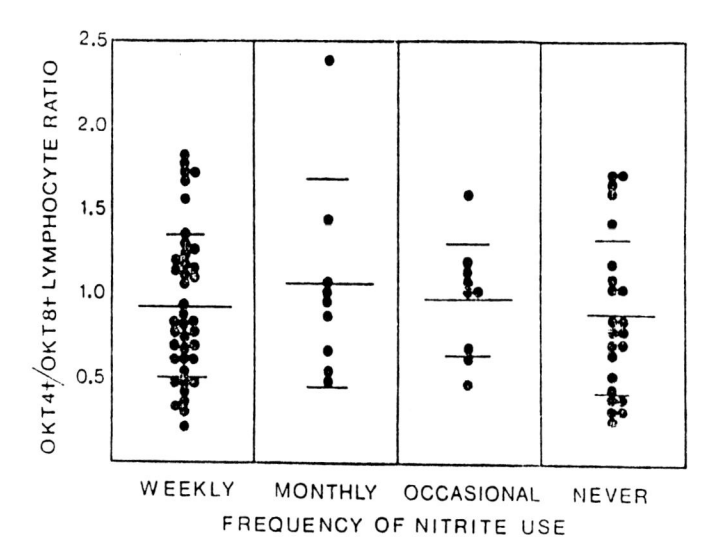

FIGURE 25–2 *OKT4:OKT8 ratio and the use of inhaled nitrites in homosexual men. The OKT4:OKT8 ratio was not related to the reported use of nitrites. Horizontal lines represent mean ± SD.*

CMV Serology

CMV antibody tests were positive in 79 of 81 homosexuals by complement fixation with titers greater than 1:16 in 63 (77.8%). Five of 20 (25%) of heterosexual controls were positive for CMV antibody, all with titers of 1:16 or less. We found no correlation between CMV antibody titers and OKT4:OKT8 ratios.

Delayed Hypersensitivity Testing

Delayed hypersensitivity skin testing was performed on 28 homosexuals. Of these, 26 had OKT4:OKT8 ratios below the normal range. Fifteen of 26 (57.7%) had at least 1 skin reaction of 5 mm or more; 7 had 2 positive reactions, and 2 had 3 positive reactions. Only 4 of 26 had reactions of 10 mm or greater. Two homosexuals with a ratio in the normal range were tested, and both had 2 positive reactions of greater than 5 mm.

Follow-Up Testing of T Cell Subset Distribution

Sixty-seven volunteers had their T lymphocyte subpopulations repeated 5 to 7 months later: 27 of 31 symptomatic and 40 of 50 asymptomatic volunteers. A significant change as defined by a change in ratio ≥0.5 in either direction occurred in 3 of 27 symptomatic repeaters, with 2 demonstrating a decrease and 1 an increase in ratio of OKT4:OKT8 cells. Of 40 asymptomatic volunteers, repeat lymphocyte subpopulations showed an increase in 9 and a decrease in 8 subjects. An increase that resulted in return to a normal ratio range (1.4 to 2.8) occurred in 6 subjects.

DISCUSSION

Patients with AIDS have been uniformly found to have a marked depression of helper/inducer T lymphocytes in the peripheral blood.[12,13] Our study was undertaken to determine the distribution of T cell subsets in homosexual men without serious illness. Similar immunologic abnormalities were found in these subjects, as in patients with full-blown AIDS, although the abnormalities were somewhat less severe.

Reduced OKT4:OKT8 ratios have been reported in a variety of diseases of noninfectious and infectious etiology. Infectious diseases associated with a reduced OKT4:OKT8 ratio include infection with CMV, HSV, EBV, influenza, and acute and chronic HBV.[14,15,16] The cause of reduced OKT4:OKT8 ratios in the homosexual volunteers studied is unknown. Whether this widespread abnormality—as measured in 81 volunteers in our study—is related to the outbreak of Kaposi's sarcoma and opportunistic infections is not known at this time. That reduced OKT4:OKT8 ratios are present in a substantial percentage of seemingly healthy homosexual men, at least in the New York City area, however, has been found by additional investigators[17,18]; that OKT4:OKT8 ratios are frequently associated with elevated titers of one or more immunoglobulins is being corroborated in our laboratory. A few conclusions, some definite but most tentative, can be made on the basis of reviewing results and correlating them to observations made by us and others in patients with full-blown AIDS.

Patients with AIDS who had Kpaosi's sarcoma or opportunistic infections have been found to have marked depression of helper-induced T lymphocytes in the peripheral blood.

The ratio of OKT4:OKT8 cells in these patients has usually been below 0.5 in our laboratory. The majority of these patients, especially those with opportunistic infections, have also been anergic to a battery of hypersensitivity skin testing agents.

Patients diagnosed with AIDS complicated by Kaposi's sarcoma or opportunistic infection frequently report prodromal symptoms of recurrent fever, weight loss, recurrent sore throats, lymphadenopathy, diarrhea, and severe fatigue during the preceding 6 to 12 months. No single diagnostic test has been identified to date that would enable a definite diagnosis of AIDS. A careful history eliciting some of the above symptoms—together with clinical findings of oral thrush and lymphadenopathy—is highly suggestive of an AIDS prodrome. A reduced level of helper-inducer T cells and a reversal of the helper/suppressor T cell ratio would substantiate a degree of immune deficiency, although the combination of these laboratory findings does not have diagnostic specificity for AIDS. A similar complex of signs, symptoms, and laboratory findings has been described with primary CMV and HSV infections as well as EBV infection (infectious mononucleosis).[19,20]

The finding of abnormal OKT4:OKT8 ratios in 82% of asymptomatic and mildly symptomatic homosexual males, with a significant trend toward lower ratios in the symptomatic subjects, suggests a progression from milder to more severe immunologic disturbances, with the greatest disturbance in patients with Kaposi's sarcoma or opportunistic infection. Stahl et al. demonstrated similar abnormal parameters in patients studied at New York University and observed in addition that the majority of patients studied had elevated levels of one or more immunoglobulin groups.[17] Abnormal T cells were similarly described by Wallace et al.[18]

The cause of the reduced T lymphocyte ratios in our homosexual subjects is unknown, and the possible relationship of the outbreak of Kaposi's sarcoma and opportunistic infection can only be assessed by a longitudinal study now in progress. The finding that the majority of the volunteers still have abnormal ratios five to seven months later suggests that immunologic abnormality is more than just a transient phenomenon.

We found that sexual promiscuity, as defined by the number of different sexual partners in the preceding year, was associated with low OKT4:OKT8 ratios. These reduced ratios may be due to a higher frequency of sexual transmitted viral infection, particularly CMV and HSV.[24] An additional factor associated with homosexual practices includes mucosal exposure to seminal plasma, which may have immunosuppressive properties, and to semen, which may lead to development of sperm antibody containing circulating immune complexes, and sperm antigenemia, which may further contribute to immunologic abnormalities.[21]

We were unable to find a relationship between the degree of helper/suppressor abnormality and chronic nitrite use (Figure 25–3). A recent publication concluded that nitrites had a causative role in suppressing T cell subsets. The effect of nitrite use may be short lived (eight hours), and we did not monitor the time of nitrite use or the time T cell subsets were performed.

Increasingly, epidemiologic observations suggest a transmissible agent as the cause of AIDS.[22,23] Whether the cause of the abnormal lymphocyte subpopulations in homosexual males is due to a transmissible agent itself or is due to factors in the homosexual lifestyle that in turn may make this population group more susceptible to this proposed transmissible agent, the finding of abnormal T cell subpopulations in 80% of healthy volunteers suggests a potentially greater problem than is presently appreciated.

Note that immunofluorescent staining of lymphocyte subpopulations with monoclonal antibodies only detects phenotypic surface markers and may not correlate with functional abnormalities. Fifteen of 26 subjects with reduced OKT4:OKT8 ratios reacted to one or more delayed hypersensitivity skin tests,

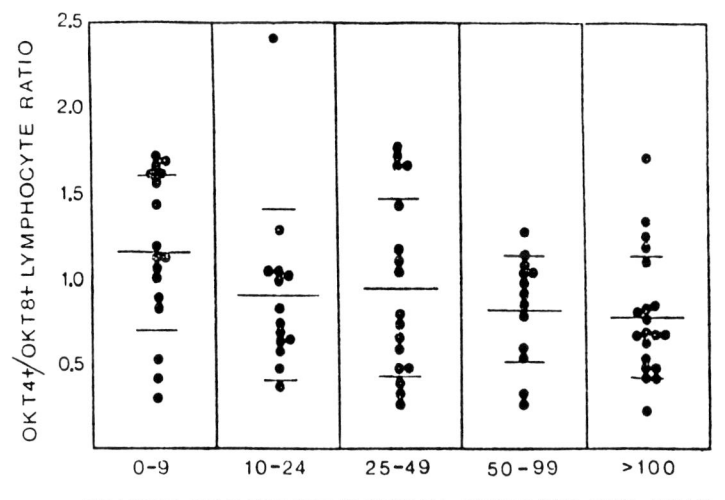

FIGURE 25–3 *OKT4:OKT8 ratios and sexual promiscuity in homosexual men. The OKT4:OKT8 ratio was higher in subjects reporting 9 or fewer different sexual partners per year than those reporting 50 to 99 partners ($P < 0.05$) and 100 or more partners ($P < 0.01$) per year. Horizontal lines represent mean ± standard deviation (SD).*

whereas virtually all patients with Kaposi's sarcoma and *Pneumocystis carinii* were anergic. Lymphocyte transformation studies performed with lymphocyte ratios by Stahl et al. indicate, however, that functional abnormality corresponds to the degree of ratio suppressors and that the majority of healthy homosexual controls also had abnormal lymphocyte function studies.[17]

Our group of homosexual volunteers may not be representative of the homosexual population of New York as a whole and a bias cannot be excluded, although we did not admit subjects with significant prodromal symptoms of AIDS into our study. Nevertheless, although the true prevalence of abnormal lymphocyte subpopulations may be lower than in our study, two other studies support the finding that it appears to be a more widespread abnormality than indicated by the numbers reported with Kaposi's sarcoma and opportunistic infection.[17,18] Longitudinal follow-up study of our group and others to determine the long-term relationship of the observed immunologic abnormality to the development of full-blown AIDS is urgently needed.

REFERENCES

1. Centers for Disease Control. Epidemiologic aspects of the current outbreak of Kaposi's sarcoma and opportunistic infections. N Engl J Med 1982;306:248.

2. Gottlieb MS, Schroff F, Schanker HM, et al. *Pseumocystis carinii* pneumonia and mucosal candidiasis in previously healthy homosexual men: Evidence of a new acquired cellular immunodeficiency. N Engl J Med 1981;305:1425.
3. Masur H, Michelis MA, Greene JB, et al. An outbreak of community-acquired *Pneumocystis carinii* pneumonia. N Engl J Med 1981;305:1431.
4. Siegal FP, Lopez C, Hammer GS, et al. Severe acquired immunodeficiency in male homosexuals, manifested by chronic perianal ulcerative herpes simplex lesions. N Engl J Med 1981;305:1439.
5. Vieira J, Frank E, Spira TJ, Landesman SH. Acquired immunodeficiency in Haitians: Opportunistic infections in previously healthy Haitian immigrants. N Engl J Med 1983;308:129.
6. Carney WP, Rubin RH, Hoffman RA, et al. Analysis of T lymphocyte subsets in cytomegalovirus mononucleosis. J Immunol 1981;126:2114.
7. Thomas HC. T-cell subsets in patients with acute and chronic HBV infection, primary biliary cirrhosis and alcohol induced liver disease. Int J Immunopharmacol 1981;3:301.
8. Penn I. Malignant lymphoma in organ transplant recipients. Transplant Proc 1981;13:736.
9. Harwood AR, Osoba D, Hofstader SL, et al. Kaposi's sarcoma in recipients of renal transplants. Am J Med 1979;67:759.
10. Kornfeld H, Vande Stouwe RA, Lange M, et al. T-lymphocyte subpopulations in homosexual men. N Engl J Med 1982;307:729.
11. Cremer NE, Hoffman M, Lennette EH. Analysis of antibody assay methods and classes of viral antibodies in serodiagnosis of cytomegalovirus infection. J Gen Clin Microbiol 1978;8:153.
12. Friedman-Kien AE, Laubenstein LJ, Rubenstein P, et al. Disseminated Kaposi's sarcoma in homosexual men. Ann Intern Med 1982;96:693.
13. Mildvan D, Mathur U, Enlow RW, et al. Opportunistic infections and immune deficiency in homosexual men. Ann Intern Med 1982;96:700.
14. Rinaldo CR Jr, Carney WP, Richter BS, et al. Mechanisms of immunosuppression in cytomegalovirus mononucleosis. J Infect Dis 1980;141:408.
15. De Waele M, Thielemans C, Van Camp BKG. Characterization of immunoregulatory T cells by EBV induced infectious mononucleosis by monoclonal antibodies. N Engl J Med 1981;304:460.
16. Corey L, Reeves WC, Holmes KK. Cellular immune response in genital herpes simplex infections. N Engl J Med 1981;299:986.
17. Stahl RE, Friedman-Kien A, Dubin R, et al. Immunological abnormalities in homosexual men. Relationship to Kaposi's sarcoma. Am J Med 1982;73:171.
18. Wallace JI, Coral FS, Rimm IJ. T-cell ratios in homosexuals. Lancet 1982;1:908.
19. Rinaldo CR Jr, Carney WP, Richter BS, et al. Mechanisms of immunosuppression in cytomegalovirus mononucleosis. J Infect Dis 1980;141:488.
20. Rasussen LE, Jordan GW, Stevens DA, Merigan TC. Lymphocyte interferon production and transformation after herpes simplex infections in humans. J Immunol 1974;112:728.
21. Witkin S, Sonnabend JA. Immune responses to spermatozoa in homosexual men. Fertil Steril 1983;39:337.
22. Centers for Disease Control. Immunodeficiency among female sexual partners of males with acquired immune deficiency syndrome (AIDS) (New York). MMWR 1983;31:697.

23. Centers for Disease Control. Acquired immune deficiency syndrome (AIDS) in prison inmates (New York). MMWR 1983;31:700.
24. Drew WL, Mintz L, Minor RC, et al. Prevalence of cytomegalovirus infection in homosexual men. J Infect Dis 1981;143:188.

Chapter 26

Immunogenetic Findings in Patients with Epidemic Kaposi's Sarcoma

Pablo Rubinstein
Mary Walker
Norman Mollen
Linda J. Laubenstein
Alvin E. Friedman-Kien

The epidemic of a disseminated, fulminant form of Kaposi's sarcoma in young homosexual men was first recognized in April 1982.[1] A series of reports published by the Centers for Disease Control (CDC) made the medical community and the general public aware of the unprecedented occurrence not only of AIDS Kaposi's sarcoma, but also of severe opportunistic infections, predominantly *Pneumocystis carinii* pneumonia, in previously healthy homosexual men.[2]

The simultaneous appearance of AIDS Kaposi's sarcoma and opportunistic infections in the same segment of the population, and their frequent coexistence in the same individual, has led to the concept that both are related in their etiology and pathogenesis. It is widely held that an initial trigger (possibly an infectious agent) reduces immunologic responsiveness and, because of the dete-

---

Authors' note: This is an unchanged version of the report originally published in the first edition of this book (1984). The methods and data presented have been extended by a great deal of subsequent literature, but are still valid. The association between EKS and HLA-DR5, although confirmed by other investigators, has become less and less significant in the New York patients. This subject is still under investigation.

Supported in part by Grants HLO9011-19 from the National Institutes of Health, RD-150 from the American Cancer Society, the Howard Gilman Foundation, Bernhill Fund, Gay Men's Health Crisis, a contract from Ortho Pharmaceuticals, and a grant from the Solomon Foundation. We are grateful to C. Stevens, M.D., for advice, much stimulating discussion, and permission to use data from the hepatitis B vaccination study.

rioration of immune surveillance mechanisms, tumors (especially Kaposi's sarcoma) or opportunistic infections are allowed to develop in genetically susceptible individuals. Thus, AIDS Kaposi's sarcoma and opportunistic infections are generally considered to be different expressions of the same acquired immunodeficiency syndrome (AIDS), even though no formal proof has emerged thus far. Suggestion of possibly transmissible etiologic factors has accumulated. Thus, several case/control studies have reported that patients with AIDS Kaposi's sarcoma and opportunistic infections are more promiscuous than most homosexual men. Contact between cases has been reported,[3,4] but the statistical significance of this finding in a highly promiscuous subgroup of homosexual men has not been rigorously evaluated. Most patients have a history of repeated viral, bacterial, and parasitic sexually transmitted disease.[5] The immunologic consequences of these repeated infections or of their treatment are unknown. Many viral and parasitic diseases are known to alter cellular immune functions. A different possibility is suggested by the high rate of exposure to so-called recreational drugs, including the suspected carcinogens amyl and butyl nitrites, that has also been found.[5]

The appearance of AIDS cases in drug addicts and possibly in hemophiliacs,[6] however, provided additional support for the idea that the AIDS epidemic is caused by an infectious agent that can be transmitted either sexually or parenterally[7] in a manner analogous to hepatitis B virus (HBV). It has since been discovered that a retrovirus, called human immunodeficiency virus (HIV), causes AIDS. Interestingly, Giraldo et al. (cited in Ref. 8) described the frequent existence of cytomegalovirus (CMV) markers and DNA in Kaposi's sarcoma tumors and postulated a pathogenic role for this virus. Furthermore, CMV infection is a well-known immunosuppressor in both humans and mice. There is also evidence of H-2 involvement in the different resistance of inbred strains of mice to CMV infection.[9-11] Thus, the situation may not be unlike that originally described in mice by Lilly et al.,[12] who showed that susceptibility to virus-induced malignancy is controlled by several genes. Because some of those genes map in or close to the major histocompatibility complex (MHC) of that species,[12] we decided to study the HLA system of patients with Kaposi's sarcoma. It was thus demonstrated that a population association exists between this disease and one of the DR antigens, DR5, an allele of the human gene homologous to the murine immune response region (IR) of the MHC.[3,5] This association has been independently confirmed.[13]

Given the involvement of the human MHC in the susceptibility to AIDS Kaposi's sarcoma, work was started on the possible mechanism of the association. Thus, we and others have reported profound alterations in the skin-test reactivity, the lymphocyte responsiveness in vitro, and the ratio between the helper-inducer and the cytotoxic-suppressor subsets of T cells. The accumulation of information on immunologic deficiency in these patients started with discussions held at the workshop on Kaposi's sarcoma sponsored by the National Institutes of Health (NIH) in September 1981.[3,5,14-19] We have also reported on the existence of high levels of circulating serum immunoglobulins and of immune complexes[3,5] in these patients that suggest the possible involvement of autoimmune reactivity.

In this chapter we review some of the observations made thus far on 65 Kaposi's sarcoma patients, report on the finding of autoantibodies to sperm and T cells, and analyze results from the repeated immunologic examination of a group of Kaposi's sarcoma patients for at least two months.

MATERIAL AND METHODS

Patients

Seventy-one individuals with biopsy-proved AIDS/Kaposi's sarcoma and 21 with classic Kaposi's sarcoma have been studied thus far for their HLA antigens. Criteria for assigning patients to the AIDS/Kaposi's sarcoma or classic Kaposi's sarcoma group include age at onset (the oldest AIDS/Kaposi's sarcoma patient was 52, the youngest classic Kaposi's sarcoma patient was 62), sexual preference (all AIDS/Kaposi's sarcoma patients were homosexual or bisexual; all classic Kaposi's sarcoma patients have been thus far strictly heterosexual) and clinical aspects (duration of symptoms before diagnosis, extent of local lesions and systemic symptoms, and clinical and epidemiologic history), as discussed previously.[3,5] Clinical evaluation of the patients included detailed dermatologic examinations as well as gatrointestinal (GI) endoscopies and radiology, routine blood chemistries and hematologic analyses, and skin challenge with the "obligatory" antigens—streptokinase-streptodornase and *Candida*. (All subjects were anergic by this criterion.) All had significant increases in the concentration of serum gammaglobulins (>2 standard deviations [SDs] over the mean for normal adult individuals), including IgM, IgG, and IgA, and all had easily detectable immune complexes in serum.

A subset of ten AIDS/Kaposi's sarcoma patients was selected for a prospective pilot study of the possible therapeutic usefulness of TP-5 (Thymopentin, ORTHO). They had very mild or inexistent systemic symptoms and were judged to allow postponement of conventional treatment. After granting informed consent, they received TP-5, 50 mg intravenously (IV) 3 times per week, for a minimum of 8 and a maximum of 12 weeks. No discernible clinical or laboratory indications of either beneficial or detrimental effects were encountered in this admittedly limited pilot trial. Minor progression of the cutaneous disease was observed in nine of the ten, and one of these nine developed opportunistic infections that required specific treatment and terminated his participation in this trial. In addition to immediate evaluation of lymphocyte functions, aliquots of these cell suspensions were kept frozen and all lectin stimulation tests were repeated on a single day on all thawed samples from the same patient.

HLA and Related Markers

Tests for a total of 52 discrete human leukocyte antigens (HLA-A, B, C, and DR) were done using a set of 180 monospecific or oligospecific antisera. For HLA-DR, the serum set used was able to discern antigens 1, 2, 3, 4, 5, 6, 7, 8, 9, and 10 and the supertypic specificities MT1, MT2, and MT3. Also, a pattern of reactivity detecting the cross-reactive form of antigens DR4 and DR5 was used. All tests were done with modified NIH microcytotoxicity test using the contrast fluorescence[20] and the two-color fluorescence tests[21] for HLA-A, B, C, and DR typing, respectively. Other genetic marker phenotypes, Factor B of the alternative pathway of complement activation, glyoxalase 1, Gm, and the third component of the complement were ascertained by conventional techniques.[22-24]

Immunohematologic Tests

Enumeration of Helper (T4 Positive) and Suppressor (T8 Positive) T Cell Subsets Counting of T3, T4, and T8 positive lymphocytes was done on Ficoll-Hypaque-separated mononuclear cells. We incubated 100 µl aliquots of a suspension containing 2×10^6 cells in phosphate buffered saline (PBS), pH 7.2, with 100 µl of empirically determined optimal dilutions of monoclonal antibodies (OKT3, OKT4, and OKT8). Directly labeled reagents were used exclusively. After 15 minutes at 37°C, the cells were washed three times in RPMI-1640 containing 0.1% of $NaNO_3$ and kept in melting ice until read. Reading was performed in a fluorescence-activated cell sorter (FACS) IV instrument (Becton Dickinson) using a simple two-parameter system: forward scatter for counting and sizing versus fluorescence intensity. The population of large monocytes was excluded by "gating" from the total lymphocyte counts, and fluorescent cells were expressed as a fraction (percentage) of the remaining lymphocytes. Typically 20,000 cells were scanned from each sample of each of the monoclonal antibodies.

Functional Studies—Lectin Stimulation Mononuclear cells separated on Ficoll-Hypaque gradients were washed and suspended to a count of 5×10^5/ml in RPMI-1640 supplemented with glutamine, HEPES, antibiotics, nonessential amino acids, and 10% fetal bovine serum (FBS). Cell suspension (100 µl) was placed in the wells of a 96-well microtiter plate. Empirically adjusted doubling dilutions of lectin (either phytohemagglutinin [PHA-M] or pokeweed mitogen [PWM]) were used so that equal volumes of three dilutions were tested on each sample: the optimum, one-half, and twice that concentration. After three or four days of culture, respectively, tritiated thymidine was added and after additional incubation the contents of each well were harvested with an automatic instrument (PHD, Cambridge), dried, and counted for beta emission in a Packard counter. Each test was done in triplicate, and the means of these triplicates were reported as uncorrected counts per minute (cpm). Samples from three normal individuals were used as controls throughout. We feel, as do others, that the means of the counts per minute for each test provide a more reliable estimate of the blastogenesis than do variously "corrected" results. For the analyses described below we have used only the counts per minute obtained with the optimal concentrations of mitogen.

Mixed Lymphocyte Culture (MLC) Tests These tests were also conducted in microtest plates with Ficoll-Hypaque separated phosphate buffered lymphocyte (PBL): 50,000 responder cells were cocultured with 50,000 stimulator cells, previously irradiated (2000 rad), in RPMI-1640 with antibiotics, HEPES, and glutamine containing 10% of normal human serum. Each test was done in triplicate. The cultures were incubated for five days, tritiated thymidine was added, and the contents were harvested 18 hours later and counted in a liquid scintillometer for beta emission.

Stimulator cells for these tests were provided by three DR-heterozygous donors who do not share haplotypes. For the analysis given below, the uncorrected counts per minute were averaged and the means used exclusively. Responsiveness in MLC tests was, however, also interpreted both by comparison with normals and by internal normalization as described previously[25] (data not shown).

Immunofluorescence Studies on Mononuclear Cells and Spermatozoa

Mononuclear cells from normal blood donors were separated from peripheral blood as before. After washing they were exposed to serum from either normal or AIDS/Kaposi's sarcoma donors. After incubation and extensive washing, they were incubated with absorbed, fluorescein-labeled, xenogeneic antibodies to human pooled immunoglobulins. (This avoids labeling of the surface immunoglobulin components of B lymphocytes). After exposure to the labeled reagent, the mononuclear cells were examined microscopically under epi-illumination with light of appropriate wavelength (490 to 500 nm) for fluorescein using selective barrier filter combinations. Labeled cells were then counted using 50× Neofluar objective. Confirmation by cytotoxicity of the results of indirect immunofluorescence tests was obtained by exposing the target cells to absorbed rabbit serum (as a source of complement) after incubation with the serum of AIDS/Kaposi's sarcoma patients or controls. Cytotoxicity was evidenced by the uptake of ethidium bromide and read as described above for HLA antibodies. Characterization of the nature of the IIF-labeled cells as T cells was accomplished by first killing all DR-positive cells with allogeneic reagents of appropriate specificity and using ethidium bromide as an indicator of cell death. Only living cells had surface fluorescence. Second, when cytotoxic OKT3 monoclonal antibodies were used instead of anti-DR, almost all the cells labeled by the AIDS/Kaposi's sarcoma serum were killed by the anti-T-cell reagent.

Semen provided by human volunteers was used for studies on spermatozoa within three hours of ejaculation. Sperm cells were separated after clotting and liquefaction of the semen and were counted and treated exactly as described above for mononuclear cells.

Elution of T Cell Binding Immunoglobulin from T Lymphocytes

Separation of this immunoglobulin was accomplished using pH 3, 0.15 m glycine buffer, on the lymphocytes of the patients. Because AIDS and Kaposi's sarcoma patients are typically lymphopenic, the yields were too small for preparatory scale separations. Lymphocyte suspensions from normal donors could, however, be substituted and used to absorb the immunoglobulin from patients' serum. Complete absorption was regularly accomplished with 5×10^7 lymphocytes/ml of serum in one hour at 22°C. Eluted immunoglobulins were assayed for binding on human PBL using the two-color fluorescence procedure to identify the different cell subsets as described above and also on cells isolated from human semen.

Analysis of Results

The means and SDs of the repeated determinations were calculated, and the coefficients of correlation (R) for all pairwise comparisons of such means computed by the standard method: $R = \text{covariance}/SD1 \times SD2$. The significance of these R values was estimated from the appropriate table (Documenta Geigy).

RESULTS

HLA Association

The only antigen with a frequency significantly different from controls was DR5, as already reported. The current data are summarized in Table 26–1.

An excess in the frequency of Bw35 was also noticed that, when appropriately corrected for the number of antigens tested, was not significant. The increase in the frequency of Bw35 was accompanied by an associated increase of Cw4: These antigens are known to maintain high linkage disequilibrium in most populations. Interestingly, the increases of Bw35 and Cw4 were independent of that of DR5 in that their joint presence in the patients was exactly as predicted from their separate gene frequencies in both normal individuals and patients (data not shown). Table 26–1 also includes data gathered independently by Nunez et al. (personal communication) on a group of homosexual patients with polyadenopathy. An identical increase of DR5 was encountered.

Table 26-1 HLA-DR frequencies (%) in patients with AIDS/Kaposi's sarcoma, classic Kaposi's sarcoma, and polyadenopathy[a]

DR	AID/Kaposi's Sarcoma[b] (N = 65)	CKS[b] (N = 21)	Polyadenopathy[c] (N = 28)	All Patients (N = 114)	Controls (N = 231)	Homosexual Men[d] (N = 76)
1	19	29	21	21	18	14
2	20	24	14	20	25	36
3	17	10	14	10	20	16
4	20	5	28	20	23	22
5	43(1)	43(2)	46(3)	44(4)	23	20
w6	19	10	17	17	15	18
7	22	24	21	22	20	34
w8	0	5	3	2	4	0

[a]Significance for difference with regard to random New York whites (N = 231): Fisher's exact probability—(1) = 0.0014, (2) = 0.044, (3) = 0.009, (4) = 0.000067; all other comparisons—nonsignificant.
[b]Patients typed at New York Blood Center.
[c]Patients typed at Hospital for Joint Diseases by Nunez A et al. (personal communication).
[d]Volunteers in the HB-vaccine trials, studied in collaboration with Dr. C. Stevens.

Antisperm Antibodies

A limited number of patients have been tested for these antibodies thus far. The results are shown in Table 26–2. All ten of the volunteers in the TP-5 study had such antibodies as defined by cytotoxicity, and in seven of them the titers were high enough to allow positive eluates to be prepared from allogeneic lymphocytes. By contrast, only eight of 20 sera from otherwise healthy homosexual men and none of eight sera from normal heterosexual men contained antisperm antibody detectable with either technique. (Very similar findings have been made with different techniques by E.V. Hess [personal communication, 1983]).

Comparisons between the Different Immunohematologic Indexes

The means and SDs of test results are given in Table 26–3. The numbers of neutrophils and of erythrocytes (RBCs) are given per cubic millimeter; those of T lymphocytes are given both in absolute numbers (N) per cubic millimeter and as a percentage of all lymphocytes, and the results of lectin stimulation and MLC tests are given in cpm. Each patient's data are presented separately. Despite the TP-5 treatment, the results of these tests were quite stable as shown by relatively small size of the variances observed. There were no identifiable time trends toward higher or lower values for any of these tests during the length of the trial.

The means of each pair of tests on the ten patients were compared by calculating the respective coefficients of correlation (R). Table 26–4 shows these R values ($\times$ 100) for all pairwise comparisons and provides support for some tentative generalizations. First, the numbers of the OKT4 and OKT8 positive T cell subsets are positively correlated ($R = 0.74$, $P < 0.01$) while their respective proportions show negative, though not significant, correlations. Thus, contrary to our expectations these T cell subsets appear to vary in the same, rather than in opposite, direction in these patients. The inversion of the normal ratio between them is, therefore, due to a more pronounced decrease of the T4 positive subset than that of the T8 positive subset while both are reduced in absolute number.

Second, and as would be expected from their reciprocally positive correlation, the numbers of both the T4 and the T8 positive subsets are highly positively

Table 26–2 Cytotoxic antibodies to sperm in the serum of AIDS/Kaposi's sarcoma patients

Samples	N	Positive (N)[a]	Titers (range)[a]
AIDS/Kaposi's sarcoma	10	10	1/2 to 1/8
Homosexual men	20	8	1/1 to 1/3
Heterosexual men	8	0	—

[a]Titers and sensitivity were lower in the immunofluorescence technique.

Immunogenetic Findings in Patients with Epidemic Kaposi's Sarcoma   411

Table 26–3 TP5 study: Means and SD

Name	Neutro-phils	OKT3 N	OKT3 %	OKT4 N	OKT4 %	OKT8 N	OKT8 %	PHA Fresh	PHA Frozen	PWM Fresh	PWM Frozen	MLC[a]	RBC	OKT4:OKT8 Ratio
BA	3,229[b]	867	61	247	17	745	52	49,400	33,700	9,800	6,100	20,300	4,400,000	0.33
	448	80	7.4	36	1.9	82	5.1	11,500	8,150	3,030	1,760	4,200	170,000	
BS	3,640	941	59	358	23	515	32	29,300	32,600	24,200	7,700	39,600	5,000,000	0.72
	464	104	11.5	93	5	195	11.3	8,800	4,150	8,700	1,430	7,650	130,000	
CO	2,839	977	60	361	22	551	34	26,800	51,900	19,600	8,400	18,400	4,140,000	0.65
	418	56	5.7	90	4.4	68	3.7	23,200	14,270	6,700	3,180	6,100	270,000	
CI	1,342	480	66	46	6	469	65	12,800	7,000	4,000	720	7,330	4,010,000	0.09
	372	28	4.9	15	1.5	56	6.8	7,140	4,240	1,700	560	2,400	150,000	
CA	1,734	1,577	68	395	17	1,099	48	25,800	39,400	8,400	3,600	24,100	5,390,000	0.35
	267	141	5.7	82	3.6	144	5.8	9,380	7,652	6,040	1,180	4,200	120,000	
FE	2,131	1,632	70	522	22	1,074	46	22,800	37,100	12,800	5,500	37,300	5,100,000	0.48
	424	178	6.9	86	3.6	301	9.5	8,980	9,984	8,500	2,229	6,400	100,000	
JN	1,295	236	40	26	4	208	35	14,800	—	5,800	—	—	3,800,000	0.11
	191	51	6.9	11	1.4	41	4.6	10,600	—	5,000	—	—	360,000	
MO	1,312	857	72	115	10	764	64	12,500	4,800	4,500	740	19,800	4,600,000	0.16
	204	82	5.3	60	4.4	49	3.8	5,900	1,300	2,400	147	4,400	130,000	
SS	1,757	552	66	99	12	433	52	27,800	17,900	8,600	2,000	—	4,070,000	0.23
	390	104	13.3	48	4.5	92	10	14,600	6,530	2,180	822	—	76,000	
WE	2,371	1,381	70	357	18	971	49	35,000	17,900	11,200	6,000	29,130	4,750,000	0.37
	632	183	9.0	91	4.4	366	15	13,800	2,420	6,020	2,252	8,900	160,000	

[a] In MLC, the number is the mean of the average response against two stimulator cells repeated six to ten times.
[b] The first number is the mean of six to ten determinations, and the second is the SD.
PHA, phytohemagglutinin; PWM, pokeweed mitogen.

Table 26-4 TP5 study: Correlation coefficients (R)[a]

	WBC	Lymph-ocytes	Neutro-phils	Mono-cytes	Plate-lets	RBC	OKT3 No.	OKT3 %	OKT4 No.	OKT4 %	OKT8 No.	OKT8 %	PHA Fresh	PHA Frozen	PWM Fresh	PWM Frozen
Lymphocytes	74x	—	—	—	—	—	—	—	—	—	—	—	—	—	—	—
Neutrophils	90[d]	38	—	—	—	—	—	—	—	—	—	—	—	—	—	—
Monocytes	14	3	13	—	—	—	—	—	—	—	—	—	—	—	—	—
Platelets	56	53	36	17	24	—	—	—	—	—	—	—	—	—	—	—
RBC	59	88[c]	29	21	—	—	—	—	—	—	—	—	—	—	—	—
OKT3																
N	65[a]	98[c]	26	6	50	88[c]	—	—	—	—	—	—	—	—	—	—
%	24	50	2	—	—	—	62x	—	—	—	—	—	—	—	—	—
OKT4																
N	84[b]	95[a]	55	−13	50	79[b]	97[c]	37	—	—	—	—	—	—	—	—
%	95[d]	81[b]	80	—	—	63[a]	40	91[c]	93[c]	—	—	—	—	—	—	—
OKT8																
N	80[b]	88[a]	15	24	40	84[a]	95[c]	73[b]	74[a]	−50	—	—	—	—	—	—
%	−45	−22	−49	—	—	−5	−6	62	−40	48	18	—	—	—	—	—
PHA																
Fresh	75[a]	37	81[b]	28	51	14	30	9	42	56	8	−22	—	—	—	—
Frozen	75[a]	64[a]	58	−31	43	31	49	58	76[b]	83[b]	16	−82[b]	44	—	—	—
PWM																
Fresh	79[b]	42	82[b]	−16	31	32	30	8	63[a]	83[b]	3	−74[a]	38	—	—	—
Frozen	95[c]	53	89[c]	−16	55	24	39	−54	73[a]	94[c]	3	−90[c]	61	88[c]	68[a]	—
MLC	69[a]	69	46	−15	12	75[b]	63[a]	2	77[b]	77[b]	42	−63[a]	27	63[a]	82[b]	56
															35	

[a] $P < 0.05$.
[b] $P < 0.01$.
[c] $P < 0.001$.
[d] R = covariance $\times$ 100.
$SD_1 \times SD_2$

correlated with the total numbers of T cells ($R = 0.97$ and 0.95, respectively both with $P < 0.001$).

Third, the expected correlation between T cell subsets and functional tests was observed in these patients. Both the number and the proportion of T4 positive cells were positively correlated with the blastogenesis induced by lectins and by allogeneic cells. Significantly negative correlations exist between the proportion (percentage) of T8 positive cells and blastogenesis. Good agreement was observed between blastogenesis results with frozen and fresh cells, although frozen cells tend to give higher R values.

Fourth, high positive R values were encountered between all T lymphocytes and between each of the two subsets with the number of erythrocytes, another unexpected finding. A positive correlation ($P < 0.01$) was also seen between the T4 positive subset and the number of granulocytes (neutrophils) that is also seen in the functional tests. The number of monocytes appeared to be unrelated to any of these subsets but platelets were positively, although not significantly, correlated with them.

Fifth, the results of lectin stimulation correlated reasonably well, given the known variability of the uncorrected results, and achieved significant values except for the fresh lymphocyte responses to PHA. Frozen-thawed and fresh cells also had high correlation coefficients; fresh cells, in general, had higher variances and lower R values.

Sixth, comparisons with the popular "OKT4:OKT8 ratio" are not given in Table 26–4, because the correlations of each of the elements of the ratios are shown. Nevertheless, the ratios were computed, and, as expected, they correlated reasonably well with the other parameters studied. Thus, for example, the R values of the ratio were positive with the blastogenesis induced on frozen and fresh cells by PWM ($R = 0.92$ and 0.97), by PHA (0.79 and 0.42), and by allogeneic cells (0.67) and with the number of neutrophils (0.83). Some of the relationships defined by each subset separately, however, are not as clear cut when using the ratio: the correlation with erythrocytes has an R of only 0.45. Similarly obscured are the correlations obtained with the total number of T cells (i.e., T3 positive), which, although positive, is not significant ($R = 0.51$).

DISCUSSION

Our initial results, suggesting that the prevalence of DR5 is significantly higher in patients with either form of Kaposi's sarcoma, have been confirmed in a larger series. The probability that this excess is due to chance is now extremely low. The finding of Nunez et al. (personal communication, 1984) that a similar association pertains to homosexual patients with the polyadenopathy syndrome appears to indicate that the same type of genetic background exists in patients who develop different types of AIDS. It would be of considerable interest to study whether DR5 is also associated with Kaposi's sarcoma, lymphomas, and opportunistic infections in iatrogenically immunosuppressed individuals. Kidney allograft recipients may be a particularly favorable group of patients, since their HLA types are usually known. Be this as it may, the implication of a DR antigen as an element in the predisposition to AIDS is consistent with the ample body of data that suggests that altered immune responsiveness is a likely pathogenetic mechanism. In this chapter we have explored two aspects of the immunologic derangement: the evidence of (auto?) immunization to antigens shared by sperm and T cells and the existence of *positive* correlations between T cells of the opposing subsets.

The search for autoantibodies was started because the T cells of AIDS/Kaposi's sarcoma patients (although not of those with classic Kaposi's sarcoma) were labeled by the antihuman immunoglobulin reagent used in the identification of B lymphocytes.[20] Because the serum was known to have consistently elevated concentrations of immunoglobulins and of immune complexes, it was hypothesized that autoimmunity to antigens expressed by T cells and perhaps others might be responsible. We found that T lymphocytes from normal individuals could be "coated" by incubation in serum from positive patients. The antibody responsible for this has only been characterized with regard to cross-reactivity with sperm, a study suggested by patients' life styles and by previous findings that demonstrated the existence of just this kind of antigenic cross-reactivity.[27] It is, furthermore, known that sperm are immunogenic and that both humoral and cellular autoimmunity result from immunization with these cells,[26,28] and the suggestion has even been made that these antisperm autoantibodies may be responsible for the immunosuppression that appears to mediate the pathogenesis of AIDS.[26]

The results of the limited subset of our patients reported in Table 26–2 agree with this suggestion in that all ten of the AIDS/Kaposi's sarcoma patients studied had antisperm antibodies. The techniques employed were low in sensitivity and the number of samples small, but there is the further indication that even healthy homosexual men may have these antibodies. These findings suggest that excessive concentrations of these antibodies may be associated with clinically relevant degrees of immunosuppression and that the homosexual male population may be at an increased risk to develop AIDS for this reason. The difference in the prevalence of these antibodies in patients and homosexual controls is significant ($X^2 = 10$, $P < 0.001$), and there are also differences in the titers. Studies on the molecular specificity of these antibodies are required before the significance of these findings may be understood.

It may be relevant to the last point to be discussed here, that autoimmunity to sperm in infertile males correlates negatively with the percentage of T cells.[27] An important reduction of these cells is known to be a feature of AIDS and has been attributed to the dramatic decrease in the number of cells of the T4 positive (helper-inducer) subset. Our data confirm and extend this finding. Note that the methods for determining the quantities of these cells are not without problems. In addition to the known variability of all indirect immunofluorescence procedures, the isolation of lymphocytes from peripheral blood yields cell suspensions with variable numbers of contaminating granulocytes and monocytes. Although it is possible to avoid including in the counts the larger of the monocytes and most granulocytes on morphologic grounds, it is obvious that some overlap must exist even when "gating" on the basis of size is done in the analysis with the FACS. The problem is even worse when visually counting cells with the fluorescence microscope. The analysis of results in our experiments is further complicated by the need to account for the weekly intervals between repeat samples, for the possible progression of the disease, and for the use of a potentially active immunomodulator, TP-5. The use of frozen lymphocytes from each bleeding, however, permits us to determine how much of the variance of the different determinations is due to technical as opposed to biologic reasons. Because of the relatively small size of the SDs computed on these repeat samples and because the means of results of the "functional" tests showed highly significant correlations with the enumeration of cell types, the several conclusions detailed in the Results section are probably warranted. Interestingly, T cell blastogenic responses to PHA are somewhat less correlated with the decrease of the T4 subset than are the T-dependent B lymphocyte responses to PWM. Serum blocking factors, however, have been detected that interfere with PHA-induced but not PWM-induced blastogenesis in some of these patients and that might cause the increase in the non-T4-correlated variance encountered here. (Rubinstein et al., unpublished observations.)

Perhaps the most interesting findings are the positive correlations observed between T4 and T8 positive cells. This positive correlation is only seen between the absolute numbers, and the expected negative relationship was found when their relative frequencies were compared. In fact, because with the techniques employed, T3 positive cells can only be either T4 *or* T8 positive, a negative correlation between the respective percentages must be encountered. For this reason, the use of relative estimates, such as the T4:T8 ratio, is not as informative. A further problem in the use of such ratios is that their variances are composites of the variances of two measurements, increasing the possibility of spurious conclusions.

The positive correlations observed between the different cell types require an explanation. It is perhaps easier to understand for the T cell subsets because they are both T cells, but the high-T-cell-correlated decrease of the neutrophils and erythrocytes portends the existence of mechanisms affecting other hematopoietic functions as well. We suggest, therefore, that the altered immunity that lies at the core of the current understanding of the pathogenesis of AIDS is one of a host of consequences of a much broader disruption of homeostasis.

REFERENCES

1. Centers for Disease Control. Kaposi's sarcoma and *Pneumocystis* pneumonia among homosexual men—New York and California. MMWR 1981;30:305.
2. Centers for Disease Control. *Pneumocystis* pneumonia. MMWR 1981;30:250.
3. Friedman-Kien AE. Disseminated Kaposi-like sarcoma syndrome in young homosexual men. J Am Acad Dermatol 1981;5:468.

4. Centers for Disease Control. A cluster of Kaposi's sarcoma and *Pneumocystis carinii* pneumonia among homosexual male residents of Los Angeles and Orange Counties, California. MMWR 1982;31:305.
5. Friedman-Kien AE, Laubenstein LJ, Rubinstein P, et al. Disseminated Kaposi's sarcoma in homosexual men. Ann Intern Med 1982;96(part 1):693.
6. Centers for Disease Control. *Pneumocystis carinii* pneumonia among persons with hemophilia A. MMWR 1982;31:365.
7. Groopman JE, Gottlieb MS. Kaposi's sarcoma: An oncologic looking glass. Nature 1982;299:103.
8. Boldogh I, Beth E, Huang ES, et al. Kaposi's sarcoma: IV. Detection of CMV DNA, CMV RNA and CMVA in tumor biopsies. Int J Cancer 1981;28:469.
9. Olding LB, Kingsbury DT, Oldstone MBA. Pathogenesis of cytomegalovirus infection. Distribution of viral products, immune complexes and autoimmunity during latent murine infection. J Gen Virol 1976;33:267.
10. Selgrade MK, Osborn JE. Role of macrophages in resistance to murine cytomegalovirus. Infect Immun 1974;10:1383.
11. Grundy JE, Mackenzie JS, Stanley NF. Influence of H-2 and non-H-2 genes on resistance to murine cytomegalovirus infection. Infect Immun 1981;32:277.
12. Lilly F, Boyse EA, Old LJ. Genetic base of susceptibility to viral leukemogenesis. Lancet 1964;2:1207.
13. Safai B, Pollack MS, Myskowsky PL, Dupont B. Increased frequency of HLA DR5 in mycosis fungoides and Kaposi's sarcoma (Abstr. 847). Fed Proc 1982;41:414.
14. Stahl R. Friedman-Kien AD, Dubin R, et al. Immune abnormalities in homosexual men with Kaposi sarcoma. Am J Med 1982;73:171.
15. Siegal FP, Lopez C, Hammer GS, et al. Severe acquired immunodeficiency in male homosexuals, manifested by chronic perianal ulcerative herpes simplex lesions. N Engl J Med 1981;305:1439.
16. Gottlieb MS, Schroff R, Schanken HM, et al. *Pneumocystis carinii* pneumonia and mucosal candidiasis in previously healthy homosexual men. N Engl J Med 1981;305:1425.
17. Masur H, Michelis MA, Greene JR, et al. An outbreak of community-acquired *Pneumocystis* pneumonia. N Engl J Med 1981;305:1431.
18. Kornfield H, Vande Stouwe RA, Lange M, et al. T-lymphocyte subpopulations in homosexual men. N Engl J Med 1982;307:729.
19. DeWys WD, Curran J, Henle W, Johnson G. Workshop on Kaposi's sarcoma: Meeting report. Cancer Treat Rep 1982;66:1387.
20. Van Rood JJ, Van Leeuwen A, Ploem JS. Simultaneous detection of two cell populations by two-colour fluorescence and application to the recognition of B-cell determinants. Nature 1976;262:795.
21. Rubinstein P, Falk C, Martin M, Suciu-Foca N. Complete HLA and Bf typing in families: I. Analysis of mixed lymphocyte culture responses and LD typing. Transplant Proc 1977;9(suppl 1):77.
22. Alper CA, Boenisch T, Watson L. Genetic polymorphism in human glycine-rich beta-glycoprotein. J Exp Med 1972;135:68.
23. Kompf J, Bissbort S, Ritter H. Red cell glyoxalase in (E.C.: 4.4.1.5.) formal genetics and linkage relations. Human-genetik 1975;28:249.
24. Alper CA, Propp RP. Genetic polymorphism of the third component of human complement (C3). J Clin Invest 1968;47:2181.
25. Rubinstein P, Falk C, Martin M, Suciu-Foca N. Complete HLA and Bf typing in

families: I. Analysis of MLC responses and ID typing with homozygous typing cells. Transplant Proc 1977;9(suppl 1):77.
26. Hurtenbach U, Shearer GM. Germ cell-induced immune suppressions in mice. J Exp Med 1982;155:1719.
27. Mathur S, Goust JM, Williamson HO, Fudenberg HH. Antigenic cross-reactivity of sperm and T-lymphocytes. Fertil Steril 1980;32:469.
28. Tung KSK, Alexander NA. Autoimmune reactions in the testes. In: Johnson AD, Gomes WR, eds. The testis, vol. IV. New York: Academic Press, 1976.

Chapter 27

Significance of Endogenous Interferon and Interferon-Induced Enzymes in Patients with AIDS

Olivia T. Preble
M. Elaine Eyster
Edward P. Gelmann
James J. Goedert

Interferons (IFNs) are a family of small proteins and glycoproteins that have antiviral properties and that can be produced by many types of cells.[1] Human IFNs are classified into three groups on the basis of their antigenic properties and their nucleic acid sequences. Alpha IFN is produced mainly by leukocytes in response to a variety of viral and nonviral stimuli. Numerous distinct subspecies of human alpha IFN, which may differ in molecular weight and biologic properties,[2] have been identified. Beta IFN is synthesized predominantly by fibroblastlike cells. Gamma or "immune" IFN is released by lymphocytes following exposure to mitogens or specific antigenic stimulation and, unlike alpha and beta IFNs, is inactivated at pH 2.

The opinions or assertions contained herein are the private views of the authors and should not be construed as official or necessarily reflecting the views of the Uniformed Services University or the Department of Defense.

We thank Annie Yeh, David Walsh, Ching Chou Yang, Elizabeth White, Sharon Rozday, and Karen Bove for excellent technical assistance, and Sophia Ward for help in preparing the manuscript. Portions of this study were supported by U.S. Public Health Service Grants CA 34994, AI 21134, and HL 32473 to Olivia T. Preble and by a grant from the Brandywine Valley Hemophilia Foundation and contracts ME 82051 and ME 82130 from the Pennsylvania Department of Health to M. Elaine Eyster.

There are a number of reasons for studying the IFN system in patients with acquired immunodeficiency syndrome (AIDS). First, although circulating IFN is rare in healthy persons, IFN can be detected in both serum and target organs of animals and humans infected naturally or experimentally with many different viruses.[1] Since AIDS has a viral etiology[3,4] and viral opportunistic infections are common in AIDS patients, one would expect detectable circulating IFN at some stage of the disease. Furthermore, IFN production is usually associated with active viral growth both in vitro and in vivo. Tests for serum IFN levels may therefore help to distinguish persons with new, acute, or reactivated infections with human immunodeficiency virus (HIV) from those who have antibody due to historic or latent infection.

Second, the relatively recent recognition that IFN treatment in vivo and in vitro can markedly affect a wide variety of humoral and cellular immune responses[5] has suggested that this family of cytokines may be involved in the development of immune disorders. Although IFNs are usually quantified in terms of their antiviral activity, alpha, beta, and gamma IFNs can each alter antibody production, cell-mediated immunity, and other functions of the immune system in ways that could exaggerate the immune disorders in patients with AIDS.[1] Furthermore, several studies[6-8] have shown that patients with active autoimmune diseases such as systemic lupus erythematosus (SLE), rheumatoid arthritis, and systemic vasculitis may have high levels of an unusual acid-labile form of alpha IFN in their serum. Lack of IFN in patients with drug-induced lupuslike syndromes suggests that this IFN may be related to the primary immune defects in autoimmune disorders,[7] and indirect evidence from mouse model systems[9-12] suggests that IFN may actually contribute to the pathogenesis of some autoimmune diseases. Early studies of AIDS showed that some of the immune abnormalities in patients with AIDS are similar to those in prototype autoimmune diseases, and several cases of apparent autoimmune thrombocytopenia in homosexual men[13,14] and hemophiliacs[15] have been described.

Finally, various human IFNs have been effective in regimens of antineoplastic therapy,[16] and several hospital centers have used natural or cloned human IFNs to treat Kaposi's sarcoma (KS) in homosexual men with AIDS.[17-20] Among the goals of these studies were evaluation of biologic responses to IFN therapy in AIDS patients and definition of parameters for predicting which patients are most likely to benefit from IFN therapy.

Initial results of tests for IFN in patients with AIDS or prodromal illnesses showed that most homosexual patients with AIDS[21,22] and each of three hemophiliacs with AIDS[23] had significant titers of an alpha IFN with biologic properties similar to the acid-labile alpha IFN in patients with prototype autoimmune diseases. This chapter will summarize more recent data on the frequency and prognostic significance of circulating alpha IFN in patients with AIDS and members of high-risk groups as well as experiments to evaluate biologic response to endogenous acid-labile alpha IFN and to therapy with exogenously administered alpha IFN in homosexual men with AIDS.

METHODS

Serum specimens from some of the homosexual subjects were obtained through Donna Mildvan (Beth Israel Medical Center, New York, NY), Alvin E. Friedman-Kien (New York University Medical Center, New York, NY), Thomas Spira (Centers for Disease Control, Atlanta), Evan Hersh and Moshe Talpaz (M.D. Anderson, Houston), Robert Biggar (National Cancer Institute [NCI], National Institutes of Health, Bethesda, MD), Martin Hirsch (Boston), Hunter Handsfield (Harborview Medical Center, Seattle), and Joseph Sonnabend (New York, NY). Samples from hemophiliacs were obtained in collaboration with Margaret Ragni and Joel Spero (University of Pittsburgh, Pittsburgh), Joan Kreiss (Harborview Medical Center, Seattle), Margaret Hilgartner (Cornell–New York Hospital, New York, NY), John Kelleher (Children's Hospital, Washington, DC), Louis Aledort (Mt. Sinai Medical Center, New York, NY), Sandor Shapiro (Jefferson Medical College, Philadelphia) and Frances Gill (Children's Hospital, Philadelphia). Serum from African patients with KS and controls were generously provided by H. Grossman and U. Hess (Kilimanjaro Christian Medical Center, Moshe, Tanzania) and John Craighead (University of Vermont, Burlington, VT). Serum and heparinized blood for isolation of peripheral blood mononuclear cells (PBMC) from homosexual men with AIDS treated at the NIH Clinical Center (Bethesda, MD) were obtained in collaboration with Henry Masur (Critical Care Medicine), Dan Longo and Ronald Steis (Medicine Branch, NCI) and Anthony Fauci and H. Clifford Lane (NIAID). All specimens were obtained with informed consent and submitted as coded samples. The presence of antibodies specific for HIV was determined by enzyme-linked immunosorbent assay (ELISA).[24,25]

IFN was assayed as described previously[6,21,23] by a semimicro method to quantitate virus-induced cytopathic effects in human GM2504 fibroblasts trisomic for chromosome 21, which carries the gene(s) for IFN receptors. The IFN titer is defined as the reciprocal of the highest dilution of sample protecting 50% of the cells. Reference human alpha, beta, and gamma IFNs were included in each assay, and results were standardized to NIH No. 023-901-527 reference human leukocyte (alpha) IFN. In this system, 100 international reference units (IU) of human alpha IFN was 500 to 1000 laboratory dilution units. To determine whether the IFN was alpha IFN, the samples were assayed in duplicate on human GM2504 fibroblasts and on bovine kidney (MDBK) cells. Reference human alpha IFN was equally active on GM2504 and MDBK cells, whereas human beta and gamma IFNs were inactive on bovine cells. This preliminary characterization was confirmed by neutralization tests using polyclonal rabbit antibodies specific for human alpha, beta, and gamma IFNs.

To test the stability of an IFN sample at pH 2, 100 μl aliquots of IFN were incubated at pH 2 for 24 hours at 4°C, returned to pH 7, and clarified by centrifugation as described previously.[6,21,23] Reference human alpha, beta, and gamma IFNs, diluted to 100 IU/ml in normal human serum (Flow Labs, Rockville, Maryland) or in IFN-negative SLE or AIDS serum, were acidified, incubated, and readjusted to pH 7 in an identical manner. Residual IFN was then assayed on GM2504 cells as described above. Reference human alpha and beta IFNs were completely stable during this procedure, whereas human gamma IFN was inactivated >30-fold.

The activity of the IFN-induced enzyme 2'-5' oligoadenylate (2-5A) synthetase was quantitated in cytoplasmic extracts of PBMC as previously described.[26] Briefly, PBMC isolated on Ficoll-hypaque gradients were stored at −70°C, lysed with NP-40 buffer, and centrifuged at 10,000 g for 15 minutes to obtain the cytoplasmic extract. 2-5A synthetase in this extract was absorbed onto polyI:polyC cellulose and incubated with adenosine triphosphate (ATP) to produce the 2-5A product.[27] The 2-5A was then quantitated by using a competition radiobinding assay[28] with ^{32}P-pCp-2-5A generously supplied by Dr. Robert H. Silverman (Uniformed Services University of the Health Sciences). Enzyme activity is expressed as pmol 2-5A synthesized per 1 mg of cytoplasmic extract protein per hour. Aliquots of an extract of IFN-treated HeLa cells were included in duplicate in each assay, and all data were normalized to an activity of 50,000 units for this reference extract. Repeat testing of several normal healthy volunteers showed that intrasubject variations of up to 50% occurred when blood was drawn on different days, so that only in vivo changes of normalized enzyme activity of ≥twofold were considered significant.

PRESENCE OF ENDOGENOUS IFN IN PATIENTS WITH AIDS

Significant levels (8 IU/ml) of circulating IFN were found in less than 2% of almost 500 sera from healthy adults (Table 27–1). These data are similar to previous studies of IFN in normal persons[29,30]; low levels of IFN in a few such sera are usually ascribed to subclinical viral infections. In contrast, IFN was detected in approximately 10% of apparently healthy, clinically asymptomatic homosexual men with a variety of past medical histories.[23,24] Retrospective analysis showed that 50% to 70% of these men had antibody to HIV, and some also had laboratory evidence of immune disorders, such as low T cell ratios. About 12% of the homosexual men with mild clinical symptoms, such as generalized unexplained lymphadenopathy, had elevated levels of serum IFN.[23] At least 70% of homosexual men with AIDS, as manifested by KS or opportunistic infections, had high levels of circulating IFN, with titers up to 100 IU/ml (see Table 27–1). Eight of 9 hemophiliacs with AIDS and two patients with transfusion-related AIDS also had high levels of circulating IFN. In addition, almost 7% of otherwise healthy multitransfused patients with hemophilia A or B had elevated levels of serum IFN. However, this category also included many children, who might be more likely than the adult controls to have a subclinical viral infection, and up to 20% of the subjects with serum IFN did not have antibody to HIV detected by ELISA. Continued prospective follow-up of these

Table 27-1 Frequency of endogenous IFN in patients with AIDS and controls

Subject Group	No. IFN+/No. Tested (≥ 8 IU/ml)	% IFN+	IFN Titer (IU/ml) (range)
Healthy heterosexual controls[a]	9/498	1.8	8–12
Homosexual men			
Asymptomatic	12/126	9.5	8–100
Lymphadenopathy	11/89	12.3	8–100
AIDS	125/165	75.6	8–100
Hemophiliacs[b]			
Asymptomatic	34/500	6.8	8–25
Lymphadenopathy	2/46	4.3	25, 50
AIDS	8/9	88.9	8–100
Transfusion-related AIDS patients	2/2	100	25, 100

[a]This group includes samples from healthy adults submitted as coded samples from several collaborators between 1980 and 1985 and samples from healthy blood donors in Orange County, CA, and Ontario, Canada, in 1984 and 1985.
[b]This group includes samples from both children and adults with hemophilia A and B attending one of eight different hemophilia centers in Washington, D.C., New York City, Philadelphia, Hershey, PA, and southern California.

patients is in progress. Only two of 46 hemophilics with lymphadenopathy were IFN positive.

These IFN levels in patients with AIDS are similar to the IFN titers found in patients being treated with 10^6 to 10^7 IU per day of exogenous alpha IFN in clinical trials of IFN therapy[31] or in patients with documented viral diseases, such as measles or influenza,[32] at the peak of IFN production. However, IFN titers rapidly decline to undetectable levels in healthy persons with viral infections,[32] and injected IFN is rapidly catabolized.[33] Prospective follow-up of numerous patients with AIDS has shown that high levels of circulating IFN may be present for months, suggesting that AIDS patients continually produce large quantities of IFN.

To evaluate the specificity of endogenous IFN in patients with AIDS or prodromal symptoms, sera from members of several "control" populations, each of which have some features in common with AIDS patients, were also tested for IFN.[34] Two of three children with *Pneumocystis carinii* pneumonia complicating immunosuppressive therapy had elevated serum IFN, but convalescent sera from these three and one additional patient were all IFN negative. Only one of 23 patients with "traditional" African or American forms of KS without AIDS had a low level of circulating IFN. Eighteen monogamous homosexual couples and most patients with chronic active infections with Epstein-Barr virus (EBV)[35] were also serum IFN negative. A few patients with antibody to HIV or T cell lymphoma had circulating gamma IFN.[34]

CHARACTERIZATION OF ENDOGENOUS IFN IN AIDS PATIENTS

Endogenous IFN in AIDS patients was characterized (Table 27-2) by testing its antiviral activity on nonhuman cells, neutralization with specific anti-IFN antibodies, and stability at pH 2. All the cloned subtypes of human alpha IFN studied so far, as well as "natural" alpha IFN, which is apparently a mixture of these subtypes, and beta IFN are stable at pH 2. Although IFNs are usually species specific, human alpha IFNs generally have significant antiviral activity on bovine cells. Almost all the many samples tested from AIDS patients had similar antiviral activity on human and bovine cells and were also neutralized (from 4-fold to >30-fold) with antibody to human alpha IFN.[21-23] Lack of complete neutralization (only fourfold to eightfold) of some samples by polyclonal antialpha antibodies also occurred with IFNs from SLE patients,[6,7] suggesting that the predominant IFN in patients with AIDS may be a normally minor component of the "natural" alpha IFN (produced by virus-stimulated lymphocytes in vitro), which was used to raise the antibodies in rabbits.

Reference alpha and beta IFNs were completely stable at pH2 for 24 hours (see Table 27-2), whereas gamma IFN was inactivated under the same conditions. IFN samples from homosexual men with AIDS or prodromal signs and from hemophiliacs with AIDS were also unstable at pH 2. All the acid-labile samples were active on bovine cells and neutralized only by antialpha IFN antibodies.[21,23] These results are similar to results with IFN from patients with SLE.[6,7] Experiments with two monoclonal anti-IFN alpha antibodies[36] extended the similarities between IFN from AIDS patients and IFN from SLE patients and

Table 27-2 Characterization of IFN in sera of AIDS patients

	IFN Titer (IU/ml)	Ratio of Titer on Human/Bovine Cells[a]	Neutralization[b] Anti α	Neutralization[b] Anti γ	Inactivation[c] at pH 2
Patients					
10 KS patients[d]	10–100	0.5–4	8–32	0	4–16
3 LA patients[d]	8–20	1–2	4–32	0	>4
3 hemophiliacs[e]	25–100	0.5–2	4–16	0	4–16
Controls					
Alpha IFN[f]	100	0.5–2	≥32	0	0
Beta IFN[f]	100	>32	0	0	0
Gamma IFN[f]	100	>32	0	≥32	>32

[a] Activity on bovine cells is characteristic of human alpha IFNs.
[b] Fold reduction of titer in samples with specific rabbit anti-IFN antibodies.
[c] Titer of pH 7 control/titer of pH 2 treated sample.
[d] All KS and LA patients were homosexual men. LA, lymphadenopathy.
[e] *All* IFN+ samples, both before and during AIDS, from these patients were completely characterized.
[f] Reference human IFNs diluted in normal human serum were used as controls in the characterization experiments.

their differences from "conventional" alpha IFNs. Although three different independently prepared "natural" human alpha IFN preparations were each completely neutralized by these monoclonal antibodies, AIDS IFNs and SLE IFNs were not affected under the same conditions.[37]

ENDOGENOUS IFN AS A PRECLINICAL MARKER FOR AIDS

The presence of an unusual alpha IFN in most AIDS patients but in a much lower proportion of persons with milder symptoms or healthy persons suggested that the appearance of circulating IFN might be useful as a preclinical marker in members of groups at risk for AIDS. Analysis of clinical records from the first group of homosexual men tested for IFN indicated that many asymptomatic patients with IFN in 1980 and 1981 progressed toward AIDS in 1982 and 1983 (Preble and Sonnabend, unpublished data). Retrospective analysis of sera from other cohorts of homosexual men with AIDS and circulating IFN showed that most had developed the IFN months before AIDS could be diagnosed clinically[24] (Preble and Handsfield, unpublished data). Prospective follow-up of initially healthy homosexual men in high-risk,[38] medium-risk (Goedert and Preble, unpublished data), and low-risk (Preble and Handsfield, unpublished data) areas has confirmed that patients may develop high levels of serum IFN more than a year before AIDS develops. These results suggest that endogenous acid-labile alpha IFN may be a negative prognostic sign in homosexual men.

Retrospective study of stored serum samples from five of the nine hemophiliacs with AIDS (see Table 27–1) showed that four of the five became serum IFN positive in the year preceding development of AIDS[24] (Eyster et al., unpublished data, 1987). One patient developed circulating IFN more than nine months before prodromal signs of AIDS appeared, such as persistent diarrhea, and IFN titers remained high until his death.[24] As with homosexual men, each of the hemophiliacs who developed IFN and then AIDS had been positive for antibody to HIV for some time. Since the appearance of circulating acid-labile alpha IFN occurred after, rather than coincident with, seroconversion, the IFN probably does not reflect a new acute infection. However, IFN may signal either reactivation of HIV or a fundamental change in the immune system of persons exposed to the virus. A prospective study of a large cohort of hemophiliacs with antibody to HIV with and without circulating IFN is in progress.

BIOCHEMICAL RESPONSE TO IFN IN AIDS PATIENTS

The enzyme $2'$-$5'$ oligoadenylate (2-5A) synthetase is specifically induced in cultured cells treated with all classes of IFN,[39] including acid-labile alpha IFN(Epstein et al., unpublished data). This enzyme has been used as an index of biologic responsiveness to IFN because it is also elevated in lymphocytes isolated from mice[40] and humans[41,42] with acute viral infections as well as lymphocytes from cancer patients undergoing IFN therapy[43,44] and patients with autoimmune diseases and circulating IFN.[45] Since various forms of human alpha IFN have been used for antineoplastic treatment of KS in AIDS patients,[17-20] experiments were done to determine if AIDS patients had a detectable biochemical response to either their endogenous acid-labile alpha IFN or to therapy with "conventional" alpha IFN.[26]

Twenty-eight patients with KS who were entered into a phase II trial of therapy with purified human lymphoblastoid alpha IFN (Wellferon, Burroughs-Wellcome, Research Triangle Park, NC) were studied.[19,26] The patients received 7.5, 15, or 25 × 10^6 units of IFN/m^2 intramuscularly (IM); serum IFN titers and 2-5A synthetase levels in PBMC were determined before, at regular intervals during, and two to four weeks after, therapy. For some of the patients, the response of isolated PBMC to IFN in vitro was tested before initiation of therapy to determine if clinical outcome could be predicted in advance of therapy. A second group of patients received therapy with recombinant-DNA-derived human alpha IFN (IFL-rA, Hoffman-LaRoche, Nutley, NJ).

PBMC from 11 healthy persons had an average of 15 units of 2-5A synthetase/1 mg protein an hour.[19] Five of the seven homosexual controls without any clinical symptoms had enzyme levels near the upper limit of normal, and two had clearly elevated 2-5A synthetase activity, with values four to five times the normal mean and twice as high as the highest enzyme level in the heterosexual controls. Although about 10% of apparently healthy homosexual men had circulating IFN (see Table 27-1), none of the homosexual controls in this particular study had detectable IFN in their serum when the PBMC were isolated. Others[46] also found high levels of synthetase in some apparently healthy homosexual men with antibody to HIV and concluded that elevated synthetase might be a poor prognostic sign in patients at risk of AIDS. When PBMC from 27 of the 28 homosexual men with KS were tested for synthetase before IFN therapy, enzyme levels ranged from normal to 50 times normal. Fifteen of the patients had very high enzyme activity, with 38 to 780 units of synthetase. Twelve of the 28 patients had endogenous acid-labile alpha IFN detectable in their serum, but not all these men had high enzyme activity, and synthetase levels were not strictly correlated with serum IFN titers.[19] However, previous studies in humans[45] and mice[40] have suggested that IFN produced locally in lymphoid organs or other tissues can induce 2-5A synthetase in circulating peripheral blood cells even in the absence of free circulating IFN. Although cytomegalovirus (CMV) infection of mice can induce IFN,[47] CMV could be isolated from urine, semen, or throat cultures from all the patients with AIDS as well as from the healthy homosexual men,[19] and CMV viremia did not correlate statistically with either circulating IFN or enzyme levels in isolated PBMC from the patients or the controls.[26]

The reasons why endogenous acid-labile alpha IFN induces 2-5A synthetase in some patients and not in others are still uncertain, but further experiments showed that PBMC from most of the homosexual men were markedly deficient in their ability to respond to "conventional" alpha IFN both in vitro and in vivo.[26] PBMC isolated from healthy controls and from 11 AIDS patients before their IFN therapy were incubated in vitro with 200 IU/ml of Wellferon. Cells from only one of seven homosexual controls, and from none of the AIDS patients, had an increase in 2-5A synthetase that was within the range found with cells from heterosexual control subjects. Twofold to sixfold decreases in enzyme level were actually seen when cells from five of the homosexual men were incubated with IFN in vitro. High endogenous levels of enzyme did not appear to be solely responsible for low levels of induction, since homosexual men with normal basal levels of 2-5A synthetase had little if any response to IFN in vitro, and the one patient with a normal induction of synthetase in vitro had fairly high basal enzyme activity.

All the patients had high titers of conventional acid-stable alpha IFN in their serum during IFN therapy; none of the patients developed detectable anti-IFN antibodies during therapy.[26] However, only three of eight patients who received 7.5×10^6 units of lymphoblastoid IFN/m^2 daily, five of 10 patients who received 15×10^6 units daily, and two of nine patients who received 25×10^6 units daily responded to the IFN therapy with significant increases in 2-5A synthetase activity in their PBMC during the first month of therapy. Increasing the dose of IFN therefore did not appreciably affect the proportion of patients with a measurable biochemical response to the IFN. Four patients who had been serum IFN-positive and who had had very high 2-5A synthetase activity before IFN therapy had dramatic *decreases* in enzyme activity during one month of IFN therapy. Five patients received additional therapy for one to six months; two had delayed increases in enzyme levels after two and three months, respectively. Similar results were obtained when another group of patients was treated with high doses of IFL-rA (Preble and Gelmann, unpublished data).

When in vitro and in vivo responses to IFN were compared, synthetase induction in cultured PBMC before IFN therapy was only a rough indicator of the 2-5A synthetase response observed in vivo during therapy. Unfortunately, it was not possible to predict clinical response to therapy on the basis of either in vitro or in vivo increases in synthetase (Table 27–3), although each patient with

Table 27–3 Clinical response and 2-5A synthetase during lymphoblastoid IFN therapy

Clinical Response[a]	No. of Patients	No. with Pretherapy Serum IFN ($\geq$ 8 IU/ml)	Change in Synthetase[b]		
			Increase	No Change	Decrease
Complete	3	0	3	0	—
Partial/minor	4	1	2	2	—
None	11	3	6	5	—
Progressive KS	9[c]	7	2	3	3
Not evaluable	1	1	—	—	1

[a]Criteria for clinical response are defined in reference 19.
[b]Increases or decreases under twofold over course of IFN therapy were considered insignificant.[19]
[c]Change could not be determined for one patient who was not tested before therapy.

a significant decrease in enzyme activity during the first month of therapy had progressive disease while receiving alpha IFN.[19,26] However, the presence of endogenous circulating alpha IFN before therapy was useful for predicting patients who would develop progressive KS during IFN therapy.[19,26] This conclusion has also been confirmed by others who treated a large group of homosexual men with recombinant alpha IFN.[20]

DISCUSSION AND CONCLUSION

The origin of endogenous acid-labile alpha IFN and its significance in the pathogenesis of AIDS is still uncertain. Both retrospective analysis and prospective follow-up studies in several laboratories have confirmed that development of endogenous acid-labile alpha IFN often precedes AIDS and may be a negative prognostic sign in both homosexual men and hemophiliacs. The fact that a similar IFN circulates in patients with prototype autoimmune diseases such as SLE may support hypotheses that AIDS has an autoimmune component. Acid-labile alpha IFN was also found in sera from infants and fetuses with congenital rubella infections,[48] and its synthesis was thought to be due to immune mechanisms or to virus-infected immune cells. In addition, an acid-labile alpha IFN may also be produced if immune cells are infected with live influenza virus.[49] Appearance of endogenous IFN may therefore signal reactivation of infection with HIV or fundamental changes in the immune status in members of high-risk groups with antibody. Experiments to test this hypothesis are in progress. In addition, the presence of endogenous alpha IFN may be a useful prognostic indicator in patients being considered for IFN therapy.

There is also indirect evidence that circulating IFN may contribute to the pathogenesis or symptoms of some autoimmune diseases. Administration of IFN or IFN inducers accelerates both the onset and severity of autoimmune disease in NZB mice,[9,10] and studies with uninfected Swiss mice and rats[11] and with mice persistently infected with lymphocytic choriomeningitis virus[12] suggest that IFN may be involved in the development of renal disorders and other manifestations of chronic diseases mediated by immune complexes. Furthermore, the side effects of IFN therapy include fever, general malaise and muscle pain, nausea or diarrhea, leukopenia, and alopecia, all of which are among the prodromal signs of AIDS. Although the immunoregulatory effects of conventional human alpha IFN are well documented,[1,2] the effects of acid-labile alpha IFN, once it appears, on the immune system are unknown.

At least half the AIDS patients tested had high basal levels of 2-5A synthetase in their PBMC. These results are consistent with other studies demonstrating that 2-5A synthetase may be a more sensitive measure of the presence of IFN than assays of serum for antiviral activity. The results are also consistent with reports of IFN-related tubuloreticular inclusions in lymphocytes from almost all AIDS patients.[50,51] However, some patients apparently did not respond biochemically to their endogenous IFN. This could be due to spreading infection with

HIV, to depletion of cells capable of responding to IFN, or to other as yet undefined factors in some patients. Furthermore, compared with PBMC from healthy heterosexual controls, cells from both homosexual controls and homosexual AIDS patients were also markedly deficient in their ability to respond to exogenous alpha IFN either in vitro or in vivo with increased 2-5A synthetase. In contrast, patients with other cancers who received therapy with much lower doses of alpha IFN developed increased 2-5A synthetase in their PBMC during the first day of therapy, and enzyme activity remained elevated throughout the course of therapy.[44] In addition, even though PBMC from healthy persons with viral infections have high synthetase activity, additional induction occurs in the cells incubated with IFN in vitro.[52] Finally, lymphoblastoid cell lines with very high (500 units) levels of endogenous synthetase activity are still capable of vigorous induction of enzyme after exposure to IFN for a few hours.[53] Although no statistical correlation was found between CMV viremia and inducibility of 2-5A synthetase, studies on the effect of HIV infection and reactivation on responsiveness to various forms of IFN are needed.

REFERENCES

1. Preble OT, Freidman RM. Interferon-induced alterations in cells: Relevance to viral and non-viral diseases. Lab Invest 1983;49:4.
2. Weck PK, Apperson S, May L, Stebbing N. Comparison of the antiviral activities of various cloned human interferon-α subtypes in mammalian cell cultures. J Gen Virol 1981;57:233.
3. Gallo RC, Salahuddin SZ, Popovic M. et al. Frequent detection and isolation of cytopathic retroviruses (HTLV-III) from patients with AIDS and at risk for AIDS. Science 1985;244:500.
4. Barre-Sinoussi F, Chermann JC, Rey F, et al. Isolation of a T-lymphotropic retrovirus from a patient at risk for acquired immune-deficiency syndrome (AIDS). Science 1983;220:868.
5. Friedman RM, Vogel SN. Interferons with special emphasis on the immune system. Adv Immunol 1983;34:97.
6. Preble OT, Black RJ, Friedman RM, et al. Systemic lupus erythematosus: Presence in human serum of an unusual acid-labile leukocyte interferon. Science 1982;216:429.
7. Preble OT, Black RJ, Klippel JH, et al. Interferon in system lupus erythematosus. In: Merigan TC, Friedman RM, Fox CF, eds. Interferons, UCLA Symposium on Molecular Cell Biology, vol. 25. New York: Academic Press, 1982; 219.
8. Hooks JJ, Jordan GW, Cupps T, et al. Multiple interferons in the circulation of patients with systemic lupus erythematosus and vasculitis. Arthritis Rheum 1982;25:396.
9. Heremans H, Billiau A, Colombatti A, et al. Interferon treatment in NZB mice: Accelerated progression of autoimmune disease. Infect Immun 1978;21:925.
10. Engleman EG, Sonnenfeld G, Dauphinee M, et al. Treatment of NZB/NZW F_1 hybrid mice with *Mycobacterium bovis* strain BCG of type II interferon preparations accelerates autoimmune diseases. Arthritis Rheum 1981;24:1296.
11. Gresser I, Morel-Maroger L, Chatelet F, et al. Delays in growth and the development

of nephritis in rats treated with interferon preparations in the neonatal period. Am J Pathol 1979;95:329.
12. Riviere Y, Gresser I, Guillon J-C, Tovey MG. Inhibition by anti-interferon serum of lymphocytic choriomeningitis virus disease in suckling mice. Proc Natl Acad Sci USA 1977;74:2135.
13. Morris L, Distenfeld A, Amorosi E, Karpatkin S. Autoimmune thrombocytopenic purpura in homosexual men. Ann Intern Med 1982;96:714.
14. Abrams DI, Kiprov DD, Goedert JJ, et al. Antibodies to human T-lymphotropic virus type III and development of the acquired immunodeficiency syndrome in homosexual men presenting with immune thrombocytopenia. Ann Intern Med 1986; 104:47.
15. Ratnoff OD, Menitove JB, Aster RH, Lederman MM. N Eng J Med 1983;308:439.
16. Steihm ER, Kronenberg LH, Rosenblatt HM, et al. Interferon: Immunobiology and clinical significance. Ann Intern Med 1982;96:80.
17. Krown SE, Real FX, Cunningham-Rundles S, et al. Preliminary observations on the effect of recombinant leukocyte A interferon in homosexual men with Kaposi's sarcoma. N Engl J Med 1983;308:1071.
18. Groopman JE, Gottlieb MS, Goodman J, et al. Recombinant alpha-2 interferon therapy for Kaposi's sarcoma associated with the acquired immunodeficiency syndrome. Ann Intern Med 1984;100:671.
19. Gelmann EP, Preble OT, Steis R, et al. Human lymphoblastoid interferon treatment of Kaposi's sarcoma in AIDS: Clinical response and prognostic parameters. Am J Med 1985;78:737.
20. Vadham-Raj S, Wong G, Gnecco C, et al. Immunological variables as predictors of prognosis in patients with Kaposi's sarcoma and the acquired immunodeficiency syndrome. Cancer Res 1986;46:417.
21. DeStefano E, Friedman RM, Friedman-Kien AE, et al. Acid-labile leukocyte interferon in homosexual man with Kaposi's sarcoma and lymphadenopathy. J Infect Dis 1982;146:451.
22. Buimovici-Klein E, Lange M, Klein RJ, et al. Is the presence of interferon predictive for AIDS? Lancet 1983;2:344.
23. Eyster ME, Goedert JJ, Poon MC, Preble OT. Acid-labile alpha interferon: A possible pre-clinical marker for AIDS in hemophiliacs. N Engl J Med 1983;309:583.
24. Sarngadharan MG, Popovic M, Bruch L, et al. Antibodies reactive with human T-lymphotropic retroviruses (HTLV-III) in the serum of patients with AIDS. Science 1984;224:506.
25. Weiss SH, Goedert JJ, Sarngadharan MG, et al. Screening test for HTLV-III (AIDS agent) antibodies: Specificity, sensitivity and applications. JAMA 1985;253:221.
26. Preble OT, Rook AH, Steis R, et al. Interferon-induced 2'-5' oligoadenylate synthetase during alpha interferon therapy in homosexual men with Kaposi's sarcoma: Marked deficiency in biochemical response to interferon in AIDS patients. J Infect Dis 1985;152:457.
27. Wells JA, Swyryd EA, Stark GR. An improved method for purifying 2',5'-oligoadenylate synthetase. J Biol Chem 1984;259:1363.
28. Knight M, Cayley PJ, Silverman RH, et al. Radioimmune, radiobinding and HPLC analysis of 2-5A and related oligonucleotides from intact cells. Nature 1980;228:189.
29. Levin S, Hahn T. Evaluation of the human interferon system in viral disease. Clin Exp Immunol 1981;46:475.
30. Sonnenfeld G, Merigan TC. The role of interferon in viral infections. Semin Immunopathol 1979;2:341.
31. Gutterman JU, Fine S, Quesada J, et al. Recombinant leukocyte A interferon: Phar-

macokinetics, single-dose tolerance and biologic effects in cancer patients. Ann Intern Med 1982;96:549.
32. Green JA, Charette RP, Yeh T-J, Smith CB. Presence of interferon in acute- and convalescent-phase sera of humans with influenza or an influenza-like illness of undetermined etiology. J Infect Dis 1982;145:837.
33. Bocci V. Pharmacokinetic studies of interferons. Pharmacol Ther 1981;13:421.
34. Preble OT, Rook AH, Quinnan GV, et al. Role of interferon in AIDS. Ann NY Acad Sci 1984;437:65.
35. Straus SE, Tosato G, Armstrong G, et al. Persisting illness and fatigue in 23 adults: Serologic and immunologic evidence for chronic active Epstein-Barr virus infection. Ann Intern Med 1985;102:7.
36. Staehelin T, Hobbs DS, Kung H-F, et al. Purification and characterization of recombinant human leukocyte interferon (IFLrA) with monoclonal antibodies. J Biol Chem 1981;256:9750.
37. Preble OT, Friedman RM. Characterization of acid-labile alpha interferon from patients with autoimmune diseases. In: deMaeyer E, Schellekens H, eds. The biology of the interferon system. New York: Elsevier, 1983;379–86.
38. Metroka CE, Sonnabend JA, Cunningham-Rundles S, Krim M. Acid-labile interferon-alpha in homosexual men: A pre-clinical marker for opportunistic infections. Abstracts of the International Conference on AIDS, Atlanta, 1985;86.
39. Revel, M. Molecular mechanisms involved in the antiviral effects of interferon. In: Gresser I, ed. Interferon I. London: Academic Press, 1979;101.
40. Schattner A, Merlin G, Shapira A, et al. Comparison of (2'-5') oligoadenylate synthetase and interferon blood levels in mice early after viral infection. J Interferon Res 1982;2:285.
41. Schattner A, Wallach D, Merlin G, et al. Assay of an interferon-induced enzyme in white blood cells as a diagnostic aid in viral diseases. Lancet 1981;2:497.
42. Williams BRG, Read SE, Freedman MH, et al. The assay of 2-5A synthetase as an indicator of interferon activity and virus infection in vivo. In: Merigan TC, Friedman RM, eds. Interferons, UCLA Symposia on Molecular and Cellular Biology, Vol. 25. New York: Academic Press, 1982;253.
43. Schattner A, Merlin G. Wallach D, et al. Monitoring of interferon therapy by assay of (2'-5') oligo isoadenylate synthetase in human peripheral blood cells. J Interferon Res 1982;1:587.
44. Merritt JA, Borden EC, Ball LA. Measurement of 2'-5' oligoadenylate synthetase during treatment with interferon alpha. J Interferon Res 1985;5:191.
45. Preble OT, Rothko K, Klippel JH, et al. Interferon-induced 2'-5' adenylate synthetase in vivo and interferon production in vitro by lymphocytes from systemic lupus patients with and without circulating interferon. J Exp Med 1983;157:2140.
46. Read SE, Williams BRG, Coates RA, et al. Elevated levels of interferon-induced 2'-5' oligoadenylate synthetase in generalized persistent lymphadenopathy and the acquired immunodeficiency syndrome. J Infect Dis 1985;152:466.
47. Kelsey DK, Overall JC Jr, Glasgow LA. Production of alpha and gamma interferons by spleen cells from cytomegalovirus-infected mice. Infect Immun 1982;36:651.
48. Lebon P, Daffos F, Checoury A, et al. Presence of an acid-labile alpha-interferon in sera from fetuses and children with congenital rubella. J Clin Microbiol 1985;21:775.
49. Balkwill FR, Griffin DB, Band HA, Beverly PCL. Immune human lymphocytes produce an acid-labile alpha-interferon. J Exp Med 1983;157:1059.
50. Anderson MG, Key P, Tovey G. Persistent lymphadenopathy in homosexual men: A clinical and ultrastructural study. Lancet 1984;1:880.
51. Grimley PM, Kang Y-H, Frederick W. Interferon-related leukocyte inclusions in

acquired immune deficiency syndrome: Localization in T cells. Am J Clin Pathol 1984;81:147.
52. Penn LJZ, Williams BRG. Interferon-induced 2-5A synthetase in human peripheral blood mononuclear cells after immunization with influenza virus and rubella virus vaccines. J Virol 1984;49:748.
53. Grimley PM, Rutherford MN, Kang YH, et al. Tubuloreticular inclusions in human lymphoma cells produced by leukocyte interferon: Dose-effect and kinetic studies related to the induction of 2'-5'A synthetase. Cancer Res 1984;144:3480.

Chapter 28

Approaches to Therapy of AIDS

Frederick P. Siegal

Management of acquired immunodeficiency syndrome (AIDS) patients presents a major challenge to the clinician, requiring expertise in virtually every medical specialty. Efforts to recognize and control the various disease manifestations require a multidisciplinary approach that has been discussed in many of its aspects in other chapters of this text. However encouraging have been recent improvements in the therapy of secondary complications of AIDS, they have ultimately all been doomed to failure. It now seems clear that direct attempts at treatment of the developing immune deficiency itself seems the only global approach to the problem, since most of the processes that arise in AIDS patients are consequent to the immune deficiency.

The AIDS retrovirus, human immunodeficiency virus (HIV), exerts profound effects on the complex systems of host defense at almost all levels of function. Although its most obvious, and perhaps principal, target is the helper T lymphocyte population expressing the T4 marker,[1-3] other cells are involved. These include monocyte-macrophages,[4] dendritic lymphoid cells involved in self-recognition and antigen presentation,[5] and cells within the central nervous system (CNS).[6-8] Some express the T4 marker, and some do not. Infection of the organism leads to profound effects on cells that have not yet been shown to be directly infected, including certain thymus-independent, non-T, large, granular lymphocytes crucial to the containment of infections with intracellular pathogens[9,10] and hematopoietic progenitor cells (colony-forming unit [CFU]-GM).[11] The histology of the thymus is profoundly affected during this infection, possibly rendering effective spontaneous reconstitution of thymus-dependent immunity a doubtful prospect (see Figures 28–1 and 28–2).

Since CDC-defined "AIDS" represents the end stage in what is clearly a protracted decline of the immune system, treatment of AIDS would best begin well in advance of the development of any secondary complications, at a time when infection with the AIDS agent has already had a demonstrable effect on

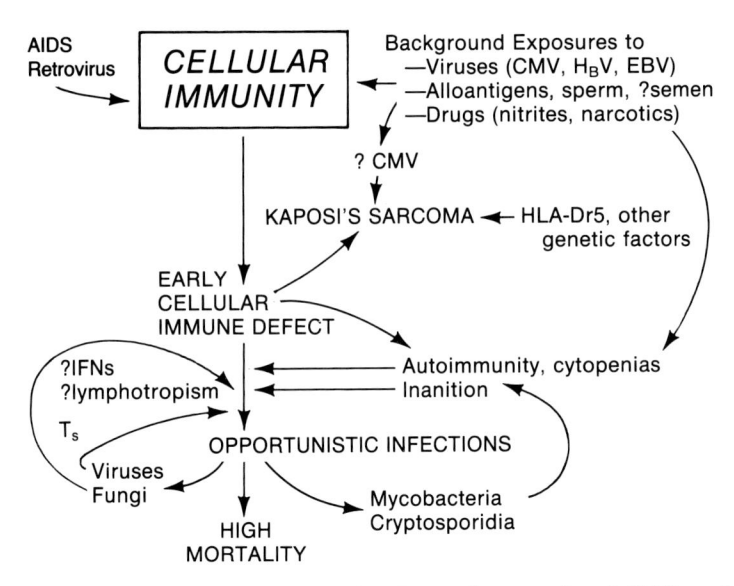

FIGURE 28-1 *Hypothetical scheme for the pathogenesis of AIDS and the relationship to Kaposi's sarcoma. The* **black box** *of cellular immunity contains the components listed in Figure 28-2. Exposure to the AIDS retrovirus, HIV, affects cellular immune mechanisms in a rather specific and profound way (see Chapter 24). This leads to subtle early defects that are still poorly defined but appear sufficient, in the presence of certain cofactors (upper right), to lead to the development of Kaposi's sarcoma in some individuals or to set off a chain of events leading to the development of opportunistic infections. The onset of serious infections with intracellular pathogens may accelerate the processes, ultimately leading to death. Some of the abnormalities perceived as being intrinsic to AIDS may instead actually be the result of secondary infections.*

the immune system. Such treatment, still largely hypothetical, would prevent the progressive decline of immune function that ultimately leads to a probably irreversible immune deficiency state.

Before the recognition of HIV as the causative agent of AIDS, treatment efforts were aimed chiefly at attaining immune reconstitution. A variety of modalities were tried (Table 28–1) without notable success. In fact, even the most vigorous attempts, including bone marrow transplantation, initiated both with and without prior conditioning regimens, failed.[12,13] These efforts were unsuccessful because some reflected a somewhat naive concept of the nature of the immune defects, because some of the agents were not particularly effective in any setting, or because the AIDS agent, although then still cloaked in mystery, was capable of destroying any activated or transplanted lymphoid elements.

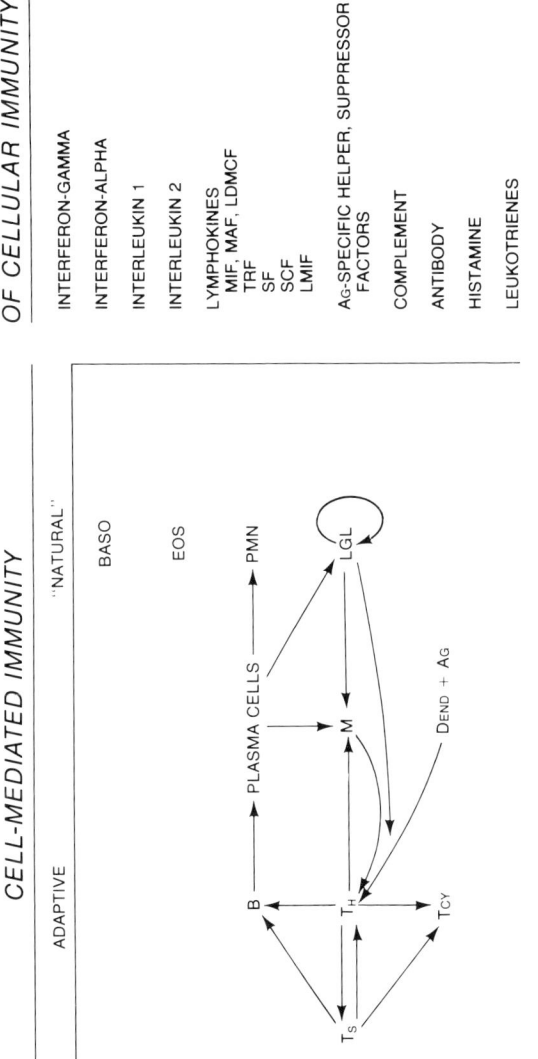

CELL-MEDIATED IMMUNITY

ADAPTIVE   "NATURAL"

BASO

EOS

B → PLASMA CELLS → PMN

LGL

M

T_S — T_H — T_{CY}

$D_{END} + A_G$

HUMORAL MEDIATORS OF CELLULAR IMMUNITY

INTERFERON-GAMMA

INTERFERON-ALPHA

INTERLEUKIN 1

INTERLEUKIN 2

LYMPHOKINES
MIF, MAF, LDMCF
TRF
SF
SCF
LMIF

A_G-SPECIFIC HELPER, SUPPRESSOR FACTORS

COMPLEMENT

ANTIBODY

HISTAMINE

LEUKOTRIENES

FIGURE 28–2 *Cellular immunity results from the interaction of diverse groups of cells with antigens. Two major classes of cells recognize foreignness, those with specific immunoglobulinlike antigen receptors that after antigen recognition are clonally selected and expanded (B and T cells that comprise adaptive immunity), and those with other receptors, the large granular lymphocytes (LGL), that can respond without prior experience with antigen. The LGL and other hematopoietic cells comprise natural immunity. All these cells communicate with one another through the lymphokines and other small molecules listed to the right of the diagram. Stimulation of cells involved in either natural or adaptive immune limbs leads to the release of interferons and other activators of macrophages and other effector cells that provide the final common pathway of cellular immunity. The model of cell-mediated immunity developed by Mackaness, in which T cell–macrophage interaction leads to enhanced stasis of intracellular pathogens, appears to account for only part of the cell-mediated immunity containing the opportunistic organisms complicating AIDS. Defects in both T-helper and LGL that interfere with activation of effector cells appear necessary before severe infectious complications arise. It is likely, because of the network that exists among these cells, that more abnormalities will develop as the disease progresses.*

Table 28–1 Efforts at immune reconstitution

Biologic Agents	Therapeutic Maneuvers
Augmenting	
Thymic hormones	Lymphocyte infusion
Transfer factor	Bone marrow transplantation
Imreg-1	
IFNs	
IL-2	
Levamisole	
Isoprinosine	
Naltrexone	
Inhibiting suppressor mechanisms	
Indomethacin	Lymphopheresis
Lithium salts	Thoracic duct drainage
Cimetidine	Extracorporeal irradiation of blood
Monoclonal antibodies	
Cyclosporin A	
Cyclophosphamide	
Other rationales	
Immune (gamma) globulins	Plasmapheresis

POSSIBLE APPROACHES TO THERAPY

Treatment of most diseases can be initiated at several levels. A direct attack on the causative agent would be the most satisfying. A variety of antiviral drugs are being investigated that are known to inhibit retroviruses. A second strategy would involve alteration of cofactors known to play a role in pathogenesis. Unfortunately, no cofactors have yet been defined. Indeed, some students of the disease have expressed the view that the only really important cofactor is the amount of time that has elapsed since the individual was infected with the virus.[14] A third tactic involves interference with inflammatory or other secondary effects of viral infection known to lead to symptoms. Efforts to interfere with hypothesized immunosuppressive or myelosuppressive viral products analogous to p15(E) associated with feline leukemia virus (FeLV) infections[15] have not been undertaken, although the existence of such molecules has been suggested. Any attempts to use immunosuppressive agents or plasmapheresis to interfere with hypothesized autoimmune pathogenetic mechanisms have either failed to affect the course of the disorder or have even hastened its course. Finally, as discussed above, attempts to interfere with the end result through immune reconstitution have been disappointing as well.

ANTIVIRAL AGENTS UNDER STUDY

The currently most promising approach to the therapy of HIV infections involves a direct attack on the AIDS virus itself. At least two potential virus-specific targets are known already. Unique to retroviruses in general is the RNA-dependent DNA polymerase (reverse transcriptase [RT]), which enables transcription of the viral RNA genome as a DNA copy and integration (as provirus) in the host cell genome. This enzyme, which human cells lack, is essential for viral replication.[16]

Another apparently special feature of the virus, one crucial to its rapid replication within cells, is the gene for a transacting protein, *tat*. The tat gene product interacts with other viral and cellular genomic and enzymatic components to greatly accelerate the transcription or translation of structural genes. Virus defective for the transactivating gene fails to replicate.[17]

Consequently, interest has focused on drugs that might interfere with RT activity and on the potential for blocking the function of the tat gene product. Strategies for antiviral therapy may ultimately involve combinations of agents directed toward both these singular features of the virus. Recent perspectives on the potential for AIDS treatment have been reviewed.[16,18,19]

REQUISITES OF A USEFUL ANTIRETROVIRAL AGENT

Several characteristics seem required of any drug to be used to inhibit the AIDS virus. Such a drug should be active in vitro, reducing the virus's ability to replicate or to cause a cytopathic effect, inhibiting formation of giant cells; capable of penetrating the blood-brain barrier, so as to gain access to any virus that has already settled within the neuraxis at the time therapy is begun; and tolerated by the patient over prolonged periods of use. Since HIV is capable of silently integrating itself into long-lived T cells and macrophages, therapy probably must continue for the patient's life. HIV will need to be chronically inhibited, since no drug seems likely to eliminate it outright. Finally, such a drug should, if possible, be administered orally or have so long a half-life in tissues that intermittent parenteral dosing is effective. Frequent parenteral administration, although possible, is clearly far more cumbersome and probably impractical for widespread chronic use.

ANTIVIRAL DRUGS IN CLINICAL TRIALS

Several drugs are known to interfere with RT of HIV. Some of these agents are relatively nonspecific inhibitors of DNA polymerases, while others are selective for RT. They are in various stages of clinical trials, but relatively little is known about their efficacy in the treatment of AIDS. Even less is known about their potential for preventing AIDS through therapy of patients not yet severely immunocompromised. Those agents considered as possibly useful are listed in Table 28-2.

HPA-23 (antimoniotungstate) was developed by the French group at Institut Pasteur as an antiviral and was used initially for the treatment of Jakob-Creutzfeld disease; from experiences in that setting, it is thought to cross the blood-brain barrier. HPA-23, given parenterally, is relatively toxic, leading regularly to thrombocytopenia, among other side effects. It is in clinical trials in France and in the United States; so far, its effects have been disappointing.[20]

Ribavirin is a relatively old, orally administered, antiviral agent that has been employed in the treatment of rhinovirus infections as well as Lassa fever. It is thought to be an inhibitor of 5' capping of viral messenger RNA, but its mechanism of action is not well defined. Preliminary studies in children with AIDS using the drug at 70 mg/kg daily initially and at half that dose later parenterally, or in longer trials at 70 mg/kg daily for 3 months orally led to no changes in clinical status or immune function. Its principal toxicity is the production of intravascular hemolysis at the high doses needed to inhibit HIV in vivo; aside from the resulting anemia, it produces CNS manifestations that can be disturbing. The presence of CNS effects suggests that ribavirin traverses the meninges. Other data[21] indicate that it does so poorly, however. Ribavirin is currently in phase 3 clinical trials in several centers.

Zidovudine (azidothymidine, [AZT, Retrovir]), 3'-azido-3'-deoxythymidine) is the first of these drugs to achieve official status as an anti-HIV agent. Zidovudine is representative of a group of 2',3'-di-deoxynucleosides that inhibit retroviral reverse transcriptase. After phosphorylation to the triphosphate, they are inserted into the growing viral DNA chain during reverse transcription of viral RNA; because the 3'hydroxy group is missing, chain termination results. It is thought that the viral RNA-dependent DNA polymerase is selectively more sensitive to this event than are cellular DNA polymerases, because the latter are better able to repair transcription errors. Another of this series of agents, di-deoxycytidine, several times more active than zidovudine in vitro, was in early clinical trial in the spring of 1987.

After preliminary phase 3 trial in 1986, zidovudine was released by the Food and Drug Administration (FDA) in early 1987 for general, if restricted, use. This agent fulfills the criteria for potential use listed above and has both antiviral and immunomodulatory effects. In a multicenter double-blind clinical trial, treated subjects with overt AIDS and AIDS-related complex (ARC) demonstrated significantly better performance status, helper T cell count, and resistance to opportunistic infectious agents, compared with placebo recipients.[23] Delayed-type hypersensitivity responses were improved in those given the drug. Preliminary evidence has emerged that zidovudine suppresses some of the CNS manifestations of HIV infections as well.[24] At the highest doses given, the clinical and laboratory improvement noted in the patients was not associated with evident antiviral effect.[25]

Table 28-2 Candidate antiviral drugs

Name	Mechanism of Action	Route of Administration	Efficacy[a]	Toxicity
AL-721	Antilipid	Oral	?	
Ansamycin	RT inhibitor	Oral	1	Hepatic, leukopenia
Antimoniotungstate (HPA-23)	RT inhibitor	Parenteral	1, 2	Hepatic, thrombocytopenia
Azidothymidine (AZT)	RT inhibitor	Oral IV	1–3	Leukopenia, neutropenia
Foscarnet	RT inhibitor	Oral	1	Renal
Ribavirin	mRNA inhibitor	IV	1, 2	Hemolysis
Suramin	RT inhibitor	Parenteral	1, 2	Renal, dermal

[a]1, inhibits virus in vitro; 2, inhibits virus in vivo; 3, affects T cell numbers or cellular immune function in vivo.

Zidovudine is associated with a number of significant side effects. It is myelosuppressive, sometimes producing a megaloblastic marrow picture of anemia and neutropenia, but it can also yield a paradoxical thrombocytosis. Nausea and vomiting, relatively severe headache, insomnia, and myalgia were seen in excess among subjects treated with active drug as compared with placebo. Based on limited experience, certain drug interactions are already known to involve decreases in glucuronidation, raising the level of active drug. Acetaminophen, nonsteroidal anti-inflammatory agents, and cimetidine should be avoided in subjects taking zidovudine. In addition, in vitro evidence for drug antagonism indicates that ribavirin should probably not be employed in combination with zidovudine, although acyclovir is synergistic.[22,26] The latter effect is currently under clinical investigation.

Ansamycin, an experimental rifampin derivative used in the treatment of *Mycobacterium avium-intracellulare* (MAI) infections, inhibits the retroviral RT and infectivity by free virus.[27] Its toxicities resemble those of the parent compound and include the production of hepatitis and leukopenia. These effects disappear when the drug is discontinued. Its safety at doses of 150 to 300 mg a day has been established in trials in AIDS patients treated for atypical mycobacteriosis. Ansamycin (like rifampin) crosses the blood-brain barrier, is administered orally, and has been well tolerated at doses of up to 750 mg daily in a small group of AIDS and ARC patients who do not have MAI infections (Siegal FP, et al., unpublished data). Its ability to inhibit HIV in vivo, or to lead to clinical or immunologic improvement in such subjects has not yet been established.

Phosphonoformic acid (Foscarnet) was developed for use in cytomegalovirus (CMV) and other herpesvirus infections but was found to retard the growth of HIV in vitro. No evidence for in vivo efficacy in HIV infections is currently available; its principal side effect appears to be nephrotoxicity.[28]

Suramin, a dye derivative related to trypan red and known for almost 60 years for its trypanosomicidal activity, was shown early to interfere with RTs.[16,29] Given parenterally and failing to cross the blood-brain barrier, in early clinical trials in AIDS patients in the United States it was found to be quite toxic, affecting skin, liver, and kidneys.[30,31] Preliminary data also suggest that the course of Kaposi's sarcoma may be worsened by its use.[32]

Of note is that serum levels equivalent to those shown in vitro to inhibit virus could be attained.[30,31] However, even though viral suppression occurred during treatment at these serum levels in about a third of patients, in none were improvements of immune function recognized. These subjects, who conformed to the CDC case definition of AIDS, had advanced immunodeficiency when treated and might not be expected to respond. But these initial data suggest that drugs capable of inhibiting HIV in vivo may not be sufficient to permit immunologic recovery. Combination of such agents with immunologic reconstitution may therefore be required. Indeed, three patients treated with suramin were later given marrow transplantation and transfusion with leukopheresis-derived cells from syngeneic donors. One of these appeared to have had an encouraging result, but two others failed to respond (see below).[32]

Future deployment of suramin as a single agent appears unlikely, both because of toxicity and its failure to enter the CNS, although there still may be a place for it in multidrug regimens. Experience with suramin emphasizes the need for careful clinical trials, since all the agents being considered can cause significant damage to recipients.

IMMUNOMODULATING AGENTS IN AIDS

A variety of drugs have been given to patients in the AIDS spectrum with the idea of augmenting immune function (see Table 28–1). These include nonsteroidal anti-inflammatory drugs (e.g., indomethacin), levamisole, isoprinosine, cimetidine, and naltrexone. The rationale for the use of these agents has varied, but none appears to augment the profoundly depressed immune systems of AIDS patients measurably. Serious clinical trials of these drugs in earlier stages of the disorder have been very limited, and none of the agents has proved efficacious.[33–36]

Trials of lymphokines have been somewhat more systematic but equally negative. Defects of interferon (IFN) production are an important component of the immune deficiency of AIDS. Consequently, infusion of IFNs might be expected to augment intracellular killing of intracellular pathogens by activating macrophages and other effector cells of cellular immunity; they might also have a direct inhibitory effect on the AIDS agent. This approach has so far proved disappointing, however. In one study, for example, the blood monocytes of patients who received recombinant gamma IFN functioned less well while receiving the lymphokine than before or after treatment.[37] The proportion of responders to alpha IFN approximates that of chemotherapy with vinblastine sulfate (Velban). It appears that those who respond are those with more minor immune deficiency, whose disease would have remained relatively indolent without treatment; a proportion of patients with KS do not rapidly progress to the development of systemic opportunistic infections.[38,39]

Defects of interleukin-2 (IL-2) production have also been described in AIDS and ARC and have prompted preliminary clinical trials of recombinant IL-2. Like IFNs, these trials have provided no evidence for any clinical use.

Indeed, it would be surprising if a single lymphokine, given by infusion, had any beneficial effect on AIDS or ARC patients. Physiologically, lymphokines are released locally at the site where the immune system recognizes a need, where the foreign antigen presents itself. The responding lymphocyte sets up a concentration gradient of a pool of lymphokines that attracts and activates cells where they are needed, but not elsewhere. The lymphokines are inactivated or absorbed rapidly in vivo, so they have no lasting toxic effects elsewhere. To duplicate effective levels by parenteral administration without activating cells essentially everywhere seems impossible. So the infusion of IL-2, IFNs, and other biologic response modifiers seems doomed to failure, except when used as direct antitumor modalities.

Agents touted as promoters of "immunoregulation" have been tried in AIDS and ARC, including polypeptide extracts or lymphocytes ("Imreg-1"), transfer factor, and various extracts of thymus or synthetic polypeptides of sequences of thymic hormones. There is little clear-cut rationale for the use of such biologic agents, and no data support any major clinical trials at present. Several of these agents have been used in uncontrolled trials for some time.

Immunosuppressive agents such as cyclosporin-A have actually been tried clinically on the probably mistaken hypothesis that the immunodepletion of AIDS is the result of an autoimmune mechanism. This approach, although gaining considerable publicity for its proponents and being enthusiastically embraced by the world media for a few brief moments, was otherwise not successful. Such efforts at treatment without sound rationale and employing drugs of major toxic potential, flying in the face of logic, deserve only contempt.

THERAPEUTIC MANEUVERS

Attempts have been made since 1981 or so to bring about immune reconstitution through the transfusion of stem cells by marrow transplantation or the provision of normal peripheral T cells by transfer of lymphoid cells obtained through leukopheresis of histocompatible donors. First allogeneic[13] and later, syngeneic[12] marrow transplantation was attempted, with and without immunosuppressive conditioning regimens. These early efforts had little positive effect and served to emphasize these patients' resistance to engraftment, suggesting the presence of a later-to-be identified etiologic agent. HIV may selectively destroy transfused lymphoid elements as they respond to environmental or alloantigens.[40]

Transplantation of marrow from a healthy identical twin into his syngeneic brother with AIDS who had been treated with suramin, followed by leukopheresis infusions, led to delayed-type hypersensitivity (DTH) skin test conversion,[32] a phenomenon previously described by the same group in another identical twin transplant recipient without benefit of an antiviral agent. In addition, this patient, who has KS, has remained free of culturable virus for several months. Two other subjects, possibly with more advanced disease, failed to respond to similar therapy. Nevertheless, the concept that transplantation in the presence of active antiviral agents might succeed survives intact.

Reconstitution of immunity, other than that which can be spontaneously achieved if an effective virustatic agent can be identified, can be expected only if immunocompetent, histocompatible, hematopoietic cells or their precursors can be provided from a healthy donor. Only then can lymphokines be delivered in an effective manner to the place they are needed.

OVERALL PHILOSOPHY OF AN APPROACH TO THE PROBLEM OF THERAPY

AIDS is a complex disorder, involving the failure of a multitude of cells and their interactions. We do not now, and probably will never, comprehend the entirety of the process. It seems dubious that therapy of this disease will succeed until ways are found to turn off the effects of the AIDS virus. As active antiviral agents are developed, synergistic combinations of drugs will most likely be needed to achieve long-term suppression. The time required to develop effective combinations will not be brief, nor will the road to their concatenation be anything but rocky. Carefully controlled studies and multicenter trials will probably be needed to develop such combinations.

Perhaps more important than the regimens developed will be the timing of their deployment. Stabilizing a declining patient should be far easier than trying to reconstitute an individual with end-stage immunodeficiency. If relatively nontoxic drugs can be found, administering them to those in the early stages of HIV infection might not only be effective in preventing the development of severe immune deficiency but could conceivably prevent, or at least reduce, the probability of transmission of the virus. One must, unfortunately, bear in mind that the virus may be prevented from proliferating by drugs only so long as the cells carrying latent virus exist in an environment containing drug. Thus, antiviral agents that fail to cross the placenta might not prevent HIV transmission to the fetus, even though they are controlling the maternal infection. Likewise, semen from a treated subject that included latently infected cells might release virus into a sexual partner not already taking an effective antiviral. Cautious optimism, at best, seems the order of the day.

REFERENCES

1. Fauci AS. Immunologic abnormalities in the acquired immunodeficiency syndrome (AIDS). Clin Res 1984,32:491.
2. Dalgleish AG, Beverley PC, Clapham PR, et al. The (T4) antigen is an essential component of the receptor for the AIDS retrovirus. Nature 1985;312:763–7.
3. Quinnan GV, Siegal JP, Epstein JS, et al. Mechanisms of T-cell functional deficiency in the acquired immunodeficiency syndrome. Ann Intern Med 1985;103:710.
4. Gyorkey F, Melnick JL, Sinkovics JG, Gyorkey P. Retrovirus resembling HTLV in macrophages of patients with AIDS (letter). Lancet 1985;1:106.
5. Armstrong JA, Horne R. Follicular dendritic cells and virus-like particles in AIDS-related lymphadenopathy. Lancet 1984;2:370–2.
6. Shaw GM, Harper ME, Hahn BH, et al. HTLV-III infection in brains of children and adults with AIDS encephalopathy. Science 1985;227:177–82.
7. Levy JA, Shimabukuro J, Hollander H, et al. Isolation of AIDS-associated retroviruses from cerebrospinal fluid and brain of patients with neurological symptoms. Lancet 1985;2:586–8.
8. Ho DD, Sarngadharan MG, Resnick L, et al. Primary human T-lymphocyte virus type III infection. Ann Intern Med 1985;103:880.
9. Lopez C, Fitzgerald PA, Siegal FP. Severe acquired immune deficiency syndrome in male homosexuals: Diminished capacity to make interferon-α in vitro associated with severe opportunistic infections. J Infect Dis 1983;148:962.
10. Siegal FP, Lopez C, Fitzgerald PA, et al. Opportunistic infections in acquired immune deficiency syndrome result from synergistic defects of both the natural and adaptive components of cellular immunity. J Clin Invest 1986;78:115.

11. Leiderman IZ, Greenberg MI, Adelsberg BR, Siegel FP. A glycoprotein inhibitor of in-vitro granulopoiesis associated with the acquired immune deficiency syndrome (AIDS). Blood 1987;70:1267–72.
12. Lane HC, Fauci AS. Immunologic reconstitution in the acquired immunodeficiency syndrome. Ann Intern Med 1985;103:714.
13. Hassett JM, Zaroulis CG, Greenberg ML, Siegel FP. Bone marrow transplantation in AIDS (letter). N Engl J Med 1983;309:665.
14. Darrow WW. Presentation, NIAID Meeting on Cofactors in AIDS, Bethesda, MD, April 7–8, 1986.
15. Teich N, Wyke J, Mak T, et al. Pathogenesis of retrovirus-induced disease. In: Weiss R, Teich N, Varmus H, Coffin J, eds. RNA tumor viruses: molecular biology of tumor viruses, ed. 2. Stony Brook, N.Y.: Cold Spring Harbor Laboratory, 1984:928.
16. Chandra P, Vogel A, Gerber T. Inhibitors of retroviral DNA polymerase: Their implication in the treatment of AIDS. Cancer Res (Suppl) 1985;45:4677s.
17. Rosen CA, Sodroski JG, Goh WC, et al. Post-transcriptional regulation accounts for the trans-activation of the human T-lymphotropic virus type III. Nature 1986; 319:555–9.
18. Hirsch MS, Kaplan JC. Prospects of therapy for infections with human T-lymphotropic virus type III. Ann Intern Med 1985; 103:750.
19. Bolognesi DP, Fischinger PJ. Prospects for treatment of human retrovirus-associated diseases. Cancer Res 45 (Suppl) 1985;4700s–705s.
20. Rozenbaum W, Dormont D, Spire B, et al. Antimoniotungstate (HPA 23) treatment of three patients with AIDS and one with prodrome (letter). Lancet 1985;1:450.
21. Blanche S, Rischer A, le Beist F, et al. Ribavirin in HTLV-III/LAV infection of infants (letter). Lancet 1986;1:863.
22. Mituya H, Broder S. Strategies for antiviral therapy in AIDS. Nature 1987;325:773.
23. Fischl MA, Richman DD, Grieco MH, et al. The efficacy of azidothymidine (AZT) in the treatment of patients with AIDS and AIDS related complex. A double blind placebo controlled trial. N Engl J Med 1987;317:184–91.
24. Yarchoan R, Berg G, Brouvers P, et al. Response of human-immune-deficiency-associated neurological disease to 3'-azido-3'-deoxycymetidine. Lancet 1987;1:132.
25. DeVita VT Jr, Broder S, Fauci AS, et al. N.I.H. conference: Developmental therapeutics and the acquired immune deficiency syndrome. Ann Intern Med 1987;106:568.
26. Vogt MW, Hartshorn KL, Furman PA, et al. Ribavirin antagonizes the effect of azidothymidine on HIV replication. Science 1987;235:1376.
27. Anand R, Moore J, Feorino P, et al. Rifabutine inhibits HTLV-III (letter). Lancet 1986;1:97.
28. Beldekas JC, Levy EM, Black P, et al. In vitro effect of foscarnet on expansion of T-cells from people with LAS and AIDS (letter). Lancet 1985;2:1128.
29. Yarchoan R, Mitsuya H, Matsushita S, Broder S. Implications of the discovery of HTLV-III for the treatment of AIDS. Cancer Res 1985;45 (Suppl): 4685s.
30. Broder S, Yarchoan R, Collins JM, et al. Effects of suramin on HTLV-III/LAV infections presenting as Kaposi's sarcoma or AIDS-related complex: Clinical pharmacology and suppression of virus replication in vivo. Lancet 1985;2:627.
31. Levine AM, Gill PS, Cohen J, et al. Suramin antiviral therapy in the acquired immunodeficiency syndrome. Ann Intern Med 1986;105:32.
32. Fauci A. Presented at the Sixth International Congress of Immunology, Toronto, Canada, July 1986.

33. Mascart-Lemone P, Huygen K, Clumeck N, et al. Stimulation of cellular function by thymopentin (TP-5) in three AIDS patients (letter). Lancet 1983;2:735.
34. Grieco MH, Reddy MM, Manvar D, et al. In-vivo immunomodulation by isoprinosine in patients with the acquired immunodeficiency syndrome and related complexes. Ann Intern Med 1984;101:206.
35. Tsang PH, Tangnavarad K, Solomon S, Bekesi JG. Modulation of T- and B-lymphocyte functions by isoprinosine in immune deficiency syndrome (AIDS). J Clin Immunol 1984;4:469.
36. Pompidou A, Delsaux MC, Telvi L, et al. Isoprinosine and Imuthiol, two potentionally active compounds in patients with AIDS-related complex symptoms. Cancer Res 1985;45 (Suppl):4671s–3s.
37. Pennington JE, Groopman JE, Small GJ, et al. Effect of intravenous recombinant gamma-interferon on the respiratory burst of blood monocytes from patients with AIDS. J Infect Dis 1986;153:609.
38. Mitsuyasu RT, Taylor JM, Glaspy J, Fahey JL. Heterogeneity of epidemic Kaposi's sarcoma. Implications for therapy. Cancer 1986:57 (Suppl):1657.
39. Krown SE, Real FX, Vadhan-Raj S, et al. Kaposi's sarcoma and the acquired immune deficiency syndrome. Treatment with recombinant interferon alpha and analysis of prognostic factors. Cancer 1986:57 (Suppl):1662.
40. Folks T, Kelly J, Benn S, et al. Susceptibility of normal human lymphocytes to infections with HTLV-III/LAV. J Immunol 1986;136:4049.

PART VI
Diagnostic Perspective

Chapter 29
AIDS: An Explanation for Its Occurrence among Homosexual Men

Joseph A. Sonnabend

The following multifactorial model was first proposed in 1983 as an explanation for the occurrence of acquired immunodeficiency syndrome (AIDS) among homosexual men that did not require the participation of a novel infectious agent. Since that time, several important observations have been made that are relevant to the process of disease acquisition then suggested. First are reports directly relating to both the environmental and biologic factors proposed as being important in the development of AIDS among homosexual men. Second, two different human retroviruses have been discovered—human immunodeficiency virus (HIV)-1 and -2—and are widely perceived as causing AIDS.

How does the multifactorial model stand up in light of these new observations? With respect to the HIVs, despite the widespread acceptance of their respective etiologic roles, these must remain conjectural as long as the following two questions (at least) remain open.

The first relates to pathogenesis and asks how HIV-1 and HIV-2 cause AIDS. While a detailed knowledge of pathogenesis is not required in order to attribute an etiologic role to a particular microorganism, the case for HIV-1 as the cause of AIDS rested on two propositions: (1) that HIV directly killed lymphocytes of the CD4 subset; and (2) that HIV is frequently associated with AIDS. Although

---

This work was supported in part by National Institutes of Health grants HD16586 and HD16587 (to Steven S. Witkin, Ph.D) and CA30196-01, American Cancer Society Grant RD-161, the Nebraska State Cigarette Tax LB 506, and the Lymphoproliferative Research Fund (to David T. Purtilo, M.D.). This presentation would not have been possible without the critical participation and support provided by Mathilde Krim, Ph.D. I am indebted to her. I am also grateful to Craig Metroka, M.D., for many useful discussions. In addition, I would like to express my appreciation to the following individuals for helping me in this work and in preparing the manuscript: Lillian Waldmann, Anne Marie Bongiovanni, Michael Jurgielski, Paul Krueger, John Donley, Terry Fonville, Harley Hackett, and Suzanne Phillips. My patients have actively participated in the studies, and I acknowledge their role as collaborators.

the mechanism of cell killing remained to be elucidated, it was assumed that HIV was directly responsible because of its tropism for CD4 lymphocytes coupled with the acceptance that the loss of this lymphocyte subset is the hallmark of AIDS. It is now known that insufficient numbers of CD4 lymphocytes are infected to account for their loss by a direct cell killing effect of HIV. Since no mechanism has been demonstrated that would account for the CD4 lymphocyte loss due to a direct cell killing action of the HIVs in vivo, other, less direct mechanisms, including HIV-induced autoimmune mechanisms, have been proposed.

It has also yet to be demonstrated how infection of a small number of CD4 lymphocytes can account for the widespread abnormalities observed in AIDS. It is now known that the tropism of HIV-1 (and presumably that of HIV-2) is not limited to lymphocytes of the CD4 subset. However, infection of B cells and of macrophages by these retroviruses, although demonstrated, has not been shown to contribute to the pathogenesis of AIDS by any mechanism.

Second, there is an alternative explanation to account for the widespread association of HIVs with AIDS that has yet to be excluded. This is that the expression of HIV—a virus that can be maintained in latency—represents an opportunistic reactivation associated with the immune dysregulation resulting from the true cause or causes of AIDS, whatever these may be, and that these causes have been associated with conditions that promote the spread of all infectious agents, pathogenic or not, that can be transmitted by blood or semen. The activation of latent microorganisms, pathogenic or not, is characteristic of AIDS. Thus the expression of HIV is an effect, rather than a cause, of AIDS.

There is no evidence to suggest that carriage of HIV as a provirus, without seroconversion or with seroconversion delayed for years after infection, is not common. If HIV is not the cause of AIDS this might be anticipated to account for the preservation of HIV in nature as well as its frequent association with AIDS. Newer genome detection techniques such as the polymerase chain reaction may indicate that carriage of HIV-1 and HIV-2 is more widespread than the distribution of AIDS (as a disease), or of HIV seropositivity. A further prediction is that HIV seropositivity found among individuals, such as organ transplant recipients, who are immunocompromised for known reasons will include some whose clinical course is no different from similar but seronegative patients.

The fact that two disparate viruses cause the same disease may not be so remarkable. Their more or less simultaneous emergence into human populations, however, would be a most improbable occurrence. There is no animal reservoir so far shown for HIV-1 or HIV-2. Thus, the likely antiquity of both HIV-1 and HIV-2 must have been associated with their preservation in nature by transmission between humans, vertical, horizontal, or both. This raises the question of why AIDS had not been recognized previously, particularly since, according to current data, HIV-1 and HIV-2 have been isolated in geographically distinct areas. The problem, of course, would be compounded if additional HIVs are isolated in yet different geographic areas.

The following model describes a process by which AIDS could have developed in homosexual men that does not require the participation of any HIV or other novel agent. The essential element of this model is that it is an interactive, multifactorial process resulting from repeated exposures, particularly rectally, to large inocula of cytomegalovirus (CMV), together with repeated exposures to multiple alloantigens contained in semen, and repeated exposures to other sexually transmitted pathogens, including *Treponema pallidum,* resulting in a cumulative impairment of cytotoxic responses against intracellular parasites, including CMV and other herpesviruses. Reactivation of Epstein-Barr virus (EBV) is an important part of the model.

It is a multifactorial model on two levels. It considers the interaction of the individual with multiple environmental factors, and it also describes how the multiple biologic effects generated within the individual by these factors can interact and produce a disease. It takes into account the environmental changes that occurred during the 1970s with respect to sexual lifestyles and the increase in the pool of sexually transmissible microorganisms, pathogenic or not, that was its consequence.

A two-stage process describing the development of AIDS is presented: an initial stage of disease acquisition, associated with repeated exposures to environmental factors, is followed by a self-perpetuating stage that no longer requires these exposures and has features of a positive feedback system. A role for interferon and possibly tumor necrosis factor in the pathogenesis has now been added.

In summary, this model illustrates how AIDS could have developed in homosexual men as a result of an interaction of known or likely biologic effects generated by repeated exposures to specific infectious and noninfectious environmental factors. Numerous reports now document the specific environmental and biologic features that were regarded as important in the 1983 model, which appears—with minor updating—below.

The occurrence in 1981 of AIDS among a group of homosexual men, predominantly in New York City, San Francisco, and Los Angeles, remains unexplained. Manifestations of the syndrome include opportunistic infections, autoimmunity, and neoplasia. Autoimmunity, once completely ignored as a component of AIDS, now receives much attention.[1,2] It is a syndrome of multiple diverse manifestations; indeed, this very heterogeneity is one of its essential features.

It had been suggested early that a new and unique transmissible agent was responsible for AIDS, thus linking the disease occurring in homosexual men with a similar syndrome seen among Haitians, intravenous (IV) drug users, and recipients of blood products.[3] This was indeed a serious assertion, and a concern for its far-reaching consequences prompted us to present our model for the genesis of the syndrome in 1983, since it does not require the person-to-person transmission of a *new* infectious agent. Rather than invoke a single common infectious etiology, this model proposes that different pathways can lead to similar disorders of immune regulation and outlines the mechanisms that may lead to AIDS in homosexual men. A group of patients who closely resemble homosexual men are renal transplant recipients, who experience the same infections, Kaposi's sarcoma (KS), and lymphomas. As is the case with the men with AIDS, renal transplant recipients have an underlying immunologic disorder, but in this instance there is no disagreement that it results from intentional immunosuppressive therapy and the effects of the allograft.

HYPOTHESIS

Any hypothesis regarding the genesis of AIDS must explain why the syndrome has occurred at this time; in short, "Why now?" It is suggested that the new element was an unprecedented level of sexual promiscuity that had developed among a subgroup of homosexual men in New York, San Francisco, Los Angeles, and some other large urban centers since the late 1960s. Homosexual patients with KS and *Pneumocystis carinii* pneumonia have reported sexual contact with an unusually large number of different partners. This has been a consistent finding in the few epidemiologic surveys that have been reported[4] and will be expanded on in later sections.

We suggest that two distinct stages may be recognized in the development of the syndrome. An initial reversible stage of disease acquisition is followed by a self-sustaining stage of disease progression. It is during the first stage that promiscuity is important, because it is associated with an accumulation of effects that will eventually lead to the second, self-sustaining stage. We believe that the cumulative effects associated with promiscuity result from repeated infection with CMV, reactivation of EBV, and immune responses to spermatozoa, as well as immune responses to alloantigens on all cellular components of semen. A role for interferon in pathogenesis is now also proposed. Each of these will be discussed in some detail.

FACTORS OF PROBABLE ETIOLOGIC IMPORTANCE IN AIDS

CMV and Immunoregulatory Defects

Infection with CMV has several effects on the immune system. There is an activation of T8 suppressor/lytic T cells, with a reduction in the helper/suppressor T cell ratio. These changes resemble those seen in persons with acute EBV infections, but unlike EBV, T subset aberrations may persist for up to one year following primary infections with CMV.[5,6] In addition, infection with CMV induces a population of monocytes with suppressor activity.[7] Autoreactive antibodies have been associated with CMV infections, as has the appearance of circulating immune complexes (CICs).[8,9] Cells infected with CMV as well as other herpesviruses express Fc receptors.[10,11] Additional observations[12] have confirmed and amplified reports on the effects of CMV noted above. CMV can act as a non-specific polyclonal B cell activator not requiring T cell help.[13] In addition, monocytes infected with CMV in vitro, as well as monocytes isolated from patients with primary CMV mononucleosis, were less able to support mitogen-induced T cell responses.[7,14,15] Monocytes infected with CMV release an inhibitor of interleukin-1; this inhibitor is a host cell protein.[12] Moreover, peripheral blood mononuclear cells infected with CMV show a depressed natural killer (NK) cell activity.[16,17]

The suggestion that CMV infection contributes to the immunologic perturbation in AIDS has now received support from at least two studies. Detels et al. noted a relationship between CMV antibody titer and T cell subset abnormalities and evidence for the acquisition of CMV infection through receptive anal intercourse.[18] Drew et al. also provide evidence for an effect of CMV infection on T cell subsets in homosexual men.[19] The recent demonstration that CMV contains a protein homologous to major histocompatibility complex (MHC) class I antigens presents another possible mechanism for an immunosuppressive effect of CMV.[20]

The following points are relevant to an association between CMV infections and sexual promiscuity:

1. CMV is excreted in saliva, urine, and semen. Viral titers are probably highest in semen.[21]
2. Asymptomatic carriage of CMV in semen may persist for over one year.[22]
3. CMV antibody has been detected in 94% of homosexual and 54% of heterosexual men attending a venereal disease (VD) clinic. The IgM isotype was detected in 57% of homosexual men, compared with 4% of heterosexual men.[23,24]
4. The prevalence of CMV viruria among homosexual men attending a VD clinic was 7% to 14%. In this study it was pointed out that the excretion rate would probably have been higher had semen been sampled.[23] It would probably also have been higher had highly promiscuous populations been selected for study.
5. Reinfection with CMV can occur. It is possible to show that a single individual may be infected with more than one strain of CMV by comparing nucleic acid fragments from different virus isolates.[24] Drew and Huang have now shown that four AIDS patients had at least two different CMV isolates from their organ cultures at autopsy.[25]

The frequency with which an individual will be reinfected with CMV is a function of both the number of different sexual contacts as well as the prevalence of CMV carriage in the population with whose members the individual interacts. We suggested that conditions had become such, at least in New York City, during the prior ten years that the prevalence of CMV carriage in populations of highly promiscuous men was at least 10% and may well have been higher.

The high rate of CMV carriage in homosexual men has been further documented in San Francisco, North Carolina, and New York State.[26,27] The carriage of CMV in semen among sexually active homosexual men in New York City, in fact, reached 40% in 1983 (Lange M, personal communication, 1986). The carriage of CMV in semen, with repeated rectal infection with high-titered inocula, is important to this model.

Reactivation of EBV

Almost all adults will have become infected with EBV, which remains latent in B cells following primary infection. EBV infects B cells, which possess receptors for the virus,[28] and has the capacity to activate B cells to immunoglobulin synthesis. EBV is thus a polyclonal activator and can act as such in the absence of T cell help.[29,30] This point is significant, since many men with AIDS show evidence of polyclonal B cell activation, and this is seen despite the virtual absence of T helper cells in some of the patients.[31] About one-third of B cells exposed in vitro can be infected by EBV, and about 10% of infected cells will be activated to immunoglobulin synthesis.[32] Among the mechanisms that have evolved to deal with this B cell infection, NK cell activity is important.[33] In addition, suppressor T cells (with a surface phenotype defined by a T8 monoclonal antibody) are activated and play a role in containing primary infections by suppressing B cell activation and proliferation.[33] In seropositive individuals, a different type of cytotoxic T cell is rapidly activated. Unlike the suppressor/lytic T cell evoked during a primary infection, these T cells (memory T cells) from seropositive individuals are specific for EBV-infected B cells.[34] These two types of T cells also differ in the kinetics of suppression of B cell activation to immunoglobulin synthesis.[34] The viral antigen-specific T cell is also HLA restricted, but while T8 cytotoxic cells recognize viral antigens on the surface of the infected cell in the context of class I MHC products, cytotoxic T cells with a T4 surface phenotype recognize antigens in the context of class II MHC products.[35] During many viral infections, HLA-restricted antigen-specific cytotoxic T cells are generated.[36]

We propose that, because of their immunosuppressive effects, CMV and possibly some other viruses cause repeated episodes of EBV reactivation. Multiple herpesvirus infections have been noted,[37] and reactivation of EBV has also been seen in some other states of immunodeficiency not directly resulting from viral infections. Administration of cyclosporin A, for example, has been associated with reactivation of EBV.[38,39] Among agents that induce EBV in vitro are corticosteroids.[40] In 1983 we found that the majority of 50 homosexual men examined showed EBV reactivation patterns (Purtilo D, Sonnabend J, unpublished data). Often, patients with AIDS develop chronic lymphadenopathy and other features of chronic infectious mononucleosis.[41]

Numerous reports now document that EBV reactivation is a common feature in homosexual men with, and at risk for, AIDS. EBV genome copies were detected in lymph node specimens from homosexual men with lymphadenopathy,[42] including those who did not demonstrate an EBV reactivation pattern, in that antibodies to EBV early antigens were absent.

Defective T cell regulation of EBV-infected B cells in AIDS was demonstrated by Birx et al.[43] and was noted and reported by us in 1983.[42]

Chang et al.[44] noted an increase in the number of EBV-infected B cells in homosexual men with lymphadenopathy. An enhanced antibody response to a broad spectrum of EBV antigens was noted by Sumaya et al.,[45] resembling that seen in reactivated EBV infections. These authors also confirmed the frequent presence of IgA anti-VCA (viral capsid antigen) antibodies we reported previously.[42]

Further evidence for EBV reactivation in AIDS-related complex (ARC) patients was provided by Ragona et al.,[46] who also demonstrated an impairment of specific anti-EBV cytotoxic responses. Asymptomatic homosexual men underwent frequent reactivation or reinfection with EBV.[47] Men who were HIV-reactive demonstrated even higher anti-EBV VCA IgG titers.

The suggestion was made that EBV may be reactivated by HIV; however, the converse could also be true, or both viruses could be reactivated by the same circumstances.

It has thus been amply demonstrated that T cell control of EBV-infected B cells is defective in AIDS patients and that EBV reactivation is frequent in AIDS and AIDS-associated conditions.

The resemblance of AIDS patients to renal transplant recipients has been mentioned. It is of great interest that in renal transplant recipients, specific T cell immunity to EBV is impaired,[48] and the lymphomas that they develop contain the EBV genome.[49] The EBV genome has now been detected in AIDS-associated lymphomas.[50]

With successive bouts of EBV reactivation, increasing numbers of B cells will be infected, some will be driven to immunoglobulin synthesis, and a variety of antibodies, possibly including some autoantibodies,[30] will be produced. Many patients show evidence of enhanced immunoglobulin synthesis, involving IgG, IgA, IgM,[51] and even IgE isotypes (Wallace J, personal communication, 1982), despite diminished T helper function. The T cell independent, polyclonal activation of B cells by EBV could explain this paradox.

The hyperimmunoglobulinemia associated with AIDS is now well documented. IgA and IgG are more frequently elevated than IgM. Increased IgD levels have also now been documented.[52] Immunoglobulin elevations may be one of the earliest AIDS-associated abnormalities demonstrable in asymptomatic homosexual men. As observed by Zolla-Pazner,[2] the hyperimmunoglobulinemia in asymptomatic homosexual men may result in part from multiple and repeated sexually transmitted infections.

A study of homosexual men selected for HIV seropositivity indicated that IgA elevations were predictive of a subsequent decline of T4 T lymphocyte numbers.[53] Our own studies have indicated an inverse correlation between T4 lymphocyte numbers and IgA levels, while IgG levels showed a positive correlation with the T8 lymphocyte subset.[54]

Polyclonal Activation of B Cells and Autoimmunity

Many AIDS patients show evidence of autoimmunity. Our finding in 1983 of positive antinuclear antibody responses in AIDS patients has been confirmed,[54] as has the occasional presence of rheumatoid factor. Antibodies reactive with T cells have also been frequently reported and are discussed later in the chapter. An antiplatelet antibody in homosexual men with idiopathic thrombo cytopenic purpura (ITP) has been described.[55] IgG anti-IgG F(ab')$_2$ antibodies have also been described in patients with AIDS or at risk for developing AIDS.[56] Autoantibodies against platelets and granulocytes were also reported by Van der Lelie et al.[57]

It has been recently proposed that autoimmunity in AIDS is induced by HIV infection, as a mechanism to explain the T cell loss in the absence of a clear-cut, direct, in vivo cytocidal effect of HIV. For example, Andrieu et al.[58] propose that because of a molecular mimicry between the HIV envelope protein and class II MHC antigens, the immune response against HIV becomes an autoimmune response against class II MHC antigens. Ziegler and Stites propose a similar autoimmune response directed at MHC class II antigens.[59] Another mechanism suggested is that free gp 120 may attach to the T4 molecule on the lymphocyte and thus present a target for antibody-dependent cytotoxic responses. There is, however, no evidence for the presence of such a mechanism in AIDS patients.

The above authors relate the development of anti-T cell autoimmunity to HIV infection. In contrast, our model proposes that anti-T cell antibodies appear as the result of multiple alloimmunization and, to some extent, as part of the polyclonal B cell activation.

It has been reported that spermatozoa express a T4 type of structure.[60] Thus, rectal insemination could induce antibodies reactive with T4 molecules as a result of exposure to spermatozoa, as well as to other cells in semen.

The best documented clinical evidence of autoimmunity is a thrombocytopenia associated with anti-platelet antibodies.[61] It is likely that the leukopenia, and some unexplained rashes frequently observed in these patients also result, at least in part, from autoimmunity. Antinuclear antibody (ANA) was found in 2 of 37 homosexual men with AIDS at a titer of 1:100, and two-thirds of these men had ANA titers of 1:10; 3 of 37 had elevated titers to (ssDNA), 4 of 37 exhibited rheumatoid factor, and 13 of 37 had circulating immune complexes by the Clq binding assay (Sonnabend J, first edition). Cryoglobulins are detectable in serum during the course of infectious mononucleosis,[62] and we would predict their presence in AIDS. An unusual acid-labile form of alpha interferon has been detected in the sera of many homosexual AIDS patients.[63-65] This type of interferon has been found in systemic lupus erythematosus and some other autoimmune diseases. Its presence in AIDS is further evidence for an autoimmune component in this disease. It is likely that additional clinical manifestations of autoimmunity will become apparent as observations are extended.

Interferon

We propose that the sustained presence of high levels of interferon plays a role in the pathogenesis of AIDS. The appearance of interferon in the sera of patients with AIDS-related conditions has been shown to carry an adverse prognostic significance for the development of the full-blown syndrome.[66,67] The AIDS-associated acid-labile alpha interferon is similar to that which appears in the sera of patients with autoimmune diseases such as SLE.[68–71] There is evidence from animal model systems that interferon may indeed contribute to the pathogenesis of disease in SLE.[72,73]

The following observations suggest that the sustained presence of high levels of interferon may contribute to the pathogenesis of AIDS:

1. Interferon selectively inhibits the T4 lymphocyte subset in vitro while exerting a slight stimulatory effect on the T8 subset.[74]
2. Interferon can activate T suppressor cells to produce a soluble immune response suppressor that may inhibit antigen-presenting macrophages.[75]
3. Interferon suppresses the proliferative response of lymphocytes to mitogens and alloantigens.[76]
4. Administration of interferon results in lymphopenia, granulocytopenia, and thrombocytopenia.[77]
5. Interferon may also inhibit lipoprotein lipase and elevate serum triglycerides and depress serum cholesterol. These changes are characteristic in AIDS. Such changes can also be induced by tumor necrosis factor or cachectin. Tumor necrosis factor levels are elevated in the sera of AIDS patients.[78]

Interferon also affects immediate hypersensitivity reactions by enhancing the release of histamine from basophils,[77] thus contributing to drug hypersensitivity and the unexplained rashes common in AIDS. Exacerbations of psoriasis, also common in AIDS, have been associated with the presence of circulating interferon.

Although interferon boosts NK cell activity in short-term exposure, prolonged treatment with interferon actually depresses NK activity.[79] Indeed, incubation of peripheral blood mononuclear cells (PBMCs) from patients with AIDS with alpha-2 interferon did not result in the enhancement of NK activity that was seen with PBMCs from healthy donors.[80] This effect could result from the fact that elevated levels of circulating alpha interferon rendered NK cells unresponsive to in vitro incubation with interferon.

Interferon increases endonuclease L activity in treated cells. On prolonged exposure to interferon, however, this enzymatic activity declines. This may account for the low endonuclease level in the PBMCs of AIDS patients.[81] The decline of endonuclease activity may be an adaptive response to prolonged exposure to interferon as may be the down regulation of interferon receptors. Interferon's antiviral activity may therefore not be fully expressed, and its toxicity may also be limited by these adaptive responses in diseases such as AIDS, which are characterized by the sustained presence of high levels of circulating interferon. In vivo correlations have shown that high interferon levels are associated with low T4 cell levels and, interestingly, with high IgA levels as well.[82]

In vivo correlations have shown that high interferon levels are associated with low T4 cell levels and, interestingly, with high IgA levels as well.[82] An increase in IgA levels appears to be an adverse prognostic marker.[53]

Finally, abnormal inclusions noted in the T lymphocytes of AIDS patients on electron microscopy can also be induced by incubating healthy lymphocytes with alpha interferon in vitro.[83]

Immune Responses to Semen

It was of interest to ask if exposure of men to multiple allogeneic semens can induce deleterious immune responses. Witkin and Sonnabend studied immune responses to spermatozoa in 18 homosexual men. Antisperm antibodies of IgG and IgA isotypes were found in 10 and 2 of the 18 men, respectively. Circulating immune complexes were elevated in two-thirds of the men, and sperm-related antigen was found in the sera of some.[84] Semen is immunogenic when deposited in the rectum.[84] Antisperm antibodies could be induced in rabbits following the careful, atraumatic introduction of pooled rabbit semen into the rectum.[85] Thus one possible factor contributing to immunologic impairment could be CICs associated with sperm-related antigens. There are antigens expressed on cells in the ejaculate, including HLA antigens and gangliosides that are shared by lymphocytes.[86] For example, spermatozoa express a ganglioside antigen, asialo GM_1, which is also present on NK cells.[87] We have now shown that antibodies to asialo GM_1 are indeed present in AIDS patients.[88] Many AIDS patients show diminished NK function.[51] Sperm-induced allogeneic immunization was associated with immune dysregulation in individuals who were anal sperm recipients.[89] In addition to the deleterious effects induced by the immune response to the components of semen, direct immunosuppressive effects of semen are well recognized.[90] It is thus possible that repeated exposure to different allogeneic semens may eventually lead to the appearance of antibodies autoreactive with T lymphocytes and NK cells. It is predictable that multiple anti-HLA antibodies will be found in promiscuous homosexual men who have never received blood transfusions. The diversity of the anti-HLA antibodies may in fact provide an objective measure of promiscuity. The fact that AIDS appears to be of only recent occurrence in homosexual men argues that exposure to allogeneic semen cannot in itself cause substantial morbidity. We propose that immune responses to semen may provide a background of immune suppression, not only promoting repeated CMV infections, but also exacerbating the resulting immunologic disorders.

Circulating Immune Complexes in AIDS

CICs have been detected in many patients with AIDS. There are now numerous reports of CICs in AIDS patients as well as in healthy homosexual men. McDougal et al.[91] showed a correlation with CICs and depressed T4 lymphocyte counts. Undoubtedly, CICs are very heterogeneous with respect to the antigenic component, and there is as yet no proof that any contribute to the development of the immune dysregulation characteristic of AIDS. In some patients, CICs may contribute to thrombocytopenia, polyserositis, arthritis, peripheral neuropathy, and nephropathy. We suggest that CICs may also contribute to the underlying immune disorder. The expression of erythrocyte C3b receptors is impaired in AIDS.[92-94] This is an important component of the mechanism for clearing CICs.

As mentioned earlier, herpesvirus infected cells may be induced to express Fc receptors.[10,11] This is of potential importance in a host with high levels of CICs. One possible mechanism by which this phenomenon might contribute to pathogenesis is that binding of CICs to Fc receptors could interfere with target recognition by cytotoxic lymphocytes.

Our additional observations have shown a clear correlation between promiscuity and the presence of CICs: 13 of 13 homosexual patients with Kaposi's sarcoma and 6 of 10 promiscuous homosexual men had CICs, whereas CICs were present in only one of eight nonpromiscuous homosexual men (Witkin S, Safai B, Krim M, Sonnabend J, unpublished observations). Undoubtedly, many different antigens participate in immune complex formation in these men. Hepatitis B, syphilis, and CMV are among the infections that are highly prevalent in these men and that can be associated with immune complexes. The association of CICs with syphilis is well documented, as is a depression of NK cell function.[95,96] Additional contributions to the CICs may appear once autoantibodies are produced. A further contribution is from sperm-related antigens, and indeed their presence in CICs in promiscuous homosexual men who have antibodies to spermatozoa has already been demonstrated.[84]

MECHANISMS OF DISEASE ACQUISITION AND TRANSITION TO A SELF-SUSTAINING STAGE

We propose that the first stage of disease acquisition is a period of frequent sexual contact with different partners in a setting in which the prevalence of CMV carriage is such that repeated infection with this virus will occur. These repeated infections are associated with an *accumulation* of effects that, in aggregate, eventually result in a switch to a self-sustaining condition characterized by an inability of cytotoxic lymphocytes to clear CMV infected cells. Antigen-specific cytotoxic T cells against CMV-infected targets have been shown to be functionally defective in AIDS.[97] The critical concept during the initial stage is that of a cumulative process involving the following:

1. An increasing level of CICs, which may react with Fc or complement receptors on some T lymphocytes and interfere with their cytotoxic function. Herpesvirus-infected cells, including CMV-infected cells, express Fc receptors and thus may bind CICs and block target recognition by cytotoxic lymphocytes.
2. The appearance in increasing concentrations of antibodies that are cross-reactive with cytotoxic T cells and NK cells. The specific targets may be regulatory or effector T cells. The consequence is impaired cytotoxicity. Antibodies reactive with T lymphocytes and NK cells may result from polyclonal B cell activation or from immunization by cross-reactive antigens present in the ejaculate.[98-101] Anti-T cell antibodies have now been repeatedly described in AIDS.
3. A diminishing ratio of T4 helper to T8 suppressor cells. The action of cytotoxic T lymphocytes would be susceptible to T8 suppression. CMV and EBV infections, as well as toxoplasmosis (which is not uncommon in AIDS), have been associated with T subset aberrations. These changes are evoked by antigens expressed on the surface of the infected cell. Persistence of infection will maintain these subset changes.

These three general influences—autoantibodies, CICs, and a decrease in T4:T8 subset ratio—conspire to inhibit an effective cytotoxic response to CMV-infected cells. The relative contribution to each might vary from patient to patient.

Eventually, the immunosuppression becomes irreversible and self-sustaining, and independent of promiscuous sexual behavior. The sustained immunoregulatory disorders impair cytotoxic responses to other intracellular parasites, which are responsible for opportunistic infections.

Figure 29–1 summarizes the mechanism of self-perpetuation in this disease; the essential feature of this second stage is an inability to mount an effective cytotoxic immune response against CMV-infected cells. This second stage has features typical of positive feedback systems.

DISCUSSION

Our model may well be less important as a representation of actual disease mechanisms than as a conceptual framework useful in formulating approaches to research on disease mechanisms and strategies toward rational intervention. In contrast to diseases resulting from infection with a single agent, this model proposes that a disease can result from sustained or repeated exposure to several different infectious and noninfectious agents that alone, as single exposures, are

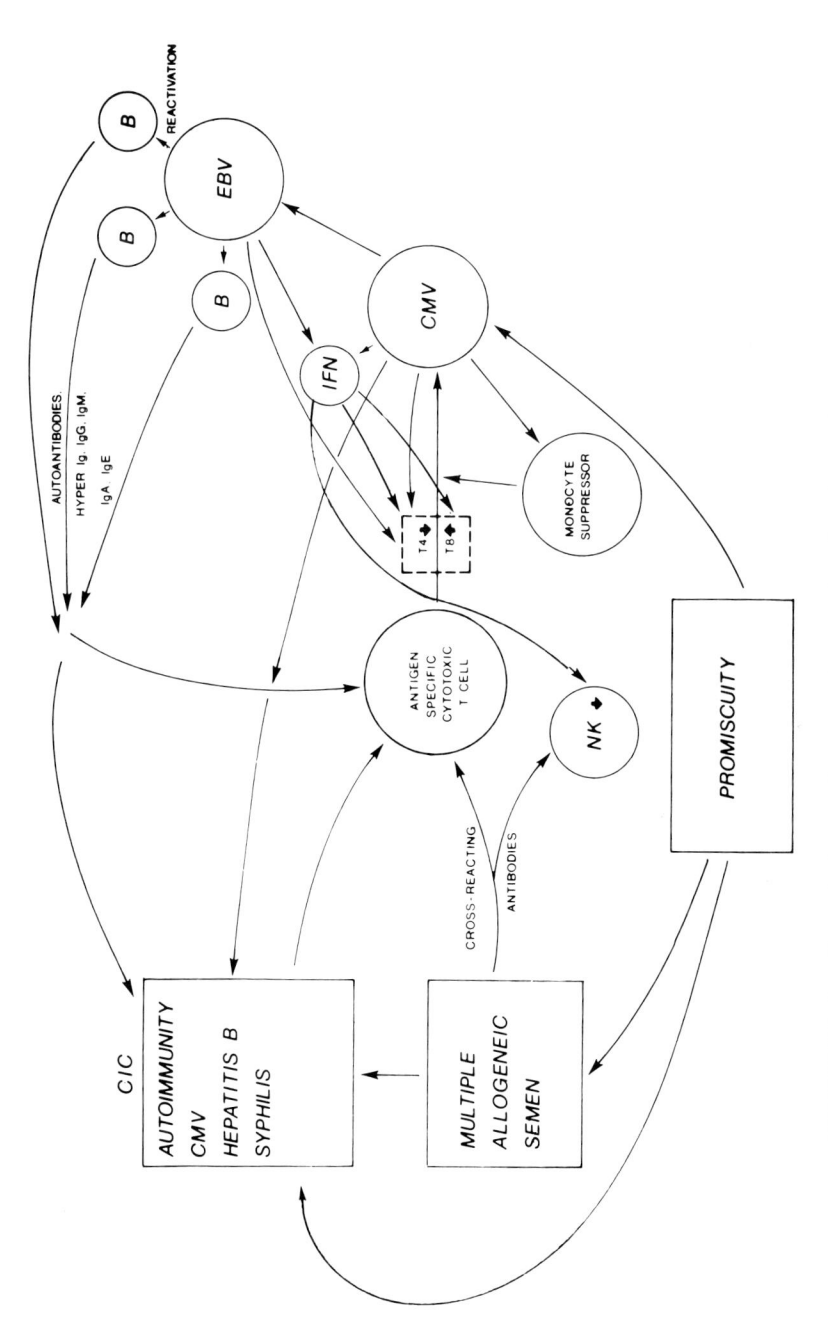

AIDS: An Explanation for Its Occurrence among Homosexual Men 461

FIGURE 29-1 *Repeated sexual contact is associated with reinfections with CMV and exposure to multiple allogeneic semens. The resulting immunoregulatory defects can become self-sustaining.*

not associated with significant morbidity. Disease develops from the combined and cumulative effects of sustained or repeated exposure to multiple factors rather than following an incubation period after infection with a single agent.

As discussed in another presentation of this model,[104] the dispersal of the elements of the immune system, the variety of different specific and nonspecific effector and regulatory functions, and the chemical diversity of the short- and long-range signals employed imply a great number and variety of vulnerable targets and therefore a susceptibility to many different influences. This model illustrates how the interaction of known or likely effects of specific environmental exposures can lead to the development of progressive immune disregulation in homosexual men repeatedly exposed to the environmental factors in question.

Many factors have been shown to have an adverse effect on immune function. If their interaction can produce disease, then we should expect to encounter more clinical immune disfunction in environments in which these factors are present in greater concentrations. One such environment was homosexual bathhouses in large urban settings in the late 1970s. Similarly, the sharing of needles by many IV-drug users provides the opportunity for frequent exposure to immunosuppressive factors. In Africa, malnutrition coupled with repeated protozoan infections constitutes an immunosuppressive burden.

As also previously discussed,[104] this multifactorial model lends itself to a formal epidemiologic analysis, which is true at two levels. First, we must have a better understanding of the environments in which AIDS develops and the ways in which affected individuals have interacted with those environments. Second, the analysis of the interactions of the various biologic effects generated by these exposures is also an appropriate and important epidemiologic undertaking.

We are aware of the conjectural nature of important aspects of this model. However, corroboration can be readily sought. For example, one can compare CMV excretion rates among different populations distinguished by different levels of promiscuity and sexual preferences and correlate these rates with the prevalence of AIDS. Perhaps the behavioral and cultural aspects that appear to be associated with the genesis of AIDS are the most troublesome; they are also critical, because they suggest an explanation for the occurrence of the syndrome at a particular time and location. Here, too, it should be possible to document whether significant changes in patterns of sexual behavior occurred in New York City in the 1970s.

Our model suggests some approaches to patient management that are of immediate practical importance. Both humoral (autoantibodies and CICs) and cellular (inversion of T4:T8 ratios and depressed NK cell activity) factors impair antiviral cytotoxic responses. Methods to remove humoral factors including interferon, such as plasmapheresis, may deserve serious consideration. There are other examples of potentially useful intervention. Cyclophosphamide may control increased immunoglobulin production, and in low dose may have an additional beneficial effect, since it preferentially inhibits T8 suppressor cells. Appropriate monoclonal antibodies may also selectively remove T8 suppressor cells. This subset also includes cytotoxic T lymphocytes, so some obvious caution is required in such an approach. These are examples of approaches to improving cytotoxic function. Any such improvement may set in motion a process leading to recovery. The hope is that some reduction in CMV antigenic load will itself lead to further improvement in immune function (Figure 29–2). Clearly, it is important to develop and test effective treatments for CMV and EBV infections.

ADDITIONAL COMMENTS ON THE QUESTION OF A SPECIFIC AGENT AS THE CAUSE OF AIDS

Traditionally, social comment in the context of a scientific communication has been regarded as inappropriate. However, in this instance, the potential for adverse social effects of a particular scientific proposal appeared so great that we believe it justified to abandon the traditional restraint on social comment. In short, if groups that already bear a heavy burden of stigmatization are perceived to carry a lethal virus capable of spreading to and decimating the population at large, the danger of consequent brutalization of such groups is only too real. This situation is even more perilous to the groups in question if there is a test that reportedly can identify apparently healthy individuals who belong to these groups, who carry the putatively lethal virus.

Because of the potential for the abuse of individuals identified as a source of contagion, it is especially important to make the distinction between hypothesis and scientific fact. Few would question the inappropriateness of creating public policy on the basis of mere conjecture. Unfortunately, in the case of AIDS such a distinction has not been made.

In addition to the social consequences, the acceptance as fact that HIV-1 and HIV-2 cause AIDS has had the following consequences:

1. Research on other etiologic factors has not been pursued.
2. Aspects of pathogenesis apparently unrelated to HIV have not been investigated. The roles of CMV and EBV infections and of sustained exposure to high levels of interferon as factors contributing to the underlying immune disregulation have yet to be explored.
3. Treatment models other than antiretroviral approaches have not been developed.
4. Patient management strategies have yet to be addressed. This issue has been virtually ignored in the belief than an effective antiretroviral approach will make these considerations redundant.

This model has attempted to describe the development of AIDS as a response to sustained or repeated environmental insults to the immune system. A two-stage mechanism of disease acquisition, the second stage having features of a positive feedback system, has been described. The details in this model have been confined to the development of AIDS in homosexual men. Analogous models can be developed for other groups.

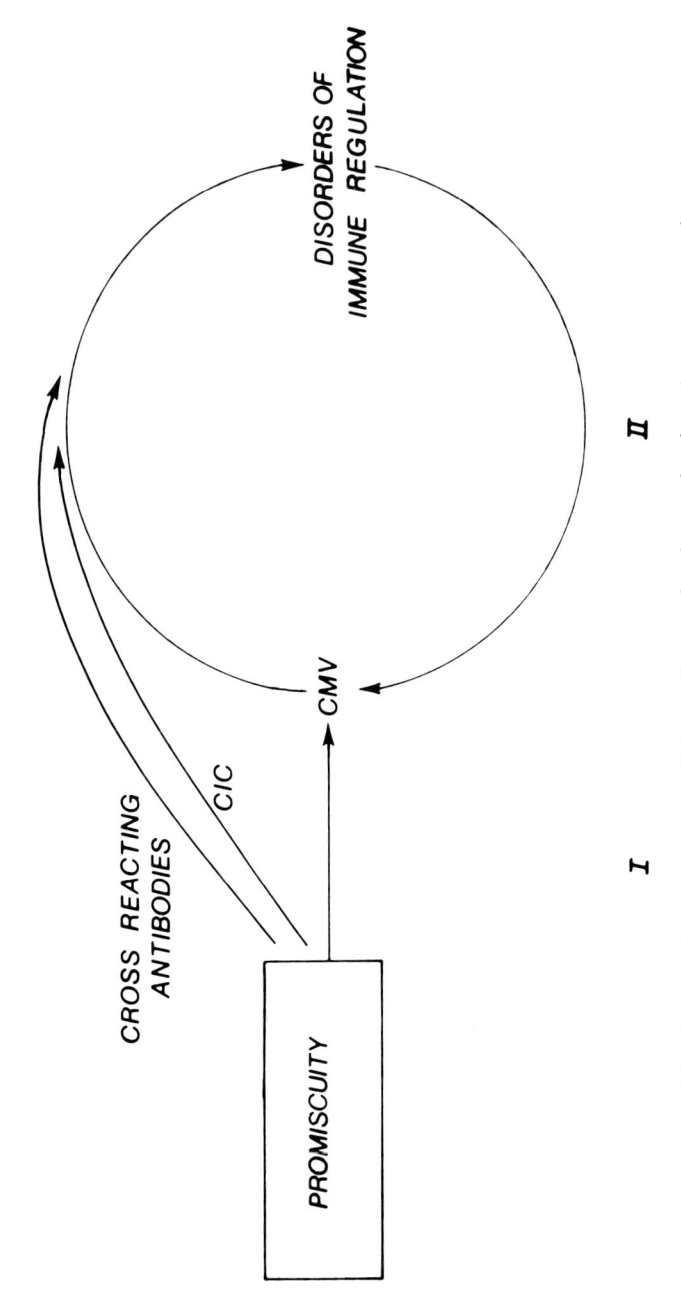

FIGURE 29–2 *A decrease in CMV antigenic load may lead to improvement in immune function.*

Although there can be little doubt that AIDS is a new phenomenon, at least in its epidemic form, among homosexual men, this cannot be said with confidence for any of the other groups. In any group, unless suspected, *P. carinii* pneumonia would not have been detected because its diagnosis required an open lung biopsy (before 1982).

The consequences of an impaired immune response may be similar, although the pathways that lead to it can be diverse. The route that we believe leads to immunosuppression in one group of patients has been the subject of this chapter. This model has also been presented elsewhere.[103–105]

REFERENCES

1. Zolla-Pazner S. B Cells in the pathogenesis of AIDS. Immunol Today 1984;5:289.
2. Zolla-Pazner S. Serology. In: Ebbesen P, Biggar RJ, Melbye M, eds. AIDS. Copenhagen: Munksgaard, 1984;151.
3. Centers for Disease Control. Acquired immune deficiency syndrome (AIDS): Precautions for clinical and laboratory staffs. MMWR 1982;31:577.
4. Marmor M, Laubenstein L, William DC, et al. Risk factors for Kaposi's sarcoma in homosexual men. Lancet 1982;1:1083.
5. Carney WP, Rubin RH, Hoffman RA, et al. Analysis of T cell subsets in cytomegalovirus mononucleosis. J Immunol 1981;126:2114.
6. Reinherz EL, O'Brien C, Rosenthal P, Schlossman SF. The cellular basis for viral induced immunodeficiency: Analysis by monoclonal antibodies. J Immunol 1980;125:1269.
7. Carney WP, Hirsch MS. Melchanisms of immunosuppression in cytomegalovirus mononucleosis: II. Virus-monocyte interactions. J Infect Dis 1981;144:47.
8. Kantor GL, Goldbey LS, Johnson BL. Immunological abnormalities induced by postperfusion cytomegalovirus infection. Ann Intern Med 1970;73:553.
9. Olding LB, Kingsburg DT, Oldstone MBA. Pathogenesis of cytomegalovirus infection. Distribution of viral products, immune complexes and autoimmunity during latent murine infection. J Gen Virol 1976;33:267.
10. Keller R, Peichel R, Goldman JN. An IgG-Fc receptor induced in cytomegalovirus-infected human fibroblasts. J Immunol 1976;116:772.
11. Rahman AA, Teschner M, Sethi KK, Brandis HE. Appearance of IgG Fc receptor(s) on cultured human fibroblasts infected with human cytomegalovirus. J Immunol 1976;117:253.
12. Sissons JG. The immunology of cytomegalovirus infection. J R Coll Physicians Lond 1986;20:40.
13. Hutt-Fletcher LM, Balachandran N, Elkins M. B Cell activation by cytomegalovirus. J Exp Med 1983;158:2171.
14. Rinaldo CR, Black PH, Hirsh MS. Interactions of virus with mononucleosis due to cytomegalovirus. J Infect Dis 1977;136:667.
15. Rinaldo CR Jr, Carney WP, Richter BS, et al. Mechanisms of immunosuppression in cytomegaloviral mononucleosis. J Infect Dis 1980;141:488.
16. Rice GP, Schrier RD, Oldstone MB. Cytomegalovirus infects human lymphocytes and monocytes: virus expression is restricted to immediate-early gene products. Proc Natl Acad Sci USA 1984;81:6134.

17. Schrier RD, Rice GP, Oldstone MB. Suppression of natural killer cell activity and T cell proliferation by fresh isolates of human cytomegalovirus. J Infect Dis 1986;153:1084.
18. Detels R, Visscher BR, Fahey JL, et al. The relation of cytomegalovirus and Epstein-Barr virus antibodies to T cell subsets in homosexually active men. JAMA 1984;251:1719.
19. Drew WL, Mills J, Levy J. Cytomegalovirus infection and abnormal T lymphocyte subset ratios in homosexual men. Ann Intern Med 1985;103:61.
20. Beck S, Barrell B. Human cytomegalovirus encodes a glycoprotein homologous to MHC class 1 antigens. Nature 1988;331:269.
21. Lang D, Kummer JF. Demonstration of cytomegalovirus in semen. N Engl J Med 1972;287:756.
22. Lang DJ, Kummer JF, Hartley DP. Cytomegalovirus in semen: Persistence and demonstration in extracellular fluids. N Engl J Med 1974;291:121.
23. Drew WL, Lawrence, Mintz L, Miner RC, et al. Prevalence of cytomegalovirus infection in homosexual men. J Infect Dis 1981;143:188.
24. Drew WL, Miner RC, Ziegler J, et al. Cytomegalovirus and Kaposi's sarcoma in young homosexual men. Lancet 1982;2:125.
25. Drew WL, Huang E. Etiology: role of cytomegalovirus. In: Ziegler JL, Dorfman R, eds. Kaposi's sarcoma. New York: Marcel Dekker, Inc., 1988;113.
26. Mintz L, Drew WL, Miner RC, et al. Cytomegalovirus infections in homosexual men. An epidemiological study. Ann Intern Med 1983;99:326.
27. Buimovici-Klein E, Lange M, Ong KR, et al. Virus isolation and immune studies in a cohort of homosexual men. J Med Virol 1988;25:371.
28. Jondal M, Klein G. Surface markers on human T and B cells. VI. Presence of Epstein-Barr virus receptors on human B lymphocytes. J Exp Med 1973;138:137.
29. Rosen A, Gergely P, Jondal M, Klein G. Polyclonal Ig production after Epstein-Barr virus infection of human leukocytes *in vitro*. Nature 1977;267:52.
30. Fong S, Vaughan JH, Tsoukas CD, et al. Selective induction of autoantibody secretion in human bone marrow by Epstein-Barr virus. J Immunol 1982;129:1941.
31. Gottlieb MS, Schrott R, Schanker HM, et al. *Pneumocystis carinii* pneumonia and mucosal candidiasis in previously healthy homosexual men. N Engl J Med 1981;305:1425.
32. Bird AG, Britton S, Ernberg I, Nilsson K. Characteristics of Epstein-Barr virus activation of human B lymphocytes. J Exp Med 1981;154:832.
33. Purtilo DT, Sakamoto K. Epstein-Barr virus and human disease: Immune responses determine the clinical and pathologic expression. Hum Pathol 1981;12:677.
34. Tosato GG, Magrath IT, Blaese RM. T cell-mediated immunoregulation of Epstein-Barr virus (EBV)-induced B lymphocyte activation in EBV seropositive and EBV seronegative individuals. J Immunol 1982;128:575.
35. Meuer SC, Schlossman SF, Reinherz, EL. Clonal analysis of human cytotoxic T lymphocytes: T4+ and T8+ effector T cells recognize products of different major histocompatibility complex regions. Proc Natl Acad Sci USA 1982;79:4590.
36. Quinan GV Jr, Kirmani N, Rook A, et al. Cytotoxic T cells in cytomegalovirus infection. N Engl J Med 1982;307:7.
37. Oill P, Fiala M, Schotterman J, et al. Cytomegalovirus mononucleosis in a healthy adult. Association with hepatitis, secondary Epstein-Barr virus antibody response and immunosuppression. Am J Med 1977;62:413.

38. Bird AG, McLachlan SM, Birtton S. Cyclosporin A promotes spontaneous outgrowth *in vitro* of Epstein-Barr virus-induced B cell lines. Nature 1981;289:300.
39. Crawford DH, Sweny P, Edwards J, et al. Long-term T cell-mediated immunity to Epstein-Barr virus in renal allograft recipients receiving cyclosporin A. Lancet 1981;1:10.
40. Magrath IT, Pizzo PA, Novikovs L, et al. Enhancement of Epstein-Barr virus replication in producer cell lines by a combination of low temperature and corticosteroids. Virology 1979;97:477.
41. Abrams D. Lymphoproliferative diseases in homosexual males. In: Purtilo DT, ed. Immune deficiency and cancer: Epstein-Barr virus and lymphoproliferative malignancies. New York: Plenum press, 1984.
42. Lipscomb H, Tatsumi E, Harada S, et al. Epstein-Barr virus and chronic lymphadenomegaly in male homosexuals with acquired immunodeficiency syndrome (AIDS). AIDS Res 1983;1:59.
43. Birx DL, Redfield RR, Tosato G. Defective regulation of Epstein-Barr virus infection in patients with acquired immunodeficiency syndrome (AIDS) or AIDS-related disorders. N Engl J Med 1986;314:874.
44. Chang RS, Thompson H, Pomeranz S. Epstein-Barr virus in homosexual men with chronic persistent generalized lymphadenopathy. J Infect Dis 1985;151:459.
45. Sumaya CV, Boswell RN, Ench Y, et al. Enhanced serological and virological findings of Epstein-Barr virus in patients with AIDS and AIDS related complex. J Infect Dis 1985;154:864.
46. Ragona G, Sirianni MC, Saddu S, et al. Evidence for disregulation in the control of Epstein-Barr virus latency in patients with AIDS related complex. Clin Exp Immunol 1986;66:17.
47. Rinaldo CR, Kingsley LA, Lyter DW, et al. Association of HTLV-III with Epstein-Barr virus infection and abnormalities of T lymphocytes in homosexual men. J Infect Dis 1986;154:556.
48. Gaston JSH, Richardson AB, Epstein MA. Epstein-Barr virus-specific T-cell memory in renal allograft recipients under long-term immunosuppression. Lancet 1982;1:923.
49. Hanto DW, Sakamoto K, Purtilo DT. The Epstein-Barr virus in the pathogenesis of post-transplant lymphoproliferative disorders. Surgery 1981;90:204.
50. Groopman JE, Sullivan JL, Mulder C, et al. Pathogenesis of B cell lymphoma in a patient with AIDS. Blood 1986;67:612.
51. Stahl RE, Friedman-Kien A, Dubin R, et al. Immunologic abnormalities in homosexual men. Am J Med 1982;73:171.
52. Chess Q, et al. Elevation of serum immunoglobulin D (IgD) in patients with the acquired immuno-deficiency syndrome (AIDS). New York Fed Proc 1983;42:6111.
53. Munoz A, Carey V, Saah AJ, et al. Predictors of decline in CD4 lymphocytes in a cohort of homosexual men infected with human immunodeficiency virus. Journal of Acquired Immune Deficiency Syndromes 1988;1:396.
54. Sonnabend JA, Witkin SS, Purtilo DT. Acquired immune deficiency syndrome (AIDS): an explanation for its occurrence among homosexual men. In: Ma P, Armstrong D, eds. The acquired immune deficiency syndrome and infections of homosexual men. New York: Yorke Medical Books, 1984;409.
55. Stricker RB, Abrams DI, Corash L, et al. Target platelet antigen in homosexual men with immune thrombocytopenia. N Engl J Med 1985;313:1375.

56. Yu JR, Lennette ET, Karpatkin S. Anti-F(ab')2 antibodies in thrombocytopenic patients at risk for acquired immunodeficiency syndrome. J Clin Invest 1986; 77:1756.
57. van der Lelie J, Lange JM, Vos JJ, et al. Autoimmunity against blood cells in human immunodeficiency-virus (HIV) infection. Br J Haematol 1987;67:109.
58. Andrieu JM, Even P, Venet A. AIDS and related syndromes as a viral-induced autoimmune disease of the immune system: an anti-MHC II disorder. Therapeutic implications. AIDS Res 1986;2:163.
59. Ziegler JL, Stites DP. Hypothesis: AIDS is an autoimmune disease directed at the immune system and triggered by a lymphotropic retrovirus. Clin Immunol Immunopathol 1986;41:305.
60. Ashida ER, Scofield VL. Lymphocyte major histocompatibility complex-encoded class II structures may act as sperm receptors. Proc Natl Acad Sci USA 1987; 84:3395.
61. Morris L, Distenfeld A, Amorosi E, et al. Autoimmune thrombocytopenic purpura (ATP) in homosexual men. Ann Intern Med 1982;96:714.
62. Charlesworth JA, Quin JW, MacDonald GJ, et al. Complement, lymphotoxins and immune complexes in infectious mononucleosis: Serial studies in uncomplicated cases. Clin Exp Immunol 1978;34:241.
63. DeStefano E, Friedman RM, Friedman-Kien AE, et al. Acid labile human leukocyte interferon in homosexual men with Kaposi's sarcoma and lymphadenopathy. J Infect Dis 1982;146:451.
64. Buimovici-Klein E, Lange M, Klein RJ, et al. Long-term follow-up of serum-interferon and its acid-stability in a group of homosexual men. AIDS Res 1986;2:99.
65. Abb J, Kochen M, Deinhardt F. Interferon production in male homosexuals with the acquired immune deficiency syndrome (AIDS) or generalized lymphadenopathy. Infection 1984;12:240.
66. Buimovici-Klein E, Lange M, Klein RJ, et al. Is presence of interferon predictive for AIDS? (letter). Lancet 1983;2:344.
67. Eyster ME, Goedert JJ, Poon MC, et al. Acid-labile alpha interferon. A possible preclinical marker for the acquired immunodeficiency syndrome in hemophilia. N Engl J Med 1983;309:583.
68. Preble OT, Black RJ, Friedman RM, et al. Systemic lupus erythematosus: presence in human serum of an unusual acid-labile leukocyte interferon. Science 1982;216:429.
69. Friedman RM, Preble OT, Black R, et al. Interferon production in patients with systemic lupus erythematosus. Arthritis Rheum 1982;25:802.
70. Hooks JJ, Jordan GW, Cupps T, et al. Multiple interferons in the circulation of patients with systemic lupus erythematosus and vasculitis. Arthritis Rheum 1982;25:396.
71. Skurkovich SV, Eremkina EI. The probable role of interferon in allergy. Ann Allergy 1975;35:356.
72. Heremans H, Billiau A, Colombatti A, et al. Interferon treatment of NZB mice: accelerated progression of autoimmune disease. Infect Immun 1978;21:925.
73. Engleman EG, Sonnenfield G, Dauphinee H, et al. Treatment of NZB/NZW F1 hybrid mice with mycobacterium bovis strain BCG or type II interferon preparations accelerates autoimmune disease. Arthritis Rheum 1981;24:1396.
74. Hokland M, Hokland P, Heron I, et al. Selective effects of alpha interferon on human T-lymphocyte subsets during mixed lymphocyte cultures. Scand J Immunol 1983;17:559.

75. Aune TM, Pierce CW. Activation of a suppressor T-cell pathway by interferon. Proc Natl Acad Sci USA 1982;79:3808.
76. Lindahl-Magnusson P, Leavy P, Gresser I. Interferon inhibits DNA synthesis induced in mouse lymphocyte suspension by phytohemagglutinin or allogeneic cells. Nature New Biol 1972;237:120.
77. Scott GM. Interferons and infectious diseases. In: Taylor-Papadimitriou J, ed. Interferons: Their impact in biology and medicine. New York: Oxford University Press, 1985.
78. Lahdevirta J, Maury CP, Teppo AM, et al. Elevated levels of circulating cachectin/tumor necrosis factor in patients with acquired immunodeficiency syndrome. Am J Med 1988;85:289.
79. Maluish AE, Ortaldo JR, Conlon JC, et al. Depression of natural killer cytotoxicity after in vivo administration of recombinant leukocyte interferon. J Immunol 1983;131:503.
80. Reddy MM, Chinoy P, Grieco MH. Differential effects of interferon-alpha 2 and interleukin-2 on natural killer cell activity in patients with acquired immune deficiency syndrome. J Biol Response Mod 1984;3:379.
81. Wu JM, Chiao JW, Maayan S. Diagnostic value of the determination of an interferon induced enzyme activity: decreased $2',5'$-oligoadenylate dependent binding protein activity in AIDS patient lymphocytes. AIDS Res 1986;2:127.
82. Sonnabend JA, Saadoun S, Grierson H, et al. Association of serum interferon with hematologic and immunologic parameters in homosexual men with AIDS and at risk for AIDS in New York City. Abstract 100. Second International Conference on AIDS June 1986. Paris.
83. Grimley PM, Kang YH, Frederick W, et al. Interferon-related leucocyte inclusions in acquired immune deficiency syndrome: localization in T cells. Am J Clin Pathol 1984;81:147.
84. Witkin S, Sonnabend JA. Immune responses to spermatozoa in homosexual men. Fertil Steril 1983;39:337.
85. Richards JM, Bedford JM, Witkin SS. Rectal insemination modifies immune responses in rabbits. Science 1984;224:390.
86. Mather S, Gaust JM, Williamson HO, et al. Cross reactivity of sperm + T lymphocyte antigens. Am J Reproductive Immunol 1981;1:113.
87. Beck BN, Gillis S, Henney CS. Display of the neutral glycolipid ganglio-N-tetraosylceramide (asialo GM 1) on cells of the natural killer and T lineages. Transplantation 1982;33:118.
88. Witkin SS, Sonnabend JA, Richards JM, et al. Induction of antibody to asialo.GM1 by spermatazoa and its occurrence in the sera of homosexual men with the acquired immune deficiency syndrome (AIDS). Clin Exp Immunol 1983;54:346.
89. Mavligit GM, Talpaz M, Hsia FT, et al. Chronic immune stimulation by sperm alloantigens. Support for the hypothesis that spermatazoa induce immune dysregulation in homosexual males. JAMA 1984;251:237.
90. James K, Hargreave TB. Immunosuppression by seminal plasma and its possible clinical significance. Immunology Today 1984;5:357.
91. McDougal JS, Hubbard M, Nicholson JKA, et al. Immune complexes in the acquired immunodeficiency syndrome (AIDS): relationship to disease manifestation, risk group, and immunologic defect. J Clin Immunol 1985;5:130.
92. Inada Y, Lange M, McKinley G et al. Hematologic correlates and the role of erythrocyte CR1(C3b receptor) in the development of AIDS. AIDS Res 1986;2:235.
93. Tausk FA, McCutchan JA, Spechko P, et al. Altered erythrocyte C3b receptor

expression, immune complexes, and complement activation in homosexual men in varying risk groups for acquired immune deficiency syndrome. J Clin Invest 1986;78:977.
94. Jouvin M-H, Rozenbaum W, Russo R, et al. Decreased expression of the C3b/C4b complement receptor (CR1) in AIDS and AIDS-related syndromes correlates with clinical subpopulations of patients with HIV infection. AIDS 1987;1:89.
95. Jensen JR, Jorgensen AS, Thestrup-Pedersen K. Depression of natural killer cell activity by syphilitic serum and immune complexes. Br J Vener Dis 1982;58:298.
96. Solling J, Solling K, Jakobsen KU. Circulating immune complexes in syphilis. Acta Derm Venereol (Stockholm) 1978;58:263.
97. Rook AH, Masur H, Lane HC, et al. Interleukin-2 enhances the depressed natural killer and cytomegalovirus-specific cytotoxic activities of lymphocytes from patients with the acquired immune deficiency syndrome. J Clin Invest 1983;72:398.
98. Kloster BE, Tomar RH, Spira TJ. Lymphocytotoxic antibodies in the acquired immune deficiency syndrome. Clin Immunol Immunopathol 1984;30:330.
99. Pruzanski W, Jacobs H, Laing LP. Lymphocytotoxic antibodies against peripheral blood B and T lymphocytes in homosexuals with AIDS and ARC. AIDS Res 1983;1:211.
100. Williams RC, Masur H, Spira TJ. Lymphocyte-reactive antibodies in acquired immune deficiency syndrome. J Clin Immunol 1984;4:118.
101. Kiprov DD, Anderson RE, Morand P, et al. Antilymphocyte antibodies and seropositivity for retroviruses in groups at high risk for AIDS. N Engl J Med 1985; 312:1517.
102. Sonnabend JA. The etiology of AIDS. AIDS Res 1984;1:1.
103. Sonnabend JA. The acquired immune deficiency syndrome: a discussion of etiologic hypotheses. AIDS Res 1984;1:107.
104. Sonnabend JA, Witkin SS, Purtilo DT. A multifactorial model for the development of AIDS in homosexual men. NY Acad Sci 1984;437:177.
105. Sonnabend JA, Witkin SS, Purtilo DT. The acquired immune deficiency syndrome and Kaposi's sarcoma in homosexual men. In: Cerimele D, ed. Kaposi's sarcoma. Jamaica, NY: Spectrum Publishers, 1985.
106. Sonnabend jA, Witkin SS, Purtilo DT. Acquired immunodeficiency syndrome: Opportunistic infections and malignancies in male homosexuals. JAMA 1983;249:2370.

Chapter 30

AIDS: An Overview

B. H. Kean

Even in a society bland to trillions in debt and billions in buyouts, the numbers are staggering:

- 5 to 10 million people infected worldwide in over 135 countries[1],
- 250,000 already dead or about to die[1],
- 1 million new cases (not infections) projected by 1993[1],
- 365,000 cases in the United States by 1992[2],
- $22 billion of cumulative costs in the United States for a total of 270,000 cases between 1980 and 1991.[3]

In terms of comparative numbers of people attacked, AIDS is not yet plague or yellow fever, but its unique malignancy and its costs are stunning. The progression of the disease—from a reduction of T-helper cells (causing those infected to be considered high-risk contacts) to the viral infection, to chronic lymphadenopathy, to opportunistic infections and the whole AIDS syndrome—is a most depressing Calvary that may take years.[4] While the rate of spread is decreasing, the total numbers of infection and disease are increasing. The key question is what percentage of those infected with the virus will develop AIDS. The estimates vary, but within five years of seroconversion, 10 to 15% are ill, by seven years 25% have AIDS and another 50% have precursors of AIDS, and some projections suggest that by 12 years all will have the disease.

Epidemics start slowly, increase explosively, and are terminated by factors intrinsic to the disease. Key considerations in analyzing epidemics are the cause, the method of transmission, and the number of nonimmune persons. Lessons can be learned only if we consider those factors in AIDS involving person-to-person transmission. As G. Smith stated, "It takes two to make a communicable disease, one to give and one to take. In an epidemic which is an affair of the herd, there must be many takers for each giver."[5] Epidemics of malaria that require the mosquito as a vector, or those of bubonic plague and typhus, which are louse-borne, are different from epidemics of influenza, poliomyelitis, syphilis—or AIDS.

From the beginning, there were those who "knew" that AIDS was caused by a virus that "originated" in Africa. In the first edition of this text, much of my overview was devoted to assembling the evidence that the cause of AIDS was a virus. The early epidemiologic and clinical data indicated that a living agent of disease was responsible for AIDS, and, since it was not visible, it had to be a virus. "At a certain point in the history of a disease sufficient evidence accumulates to justify informed speculation on the nature of the agent—long before its isolation or proper definition. . . . The agent is a virus."[6,7]

Why Africa? Justifiably or not, many think of that continent as a repository of ancient, occult diseases. Yellow fever, the hepatitis group, the Bunyamwera group, the Rift Valley viruses, the Simbu group, the Bwanba groups, Lassa fever, and others with exotic names have raised our awareness of the reservoir of viral diseases in Africa. Other parts of the world, from Siberia to the Falklands, have their own groups of viruses, but the report that Kaposi's sarcoma was found in an inordinately large number of patients with AIDS focused attention immediately on that part of the world where the tumor is commonly seen: Africa.

Those who have practiced only in North America remember Kaposi's sarcoma from the rare case presented at a clinical pathologic or dermatologic conference. It is more prevalent in the Balkans and some central European countries, but, even there, it is rare. The situation in Africa, however, is different. In 1962 and 1963, we visited Central Africa in an effort to determine whether some reasonable relationship could be established between Burkitt's tumor and malaria. At that time, our attention was drawn by pathologists to the presence of an "African" tumor, Kaposi's sarcoma.

In 1965, Reynolds et al.[8] published a report on 70 cases of histologically proved cases of Kaposi's sarcoma seen during a 38-year period at Mayo Clinic (most were referred from different parts of the country). But workers in Africa had seen many more. For example, Murray and Lothe[9] reported on almost 500 cases seen by them in Kampala during a 37-year period.

If the AIDS syndrome was indeed due to a virus, and if Kaposi's sarcoma was an integral part of that syndrome, then there was no escaping the notion that we were dealing with an African disease. (There is irony in the fact that the common Kaposi's sarcoma of Africa may differ from the variety found in patients with AIDS.)

Haiti was a detour. In 1981, Jean Pape (personal communication) drew our attention to three unusual patients with intractable diarrhea of a variety that had not been seen before in Haiti. The implication was that they had a form of intestinal tuberculosis. There is little doubt now but that the three died of AIDS, that the diarrhea was caused by a "new" parasite, *Cryptosporidium,* and that the tuberculosis was caused by *Mycobacterium avium intracellularae* (MAI). The large number of AIDS cases that appeared among Haitians in Miami, Port-au-Prince, and elsewhere suggested a special connection between that country and the disease. Just as the incontrovertible data indicating that AIDS was a disease of homosexuals initially aroused emotional ire, so the "chauvinistic" accusation against Haiti beclouded a simple unexpected observation.*

AIDS in Haiti was a new disease, as it was in New York. There were no large numbers of cases of Kaposi's sarcoma on file, and certainly the dermatologists and pathologists of that country would not have missed it. How did AIDS get from Africa to either New York or Haiti? Did Haiti send AIDS to New York, or did New York bring it to Haiti? That there was an intensive homosexual exchange between Haiti and New York City had been well known for some time. Planeloads of gays from New York City and from Canada flew to Port-au-Prince for vacations with male prostitutes who were young, cheap, and available—an unhappy consequence of the island's poverty. The early denials of homosexuality in the Haitian population were greeted skeptically by those who knew of the Haitian hotels that resembled the "baths" in New York City.

Part of the mystery may be explained by the hegira during the 1960s and 1970s, in which several thousand Haitians went to mid-Africa as specialists in agriculture and other enterprises. A certain number of this group returned to Haiti; one may speculate that the disease was then seeded into the Haitian population and then transmitted to visitors from the United States. Other routes certainly are possible. Some of the AIDS in Europe, e.g., Belgium, may have been brought there from Africa by these displaced Haitians. (No country is immune. In this hemisphere, Canada and Brazil are quickly catching up to Haiti.)

The epidemiologic route, therefore, may be relatively simple: longstanding, chronic, viral disease in the African population, somewhat more common in men than in women but found in both; transmitted to Haitians a decade or two ago during a migration (the customary route for the transmission of epidemic disease); and finally, the seeding of the virus into the homosexual population of New York City. ("Most epidemics or pandemics are probably due to strayed parasites"—Theobald Smith.[5])

Whether AIDS went from New York to Haiti or Haiti to New York is of little consequence compared with the bigger problem: Why did it suddenly become so virulent? What accounted for the transformation of an unrecognized virus—a bland virus, an old virus, a disseminated virus, a bisexual virus—into an epidemic virus? The explanation may be simple, and brings us back to first principles of biology and virology: attenuation by slow passage and increase of virulence by rapid passage.

That is what may have happened with the viral agent of AIDS. When HIV was introduced into a community where the sexual habits were such that the agent could be transmitted very quickly, its virulence increased and it became the killer virus we know it to be. This theory will suffice until a better one appears. (It is difficult for most of us to believe that practices in a limited group would permit sexual exposure to 5, 10, or 20 or more individuals in a day or in a weekend, yet reports of this kind of automatic sex are well documented.)

---

*The bizarre reactions of individuals and populations to a devastating plague are recorded in almost revolting detail by Hecker.[10]

Migrations from remote areas to urban centers and the common use of blood transfusions helped the spread of HIV.[11]

The secondary invaders demand attention.[12,13] Why some and not others? Which represent coincidental infection and which predispose to others?

VIRUSES

Whether the viruses—herpes, cytomegalovirus (CMV), Epstein-Barr virus (EBV), hepatitis B virus (HBV)—are secondary invaders or are in reality cohorts in the same body of infected individuals is not known. Since the prevalence of these viruses in the gay population is so great, it is difficult at the moment to consider them as other than fellow travelers in those who also acquire HIV. That viruses can reduce immunity to other diseases was first reported by Von Pirquet,[14] who noted that a large percentage of his patients who were tuberculin-positive on skin test became tuberculin-negative following an attack of measles.

BACTERIA

The bacteria require another explanation. The bacteria that have been most prominent in AIDS—MAI, *Shigella* sp., *Salmonella* sp., *Campylobacter* sp., *Hemophilus* sp.—are not the usual bacterial flora. Where are the pneumococci, the streptococci, the staphylococci, and the meningococci? Only 10% of the cases of opportunistic pneumonia are caused by the common bacteria; 90% are caused by *Pneumocystis carinii*.[15] Why mycobacteria of the unusual varieties rather than *M. tuberculosis*? Yes, it is possible to find instances of the more common bacteria as destroyers in the disease, but one cannot fail to be struck by the rarity of the common and the frequency of the rare in AIDS.

RICKETTSIA

These organisms have remained "silent," for the most part, but the related *Chlamydia* have been prominent in AIDS.

FUNGI

The fungi common in patients with AIDS—*Candida albicans, Cryptococcus neoformans, Aspergillus fumigatus,* and so on—cannot be called rare, but why these particular fungi are prominent in patients with AIDS is not known. Histoplasmosis has been reported, but it "should" be more common in AIDS than it is.

PARASITES

The most startling phenomenon is in the field of parasitology. Many of the premier U.S. medical schools spend only a few hours on the parasites of humans; AIDS may soon force a major change in their curricula. That *P. carinii* attacked the very old, the very young, and the immunosuppressed has been known for some time. But that some members of the house staff would see more patients with pneumonia due to pneumocystis rather than pneumococcus could not have been predicted.[16]

Toxoplasmosis has long been a problem in those who were immunosuppressed, especially in patients being treated for disseminated cancer. Why the disease presents clinically as a brain tumor was not understood. The debate was simply whether the immunosuppression revealed a preexisting disease or whether the immunosuppressed were more susceptible to acquiring the infection. At present, evidence suggests that in AIDS a preexisting infection is "revealed" and becomes disseminated, often with localization in the brain, during immunosuppression of the patient.

Cryptosporidiosis was not known as a disease of humans until less than a decade ago. How it was missed during the 300 years of microscopic coprology since Leewenhoek first saw *Giardia lamblia* will always be a mystery. The appearance of the "new parasite" in the AIDS patients stimulated enough excitement and study that a whole new body of information regarding the nature and distribution of the parasite has been created quickly.

More perplexing than those parasites that are found so frequently in AIDS is the virtual absence of those that might have been expected to be prominent. For a decade, an epidemic of amebiasis and giardiasis had decimated the health of the gay population in New York, San Francisco, and elsewhere. Improperly diagnosed, improperly treated, and improperly prevented, as many as half the active gays became infected and reinfected.[17] Constructive efforts to involve the public health authorities produced only resentment and invective; the patients continued to be "ripped off." Yet amebiasis, which can be exacerbated under steroid therapy, and the clinical syndrome of giardiasis, which is often severe in patients with hypogammaglobulinemia, have not been featured in the AIDS syndrome. Amebic abscess of the liver has not been a problem. Malaria should have killed some of the Haitians, but it didn't. *Strongyloides stercoralis* dissemination with septic shock has been reported in AIDS, but certainly not often. One can only conclude that the lost immunologic element that permits so many opportunistic infections in AIDS is discriminatory and that patients are protected against many infections by the other biologic mechanisms, both serologic and cellular.[18]

It is certain that the epidemic of AIDS will peak and subside—with or without scientific intervention—as have all epidemics, but whether the damage to our society is already calculable or whether it will reach yet unimagined dimensions is not clear.

Our course is certain: a multivalent attack on all aspects of AIDS. Our main resources are three, but none has been marshalled adequately, although, since the first edition of this book, vast improvements are apparent as the immensity of the problem is being more widely appreciated:

1. The National Institutes of Health (NIH). Although impressive sums have been allotted to in-house research, the needs are almost open-ended.
2. Medical schools and universities. Standard grant systems remain in place, but are being modified to reduce lag times.
3. Biomedical industry. A score of the finest biomedical scientists are "in industry." Many are working on projects to enhance the profitability of public companies. More must be persuaded to divert their activities to AIDS, and the companies for which they work must be compensated for their diversion. Only the government can do this. The national emergency demands it.

As one reads the mounting literature on AIDS, a subtle note of optimism can be recognized, although prospects for those already sick with AIDS remain poor. A dozen channels for prevention have already been opened, with the word *condom* being spelled in grammar school classrooms. Prospects for a vaccine are increasing as the nature of the virus is unravelled.[19] The origin of the AIDS virus and its genetic relationship with HIV-2 in humans and SIV in the non-human primates of Africa is beautifully described by Essex and Kanki[20] who suggest that this type of knowledge "will help in the design of vaccines to prevent infection with HIVs."

When the AIDS epidemic is over, our knowledge of infection, tumor, and immunity will have taken a series of quantum leaps. Medicine will never be the same.

REFERENCES

1. Mann JM, Chin J, Piot P, Quinn T. The international epidemiology of AIDS. Scientific American 1988;Oct.:82.
2. Heyward WL, Curran JW. The epidemiology of AIDS in the U.S. Scientific American 1988;Oct.:72.
3. Bloom DE, Carliner G. The economic impact of AIDS in the United States. Science 1988;239:604.
4. Redfield RR, Wright DC, Tramont EC. Special report: The Walter Reed Staging Classification for HTLV-III/LAV infection. N Engl J Med 1986;314:131.
5. Smith G. Plague on us. New York: The Commonwealth Fund, 1941.
6. Kean BH. The biological range of the acquired immune deficiency syndrome. In: Ma P, Armstrong D, eds. AIDS and infections of homosexual men. New York: Yorke, 1984.
7. Gallo RC, Salahuddin SZ, Popovic M, et al. Frequent detection and isolation of cytopathic retroviruses (HTLV-III) from patients with AIDS and at risk for AIDS. Science 1984;224:550.
8. Reynolds W, Winkelmann RK, Soule EH. Kaposi's sarcoma: A clinicopathologic study with particular reference to its relationship to the reticuloendothelial system. Medicine 1965;44:419.

9. Murray JF, Lothe F. The histopathology of Kaposi's sarcoma. Acta Unio Internat Contra Cancrum 1962;18:413.
10. Hecker JFC. The epidemics of the Middle Ages. London: George Woodfall and Son, 1844.
11. Gallo RC, Montagnier L. AIDS in 1988. Scientific American 1988;Oct.:41.
12. Lerner CW, Tapper ML. Opportunistic infection complicating acquired immune deficiency syndrome. Clinical features of 25 cases. Medicine 1984;63:155.
13. Fauci AS, Macher AM, Longo DL, et al. Acquired immunodeficiency syndrome: epidemiologic, clinical, immunologic, and therapeutic considerations. Ann Intern Med 1984;100:92.
14. Von Pirquet C. Das verhalten das kutanen tuberkulin reaktion währent der masem. Dtsch Med Wochenschr 1908;34:1297.
15. Polsky B, Gold JWM, Whimby E, et al. Bacterial pneumonia in patients with the acquired immunodeficiency syndrome. Ann Intern Med 1986;104:38.
16. Wachter RM. The impact of acquired immunodeficiency syndrome on medical residency training. N Engl J Med 1986;314:177.
17. Kean BH, William DC, Luminais SK. Epidemic of amoebiasis and giardiasis in a biased population. Br J Vener Dis 1979;55:375.
18. Laurence J. The immune systems in AIDS. Sci Am 1985;253:84.
19. Francis DP, Petricciani JC. The prospects for and pathways toward a vaccine for AIDS. N Engl J Med 1985;313:1586.
20. Essex M, Kanki PJ. The origins of the AIDS virus. Scientific American 1988;Oct:64.

APPENDIX A

Recommendations for Prevention of HIV Transmission in Health Care Settings

MMWR Supplement

Introduction

Human immunodeficiency virus (HIV), the virus that causes acquired immunodeficiency syndrome (AIDS), is transmitted through sexual contact and exposure to infected blood or blood components and perinatally from mother to neonate. HIV has been isolated from blood, semen, vaginal secretions, saliva, tears, breast milk, cerebrospinal fluid, amniotic fluid, and urine and is likely to be isolated from other body fluids, secretions, and excretions. However, epidemiologic evidence has implicated only blood, semen, vaginal secretions, and possibly breast milk in transmission.

The increasing prevalence of HIV increases the risk that health-care workers will be exposed to blood from patients infected with HIV, especially when blood and body-fluid precautions are not followed for all patients. Thus, this document emphasizes the need for health-care workers to consider **all** patients as potentially infected with HIV and/or other blood-borne pathogens and to adhere rigorously to infection-control precautions for minimizing the risk of exposure to blood and body fluids of all patients.

The recommendations contained in this document consolidate and update CDC recommendations published earlier for preventing HIV transmission in health-care settings: precautions for clinical and laboratory staffs (*1*) and precautions for health-care workers and allied professionals (*2*); recommendations for preventing HIV transmission in the workplace (*3*) and during invasive procedures (*4*); recommendations for preventing possible transmission of HIV from tears (*5*); and recommendations for providing dialysis treatment for HIV-infected patients (*6*). These recommendations also update portions of the "Guideline for Isolation Precautions in Hospitals" (*7*) and reemphasize some of the recommendations contained in "Infection Control Practices for Dentistry" (*8*). The recommendations contained in this document have been developed for use in health-care settings and emphasize the need to treat blood and other body fluids from **all** patients as potentially infective. These same prudent precautions also should be taken in other settings in which persons may be exposed to blood or other body fluids.

Definition of Health-Care Workers

Health-care workers are defined as persons, including students and trainees, whose activities involve contact with patients or with blood or other body fluids from patients in a health-care setting.

Health-Care Workers with AIDS

As of July 10, 1987, a total of 1,875 (5.8%) of 32,395 adults with AIDS, who had been reported to the CDC national surveillance system and for whom occupational information was available, reported being employed in a health-care or clinical laboratory setting. In comparison, 6.8 million persons—representing 5.6% of the U.S. labor force—were employed in health services. Of the health-care workers with AIDS, 95% have been reported to exhibit high-risk behavior; for the remaining 5%, the means of HIV acquisition was undetermined. Health-care workers with AIDS were significantly more likely than other workers to have an undetermined risk (5% versus 3%, respectively). For both health-care workers and non-health-care workers with AIDS, the proportion with an undetermined risk has not increased since 1982.

AIDS patients initially reported as not belonging to recognized risk groups are investigated by state and local health departments to determine whether possible risk factors exist. Of all health-care workers with AIDS reported to CDC who were initially characterized as not having an identified risk and for whom follow-up information was available, 66% have been reclassified because risk factors were identified or because the patient was found not to meet the surveillance case definition for AIDS. Of the 87 health-care workers currently categorized as having no identifiable risk, information is incomplete on 16 (18%) because of death or refusal to be interviewed; 38 (44%) are still being investigated. The remaining 33 (38%) health-care workers were interviewed or had other follow-up information available. The occupations of these 33 were as follows: five physicians (15%), three of whom were surgeons; one dentist (3%); three nurses (9%); nine nursing assistants (27%); seven housekeeping or maintenance workers (21%); three clinical laboratory technicians (9%); one therapist (3%); and four others who did not have contact with patients (12%). Although 15 of these 33 health-care workers reported parenteral and/or other non-needlestick exposure to blood or body fluids from patients in the 10 years preceding their diagnosis of AIDS, none of these exposures involved a patient with AIDS or known HIV infection.

Risk to Health-Care Workers of Acquiring HIV in Health-Care Settings

Health-care workers with documented percutaneous or mucous-membrane exposures to blood or body fluids of HIV-infected patients have been prospectively evaluated to determine the risk of infection after such exposures. As of June 30, 1987, 883 health-care workers have been tested for antibody to HIV in an ongoing surveillance project conducted by CDC (9). Of these, 708 (80%) had percutaneous exposures to blood, and 175 (20%) had a mucous membrane or an open wound contaminated by blood or body fluid. Of 396 health-care workers, each of whom had only a convalescent-phase serum sample obtained and tested $\geqslant$90 days postexposure, one—for whom heterosexual transmission could not be ruled out—was seropositive for HIV antibody. For 425 additional health-care workers, both acute- and convalescent-phase serum samples were obtained and tested; none of 74 health-care workers with nonpercutaneous exposures seroconverted, and three (0.9%) of 351 with percutaneous exposures seroconverted. None of these three health-care workers had other documented risk factors for infection.

Two other prospective studies to assess the risk of nosocomial acquisition of HIV infection for health-care workers are ongoing in the United States. As of April 30, 1987, 332 health-care workers with a total of 453 needlestick or mucous-membrane exposures to the blood or other body fluids of HIV-infected patients were tested for HIV antibody at the National Institutes of Health (*10*). These exposed workers included 103 with needlestick injuries and 229 with mucous-membrane exposures; none had seroconverted. A similar study at the University of California of 129 health-care workers with documented needlestick injuries or mucous-membrane exposures to blood or other body fluids from patients with HIV infection has not identified any seroconversions (*11*). Results of a prospective study in the United Kingdom identified no evidence of transmission among 150 health-care workers with parenteral or mucous-membrane exposures to blood or other body fluids, secretions, or excretions from patients with HIV infection (*12*).

In addition to health-care workers enrolled in prospective studies, eight persons who provided care to infected patients and denied other risk factors have been reported to have acquired HIV infection. Three of these health-care workers had needlestick exposures to blood from infected patients (*13-15*). Two were persons who provided nursing care to infected persons; although neither sustained a needlestick, both had extensive contact with blood or other body fluids, and neither observed recommended barrier precautions (*16,17*). The other three were health-care workers with non-needlestick exposures to blood from infected patients (*18*). Although the exact route of transmission for these last three infections is not known, all three persons had direct contact of their skin with blood from infected patients, all had skin lesions that may have been contaminated by blood, and one also had a mucous-membrane exposure.

A total of 1,231 dentists and hygienists, many of whom practiced in areas with many AIDS cases, participated in a study to determine the prevalence of antibody to HIV; one dentist (0.1%) had HIV antibody. Although no exposure to a known HIV-infected person could be documented, epidemiologic investigation did not identify any other risk factor for infection. The infected dentist, who also had a history of sustaining needlestick injuries and trauma to his hands, did not routinely wear gloves when providing dental care (*19*).

Precautions To Prevent Transmission of HIV

Universal Precautions

Since medical history and examination cannot reliably identify all patients infected with HIV or other blood-borne pathogens, blood and body-fluid precautions should be consistently used for **all** patients. This approach, previously recommended by CDC (*3,4*), and referred to as "universal blood and body-fluid precautions" or "universal precautions," should be used in the care of **all** patients, especially including those in emergency-care settings in which the risk of blood exposure is increased and the infection status of the patient is usually unknown (*20*).

1. All health-care workers should routinely use appropriate barrier precautions to prevent skin and mucous-membrane exposure when contact with blood or other body fluids of any patient is anticipated. Gloves should be worn for touching blood and body fluids, mucous membranes, or non-intact skin of all patients, for handling items or surfaces soiled with blood or body fluids, and for performing venipuncture and other vascular access procedures. Gloves should be changed after contact with each patient. Masks and protective eyewear or face shields should be worn during procedures that are likely to generate droplets of blood or other body fluids to prevent exposure of mucous membranes of the mouth, nose, and eyes. Gowns or aprons should be worn during procedures that are likely to generate splashes of blood or other body fluids.
2. Hands and other skin surfaces should be washed immediately and thoroughly if contaminated with blood or other body fluids. Hands should be washed immediately after gloves are removed.
3. All health-care workers should take precautions to prevent injuries caused by needles, scalpels, and other sharp instruments or devices during procedures; when cleaning used instruments; during disposal of used needles; and when handling sharp instruments after procedures. To prevent needlestick injuries, needles should not be recapped, purposely bent or broken by hand, removed from disposable syringes, or otherwise manipulated by hand. After they are used, disposable syringes and needles, scalpel blades, and other sharp items should be placed in puncture-resistant containers for disposal; the puncture-resistant containers should be located as close as practical to the use area. Large-bore reusable needles should be placed in a puncture-resistant container for transport to the reprocessing area.
4. Although saliva has not been implicated in HIV transmission, to minimize the need for emergency mouth-to-mouth resuscitation, mouthpieces, resuscitation bags, or other ventilation devices should be available for use in areas in which the need for resuscitation is predictable.
5. Health-care workers who have exudative lesions or weeping dermatitis should refrain from all direct patient care and from handling patient-care equipment until the condition resolves.
6. Pregnant health-care workers are not known to be at greater risk of contracting HIV infection than health-care workers who are not pregnant; however, if a health-care worker develops HIV infection during pregnancy, the infant is at risk of infection resulting from perinatal transmission. Because of this risk, pregnant health-care workers should be especially familiar with and strictly adhere to precautions to minimize the risk of HIV transmission.

Implementation of universal blood and body-fluid precautions for **all** patients eliminates the need for use of the isolation category of "Blood and Body Fluid Precautions" previously recommended by CDC (7) for patients known or suspected to be infected with blood-borne pathogens. Isolation precautions (e.g., enteric, "AFB" [7]) should be used as necessary if associated conditions, such as infectious diarrhea or tuberculosis, are diagnosed or suspected.

Precautions for Invasive Procedures

In this document, an invasive procedure is defined as surgical entry into tissues, cavities, or organs or repair of major traumatic injuries 1) in an operating or delivery room, emergency department, or outpatient setting, including both physicians' and dentists' offices; 2) cardiac catheterization and angiographic procedures; 3) a vaginal or cesarean delivery or other invasive obstetric procedure during which bleeding may occur; or 4) the manipulation, cutting, or removal of any oral or perioral tissues, including tooth structure, during which bleeding occurs or the potential for bleeding exists. The universal blood and body-fluid precautions listed above, combined with the precautions listed below, should be the minimum precautions for **all** such invasive procedures.

1. All health-care workers who participate in invasive procedures must routinely use appropriate barrier precautions to prevent skin and mucous-membrane contact with blood and other body fluids of all patients. Gloves and surgical masks must be worn for all invasive procedures. Protective eyewear or face shields should be worn for procedures that commonly result in the generation of droplets, splashing of blood or other body fluids, or the generation of bone chips. Gowns or aprons made of materials that provide an effective barrier should be worn during invasive procedures that are likely to result in the splashing of blood or other body fluids. All health-care workers who perform or assist in vaginal or cesarean deliveries should wear gloves and gowns when handling the placenta or the infant until blood and amniotic fluid have been removed from the infant's skin and should wear gloves during post-delivery care of the umbilical cord.
2. If a glove is torn or a needlestick or other injury occurs, the glove should be removed and a new glove used as promptly as patient safety permits; the needle or instrument involved in the incident should also be removed from the sterile field.

Precautions for Dentistry*

Blood, saliva, and gingival fluid from **all** dental patients should be considered infective. Special emphasis should be placed on the following precautions for preventing transmission of blood-borne pathogens in dental practice in both institutional and non-institutional settings.

1. In addition to wearing gloves for contact with oral mucous membranes of all patients, all dental workers should wear surgical masks and protective eyewear or chin-length plastic face shields during dental procedures in which splashing or spattering of blood, saliva, or gingival fluids is likely. Rubber dams, high-speed evacuation, and proper patient positioning, when appropriate, should be utilized to minimize generation of droplets and spatter.
2. Handpieces should be sterilized after use with each patient, since blood, saliva, or gingival fluid of patients may be aspirated into the handpiece or waterline. Handpieces that cannot be sterilized should at least be flushed, the outside surface cleaned and wiped with a suitable chemical germicide, and then rinsed. Handpieces should be flushed at the beginning of the day and after use with each patient. Manufacturers' recommendations should be followed for use and maintenance of waterlines and check valves and for flushing of handpieces. The same precautions should be used for ultrasonic scalers and air/water syringes.

*General infection-control precautions are more specifically addressed in previous recommendations for infection-control practices for dentistry (8).

3. Blood and saliva should be thoroughly and carefully cleaned from material that has been used in the mouth (e.g., impression materials, bite registration), especially before polishing and grinding intra-oral devices. Contaminated materials, impressions, and intra-oral devices should also be cleaned and disinfected before being handled in the dental laboratory and before they are placed in the patient's mouth. Because of the increasing variety of dental materials used intra-orally, dental workers should consult with manufacturers as to the stability of specific materials when using disinfection procedures.
4. Dental equipment and surfaces that are difficult to disinfect (e.g., light handles or X-ray-unit heads) and that may become contaminated should be wrapped with impervious-backed paper, aluminum foil, or clear plastic wrap. The coverings should be removed and discarded, and clean coverings should be put in place after use with each patient.

Precautions for Autopsies or Morticians' Services

In addition to the universal blood and body-fluid precautions listed above, the following precautions should be used by persons performing postmortem procedures:
1. All persons performing or assisting in postmortem procedures should wear gloves, masks, protective eyewear, gowns, and waterproof aprons.
2. Instruments and surfaces contaminated during postmortem procedures should be decontaminated with an appropriate chemical germicide.

Precautions for Dialysis

Patients with end-stage renal disease who are undergoing maintenance dialysis and who have HIV infection can be dialyzed in hospital-based or free-standing dialysis units using conventional infection-control precautions (21). Universal blood and body-fluid precautions should be used when dialyzing **all** patients.

Strategies for disinfecting the dialysis fluid pathways of the hemodialysis machine are targeted to control bacterial contamination and generally consist of using 500-750 parts per million (ppm) of sodium hypochlorite (household bleach) for 30-40 minutes or 1.5%-2.0% formaldehyde overnight. In addition, several chemical germicides formulated to disinfect dialysis machines are commercially available. None of these protocols or procedures need to be changed for dialyzing patients infected with HIV.

Patients infected with HIV can be dialyzed by either hemodialysis or peritoneal dialysis and do not need to be isolated from other patients. The type of dialysis treatment (i.e., hemodialysis or peritoneal dialysis) should be based on the needs of the patient. The dialyzer may be discarded after each use. Alternatively, centers that reuse dialyzers—i.e., a specific single-use dialyzer is issued to a specific patient, removed, cleaned, disinfected, and reused several times on the same patient only—may include HIV-infected patients in the dialyzer-reuse program. An individual dialyzer must never be used on more than one patient.

Precautions for Laboratories[†]

Blood and other body fluids from **all** patients should be considered infective. To supplement the universal blood and body-fluid precautions listed above, the following precautions are recommended for health-care workers in clinical laboratories.

[†]Additional precautions for research and industrial laboratories are addressed elsewhere (22,23).

1. All specimens of blood and body fluids should be put in a well-constructed container with a secure lid to prevent leaking during transport. Care should be taken when collecting each specimen to avoid contaminating the outside of the container and of the laboratory form accompanying the specimen.
2. All persons processing blood and body-fluid specimens (e.g., removing tops from vacuum tubes) should wear gloves. Masks and protective eyewear should be worn if mucous-membrane contact with blood or body fluids is anticipated. Gloves should be changed and hands washed after completion of specimen processing.
3. For routine procedures, such as histologic and pathologic studies or microbiologic culturing, a biological safety cabinet is not necessary. However, biological safety cabinets (Class I or II) should be used whenever procedures are conducted that have a high potential for generating droplets. These include activities such as blending, sonicating, and vigorous mixing.
4. Mechanical pipetting devices should be used for manipulating all liquids in the laboratory. Mouth pipetting must not be done.
5. Use of needles and syringes should be limited to situations in which there is no alternative, and the recommendations for preventing injuries with needles outlined under universal precautions should be followed.
6. Laboratory work surfaces should be decontaminated with an appropriate chemical germicide after a spill of blood or other body fluids and when work activities are completed.
7. Contaminated materials used in laboratory tests should be decontaminated before reprocessing or be placed in bags and disposed of in accordance with institutional policies for disposal of infective waste (24).
8. Scientific equipment that has been contaminated with blood or other body fluids should be decontaminated and cleaned before being repaired in the laboratory or transported to the manufacturer.
9. All persons should wash their hands after completing laboratory activities and should remove protective clothing before leaving the laboratory.

Implementation of universal blood and body-fluid precautions for **all** patients eliminates the need for warning labels on specimens since blood and other body fluids from all patients should be considered infective.

Environmental Considerations for HIV Transmission

No environmentally mediated mode of HIV transmission has been documented. Nevertheless, the precautions described below should be taken routinely in the care of **all** patients.

Sterilization and Disinfection

Standard sterilization and disinfection procedures for patient-care equipment currently recommended for use (25,26) in a variety of health-care settings—including hospitals, medical and dental clinics and offices, hemodialysis centers, emergency-care facilities, and long-term nursing-care facilities—are adequate to sterilize or disinfect instruments, devices, or other items contaminated with blood or other body fluids from persons infected with blood-borne pathogens including HIV (21,23).

Instruments or devices that enter sterile tissue or the vascular system of any patient or through which blood flows should be sterilized before reuse. Devices or items that contact intact mucous membranes should be sterilized or receive high-level disinfection, a procedure that kills vegetative organisms and viruses but not necessarily large numbers of bacterial spores. Chemical germicides that are registered with the U.S. Environmental Protection Agency (EPA) as "sterilants" may be used either for sterilization or for high-level disinfection depending on contact time.

Contact lenses used in trial fittings should be disinfected after each fitting by using a hydrogen peroxide contact lens disinfecting system or, if compatible, with heat (78 C-80 C [172.4 F-176.0 F]) for 10 minutes.

Medical devices or instruments that require sterilization or disinfection should be thoroughly cleaned before being exposed to the germicide, and the manufacturer's instructions for the use of the germicide should be followed. Further, it is important that the manufacturer's specifications for compatibility of the medical device with chemical germicides be closely followed. Information on specific label claims of commercial germicides can be obtained by writing to the Disinfectants Branch, Office of Pesticides, Environmental Protection Agency, 401 M Street, SW, Washington, D.C. 20460.

Studies have shown that HIV is inactivated rapidly after being exposed to commonly used chemical germicides at concentrations that are much lower than used in practice (*27-30*). Embalming fluids are similar to the types of chemical germicides that have been tested and found to completely inactivate HIV. In addition to commercially available chemical germicides, a solution of sodium hypochlorite (household bleach) prepared daily is an inexpensive and effective germicide. Concentrations ranging from approximately 500 ppm (1:100 dilution of household bleach) sodium hypochlorite to 5,000 ppm (1:10 dilution of household bleach) are effective depending on the amount of organic material (e.g., blood, mucus) present on the surface to be cleaned and disinfected. Commercially available chemical germicides may be more compatible with certain medical devices that might be corroded by repeated exposure to sodium hypochlorite, especially to the 1:10 dilution.

Survival of HIV in the Environment

The most extensive study on the survival of HIV after drying involved greatly concentrated HIV samples, i.e., 10 million tissue-culture infectious doses per milliliter (*31*). This concentration is at least 100,000 times greater than that typically found in the blood or serum of patients with HIV infection. HIV was detectable by tissue-culture techniques 1-3 days after drying, but the rate of inactivation was rapid. Studies performed at CDC have also shown that drying HIV causes a rapid (within several hours) 1-2 log (90%-99%) reduction in HIV concentration. In tissue-culture fluid, cell-free HIV could be detected up to 15 days at room temperature, up to 11 days at 37 C (98.6 F), and up to 1 day if the HIV was cell-associated.

When considered in the context of environmental conditions in health-care facilities, these results do not require any changes in currently recommended sterilization, disinfection, or housekeeping strategies. When medical devices are contaminated with blood or other body fluids, existing recommendations include the cleaning of these instruments, followed by disinfection or sterilization, depending on the type of medical device. These protocols assume "worst-case" conditions of extreme virologic and microbiologic contamination, and whether viruses have been inactivated after drying plays no role in formulating these strategies. Consequently, no changes in published procedures for cleaning, disinfecting, or sterilizing need to be made.

Housekeeping

Environmental surfaces such as walls, floors, and other surfaces are not associated with transmission of infections to patients or health-care workers. Therefore, extraordinary attempts to disinfect or sterilize these environmental surfaces are not necessary. However, cleaning and removal of soil should be done routinely.

Cleaning schedules and methods vary according to the area of the hospital or institution, type of surface to be cleaned, and the amount and type of soil present. Horizontal surfaces (e.g., bedside tables and hard-surfaced flooring) in patient-care areas are usually cleaned on a regular basis, when soiling or spills occur, and when a patient is discharged. Cleaning of walls, blinds, and curtains is recommended only if they are visibly soiled. Disinfectant fogging is an unsatisfactory method of decontaminating air and surfaces and is not recommended.

Disinfectant-detergent formulations registered by EPA can be used for cleaning environmental surfaces, but the actual physical removal of microorganisms by scrubbing is probably at least as important as any antimicrobial effect of the cleaning agent used. Therefore, cost, safety, and acceptability by housekeepers can be the main criteria for selecting any such registered agent. The manufacturers' instructions for appropriate use should be followed.

Cleaning and Decontaminating Spills of Blood or Other Body Fluids

Chemical germicides that are approved for use as "hospital disinfectants" and are tuberculocidal when used at recommended dilutions can be used to decontaminate spills of blood and other body fluids. Strategies for decontaminating spills of blood and other body fluids in a patient-care setting are different than for spills of cultures or other materials in clinical, public health, or research laboratories. In patient-care areas, visible material should first be removed and then the area should be decontaminated. With large spills of cultured or concentrated infectious agents in the laboratory, the contaminated area should be flooded with a liquid germicide before cleaning, then decontaminated with fresh germicidal chemical. In both settings, gloves should be worn during the cleaning and decontaminating procedures.

Laundry

Although soiled linen has been identified as a source of large numbers of certain pathogenic microorganisms, the risk of actual disease transmission is negligible. Rather than rigid procedures and specifications, hygienic and common-sense storage and processing of clean and soiled linen are recommended (26). Soiled linen should be handled as little as possible and with minimum agitation to prevent gross microbial contamination of the air and of persons handling the linen. All soiled linen should be bagged at the location where it was used; it should not be sorted or rinsed in patient-care areas. Linen soiled with blood or body fluids should be placed and transported in bags that prevent leakage. If hot water is used, linen should be washed with detergent in water at least 71 C (160 F) for 25 minutes. If low-temperature($\leqslant$70 C [158 F]) laundry cycles are used, chemicals suitable for low-temperature washing at proper use concentration should be used.

Infective Waste

There is no epidemiologic evidence to suggest that most hospital waste is any more infective than residential waste. Moreover, there is no epidemiologic evidence that hospital waste has caused disease in the community as a result of improper disposal. Therefore, identifying wastes for which special precautions are indicated is largely a matter of judgment about the relative risk of disease transmission. The most practical approach to the management of infective waste is to identify those wastes with the potential for causing infection during handling and disposal and for which some special precautions appear prudent. Hospital wastes for which special precautions appear prudent include microbiology laboratory waste, pathology waste, and blood specimens or blood products. While any item that has had contact with blood, exudates, or secretions may be potentially infective, it is not usually considered practical or necessary to treat all such waste as infective (*23,26*). Infective waste, in general, should either be incinerated or should be autoclaved before disposal in a sanitary landfill. Bulk blood, suctioned fluids, excretions, and secretions may be carefully poured down a drain connected to a sanitary sewer. Sanitary sewers may also be used to dispose of other infectious wastes capable of being ground and flushed into the sewer.

Implementation of Recommended Precautions

Employers of health-care workers should ensure that policies exist for:
1. Initial orientation and continuing education and training of all health-care workers—including students and trainees—on the epidemiology, modes of transmission, and prevention of HIV and other blood-borne infections and the need for routine use of universal blood and body-fluid precautions for **all** patients.
2. Provision of equipment and supplies necessary to minimize the risk of infection with HIV and other blood-borne pathogens.
3. Monitoring adherence to recommended protective measures. When monitoring reveals a failure to follow recommended precautions, counseling, education, and/or re-training should be provided, and, if necessary, appropriate disciplinary action should be considered.

Professional associations and labor organizations, through continuing education efforts, should emphasize the need for health-care workers to follow recommended precautions.

Serologic Testing for HIV Infection

Background

A person is identified as infected with HIV when a sequence of tests, starting with repeated enzyme immunoassays (EIA) and including a Western blot or similar, more specific assay, are repeatedly reactive. Persons infected with HIV usually develop antibody against the virus within 6-12 weeks after infection.

The sensitivity of the currently licensed EIA tests is at least 99% when they are performed under optimal laboratory conditions on serum specimens from persons infected for ≥12 weeks. Optimal laboratory conditions include the use of reliable reagents, provision of continuing education of personnel, quality control of procedures, and participation in performance-evaluation programs. Given this performance, the probability of a false-negative test is remote except during the first several weeks after infection, before detectable antibody is present. The proportion of infected persons with a false-negative test attributed to absence of antibody in the early stages of infection is dependent on both the incidence and prevalence of HIV infection in a population (Table 1).

The specificity of the currently licensed EIA tests is approximately 99% when repeatedly reactive tests are considered. Repeat testing of initially reactive specimens by EIA is required to reduce the likelihood of laboratory error. To increase further the specificity of serologic tests, laboratories must use a supplemental test, most often the Western blot, to validate repeatedly reactive EIA results. Under optimal laboratory conditions, the sensitivity of the Western blot test is comparable to or greater than that of a repeatedly reactive EIA, and the Western blot is highly specific when strict criteria are used to interpret the test results. The testing sequence of a repeatedly reactive EIA and a positive Western blot test is highly predictive of HIV infection, even in a population with a low prevalence of infection (Table 2). If the Western blot test result is indeterminant, the testing sequence is considered equivocal for HIV infection.

TABLE 1. Estimated annual number of patients infected with HIV not detected by HIV-antibody testing in a hypothetical hospital with 10,000 admissions/year*

Beginning prevalence of HIV infection	Annual incidence of HIV infection	Approximate number of HIV-infected patients	Approximate number of HIV-infected patients not detected
5.0%	1.0%	550	17-18
5.0%	0.5%	525	11-12
1.0%	0.2%	110	3-4
1.0%	0.1%	105	2-3
0.1%	0.02%	11	0-1
0.1%	0.01%	11	0-1

*The estimates are based on the following assumptions: 1) the sensitivity of the screening test is 99% (i.e., 99% of HIV-infected persons with antibody will be detected); 2) persons infected with HIV will not develop detectable antibody (seroconvert) until 6 weeks (1.5 months) after infection; 3) new infections occur at an equal rate throughout the year; 4) calculations of the number of HIV-infected persons in the patient population are based on the mid-year prevalence, which is the beginning prevalence plus half the annual incidence of infections.

When this occurs, the Western blot test should be repeated on the same serum sample, and, if still indeterminant, the testing sequence should be repeated on a sample collected 3-6 months later. Use of other supplemental tests may aid in interpreting of results on samples that are persistently indeterminant by Western blot.

Testing of Patients

Previous CDC recommendations have emphasized the value of HIV serologic testing of patients for: 1) management of parenteral or mucous-membrane exposures of health-care workers, 2) patient diagnosis and management, and 3) counseling and serologic testing to prevent and control HIV transmission in the community. In addition, more recent recommendations have stated that hospitals, in conjunction with state and local health departments, should periodically determine the prevalence of HIV infection among patients from age groups at highest risk of infection (32).

Adherence to universal blood and body-fluid precautions recommended for the care of all patients will minimize the risk of transmission of HIV and other blood-borne pathogens from patients to health-care workers. The utility of routine HIV serologic testing of patients as an adjunct to universal precautions is unknown. Results of such testing may not be available in emergency or outpatient settings. In addition, some recently infected patients will not have detectable antibody to HIV (Table 1).

Personnel in some hospitals have advocated serologic testing of patients in settings in which exposure of health-care workers to large amounts of patients' blood may be anticipated. Specific patients for whom serologic testing has been advocated include those undergoing major operative procedures and those undergoing treatment in critical-care units, especially if they have conditions involving uncontrolled bleeding. Decisions regarding the need to establish testing programs for patients should be made by physicians or individual institutions. In addition, when deemed appropriate, testing of individual patients may be performed on agreement between the patient and the physician providing care.

In addition to the universal precautions recommended for all patients, certain additional precautions for the care of HIV-infected patients undergoing major surgical operations have been proposed by personnel in some hospitals. For example, surgical procedures on an HIV-infected patient might be altered so that hand-to-hand passing of sharp instruments would be eliminated; stapling instruments rather than

TABLE 2. Predictive value of positive HIV-antibody tests in hypothetical populations with different prevalences of infection

	Prevalence of infection	Predictive value of positive test[*]
Repeatedly reactive enzyme immunoassay (EIA)[†]	0.2%	28.41%
	2.0%	80.16%
	20.0%	98.02%
Repeatedly reactive EIA followed by positive Western blot (WB)[§]	0.2%	99.75%
	2.0%	99.97%
	20.0%	99.99%

[*]Proportion of persons with positive test results who are actually infected with HIV.
[†]Assumes EIA sensitivity of 99.0% and specificity of 99.5%.
[§]Assumes WB sensitivity of 99.0% and specificity of 99.9%.

hand-suturing equipment might be used to perform tissue approximation; electrocautery devices rather than scalpels might be used as cutting instruments; and, even though uncomfortable, gowns that totally prevent seepage of blood onto the skin of members of the operative team might be worn. While such modifications might further minimize the risk of HIV infection for members of the operative team, some of these techniques could result in prolongation of operative time and could potentially have an adverse effect on the patient.

Testing programs, if developed, should include the following principles:

- Obtaining consent for testing.
- Informing patients of test results, and providing counseling for seropositive patients by properly trained persons.
- Assuring that confidentiality safeguards are in place to limit knowledge of test results to those directly involved in the care of infected patients or as required by law.
- Assuring that identification of infected patients will not result in denial of needed care or provision of suboptimal care.
- Evaluating prospectively 1) the efficacy of the program in reducing the incidence of parenteral, mucous-membrane, or significant cutaneous exposures of health-care workers to the blood or other body fluids of HIV-infected patients and 2) the effect of modified procedures on patients.

Testing of Health-Care Workers

Although transmission of HIV from infected health-care workers to patients has not been reported, transmission during invasive procedures remains a possibility. Transmission of hepatitis B virus (HBV)—a blood-borne agent with a considerably greater potential for nosocomial spread—from health-care workers to patients has been documented. Such transmission has occurred in situations (e.g., oral and gynecologic surgery) in which health-care workers, when tested, had very high concentrations of HBV in their blood (at least 100 million infectious virus particles per milliliter, a concentration much higher than occurs with HIV infection), and the health-care workers sustained a puncture wound while performing invasive procedures or had exudative or weeping lesions or microlacerations that allowed virus to contaminate instruments or open wounds of patients (*33,34*).

The hepatitis B experience indicates that only those health-care workers who perform certain types of invasive procedures have transmitted HBV to patients. Adherence to recommendations in this document will minimize the risk of transmission of HIV and other blood-borne pathogens from health-care workers to patients during invasive procedures. Since transmission of HIV from infected health-care workers performing invasive procedures to their patients has not been reported and would be expected to occur only very rarely, if at all, the utility of routine testing of such health-care workers to prevent transmission of HIV cannot be assessed. If consideration is given to developing a serologic testing program for health-care workers who perform invasive procedures, the frequency of testing, as well as the issues of consent, confidentiality, and consequences of test results—as previously outlined for testing programs for patients—must be addressed.

Management of Infected Health-Care Workers

Health-care workers with impaired immune systems resulting from HIV infection or other causes are at increased risk of acquiring or experiencing serious complications of infectious disease. Of particular concern is the risk of severe infection following exposure to patients with infectious diseases that are easily transmitted if appropriate precautions are not taken (e.g., measles, varicella). Any health-care worker with an impaired immune system should be counseled about the potential risk associated with taking care of patients with any transmissible infection and should continue to follow existing recommendations for infection control to minimize risk of exposure to other infectious agents (7,35). Recommendations of the Immunization Practices Advisory Committee (ACIP) and institutional policies concerning requirements for vaccinating health-care workers with live-virus vaccines (e.g., measles, rubella) should also be considered.

The question of whether workers infected with HIV—especially those who perform invasive procedures—can adequately and safely be allowed to perform patient-care duties or whether their work assignments should be changed must be determined on an individual basis. These decisions should be made by the health-care worker's personal physician(s) in conjunction with the medical directors and personnel health service staff of the employing institution or hospital.

Management of Exposures

If a health-care worker has a parenteral (e.g., needlestick or cut) or mucous-membrane (e.g., splash to the eye or mouth) exposure to blood or other body fluids or has a cutaneous exposure involving large amounts of blood or prolonged contact with blood—especially when the exposed skin is chapped, abraded, or afflicted with dermatitis—the source patient should be informed of the incident and tested for serologic evidence of HIV infection after consent is obtained. Policies should be developed for testing source patients in situations in which consent cannot be obtained (e.g., an unconscious patient).

If the source patient has AIDS, is positive for HIV antibody, or refuses the test, the health-care worker should be counseled regarding the risk of infection and evaluated clinically and serologically for evidence of HIV infection as soon as possible after the exposure. The health-care worker should be advised to report and seek medical evaluation for any acute febrile illness that occurs within 12 weeks after the exposure. Such an illness—particularly one characterized by fever, rash, or lymphadenopathy—may be indicative of recent HIV infection. Seronegative health-care workers should be retested 6 weeks post-exposure and on a periodic basis thereafter (e.g., 12 weeks and 6 months after exposure) to determine whether transmission has occurred. During this follow-up period—especially the first 6-12 weeks after exposure, when most infected persons are expected to seroconvert—exposed health-care workers should follow U.S. Public Health Service (PHS) recommendations for preventing transmission of HIV (36,37).

No further follow-up of a health-care worker exposed to infection as described above is necessary if the source patient is seronegative unless the source patient is at high risk of HIV infection. In the latter case, a subsequent specimen (e.g., 12 weeks following exposure) may be obtained from the health-care worker for antibody testing. If the source patient cannot be identified, decisions regarding appropriate follow-up should be individualized. Serologic testing should be available to all health-care workers who are concerned that they may have been infected with HIV.

If a patient has a parenteral or mucous-membrane exposure to blood or other body fluid of a health-care worker, the patient should be informed of the incident, and the same procedure outlined above for management of exposures should be followed for both the source health-care worker and the exposed patient.

References
1. CDC. Acquired immunodeficiency syndrome (AIDS): Precautions for clinical and laboratory staffs. MMWR 1982;31:577-80.
2. CDC. Acquired immunodeficiency syndrome (AIDS): Precautions for health-care workers and allied professionals. MMWR 1983;32:450-1.
3. CDC. Recommendations for preventing transmission of infection with human T-lymphotropic virus type III/lymphadenopathy-associated virus in the workplace. MMWR 1985;34:681-6, 691-5.
4. CDC. Recommendations for preventing transmission of infection with human T-lymphotropic virus type III/lymphadenopathy-associated virus during invasive procedures. MMWR 1986;35:221-3.
5. CDC. Recommendations for preventing possible transmission of human T-lymphotropic virus type III/lymphadenopathy-associated virus from tears. MMWR 1985;34:533-4.
6. CDC. Recommendations for providing dialysis treatment to patients infected with human T-lymphotropic virus type III/lymphadenopathy-associated virus infection. MMWR 1986;35:376-8, 383.
7. Garner JS, Simmons BP. Guideline for isolation precautions in hospitals. Infect Control 1983;4 (suppl) :245-325.
8. CDC. Recommended infection control practices for dentistry. MMWR 1986;35:237-42.
9. McCray E, The Cooperative Needlestick Surveillance Group. Occupational risk of the acquired immunodeficiency syndrome among health care workers. N Engl J Med 1986;314:1127-32.
10. Henderson DK, Saah AJ, Zak BJ, et al. Risk of nosocomial infection with human T-cell lymphotropic virus type III/lymphadenopathy-associated virus in a large cohort of intensively exposed health care workers. Ann Intern Med 1986;104:644-7.
11. Gerberding JL, Bryant-LeBlanc CE, Nelson K, et al. Risk of transmitting the human immunodeficiency virus, cytomegalovirus, and hepatitis B virus to health care workers exposed to patients with AIDS and AIDS-related conditions. J Infect Dis 1987;156:1-8.
12. McEvoy M, Porter K, Mortimer P, Simmons N, Shanson D. Prospective study of clinical, laboratory, and ancillary staff with accidental exposures to blood or other body fluids from patients infected with HIV. Br Med J 1987;294:1595-7.
13. Anonymous. Needlestick transmission of HTLV-III from a patient infected in Africa. Lancet 1984;2:1376-7.
14. Oksenhendler E, Harzic M, Le Roux JM, Rabian C, Clauvel JP. HIV infection with seroconversion after a superficial needlestick injury to the finger. N Engl J Med 1986;315:582.
15. Neisson-Vernant C, Arfi S, Mathez D, Leibowitch J, Monplaisir N. Needlestick HIV seroconversion in a nurse. Lancet 1986;2:814.
16. Grint P, McEvoy M. Two associated cases of the acquired immune deficiency syndrome (AIDS). PHLS Commun Dis Rep 1985;42:4.
17. CDC. Apparent transmission of human T-lymphotropic virus type III/lymphadenopathy-associated virus from a child to a mother providing health care. MMWR 1986;35:76-9.
18. CDC. Update: Human immunodeficiency virus infections in health-care workers exposed to blood of infected patients. MMWR 1987;36:285-9.
19. Kline RS, Phelan J, Friedland GH, et al. Low occupational risk for HIV infection for dental professionals [Abstract]. In: Abstracts from the III International Conference on AIDS, 1-5 June 1985. Washington, DC: 155.
20. Baker JL, Kelen GD, Sivertson KT, Quinn TC. Unsuspected human immunodeficiency virus in critically ill emergency patients. JAMA 1987;257:2609-11.
21. Favero MS. Dialysis-associated diseases and their control. In: Bennett JV, Brachman PS, eds. Hospital infections. Boston: Little, Brown and Company, 1985:267-84.

22. Richardson JH, Barkley WE, eds. Biosafety in microbiological and biomedical laboratories, 1984. Washington, DC : US Department of Health and Human Services, Public Health Service. HHS publication no. (CDC) 84-8395.
23. CDC. Human T-lymphotropic virus type III/lymphadenopathy-associated virus: Agent summary statement. MMWR 1986;35:540-2, 547-9.
24. Environmental Protection Agency. EPA guide for infectious waste management. Washington, DC :U.S. Environmental Protection Agency, May 1986 (Publication no. EPA/530-SW-86-014).
25. Favero MS. Sterilization, disinfection, and antisepsis in the hospital. In: Manual of clinical microbiology. 4th ed. Washington, DC: American Society for Microbiology, 1985;129-37.
26. Garner JS, Favero MS. Guideline for handwashing and hospital environmental control, 1985. Atlanta: Public Health Service, Centers for Disease Control, 1985. HHS publication no. 99-1117.
27. Spire B, Montagnier L, Barré-Sinoussi F, Chermann JC. Inactivation of lymphadenopathy associated virus by chemical disinfectants. Lancet 1984;2:899-901.
28. Martin LS, McDougal JS, Loskoski SL. Disinfection and inactivation of the human T lymphotropic virus type III/lymphadenopathy-associated virus. J Infect Dis 1985; 152:400-3.
29. McDougal JS, Martin LS, Cort SP, et al. Thermal inactivation of the acquired immunodeficiency syndrome virus-III/lymphadenopathy-associated virus, with special reference to antihemophilic factor. J Clin Invest 1985;76:875-7.
30. Spire B, Barré-Sinoussi F, Dormont D, Montagnier L, Chermann JC. Inactivation of lymphadenopathy-associated virus by heat, gamma rays, and ultraviolet light. Lancet 1985;1:188-9.
31. Resnik L, Veren K, Salahuddin SZ, Tondreau S, Markham PD. Stability and inactivation of HTLV-III/LAV under clinical and laboratory environments. JAMA 1986;255:1887-91.
32. CDC. Public Health Service (PHS) guidelines for counseling and antibody testing to prevent HIV infection and AIDS. MMWR 1987;3:509-15..
33. Kane MA, Lettau LA. Transmission of HBV from dental personnel to patients. J Am Dent Assoc 1985;110:634-6.
34. Lettau LA, Smith JD, Williams D, et. al. Transmission of hepatitis B with resultant restriction of surgical practice. JAMA 1986;255:934-7.
35. Williams WW. Guideline for infection control in hospital personnel. Infect Control 1983;4 (suppl) :326-49.
36. CDC. Prevention of acquired immune deficiency syndrome (AIDS): Report of inter-agency recommendations. MMWR 1983;32:101-3.
37. CDC. Provisional Public Health Service inter-agency recommendations for screening donated blood and plasma for antibody to the virus causing acquired immunodeficiency syndrome. MMWR 1985;34:1-5.

APPENDIX B

Biosafety Level Criteria: Laboratory and Vertebrate Animal

MMWR Supplement

Biosafety Level 2

Biosafety Level 2 is similar to Level 1 and is suitable for work involving agents that represent a moderate hazard for personnel and the environment. It differs in that a) laboratory personnel have specific training in handling pathogenic agents and are directed by competent scientists, b) access to the laboratory is limited when work is being conducted, and c) certain procedures in which infectious aerosols are created are conducted in biological safety cabinets or other physical containment equipment.

The following standard and special practices, safety equipment, and facilities apply to agents assigned to Biosafety Level 2:

A. Standard microbiological practices
1. Access to the laboratory is limited or restricted by the laboratory director when work with infectious agents is in progress.
2. Work surfaces are decontaminated at least once a day and after any spill of viable material.
3. All Infectious liquid or solid waste is decontaminated before being disposed of.
4. Mechanical pipetting devices are used; mouth pipetting is prohibited.
5. Eating, drinking, smoking, and applying cosmetics are not permitted in the work area. Food must be stored in cabinets or refrigerators designed and used for this purpose only. Food storage cabinets or refrigerators should be located outside the work area.
6. Persons are to wash their hands when they leave the laboratory after handling infectious material or animals.
7. All procedures are performed carefully to minimize the creation of aerosols.

B. Special practices
1. Contaminated materials that are to be decontaminated away from the laboratory are placed in a durable, leakproof container that is closed before being removed from the laboratory.
2. The laboratory director limits access to the laboratory. In general, persons who are at increased risk of acquiring infection or for whom infection may be unusually hazardous are not allowed in the laboratory or animal rooms. The director has the final responsibility for assessing each circumstance and determining who may enter or work in the laboratory.
3. The laboratory director establishes policies or procedures whereby only persons who have been advised of the potential hazard and who meet any specific entry requirements (e.g., vaccination) enter the laboratory or animal rooms.
4. When an infectious agent being worked with in the laboratory requires special provisions for entry (e.g., vaccination), a hazard warning sign that

incorporates the universal biohazard symbol is posted on the access door to the laboratory work area. The hazard warning sign identifies the infectious agent, lists the name and telephone number of the laboratory director or other responsible person(s), and indicates the special requirement(s) for entering the laboratory.
5. An insect and rodent control program is in effect.
6. Laboratory coats, gowns, smocks, or uniforms are worn while in the laboratory. Before leaving the laboratory for nonlaboratory areas (e.g., cafeteria, library, administrative offices), this protective clothing is removed and left in the laboratory or covered with a clean coat not used in the laboratory.
7. Animals not involved in the work being performed are not permitted in the laboratory.
8. Special care is taken to avoid having skin be contaminated with infectious material; gloves should be worn when handling infected animals and when skin contact with infectious material is unavoidable.
9. All waste from laboratories and animal rooms is appropriately decontaminated before disposal.
10. Hypodermic needles and syringes are used only for parenteral injection and aspiration of fluids from laboratory animals and diaphragm bottles. Only needle-locking syringes or disposable syringe-needle units (i.e., the needle is integral to the syringe) are used for the injection or aspiration of infectious fluid. Extreme caution should be used when handling needles and syringes to avoid autoinoculation and the generation of aerosols during use and disposal. A needle should not be bent, sheared, replaced in the sheath or guard, or removed from the syringe following use. The needle and syringe should be promptly placed in a puncture-resistant container and decontaminated, preferably by autoclaving, before discard or reuse.
11. Spills and accidents that result in overt exposures to infectious material are immediately reported to the laboratory director. Medical evaluation, surveillance, and treatment are provided as appropriate, and written records are maintained.
12. When appropriate, considering the agent(s) handled, baseline serum samples for laboratory and other at-risk personnel are collected and stored. Additional serum specimens may be collected periodically, depending on the agents handled or on the function of the facility.
13. A biosafety manual is prepared or adopted. Personnel are advised of special hazards and are required to read instructions on practices and procedures and to follow them.

C. **Containment equipment**
Biological safety cabinets (Class I or II) or other appropriate personal-protection or physical-containment devices are used when:
1. Procedures with a high potential for creating infectious aerosols are conducted. These may include centrifuging, grinding, blending, vigorous shaking or mixing, sonic disruption, opening containers of infectious materials whose internal pressures may be different from ambient pressures, inoculating animals intranasally, and harvesting infected tissues from animals or eggs.
2. High concentrations or large volumes of infectious agents are used. Some types of materials may be centrifuged in the open laboratory if sealed heads

or centrifuge safety cups are used and if the containers are opened only in a biological safety cabinet.
D. Laboratory facilities
1. The laboratory is designed so that it can be easily cleaned.
2. Bench tops are impervious to water and resistant to acids, alkalis, organic solvents, and moderate heat.
3. Laboratory furniture is sturdy, and spaces between benches, cabinets, and equipment are accessible for cleaning.
4. Each laboratory contains a sink for hand washing.
5. If the laboratory has windows that open, they are fitted with fly screens.
6. An autoclave for decontaminating infectious laboratory wastes is available.

Biosafety Level 3

Biosafety Level 3 is applicable to clinical, diagnostic, teaching, research, or production facilities in which work is done with indigenous or exotic agents that may cause serious or potentially lethal disease as a result of exposure by inhalation. Laboratory personnel have specific training in handling pathogenic and/or potentially lethal agents and are supervised by competent scientists who are experienced in working with these agents. All procedures involving the manipulation of infectious material are conducted within biological safety cabinets or other physical containment devices or by personnel wearing appropriate personal-protection clothing and devices. The laboratory has special engineering and design features. It is recognized, however, that many existing facilities may not have all the facility safeguards recommended for Biosafety Level 3 (e.g., access zone, sealed penetrations, and directional airflow). In these circumstances, acceptable safety may be achieved for routine or repetitive operations (e.g., diagnostic procedures involving the propagation of an agent for identification, typing, and susceptibility testing) in laboratories in which facility features satisfy Biosafety Level 2 recommendations if the recommended "Standard Microbiological Practices," "Special Practices," and "Containment Equipment" for Biosafety Level 3 are rigorously followed. The decision to implement this modification of Biosafety Level 3 recommendations should be made only by the laboratory director.

The following standard and special safety practices, equipment, and facilities apply to agents assigned to Biosafety Level 3:

A. Standard microbiological practices
1. Work surfaces are decontaminated at least once a day and after any spill of viable material.
2. All infectious liquid or solid waste is decontaminated before being disposed of.
3. Mechanical pipetting devices are used; mouth pipetting is prohibited.
4. Eating, drinking, smoking, storing food, and applying cosmetics are not permitted in the work area.
5. Persons wash their hands after handling infectious materials and animals and every time they leave the laboratory.
6. All procedures are performed carefully to minimize the creation of aerosols.

B. Special practices
1. Laboratory doors are kept closed when experiments are in progress.

2. Contaminated materials that are to be decontaminated at a site away from the laboratory are placed in a durable, leakproof container that is closed before being removed from the laboratory.
3. The laboratory director controls access to the laboratory and limits access only to persons whose presence is required for program or support purposes. Persons who are at increased risk of acquiring infection or for whom infection may be unusually hazardous are not allowed in the laboratory or animal rooms. The director has the final responsibility for assessing each circumstance and determining who may enter or work in the laboratory.
4. The laboratory director establishes policies and procedures whereby only persons who have been advised of the potential biohazard, who meet any specific entry requirements (e.g., vaccination), and who comply with all entry and exit procedures enter the laboratory or animal rooms.
5. When infectious materials or infected animals are present in the laboratory or containment module, a hazard warning sign (incorporating the universal biohazard symbol) is posted on all laboratory and animal-room access doors. The hazard warning sign identifies the agent, lists the name and telephone number of the laboratory director or other responsible person(s), and indicates any special requirements for entering the laboratory, such as the need for vaccinations, respirators, or other personal-protection measures.
6. All activities involving infectious materials are conducted in biological safety cabinets or other physical-containment devices within the containment module. No work is conducted in open vessels on the open bench.
7. The work surfaces of biological safety cabinets and other containment equipment are decontaminated when work with infectious materials is finished. Plastic-backed paper toweling used on nonperforated work surfaces within biological safety cabinets facilitates clean-up.
8. An insect and rodent control program is in effect.
9. Laboratory clothing that protects street clothing (e.g., solid-front or wrap-around gowns, scrub suits, coveralls) is worn in the laboratory. Laboratory clothing is not worn outside the laboratory, and it is decontaminated before being laundered.
10. Special care is taken to avoid skin contamination with infectious materials; gloves are worn when handling infected animals and when skin contact with infectious materials is unavoidable.
11. Molded surgical masks or respirators are worn in rooms containing infected animals.
12. Animals and plants not related to the work being conducted are not permitted in the laboratory.
13. All waste from laboratories and animal rooms is appropriately decontaminated before being disposed of.
14. Vacuum lines are protected with high-efficiency particulate air (HEPA) filters and liquid disinfectant traps.
15. Hypodermic needles and syringes are used only for parenteral injection and aspiration of fluids from laboratory animals and diaphragm bottles. Only needle-locking syringes or disposable syringe-needle units (i.e., the needle

is integral to the syringe) are used for the injection or aspiration of infectious fluids. Extreme caution is used when handling needles and syringes to avoid autoinoculation and the generation of aerosols during use and disposal. A needle should not be bent, sheared, replaced in the sheath or guard, or removed from the syringe following use. The needle and syringe should be promptly placed in a puncture-resistant container and decontaminated, preferably by autoclaving, before being discarded or reused.
16. Spills and accidents that result in overt or potential exposures to infectious material are immediately reported to the laboratory director. Appropriate medical evaluation, surveillance, and treatment are provided, and written records are maintained.
17. Baseline serum samples for all laboratory and other at-risk personnel are collected and stored. Additional serum specimens may be collected periodically, depending on the agents handled or the function of the laboratory.
18. A biosafety manual is prepared or adopted. Personnel are advised of special hazards and are required to read instructions on practices and procedures and to follow them.

C. **Containment equipment**

Biological safety cabinets (Class I, II, or III) or other appropriate combinations of personal-protection or physical-containment devices (e.g., special protective clothing, masks, gloves, respirators, centrifuge safety cups, sealed centrifuge rotors, and containment caging for animals) are used for all activities with infectious materials that pose a threat of aerosol exposure. These include: manipulation of cultures and of clinical or environmental material that may be a source of infectious aerosols; the aerosol challenge of experimental animals; harvesting of tissues or fluids from infected animals and embryonated eggs; and necropsy of infected animals.

D. **Laboratory facilities**
1. The laboratory is separated from areas that are open to unrestricted traffic flow within the building. Passage through two sets of doors is the basic requirement for entry into the laboratory from access corridors or other contiguous areas. Physical separation of the high-containment laboratory from access corridors or other laboratories or activities may also be provided by a double-doored clothes-change room (showers may be included), airlock, or other access facility that requires passing through two sets of doors before entering the laboratory.
2. The interior surfaces of walls, floors, and ceilings are water resistant so that they can be easily cleaned. Penetrations in these surfaces are sealed or capable of being sealed to facilitate decontaminating the area.
3. Bench tops are impervious to water and resistant to acids, alkalis, organic solvents, and moderate heat.
4. Laboratory furniture is sturdy, and spaces between benches, cabinets, and equipment are accessible for cleaning.
5. Each laboratory contains a sink for washing hands. The sink is foot, elbow, or automatically operated and is located near the laboratory exit door.
6. Windows in the laboratory are closed and sealed.
7. Access doors to the laboratory or containment module are self-closing.

8. An autoclave for decontaminating laboratory wastes is available, preferably within the laboratory.
9. A ducted exhaust-air ventilation system is provided. This system creates directional airflow that draws air into the laboratory through the entry area. The exhaust air is not recirculated to any other area of the building, is discharged to the outside, and is dispersed away from occupied areas and air intakes. Personnel must verify that the direction of the airflow is proper (i.e., into the laboratory). The exhaust air from the laboratory room can be discharged to the outside without being filtered or otherwise treated.
10. The HEPA-filtered exhaust air from Class I or CLass II biological safety cabinets is discharged directly to the outside or through the building exhaust system. Exhaust air from Class I or II biological safety cabinets may be recirculated within the laboratory if the cabinet is tested and certified at least every 12 months. If the HEPA-filtered exhaust air from Class I or II biological safety cabinets is to be discharged to the outside through the building exhaust system, it is connected to this system in a manner (e.g., thimble-unit connection) that avoids any interference with the air balance of the cabinets or building exhaust system.

VERTEBRATE ANIMAL BIOSAFETY LEVEL CRITERIA
Animal Biosafety Level 2
A. Standard practices
1. Doors to animal rooms open inward, are self-closing, and are kept closed when infected animals are present.
2. Work surfaces are decontaminated after use or spills of viable materials.
3. Eating, drinking, smoking, and storing of food for human use are not permitted in animal rooms.
4. Personnel wash their hands after handling cultures and animals and before leaving the animal room.
5. All procedures are carefully performed to minimize the creation of aerosols.
6. An insect and rodent control program is in effect.

B. Special practices
1. Cages are decontaminated, preferably by autoclaving, before being cleaned and washed.
2. Surgical-type masks are worn by all personnel entering animal rooms housing nonhuman primates.
3. Laboratory coats, gowns, or uniforms are worn while in the animal room. This protective clothing is removed before leaving the animal facility.
4. The laboratory or animal-facility director limits access to the animal room only to personnel who have been advised of the potential hazard and who need to enter the room for program or service purposes when work is in progress. In general, persons who may be at increased risk of acquiring

infection or for whom infection might be unusually hazardous are not allowed in the animal room.
5. The laboratory or animal-facility director establishes policies and procedures whereby only persons who have been advised of the potential hazard and who meet any specific requirements (e.g., vaccination) may enter the animal room.
6. When an infectious agent in use in the animal room requires special-entry provisions (e.g., vaccination), a hazard warning sign (incorporating the universal biohazard symbol) is posted on the access door to the animal room. The hazard warning sign identifies the infectious agent, lists the name and telephone number of the animal-facility supervisor or other responsible person(s), and indicates the special requirement(s) for entering the animal room.
7. Special care is taken to avoid contaminating skin with infectious material; gloves should be worn when handling infected animals and when skin contact with infectious materials is unavoidable.
8. All waste from the animal room is appropriately decontaminated—preferably by autoclaving—before being disposed of. Infected animal carcasses are incinerated after being transported from the animal room in leakproof, covered containers.
9. Hypodermic needles and syringes are used only for the parenteral injection or aspiration of fluids from laboratory animals and diaphragm bottles. Only needle-locking syringes or disposable syringe-needle units (i.e., the needle is integral to the syringe) are used for the injection or aspiration of infectious fluids. A needle should not be bent, sheared, replaced in the sheath or guard, or removed from the syringe following use. The needle and syringe should be promptly placed in a puncture-resistant container and decontaminated, preferably by autoclaving, before being discarded or reused.
10. If floor drains are provided, the drain taps are always filled with water or a suitable disinfectant.
11. When appropriate, considering the agents handled, baseline serum samples from animal-care and other at-risk personnel are collected and stored. Additional serum samples may be collected periodically, depending on the agents handled or the function of the facility.

C. Containment equipment

Biological safety cabinets, other physical-containment devices, and/or personal-protection devices (e.g., respirators, face shields) are used when procedures with a high potential for creating aerosols are conducted. These include necropsy of infected animals, harvesting of infected tissues or fluids from animals or eggs, intranasal inoculation of animals, and manipulation of high concentrations or large volumes of infectious materials.

D. Animal facilities

1. The animal facility is designed and constructed to facilitate cleaning and housekeeping.
2. A sink for washing hands is available in the room that houses infected animals.
3. If the animal facility has windows that open, they are fitted with fly screens.

4. It is recommended, but not required, that the direction of airflow in the animal facility is inward and that exhaust air is discharged to the outside without being recirculated to other rooms.
5. An autoclave that can be used for decontaminating infectious laboratory waste is available in the same building that contains the animal facility.

Animal Biosafety Level 3
A. Standard practices
1. Doors to animal rooms open inward, are self-closing, and are kept closed when work with infected animals is in progress.
2. Work surfaces are decontaminated after use or after spills of viable materials.
3. Eating, drinking, smoking, and storing of food for human use are not permitted in the animal room.
4. Personnel wash their hands after handling cultures or animals and before leaving the laboratory.
5. All procedures are carefully performed to minimize the creation of aerosols.
6. An insect and rodent control program is in effect.

B. Special practices
1. Cages are autoclaved before bedding is removed and before they are cleaned and washed.
2. Surgical-type masks or other respiratory protection devices (e.g., respirators) are worn by personnel entering rooms that house animals infected with agents assigned to Biosafety Level 3.
3. Wrap-around or solid-front gowns or uniforms are worn by personnel entering the animal room. Front-button laboratory coats are unsuitable. Protective gowns must remain in the animal room and must be decontaminated before being laundered.
4. The laboratory director or other responsible person limits access to the animal room only to personnel who have been advised of the potential hazard and who need to enter the room for program or service purposes when infected animals are present. In general, persons who may be at increased risk of acquiring infection or for whom infection might be unusually hazardous are not allowed in the animal room.
5. The laboratory director or other responsible person establishes policies and procedures whereby only persons who have been advised of the potential hazard and meet any specific requirements (e.g., vaccination) may enter the animal room.
6. Hazard warning signs (incorporating the universal biohazard warning symbol) are posted on access doors to animal rooms containing animals infected with agents assigned to Biosafety Level 3 are present. The hazard warning sign should identify the agent(s) in use, list the name and telephone number of the animal room supervisor or other responsible person(s), and indicate any special conditions of entry into the animal room (e.g., the need for vaccinations or respirators).
7. Personnel wear gloves when handling infected animals. Gloves are removed aseptically and autoclaved with other animal room waste before being disposed of or reused.

8. All wastes from the animal room are autoclaved before being disposed of. All animal carcasses are incinerated. Dead animals are transported from the animal room to the incinerator in leakproof, covered containers.
9. Hypodermic needles and syringes are used only for gavage or parenteral injection or aspiration of fluids from laboratory animals and diaphragm bottles. Only needle-locking syringes or disposable syringe-needle units (i.e., the needle is integral to the syringe) are used. A needle should not be bent, sheared, replaced in the sheath or guard, or removed from the syringe following use. The needle and syringe should be promptly placed in a puncture-resistant container and decontaminated, preferably by autoclaving, before being discarded or reused. When possible, cannulas should be used instead of sharp needles (e.g., gavage).
10. If floor drains are provided, the drain traps are always filled with water or a suitable disinfectant.
11. If vacuum lines are provided, they are protected with HEPA filters and liquid disinfectant traps.
12. Boots, shoe covers, or other protective footwear and disinfectant footbaths are available and used when indicated.

C. Containment equipment
1. Personal-protection clothing and equipment and/or other physical-containment devices are used for all procedures and manipulations of infectious materials or infected animals.
2. The risk of infectious aerosols from infected animals or their bedding can be reduced if animals are housed in partial-containment caging systems, such as open cages placed in ventilated enclosures (e.g., laminar-flow cabinets), solid-wall and -bottom cages covered by filter bonnets, or other equivalent primary containment systems.

D. Animal facilities
1. The animal facility is designed and constructed to facilitate cleaning and housekeeping and is separated from areas that are open to unrestricted personnel traffic within the building. Passage through two sets of doors is the basic requirement for entry into the animal room from access corridors or other contiguous areas. Physical separation of the animal room from access corridors or from other activities may also be provided by a double-doored clothes change room (showers may be included), airlock, or other access facility that requires passage through two sets of doors before entering the animal room.
2. The interior surfaces of walls, floors, and ceilings are water resistant so that they can be cleaned easily. Penetrations in these surfaces are sealed or capable of being sealed to facilitate fumigation or space decontamination.
3. A foot, elbow, or automatically operated sink for hand washing is provided near each animal-room exit door.
4. Windows in the animal room are closed and sealed.
5. Animal room doors are self-closing and are kept closed when infected animals are present.
6. An autoclave for decontaminating wastes is available, preferably within the animal room. Materials to be autoclaved outside the animal room are transported in a covered, leakproof container.

7. An exhaust-air ventilation system is provided. This system creates directional airflow that draws air into the animal room through the entry area. The building exhaust can be used for this purpose if the exhaust air is not recirculated to any other area of the building, is discharged to the outside, and is dispersed away from occupied areas and air intakes. Personnel must verify that the direction of the airflow is proper (i.e., into the animal room). The exhaust air from the animal room that does not pass through biological safety cabinets or other primary containment equipment can be discharged to the outside without being filtered or otherwise treated.
8. The HEPA-filtered exhaust air from Class I or Class II biological safety cabinets or other primary containment devices is discharged directly to the outside or through the building's exhaust system. Exhaust air from these primary containment devices may be recirculated within the animal room if the cabinet is tested and certified at least every 12 months. If the HEPA-filtered exhaust air from Class I or Class II biological safety cabinets is discharged to the outside through the building exhaust system, it is connected to this system in a manner (e.g., thimble-unit connection) that avoids any interference with the air balance of the cabinets or building exhaust system.

APPENDIX C

CDC Cautionary Notice for All Human-Serum-Derived Reagents Used as Controls

MMWR Supplement

CDC cautionary notice for all human-serum-derived reagents used as controls:

> **WARNING**: Because no test method can offer complete assurance that laboratory specimens do not contain HIV, hepatitis B virus, or other infectious agents, this specimen should be handled at the BSL 2 as recommended for any potentially infectious human serum or blood specimen in the CDC-NIH manual, *Biosafety in Microbiological and Biomedical Laboratories*, 1984, pages 11-13.

If additional statements describing the results of any heat treatment or serologic procedure(s) already performed on the human-serum reagent or control are used in conjunction with the above cautionary notice, these statements should be worded so as not to diminish the impact of the warning that emphasizes the need for universal precautions.

References
1. Richardson JH, Barkley WE, eds. Biosafety in microbiological and biomedical laboratories, 1984. Washington, DC: Public Health Service, 1984; DHHS publication no. (CDC)84-8395.
2. CDC. Human T-lymphotropic virus type III/lymphadenopathy-associated virus agent summary statement. MMWR 1986;35:540-2, 547-9.
3. CDC. Recommendations for prevention of HIV transmission in health-care settings. MMWR 1987;36(suppl 2):3S-18S.
4. Isenberg HD, Washington JA, Balows A, Sonnenwirth AC. Collection, handling and processing of specimens. In: Lennette EH, Balows A, Hausler WJ, Shadomy HJ, eds. Manual of clinical microbiology, 4th ed. Washington, DC: American Society for Microbiology, 1985:73-98.
5. CDC. Acquired immune deficiency syndrome (AIDS): precautions for clinical and laboratory workers. MMWR 1982;32:577-80.
6. CDC. Recommendations for preventing transmission of infection with human T-lymphotropic virus type III/lymphadenopathy-associated virus in the workplace. MMWR 1985;34:681.
7. CDC. Recommendations for preventing transmission of infection with human T-lymphotropic virus type III/lymphadenopathy-associated virus during invasive procedures. MMWR 1986;35:221-3.
8. CDC. Recommendations for preventing transmission of infection with human T-lymphotropic virus type III/lymphadenopathy-associated virus in the workplace. MMWR 1985;34:682-6, 691-5.
9. U.S. Department of Health and Human Services, Public Health Service. Joint advisory notice: HBV/HIV. Federal Register 1987;52 (October 30): 41818-24.

10. CDC. Update: evaluation of human T-lymphotropic virus type III/lymphadenopathy-associated virus infection in health-care personnel—United States. MMWR 1985;34:575-8.
11. CDC. Human immunodeficiency virus infections in health-care workers exposed to blood of infected patients. MMWR 1987;36:285-9.
12. Anonymous. Needlestick transmission of HTLV-III from a patient infected in Africa. Lancet 1984;2:1376-7.
13. Stricof RL, Morse DL. HTLV-III/LAV seroconversion following a deep intramuscular needlestick injury. New Engl J Med 1986;314:1115.
14. McCray E, Cooperative Needlestick Study Group. Occupational risk of the acquired immunodeficiency syndrome among health-care workers. N Engl J Med 1986;314:1127-32.
15. Weiss SH, Saxinger WC, Richtman D, et al. HTLV-III infection among health-care workers: association with needlestick injuries. JAMA 1985;254:2089-93.
16. Henderson DK, Saah AJ, Zak BJ, et al. Risk of nosocomial infection with human T-cell lymphotropic virus type III/lymphadenopathy-associated virus in a large cohort of intensively exposed health care workers. Ann Intern Med 1986;104:644-7.
17. Gerberding JL, Bryant-Le Blanc CE, Nelson K, et al. Risk of transmitting the human immunodeficiency virus, cytomegalovirus, and hepatitis B virus to health-care workers exposed to patients with AIDS and AIDS-related conditions. J Infect Dis 1987;156:1-8.
18. Weiss SH, Goedert JJ, Gartner S, et al. Risk of human immunodeficiency virus (HIV-1) infection among laboratory workers. Science 1988;239:68-71.
19. U.S. Department of Health and Human Services, Public Health Service. Biosafety guidelines for use of HTLV-III and related viruses. Federal Register 1984 (October 16);49:40556.
20. U.S. Environmental Protection Agency. EPA guide for infectious waste management. Washington, DC: U.S. Environmental Protection Agency, 1986; Publication no. EPA/530-5W-86-014.
21. Favero MS. Sterilization, disinfection and antisepsis in the hospital. In: Lennette EH, Balows A, Hausler WJ, Shadomy HJ, eds. Manual of clinical microbiology, 4th ed. Washington, DC: American Society for Microbiology: 1985;129-37.
22. Martin LS, McDougal JS, Loskoski SL. Disinfection and inactivation of the human T lymphotropic virus type III/lymphadenopathy-associated virus. J Infect Dis 1985:152:400-3.
23. Resnick L, Veren K, Salahuddin, SZ, Tondreau S, Markham PD. Stability and inactivation of HTLV-III/LAV under clinical and laboratory environments. JAMA 1986;255:1887-91.
24. Favero MS, Petersen NJ, Bond WW. Transmission and control of laboratory-acquired hepatitis infection. In: Miller BM, Groschel DHM, Richardson JH, et al., eds. Laboratory safety: principles and practice. Washington, DC: American Society for Microbiology, 1986:49-58.
25. CDC. Public Health Service guidelines for counseling and antibody testing to prevent HIV infections and AIDS. MMWR 1987;36:509-15.
26. Ronalds CJ, Grint PCA, Kangro HD. Disinfection and inactivation of HTLV-III/LAV [Letter]. J Infect Dis 1986;153:996.
27. Evans RP, Shanson DC. Effect of heat on serologic tests for hepatitis B and syphilis and on aminoglycoside assays [Letter]. Lancet 1985;1:1458.
28. Van den Akker R, Hekker AC, Osterhaus ADME. Heat inactivation of serum may interfere with HTLV-III/LAV serology [Letter]. Lancet 1985;2:672.
29. Mortimer PP, Parry JV, Mortimer JY. Which anti-HTLV III/LAV assays for screening and confirmatory testing? Lancet 1985;2:873-7.
30. Jungkind DL, DiRenzo SA, Young SJ. Effect of using heat-inactivated serum with the Abbott human T-cell lymphotropic virus type III antibody test. J Clin Microbiol 1986;23:381-2.
31. Goldie DJ, McConnell AA, Cooke PR. Heat treatment of whole blood and serum before chemical analysis [Letter]. Lancet 1985;1:1161.
32. Lai L, Ball G, Stevens J, Shanson D. Effect of heat treatment of plasma and serum on biochemical indices [Letter]. Lancet 1985;1:1457-8.
33. CDC. Additional recommendations to reduce sexual and drug abuse-related transmission of human T-lymphotropic virus type III/lymphadenopathy-associated virus. MMWR 1986;35:152-5.
34. CDC. Revision of the case definition of acquired immunodeficiency syndrome for national reporting—United States. MMWR 1985;34:373-5.
35. CDC. Diagnosis and management of mycobacterial infection and disease in persons with human T-lymphotropic virus type III/lymphadenopathy-associated virus infection. MMWR 1986;35:448-52.
36. CDC. Revision of the CDC surveillance case definition for acquired immunodeficiency syndrome. MMWR 1987;36(suppl 1):1S-15S.

Index

Page numbers in italics refer to figures; page numbers followed by t indicate tabular material.

Acanthamoeba, 183
　meningoencephalitis and, laboratory diagnosis of, 185
Acanthamoeba castellanii, 185
Acanthamoeba polyphaga, 182, 185
Accessory cells, in AIDS, function of, *316,* 316–317
Acquired immunodeficiency syndrome (AIDS). *See also* AIDS-related complex; Human immunodeficiency virus
　bacteria and, 474
　CDC surveillance case definition for, 223–236, *224*
　　with laboratory evidence against HIV infection, 228
　　with laboratory evidence for HIV infection, 226–228
　　without laboratory evidence regarding HIV infection, 225–226
　in children, 243, 296–303
　　CDC definition of, 301
　　definition of, 225
　　transmission of, 302
　CMV infection in, 121–123, 122t
　cryptosporidiosis in, 81–82
　cytotoxic T lymphocytes in, 219–320, *320*
　definition of, 237
　in children, 225, 301
　early studies suggesting sexual transmission of, 240–241
　in Europe, 311–324, 312t
　　prevalence of HIV antibodies and, 313–314
　fungi and, 474
　gay bowel syndrome and, 54–56, *55–58*
　in health-care workers, 243, 480
　management of, 492
　immunodeficiency of, 314–319
　　active suppression of proliferative responses by AIDS cells or soluble factors and, 317–318, *318*
　　function of AIDS accessory cells and, *316,* 316–317
　　function of T cell subsets from patients with AIDS and, 314–316, *315*
　　mechanisms of immune suppression in, 373–381, 375–379t, *380*
　　role of cytokines for decreased transformation responses of AIDS cells and, 318–319
　immunological responses in, 383–388
　　B lymphocyte deficiencies and, 384–385
　　immunologic responses to HIV and, 387–388
　　interferon and, 385–387
　　natural killer cells and, 385
　　susceptibility to opportunistic infections and, 387

507

508   AIDS and Infections of Homosexual Men

T cell-mediated immunity and, 383–384
incidence and mortality and, 238, 238–240t, 240
laboratory diagnosis of, 148, 155–156
   HIV serology and, 155–156
multifactorial model for occurrence among homosexual men, 449–465
   circulating immune complexes and, 459
   CMV and immunoregulatory defects and, 452–454
   immune responses to semen and, 458–459
   interferon and, 457–458
   mechanisms of disease acquisition and transition to self-sustaining stage and, 459–460, 461
   polyclonal activation of B cells and autoimmunity and, 456–457
   reactivation of EBV and, 454–456
   specific agent as cause of AIDS and, 463, 465
opportunistic infections in. See Opportunistic infections; *specific infections*
parasites and, 475–476
pathogenesis of, 449–451
prevention of, 244–245
in prisoners, 305–309, 306t, 307t
prognostic factors for development of, 321
in prostitutes, 285–294
   antibody to asialo GM1 and, 290
   circulating immune complex assay and, 291
   former drug-abusing women and, 292–294
   lymphocyte subsets and, 290
   sperm antibody assay and, 290
rickettsia and, 474
significance of interferon and interferon-induced enzymes in, 419–429
   biochemical response to IFN and, 425–428, 427t
   characterization of endogenous IFN in, 424t, 424–425

endogenous IFN as preclinical marker and, 425
presence of endogenous IFN in AIDS and, 422–423, 423t
study methods for, 421–422
therapeutic approaches to, 433–443, 434, 435, 436t
   antiviral agents under study for, 437
   clinical trials of antiviral agents for, 437–438, 439t, 440–441
   immunomodulating agents in, 441–442
   overall philosophy and, 442–443
   requisites of useful antiretroviral agents for, 437
   therapeutic maneuvers and, 442
transfusion-associated, 243
viruses and, 474
Actinomycin D (dactinomycin), in Kaposi's sarcoma, 361, 362
Acyclovir
   in *Cryptosporidium* infections, 348, 349
   in *Herpes simplex* infections, 53, 111, 115, 330, 342
   in *Herpes zoster* infections, 342
ADCC. See Antibody-dependent cellular cytotoxicity
Adenoviral infections, laboratory diagnosis of, 190
Africa, as source of AIDS epidemic, 472
Age, Kaposi's sarcoma and, 253
AIDS. See Acquired immunodeficiency syndrome
AIDS dementia, 268, 269, 332
AIDS-related complex (ARC)
   cryptosporidiosis in, 81
   demyelinating polyneuropathies in, 270
   mononeuropathy multiplex in, 270
Algal infection, opportunistic, laboratory diagnosis of, 188
Alopecia, in syphilis, 18
Alpha-diflouromethylornithine (DFMO), in *Cryptosporidium* infections, 348
Alternaria, 187
Amebiasis. See *Entamoeba histolytica*
Amikacin, in MAI, 340
Amitriptyline (Elavil), in peripheral neuropathies associated with AIDS, 270

Amoxicillin, in salmonella, 330
Amphotericin B
  in cryptococcal infections, 331, 349
  in toxoplasmosis, 347
Ampicillin
  in infections taking advantage of B-cell defects, 333
  in *Listeria* infections of CNS, 277
  in *Neisseria* infections, 34, 335
  in salmonella, 330
Anal canal, laceration of, 51
Anal fissures, 50–51
Angiomatosis, epithelioid, 183
Ansamycin
  in AIDS, 440
  in bacillemia, 341
  in MAI, 329, 340
Antibody(ies)
  antisperm
    Kaposi's sarcoma and, 410, 410t
    among prostitutes, 290
  asialo GM1, among prostitutes, 290
  autoantibodies and, Kaposi's sarcoma and, 414
Antibody-dependent cellular cytotoxicity (ADCC), in AIDS, 388
Antibody test
  diagnosis of STDs without diarrhea and, 156–157
  direct fluorescent, 173–174
Antigen(s)
  associated with immunodiagnostic tests, in AIDS, 211–212
  serologically determined, in AIDS, 207–211
Antigen capture assay, for HIV, 155, 157–163
  direct demonstration of HIV and, 159
  HIV culture and, 159–163
Antigen test, 157–168
  Condyloma acuminatum and, 168
  direct, identification of *Chlamydia* by, 142
  direct demonstration of HIV and, 159
  herpesviruses and, 163–167
  HIV culture and, 159–163
  Molluscum contagiosum and, 167
  viral hepatitis and, 167

Antisperm antibodies
  Kaposi's sarcoma and, 410, 410t
  among prostitutes, 290
Antiviral agents
  for AIDS therapy, 437
    clinical trials of, 437–438, 439t, 440–441
    requisites of, 437
  in *Herpes simplex* infections, 111
  in Kaposi's sarcoma, 365
    antiretrovirus agents and, 365
    immune modulators with, 365–366
Arabinosyl cytosine (Ara-C; cytosine arabinoside)
  in non-Hodgkin's lymphoma, 280
  in PML, 342
  in viral infections, 342–343
ARC. *See* AIDS-related complex
Arsenic, in Kaposi's sarcoma, 359
art gene, 208
Asialo GM1 antibody, among prostitutes, 290
Aspergillus, 187
Atabrine (quinacrine hydrochloride), in giardiasis, 74
Autoantibodies, Kaposi's sarcoma and, 414
Autoimmune diseases, interferon and, 428
Autoimmunity
  cellular, Kaposi's sarcoma and, 414
  etiology of AIDS and, 456–457
Autopsies, precautions to prevent transmission of HIV and, 484
Azathioprine, in Kaposi's sarcoma, 356
Azidothymidine (AZT; Retrovir; Zidovudine)
  in AIDS, 438, 440
  in HIV encephalopathy, 268
  in Kaposi's sarcoma, 365
    interferon with, 365–366

B cell(s)
  deficiencies of, in AIDS, 384–385
  polyclonal activation of, 456–457
B-cell defects, infections taking advantage of, 332–333
Bacillemia, treatment of, 341
Bactec blood culture system, 183

Bacterial infections. *See also specific infections*
  associated with diarrhea, laboratory diagnosis of, 168–169
  in children, 303
  without diarrhea, laboratory diagnosis of, 132–147
  enteric pathogens and, 8
  neurologic manifestations of, 277
  opportunistic, laboratory diagnosis of, 187–188
  treatment of, 340–341
Bartonella, 183
BCNU. *See* 1,3–bis(B-chloroethyl)-1–nitrosurea
BFP. *See* Biologic false-positive reaction
Bichloracetic acid, in condyloma acuminata, 52
Biologic false-positive (BFP) reaction, syphilis and, 19
Biosafety level criteria, laboratory and vertebrate animal, 495–504
  level 2, 495–497, 500–502
  level 3, 497–500, 502–504
1,3–Bis(B-chloroethyl)-1–nitrosurea (BCNU), in Kaposi's sarcoma, 363
1,2 Bis(3,5–dioxopiperazine-1–yl)propane (Razoxane), in Kaposi's sarcoma, 363
Blastocystis hominis, laboratory diagnosis of, 176
Blastomyces, 187
Bleomycin, in Kaposi's sarcoma, 362
Blood donors, screening of, 244
Blood spills, precautions to prevent transmission of HIV and, 487
Blood transfusions, AIDS associated with, 243
Body fluid spills, precautions to prevent transmission of HIV and, 487
Bone marrow transplantation
  in AIDS, 442
  in Kaposi's sarcoma, 366
Botryomycosis, 182
Brain
  abscesses of, in AIDS, 332
  HIV in, in children, 303
  toxoplasmosis of, presumptive diagnostic criteria for, 236

Bronchoalveolar lavage, in *Pneumocystis carinii* pneumonia, 183

Caffeine culture and medium, 183
Calcium codylate, in Kaposi's sarcoma, 359
Calcofluor white fluorescent stain, 183
Calymmatobacterium granulomatis, diagnosis of, 146–147
Campylobacter, 8, 59, 169, 182
  diarrhea and, 61–64
Campylobacter cinadei, 8, 169
Campylobacter fennelliae, 8, 169
Campylobacter fetus, 61, 63
Campylobacter intestinalis, 169
Campylobacter jejuni, 8, 62–63, 169
Campylobacter-like organisms (CLOs), 8, 59, 63–64, 169
Candida, 330–331
  definitive diagnostic method for, 233
  of esophagus, presumptive diagnostic criteria for, 235
  laboratory diagnosis of, 147
  treatment of, 331
Candida albicans, 186
  diagnosis of, 147
  treatment of, 350
Candida parapsilopsis, 186
Candida tropicalis, 186
Carbamazepine (Tegretol), in peripheral neuropathies associated with AIDS, 270
Carbarsone (Pulvule), in amebiasis, 73
Carbohydrate fermentation, using cystine tryptophane peptone agar, identification of gonococci with, 135
Cat-scratch disease bacillus, 183, 187
  laboratory diagnosis of, 188, *189*
CDC. *See* Centers for Disease Control
Cefoperazone, in salmonella, 330
Ceftriaxone
  in *Neisseria* infections, 34, 35
  in salmonella, 330
Cefuroxime, in infections taking advantage of B-cell defects, 333
Centers for Disease Control (CDC)
  guidelines for syphilis therapy and, 20
  pediatric AIDS defined by, 301

Central nervous system. *See* Brain; Dementia; Neurologic complications
Cerebrospinal fluid (CSF), examination of, in syphilis, 20, 21
Cerebrovascular disease, in AIDS, 281, 281
Chancres. *See* Syphilis
Chancroid. *See* Hemophilus ducreyi
Chemotherapy. *See also specific drugs and drug types*
  in Kaposi's sarcoma, 359–360
Children
  AIDS in, 243, 296–303
    definition of, 225, 301
    transmission of, 302
  Kaposi's sarcoma in, 303
Chlamydia
  etiology and epidemiology of, 7
  laboratory diagnosis of, 138–139, 139t, 140t, 141t, 142–143
Chlamydia trachomatis, 5
  LGV and non-LGV strains of, 7
  rectal, 7, 39–44, 40t
    study methodology for, 39–40
    study results and, 40–42, 41t, 42, 42t, 43
  treatment of, 54
  urethral, 7, 39
    identification of, 138–139, 142–143
Chlamydiazime test, identification of *Chlamydia* by, 142
Chorioretinitis, CMV infections and, 329
CICs. *See* Circulating immune complexes
CIE. *See* Counter-immuno-electrophoresis
Ciprofloxacin
  in MAI, 340
  in salmonella, 330
Circulating immune complexes (CICs)
  in AIDS, 459
  among prostitutes, 291
Clindamycin, in toxoplasmosis, 275, 332, 346, 347, 348
Clofazimine (Lamprene)
  in bacillemia, 341
  in MAI, 329, 340–341
CLOs. *See* Campylobacter-like organisms
Clotting-factor concentrates, heat-treated, 244
CMV. *See* Cytomegalovirus

Coagglutination tests, 135, 137
Coccidiodomycosis, definitive diagnostic methods for, 233
Coccidioides immitis, 176, 187
Coccidiosis. *See Cryptosporidium; Isospora belli*
Colitis, 4
Condyloma acuminata
  etiology and epidemiology of, 6–7
  laboratory diagnosis of, 168
  treatment of, 52–53, 53
Contact lenses, disinfection of, 486
Corynebacterium equi, 182
Corynebacterium pseudodiphtheriticum, 182
Counter-immuno-electrophoresis (CIE), diagnosis of giardiasis and, 176
Cryosurgery, in Kaposi's sarcoma, 357
Cryptococcosis
  definitive diagnostic methods for, 233
  neurologic manifestations of, 275–277, 278
Cryptococcus neoformans, 176, 331
  treatment of, 331, 349–350
Cryptosporidiosis, 56
  in AIDS, 475
  definitive diagnostic method for, 233
  immune modulation and, 374
  laboratory diagnosis of, 175, 184–185
Cryptosporidium, 77–86, 331
  AIDS and, 81–82
  diagnosis of, 184
  epidemiology of, 84–85
  in immunocompetent individuals, 80
  in immunocompromised individuals, without AIDS, 81
  pathogenesis of, 83
  taxonomy and life cycle and, 77–80, 78, 79
  transmission of, 82–83, 83
  treatment of, 85–86, 331, 348–349
CSF. *See* Cerebrospinal fluid
Cunninghamella, 187
Cunninghamella bertholletiae, 187
Cyclophosphamide, in Kaposi's sarcoma, 356, 364
Cycloserine, in MAI, 329, 340
Cyclosporin-A, in AIDS, 442

Cytokines, role for decreased transformation responses of AIDS cells, 318–319
Cytomegalovirus (CMV), 119–127, 120t, 121t, 328–329
　in AIDS, 121–123, 122t
　　serology and, 393, 396
　definitive diagnostic method for, 233
　etiology of AIDS and, 452–454
　in Kaposi's sarcoma, 124–127, 261
　　demonstration of CMV genome and antigens in Kaposi's sarcoma tissue and, 125–126
　　epidemiology of, 126t, 126–127, 127t
　　oncogenic potential and, 124t, 124–125
　　serologic association and, 125
　mechanisms of acquisition and transition to self-sustaining stage and, 459–460, 461
　neurologic manifestations of, 271, 271–272
　in *Pneumocystis carinii* pneumonia, 123t, 123–124
　retinitis and, presumptive diagnostic criteria for, 235
　treatment of, 55, 328–329
Cytoplasmic immunofluorescence test, antigen detection with, 212
Cytosine arabinoside (arabinosyl cytosine; Ara-C)
　in non-Hodgkin's lymphoma, 280
　in PML, 342
　in viral infections, 342–343

Dactinomycin (actinomycin D), in Kaposi's sarcoma, 361, 362
Dapsone, in Kaposi's sarcoma, 365
Dark-field microscopy, in diagnosis of syphilis, 19
Decadron, in toxoplasmosis, 346
Delayed hypersensitivity, in AIDS, 393, 396
Dementia, in AIDS, 268, 269, 332
　definitive diagnostic methods for, 234
Demyelinating polyneuropathies, in ARC, 270
Denmark, incidence of AIDS in, 313

Dentistry, precautions to prevent transmission of HIV and, 483–484
DFAT test, identification of *Chlamydia* by, 142
DFMO (alpha-diflouromethylornithine), in *Cryptosporidium* infections, 348
DHPG. See Gancyclovir
Diagnosis. See also Laboratory diagnosis
　definitive, for diseases indicative of AIDS, 233–234
　presumptive, of diseases indicative of AIDS, 235–236
Dialysis, precautions to prevent transmission of HIV and, 484
Diarrhea, 47–91. See also specific diseases
　bacterial, 59–65
　　Campylobacter and, 61–64
　　laboratory diagnosis of, 168–169
　　Salmonella and, 64–65
　　Shigella and, 60–61
　parasitic, laboratory diagnosis of, 169–176
Dientamoeba fragilis, 74
Diiodohydroxyquin (Iodoquinol), in amebiasis, 72
Dilantin, in toxoplasmosis, 346
Diloxanide furonate, in amebiasis, 72
Dimethyl-imidazole-triazeno-carboxamide (DTIC), in Kaposi's sarcoma, 363
Direct antigen tests, identification of *Chlamydia* by, 142
Direct fluorescent antibody tests, 173–174
Disinfection, precautions to prevent transmission of HIV and, 485–486
Doxorubicin, in Kaposi's sarcoma, 362
Drug abuse, among women, 292–294
DTIC. See Dimethyl-imidazole-triazeno-carboxamide
Dupont CMV Nick Translation kit, 166
Dupont Isolator, 183, 340
Dupont strip, for HIV, 157

EBV. See Epstein-Barr virus
EIAs. See Enzyme immunoassays
Elavil (amitriptyline), in peripheral neuropathies associated with AIDS, 270
Electrocoagulation, in condyloma acuminata, 52–53

Electron microscopy, HIV identification and, 162
ELISA. *See* Enzyme-linked immunosorbent assay
Encephalitis
  CMV, 271, 271–272
  Herpes simplex, 272
Encephalitozoon, 186
Encephalopathy, 268, 269
  in children, 303
  definitive diagnostic methods for, 234
Endolimax nana, laboratory diagnosis of, 176
Entamoeba histolytica, 8, 70–73
  diagnosis of, 71–72
  laboratory diagnosis of, 174–175
  treatment of, 72–73
Enteritis, 4
Enterobiasis, laboratory diagnosis of, 176
Enterocolitis, CMV infections and, 329
env gene, 208–209, 210
Enzyme immunoassays (EIAs), 489
  for HIV, 155, 156
  identification of *Chlamydia* by, 142
Enzyme-linked immunosorbent assay (ELISA)
  blood donor testing and, 244
  Herpes simplex virus and, 164
Epidemics, 471–472
Epidemiology. *See also* Immunologic abnormalities, epidemiologic observations of
  of *Chlamydia* infections, 7
  CMV involvement in Kaposi's sarcoma and, 126t, 126–127, 127t
  of condylomata acuminata, 6–7
  of Cryptosporidiosis, 84–85
  of gastrointestinal infections, 4–5, 8
  of hepatitis A and B, 7–8
  of *Herpes simplex* infections, 6, 112
  of Kaposi's sarcoma, 252–262
    age and, 253
    geographic location and race and, 252–253
    incidence and, 252
    sex and, 253
  of *Neisseria gonorrhoeae* infections, 5–6, 26–28, 27t, 29t

  of *Neisseria meningitidis* infections, 28, 30, 30t
  of nongonococcal urethritis, 7
  of *Treponema pallidum* infections, 6
Epithelioid angiomatosis, 183
Epstein-Barr virus (EBV)
  etiology of AIDS and, 454–456
  laboratory diagnosis of, 190
Erythromycin
  in amebiasis, 71, 73
  in *Chlamydia trachomatis* infections, 54
  in syphilis, 20
Esophagitis, candida, 331
  presumptive diagnostic criteria for, 235
  treatment of, 350
Ethambutol
  in bacillemia, 341
  in MAI, 329, 340
Ethionamide, in MAI, 329, 340
Etoposide, in Kaposi's sarcoma, 361–362
Europe, AIDS in, 311–314, 312t

False-positive reaction, biologic, syphilis and, 19
Fansidar (sulfadoxine-pyrimethamine), in *Pneumocystis carinii* pneumonia, 345
Flagyl (metronidazole)
  in amebiasis, 72
  in giardiasis, 74
Fluconazole, in cryptococcal infections, 331, 349
5 Flucytosine (5–FC), in cryptococcal infections, 331, 349
Folinic acid, in *Toxoplasma gondii* infections, 332, 346
Foreign body, retained, 51–52
Formalin-acetate method, for stool concentration, 174
Foscarnet (phosphonoformate)
  in AIDS, 440
  in CMV infections, 329
Fowler's solution, in Kaposi's sarcoma, 359
France, incidence of AIDS in, 314
FTA-ABS test, diagnosis of syphilis and, 19, 20, 145
Fungal infections. *See also specific infections*

without diarrhea, laboratory diagnosis of, 147
opportunistic, laboratory diagnosis of, 186–187
treatment of, 349–350
Furazolidone, in *Cryptosporidium* infections, 348, 349

gag gene, 207
Gancyclovir (DHPG), in viral infections, 342
   CMV and, 272, 329
Gastrointestinal infections. *See also specific infections*
   etiology and epidemiology of, 4–5
Gay bowel syndrome, 5, 49–57, 168
   AIDS and, 54–56, 55–58
   infections and, 52–54, 53
   problems with term, 49
   trauma and, 50–52
Gene probe, 183
Generic probe, 188
Genetic factors, in Kaposi's sarcoma, 261
Germany, incidence of AIDS in, 314
Germicides, preventing transmission of HIV and, 486
Giardia lamblia, 8, 73–74
   diagnosis of, 73, 176
   treatment of, 74
Gonochek, 138
GonoGen test, 135
Gonorrhea. *See Neisseria gonorrhoeae*
Gonozyme test, 138
Granuloma inguinale, laboratory diagnosis of, 146–147

Hair loss, in syphilis, 18
Haiti, AIDS epidemic and, 472–473
Health-care workers
   with AIDS, 243, 480
      management of, 492
   definition of, 479
   risk of acquiring HIV and, 480–481
Heat-treated clotting-factor concentrates, 244
Hemophilus ducreyi
   diagnosis of, 145–146, 146t
   laboratory diagnosis of, 145–146, 146t
Hemophilus influenzae pneumonia, treatment of, 341

Hemophilus parainfluenzae, 182
Hepatitis, syphilitic, 15
Hepatitis A
   etiology and epidemiology of, 7–8
   laboratory diagnosis of, 167
Hepatitis B
   in children, 303
   etiology and epidemiology of, 7–8
   laboratory diagnosis of, 167
   transmission of, as model for AIDS transmission, 99–105, *100–104*
   treatment of, 53
Herpes simplex, 5, 109–115, 330
   clinical disease and, 113–115, 114t
   diagnosis of, 164–167
      definitive methods for, 233
   etiology and epidemiology of, 6, 112
   pathogenesis of, 112–113, 113t
   treatment of, 53, 55, 55–56, 330, 342
   viruses and, 109–111, *110, 111*
Herpes virus
   laboratory diagnosis of, 163–167
      herpesvirus 6 and, 190
   neurologic manifestations of, 272
Herpes zoster, 176
   treatment of, 342
Histoplasma
   definitive diagnostic methods for, 233
   treatment of, 350
Histoplasma capsulatum, 176, 187
HIV. *See* Human immunodeficiency virus
HIV dementia, 268, *269*, 332
   definitive diagnostic methods for, 234
HIV encephalopathy, 268, 269
   in children, 303
   definitive diagnostic methods for, 234
HIV SNAP probe kit, 163
HIV wasting syndrome, definitive diagnostic methods for, 234
HLA antigens, Kaposi's sarcoma and, 404–405, 406, 408, 409t
Housekeeping, precautions to prevent transmission of HIV and, 487
HPA-23 (antimoniotungstate), in AIDS, 438
HTLV-1, 205–206, *206*
HTLV-2, 205, *206*
HTLV-3, 205, 206, *206*
Human immunodeficiency virus (HIV), 148, 155–156, 205–216

antigens detected with immunodiagnostic tests and, 211–212
culture of, 159–163
direct demonstration of, 159
immunologic responses to, 387–388
incubation period for, 303
management of exposures to, 492–493
secretory immune response to, 214–216
serologically determined antigens and, 207–211
survival in environment, 486–487
Human immunodeficiency virus (HIV) infections, 241–242
　AIDS and, 241–242
　　prevention of, 244–245
　CDC surveillance case definition for AIDS and
　　with laboratory evidence against HIV infection, 228
　　with laboratory evidence for HIV infection, 226–228
　　without laboratory evidence regarding HIV infection, 225–226
　inconclusive laboratory evidence for, 232
　laboratory evidence against, 228, 231
　laboratory evidence for, 226–228, 231
　modes of transmission of, 242–243
　neurologic disease induced by, 267–271
　peripheral neuropathies associated with, 270–271
　persistence of, 242
　prevention of transmission in health care settings, 479–493
　　cleaning and decontaminating spills of blood or body fluids and, 487
　　health-care workers with AIDS and, 480
　　housekeeping and, 487
　　implementation of precautions and, 488
　　infective waste and, 488
　　laundry and, 487–488
　　management of exposures and, 492–493
　　management of infected health-care workers and, 492
　　precautions for autopsies or morticians' services and, 484
　　precautions for dentistry and, 483–484
　　precautions for dialysis and, 484
　　precautions for invasive procedures and, 482–483
　　precautions for laboratories and, 484–485
　　risk to health-care workers and, 480–481
　　serologic testing for HIV infection and, 489t, 489–491, 490t
　　sterilization and disinfection and, 485–486
　　survival of HIV in environment and, 486–487
　　universal precautions for, 481–482
Human papilloma virus. See Condylomata acuminata
Humatin (paromomycin), in amebiasis, 72
Hypergammaglobulinemia, in children, 303
Hyperimmune bovine colostrum, in cryptosporidiosis, 86
Hyperimmunoglobulinemia, in AIDS, 455
Hypersensitivity, delayed, in AIDS, 393, 396
Hypoglycemia, pentamidine and, 344

IDEIA test, identification of *Chlamydia* by, 142–143
IFA. See Immunofluorescence
IFNs. See Interferons
IL-2. See Interleukin-2
Immulok, 165
Immune modulators
　in AIDS, 441–442
　in Kaposi's sarcoma, 357
　　antiviral drugs with, 365–366
Immune stimulation, in Kaposi's sarcoma, 364–365
Immunocompetent individuals, cryptosporidiosis in, 80
Immunocompromised individuals, cryptosporidiosis in, 81
Immunofluorescence (IFA)
　HIV identification and, 161–162
　membrane, antigen detection with, 212
Immunoglobulin, T cell binding, Kaposi's sarcoma and, 408
Immunoglobulin A, secretory, 214

Immunohematologic tests, in Kaposi's sarcoma, 406–407
Immunologic abnormalities
  of AIDS. *See* Acquired immunodeficiency syndrome, immunodeficiency of
  associated with Kaposi's sarcoma, 260
  epidemiologic observations of, 391–399
    CMV serology and, 396
    delayed hypersensitivity testing and, 396
    distribution of T cell subsets and, 394, *394*, 395t, 396
    follow-up testing of T cell subset distribution and, 396–397
    materials and methods for, 392–393
    symptoms and, 393–394
  immunoregulatory, etiology of AIDS and, 452–454
Immunosuppressive agents, in AIDS, 442
Indirect fluorescent antibody tests, 173–174
Infants, AIDS in, 243
Infective waste, precautions to prevent transmission of HIV and, 488
Interferons (IFNs)
  in AIDS, 385–387, 419–429, 441
    biochemical response to IFN in AIDS patients and, 425–428, 427t
    characterization of endogenous IFN and, 424t, 424–425
    endogenous IFN as preclinical marker for AIDS and, 425
    endogenous IFN in AIDS patients and, 422–423, 423t
    etiology of AIDS and, 457–458
    study methods and, 421–422
  in bacillemia, 341
  immune modulation and, 377–380
  in Kaposi's sarcoma, 357, 364–365
    azidothymidine with, 365–366
Interleukin-2 (IL-2), in AIDS, 441
Invasive procedures, precautions to prevent transmission of HIV and, 482-483
Iodoquinol (diiodohydroxyquin), in amebiasis, 72
Isoniazid
  in bacillemia, 341
  in bacterial infections, 340, 341

Isoprinosine, in Kaposi's sarcoma, 365
Isospora belli, 86, 87, 88
  diagnosis of, 175
    definitive method for, 233

Kaposi's sarcoma (KS), 56, *56–57,* 251–262
  African, 356
  background of, 355–357
  cell of origin and etiology of, 261
  in children, 303
  classic, 355–356
  classification of, 259–260
  clinical manifestations and course of, 253–256, *254–257*
  CMV infection in, 124–127
    demonstration of CMV genome and antigens in Kaposi's sarcoma tissue and, 125–126
    epidemiology of, 126t, 126–127, 127t
    oncogenic potential and, 124t, 124–125
    serologic association and, 125
  conditions associated with, 260–261
  definitive diagnostic method for, 233
  epidemic, 356–357
    antisperm antibodies and, 410, 410t
    comparison of immunohematologic indexes and, 410, 411t, 412t, 413
    elution of T cell binding immunoglobulin from T lymphocytes and, 408
    HLA association and, 408, 409t
    immunofluorescence studies on mononuclear cells and spermatozoa and, 407–408
    immunogenetic findings in, 403–415
    immunohematologic tests and, 406–407
    opportunistic infections and, 403–404
  epidemiology of, 252–262
    age and, 253
    geographic location and race and, 252–253
    incidence and, 252
    sex and, 253
  histopathology of, 257–259, *258, 259*
  history of, 251–252

immune modulation and, 376
in immunosuppressed patients, 356
laboratory findings in, 261
lymphadenopathic, 256
neurologic manifestations of, 280
presumptive diagnostic criteria for, 235
treatment of, 355–366
  background of, 356–357
  BCNU in, 363
  biologic-response modifiers in, 364–365
  bleomycin in, 362
  chemotherapy in, 359–360
  dactinomycin in, 362
  DTIC in, 363
  future directions in, 365–366
  miscellaneous anticancer drugs in, 363–364
  miscellaneous drugs in, 365
  radiotherapy in, 357–359
  Vinca alkaloids in, 360–362
Ketoconazole
  in *Candida* infections, 331
  in cryptococcal infections, 350
  in *Cryptosporidium* infections, 348
KS. *See* Kaposi's sarcoma

Laboratory(ies), precautions to prevent transmission of HIV and, 484–485
Laboratory diagnosis, 131–190, 133t, 134t
  of opportunistic infections with AIDS, 176–190, 177–182t
    algal infection and, 188
    bacterial infections and, 187–188
    fungal infections and, 186–187
    parasitic infections and, 183–186
    viral infections and, 189–190
  of sexually transmitted diseases associated with diarrhea, 168–176
    bacterial infections and, 168–169
    parasitic infections and, 169–176
  of sexually transmitted diseases without diarrhea, 132–168
    antibody test and, 156–157
    antigen test and, 157–168
    bacterial infections and, 132–147
    fungal infections and, 147
    parasitic infections and, 147
    viral infections and, 148–156

Lamprene (clofazimine)
  in bacillemia, 341
  in MAI, 329, 340–341
Laundry, precautions to prevent transmission of HIV and, 487–488
Lectin stimulation, in Kaposi's sarcoma, 406–407
Leishmaniasis, rectal, 182
Leukoencephalopathy, multifocal, progressive. *See* Progressive multifocal leukoencephalopathy
LGV. *See* Lymphogranuloma venereum
Listeria monocytogenes, of central nervous system, 182, 277
Lung biopsy, in *Pneumocystis carinii* pneumonia, 183–184
Lymphadenopathy, in AIDS, 55
  immune modulation and, 377–380
  in syphilis, 15, 18, 54
Lymphocyte subpopulations. *See also* B cell(s); T cell(s)
  in AIDS, 393
    distribution of, 394, *394,* 395t, 396, 396–397
  among prostitutes, 290
Lymphogranuloma venereum (LGV), 54
  identification of, 144
  laboratory diagnosis of, 144
  treatment of, 54
Lymphoid hyperplasia, definitive diagnostic method for, 233
Lymphoid pneumonia
  definitive diagnostic method for, 233
  presumptive diagnostic criteria for, 236
Lymphoma
  of central nervous system, primary, 279, *280*
  definitive diagnostic method for, 233
  non-Hodgkin's, systemic, neurologic manifestations of, 280
Lymphopenia, in children, 303
Lymphoreticular tumors, associated with Kaposi's sarcoma, 260

Maculopathy, vacuolar, 270
MAI. *See Mycobacterium avium-intracellulare*
Major histocompatibility complex (MHC), Kaposi's sarcoma and, 404

Malignancies. *See also specific diseases*
  primary, second, associated with Kaposi's sarcoma, 260
MCK. *See* Modified Cold Kinyoun
Membrane immunofluorescence test, antigen detection with, 212
Meningitis
  aseptic, associated with HIV infection, 267–268
  cryptococcal, 186–187, 277, 331
    treatment of, 349–350
Meningococcal infections. *See Neisseria meningitidis*
Methotrexate, in non-Hodgkin's lymphoma, systemic, 280
Metronidazole (Flagyl)
  in amebiasis, 72
  in giardiasis, 74
MHA test, syphilis and, 19–20
MHC. *See* Major histocompatibility complex
Microimmunofluorescent (MFI) test, identification of *Chlamydia* by, 143
Microsporidia, 89, 89–91, 182
  laboratory diagnosis of, 175, 186
Mixed lymphocyte culture (MLC) tests, in Kaposi's sarcoma, 407
Modified Cold Kinyoun (MCK), 173
Molds, laboratory diagnosis of, 187
Molluscum contagiosum, laboratory diagnosis of, 167
Mononeuropathy multiplex, in ARC, 270
Mononuclear cells
  immunofluorescence studies on, Kaposi's sarcoma and, 407–408
  peripheral blood cells and, interferon and, 421, 426–427
Morticians' services, precautions to prevent transmission of HIV and, 484
Mucorales, 187
Mycobacterial probe, 188
Mycobacterium
  definitive diagnostic method for, 233
  laboratory diagnosis of, 187–188
  neurologic manifestations of, 277
  presumptive diagnostic criteria for, 235
Mycobacterium avium-intracellulare (MAI), 182, 187–188, 277
  treatment of, 329, 340–341

Mycobacterium kansasii, 176
Mycobacterium tuberculosis, 182, 187–188
  treatment of, 340
Mycoplasma, identification of, 144
Myelopathy, vacuolar, 270

Natural killer (NK) cells
  in AIDS, 385
  interferon and, 457
Neisseria gonorrhoeae, 5–6, 25–26
  AIDS and other HIV infections and, 36
  of anal canal, 27
  anorectal, 5, 31
  clinical spectrum of, 30–32
  decline in incidence of, 28
  diagnosis of, 32–34
    laboratory studies in, 132, 135, 135t, 136t, 137, 137–138
  dissemination of, 31–32
  epidemiology of, 5–6, 26–28, 27t, 29t
  etiology of, 5–6
  mode of transmission of, 26
  pharyngeal, 5–6, 27, 31
  prevalence of, 26
  rectal, 5, 31
  treatment of, 34–35, 35t, 52
  urethral, 5, 27, 30
Neisseria meningitidis, 25–26
  AIDS and other HIV infections and, 36
  of anal canal, 28, 30
  anorectal, 31
  clinical spectrum of, 30–32
  diagnosis of, 32–34
  dissemination of, 31–32
  epidemiology of, 28, 30, 30t
  laboratory diagnosis of, 138
  oropharyngeal, 28
  prevalence of, 26
  treatment of, 34–35, 35t
  urethral, 28, 30–31
Neoplastic disease. *See also specific diseases*
  affecting nervous system, in AIDS, 279–281
Neurologic complications, 265–281, 266t. *See also* Brain; Dementia
  HIV-induced neurologic disease and, 267–271

neoplastic disease affecting nervous system and, 279–281
neuropathies and
  in ARC, 270
  autonomic, in AIDS, 270–271
  peripheral, associated with HIV infection, 270–271
neuropathogenesis and, 265, 267
nonviral infectious diseases affecting nervous system and, 273–279
of syphilis, 20–21, 279
viral diseases affecting nervous system and, 271–273
Neurosyphilis, 279
  treatment of, 20–21
Neurotoxicity, of *Vinca* alkaloids, 360
Nitrogen mustard, in Kaposi's sarcoma, 359
NK. See Natural killer cells
Nosema cuniculi, 186
Nucleic acid probe, HIV identification and, 162–163
Nystatin, in cryptococcal infections, 350

OI. See Opportunistic infections
2'-5' Oligodenylate (2–5A) synthetase, in AIDS, 425–428, 427t
Opportunistic infections (OI), 321. See also *specific infections*
  in AIDS, 325–333, 386
    epidemiologic observations of, 391–399
    immune defects and associated complications and, 326–327
    susceptibility to, 387
  associated with Kaposi's sarcoma, 261, 403–404
  immune modulation and, 374
  laboratory diagnosis of, 176–190, 177–182t
    parasitic infections and, 183–186
  taking advantage of B-cell defects, 332–333
  treatment of, 337–350, 338–339t, 361, 362, 364
    bacterial infections and, 340–341
    Cryptosporidium and, 348–349
    fungal infections and, 349–350
    protozoal infections and, 343–345
    toxoplasmosis and, 345–348
    viral infections and, 341–343
orf gene, 210–211

Parasitic infections, 69–75. See also *specific infections*
  AIDS and enteric protozoa and, 70
  associated with diarrhea, laboratory diagnosis of, 169–176
  without diarrhea, laboratory diagnosis of, 147
  Dientamoeba fragilis and, 74
  intestinal, etiology and epidemiology of, 8
  opportunistic, laboratory diagnosis of, 183–186
  patient education and, 74–75
Paromomycin (Humatin), in amebiasis, 72
Patient education, parasitic infections and, 74–75
PBMC. See Peripheral blood mononuclear cells
Pediculosis, laboratory diagnosis of, 147
Penicillin G, in syphilis, 20–21
Pentamidine
  in infections taking advantage of B-cell defects, 333
  in *Pneumocystis carinii* pneumonia, 328, 341, 344–345
  in toxoplasmosis, 346
Peripheral blood mononuclear cells (PBMC), interferon and, 421, 426–427
Peripheral neuropathies, associated with HIV infection, 270–271
Phadebact test, 135, 137
Phosphonoformic acid (Foscarnet)
  in AIDS, 440
  in CMV infections, 329
Phthiriasis, laboratory diagnosis of, 147
Plaque assay, HIV identification and, 162
Plasmodia, 182
PML. See Progressive multifocal leukoencephalopathy
Pneumocystis carinii pneumonia, 176, 321, 328, 475
  CMV infection in, 123t, 123–124
  definitive diagnostic method for, 233
  laboratory diagnosis of, 183–184

presumptive diagnostic criteria for, 236
treatment of, 55, 328, 341, 343–345
Pneumonia. *See also Pneumocystis carinii* pneumonia
bacterial, treatment of, 341
lymphoid
definitive diagnostic method for, 233
presumptive diagnostic criteria for, 236
Pneumonitis
chronic, in children, 303
CMV infections and, 329
Podophyllin, in condyloma acuminata, 52
pol gene, 207–208
Policies, for prevention of transmission of HIV, 488
Polyneuropathies, demyelinating, in ARC, 270
Prednisone, in Kaposi's sarcoma, 356
Prisoners, AIDS in, 305–309, 306t, 307t
Probenecid, in syphilis, 21
Proctitis, 4
Chlamydia trachomatis and. *See Chlamydia trachomatis* infections, rectal
gonorrheal, 52
Herpes simplex, 113–114
pathogens causing, 5
Proctocolitis, pathogens causing, 5
Progressive multifocal leukoencephalopathy (PML), 332
definitive diagnostic method for, 233
laboratory diagnosis of, 189
neurologic manifestations of, 272–273, 273–274
treatment of, 342
Proliferative responses, active suppression of, by AIDS cells or soluble factors, 317–318, *318*
Prototheca wickerhamii, 182
laboratory diagnosis of, 188
Protozoal infections. *See also* Parasitic infections; *specific infections*
treatment of, 343–345
Pruritus, in Kaposi's sarcoma, 253
Pseudallescheria, 187
Pulvule (Carbarsone), in amebiasis, 73
Pyrazinamide, in bacterial infections, 340
Pyrimethamine, in toxoplasmosis, 275, 332, 346, 347–348

QuadFERM test, 138
Quinacrine hydrochloride (Atabrine), in giardiasis, 74

Radiation therapy, in Kaposi's sarcoma, 357–359
RapID NH, 138
Razoxane (1,2 bis(3,5–dioxopiperazine-1–yl)propane), in Kaposi's sarcoma, 363
Retinitis, CMV, presumptive diagnostic criteria for, 235
Retrovir (azidothymidine; AZT; Zidovudine)
in AIDS, 438, 440
in HIV encephalopathy, 268
Reverse transcriptase (RT)
antiviral agents and, 437
HIV identification and, 161
Ribavarin
in AIDS, 438
in Kaposi's sarcoma, 365
Rifampin, in bacterial infections, 340
RIM-N Kit, 137–138
RIN-Test, 138
RIPA assay, 212
RT. *See* Reverse transcriptase

Salmonella, 8, 59, 330
definitive diagnostic method for, 233
diarrhea and, 64–65
treatment of, 330
Salmonella enteritidis, 64
Salmonella typhi, 64, 65
Salmonella typhimurium, treatment of, 341
Sarcoptes scabieri, diagnosis of, 147
Second primary malignancies, associated with Kaposi's sarcoma, 260
Secretory immunoglobulin A, 214
Semen, immune responses to, 458–459
antisperm antibodies and, 290, 410, 410t
Serologic testing
for HIV, 155–156
precautions to prevent transmission of HIV and, 489t, 489–490, 490t
for syphilis, 19–20
Sex, Kaposi's sarcoma and, 253

Sexually transmitted diseases (STDs). *See also specific diseases*
  risk factors for, 4
Shigella, 8, 59
  diarrhea and, 60–61
Skin nodules, laboratory diagnosis of, 185
SNAP herpes simplex probes, 165
Sodium hypochlorite, as disinfectant, 486
sor gene, 208
Spectinomycin, in *Neisseria* infections, 35, 52
Sperm antibodies
  Kaposi's sarcoma and, 410, 410t
  among prostitutes, 290
Spermatozoa, immunofluorescence studies on, Kaposi's sarcoma and, 407–408
Spiramycin, in *Cryptosporidium* infections, 86, 348
Sporotrichum schenckii, 187
Sporotrix schenckii, 176
STDs. *See* Sexually transmitted diseases
Sterilization, precautions to prevent transmission of HIV and, 485–486
Streptococcus pneumoniae pneumonia, treatment of, 341
Streptomycin, in bacterial infections, 340
Strongyloides, 182
Sucrose flotation, for stool concentration, 174
Sulfadiazine, in toxoplasmosis, 275, 332, 346, 347–348
Sulfadoxine-pyrimethamine (Fansidar), in *Pneumocystis carinii* pneumonia, 345
Sulfamethoxazole. *See also* Trimethoprim-sulfamethoxazole
  allergic reactions to, 321
Sulfonamides, in amebiasis, 71
Suramin, in AIDS, 440–441
Switzerland, incidence of AIDS in, 314
Syphilis. *See Treponema pallidum*
Systemic lupus erythematosis, associated with Kaposi's sarcoma, 260

T cell(s)
  cytotoxic, in AIDS, 319–320, *320*
  elution of T cell binding immunoglobulin from, Kaposi's sarcoma and, 408

T cell binding immunoglobulin, elution from T lymphocytes, Kaposi's sarcoma and, 408
T cell-mediated immunity, in AIDS, 383–384
T cell subsets
  in AIDS, function of, 314–316, *315*
  in Kaposi's sarcoma, enumeration of, 406
tat gene, 208, 437
Tegretol (carbamazepine), in peripheral neuropathies associated with AIDS, 270
Tetracycline
  in amebiasis, 71, 73
  in *Chlamydia trachomatis* infections, 44, 54
  in *Neisseria* infections, 34
  in syphilis, 20
Thrush. *See Candida*
Thymopentin (TP-5), in Kaposi's sarcoma, 405
Tissue culture, *Herpes simplex* virus and, 165
Toxoplasma gondii, 331–332
  in AIDS, 475
  of brain, presumptive diagnostic criteria for, 236
  definitive diagnostic method for, 233
  laboratory diagnosis of, 185
  neurologic manifestations of, 273, 275, 276
  treatment of, 332, 345–348
Transactivation, 208
Transformation responses, of AIDS cells, decreased, role of cytokines for, 318–319
Transfusions, AIDS associated with, 243
Trauma, gay bowel syndrome and, 50–52
Treponema pallidum, 13–21
  anorectal chancres in, 6
  case presentations and, 13, 14t, 15–16, *16*
  chancres in, 6, 15, 17, 54
  clinical manifestations of, *17*, 17–18, *18*
  diagnosis of, 19–20, 144–145
    direct dark-field examination and, 145

serologic tests and, 145
etiology and epidemiology of, 6
primary, 17
secondary, 17, 17–18, 18
neurologic manifestations of, 15
treatment of, 20–21, 53–54
Triaziquone (2,3,5–tris 1–azire-dinye-p-benzoquinone), in Kaposi's sarcoma, 359–360
Trichomonas vaginalis, diagnosis of, 147
Trichosporon, 186
Trimethoprim-sulfamethoxazole
in *Cryptosporidium* infections, 331
in infections taking advantage of B-cell defects, 333
in *Pneumocystis carinii* pneumonia, 328, 344, 345
in toxoplasmosis, 346, 347
Trimetrexate, in *Pneumocystis carinii* pneumonia, 328
2,3,5–Tris 1–azire-dinye-p-benzoquinone (Triaziquone), in Kaposi's sarcoma, 359–360
Truant's stain, 173
Tuberculosis, 329–330
definitive diagnostic method for, 233
treatment of, 329–330
Tumor necrosis factor, in bacillemia, 341
Tunicamycin, treatment of HIV-infected cells with, 209
Tzanck smear, preparation of, 164

Ultranebulizer, 183
United Kingdom, incidence of AIDS in, 314
Ureaplasma urealyticum
identification of, 138
laboratory diagnosis of, 144
Urethritis
chlamydial, 7, 39
identification of, 138–139, 142–143

Neisseria gonorrhoeae and, 5, 27, 30
Neisseria meningitidis and, 28, 30–31
nongonococcal, etiology and epidemiology of, 7

Vacuolar myelopathy, 270
Varicella zoster, laboratory diagnosis of, 190
Venereal Disease Research Laboratory (VDRL) test, syphilis and, 20
Vidarabine, in *Herpes zoster* infections, 342
Vinca alkaloids, in Kaposi's sarcoma, 359, 360–362
Viral DNA probe, 165
Viral infections. *See also specific infections*
without diarrhea, laboratory diagnosis of, 148–156
opportunistic, laboratory diagnosis of, 189–190
treatment of, 341–343

Wart(s). *See* Condyloma acuminata
Warthin Starry stain, 183
Waste, precautions to prevent transmission of HIV and, 488
Wasting syndrome, definitive diagnostic methods for, 234
Western blot test, 155, 156, 489–490
antigen detection with, 211–212

Yeast infections, laboratory diagnosis of, 186–187

Zidovudine (azidothymidine; AZT; Retrovir)
in AIDS, 438, 440
in HIV encephalopathy, 268

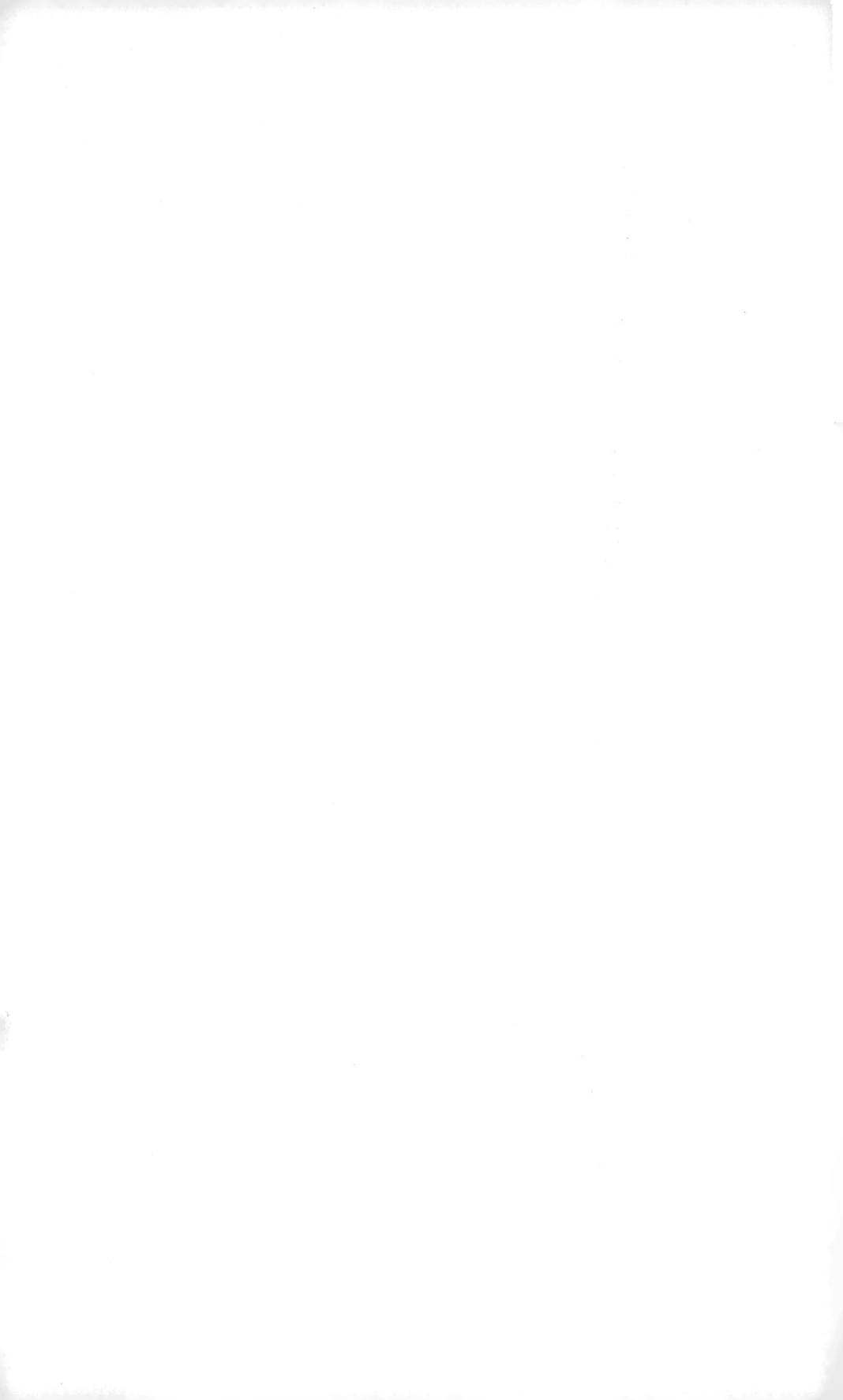